Methods in Pharmacology and Toxicology

For further volumes:
http://www.springer.com/series/7653

Nanomaterials in Pharmacology

Edited by

Zheng-Rong Lu

Department of Biomedical Engineering, Case Western Reserve University, Cleveland, OH, USA

Shinji Sakuma

Laboratory of Drug Delivery System, Faculty of Pharmaceutical Sciences, Setsunan University, Hirakata, Osaka, Japan

Humana Press

Editors
Zheng-Rong Lu
Department of Biomedical Engineering
Case Western Reserve University
Cleveland, OH, USA

Shinji Sakuma
Laboratory of Drug Delivery System
Faculty of Pharmaceutical Sciences
Setsunan University
Hirakata, Osaka, Japan

ISSN 1557-2153 ISSN 1940-6053 (electronic)
Methods in Pharmacology and Toxicology
ISBN 978-1-4939-3120-0 ISBN 978-1-4939-3121-7 (eBook)
DOI 10.1007/978-1-4939-3121-7

Library of Congress Control Number: 2015947788

Springer New York Heidelberg Dordrecht London

Printed on acid-free paper

Humana Press is a brand of Springer
Springer Science+Business Media LLC New York is part of Springer Science+Business Media (www.springer.com)

Preface

Nanomaterials have played a significant role in pharmacology. Proteins and nucleic acids are nanosized building blocks of life and have been used as therapeutics in treating human diseases. Advancements in molecular biology and biotechnology have led to the clinical development and application of numerous nanosized biologics, including proteins and nucleic acids, in treating human diseases. Although non-biological nanomaterials were used as therapeutics long before modern science in human history, recent development of nanotechnology has resulted in a stockpile of novel synthetic nanomaterials with unique properties and functions. These nanomaterials can be used as new therapeutics or as vehicles to modify and enhance the efficacy of existing therapeutics. A number of nanosized drug delivery systems and therapeutics based on synthetic nanomaterials are currently approved for clinical use or in clinical development. It is expected that safer nanomaterials will also be available in pharmacological applications.

Nanomaterials in Pharmacology aims to introduce nanomaterials as a new therapeutic regimen in treating human diseases. There have been explosive expansions of research activities in the fields of nanotechnology and nanomedicine in recent years. Various nanomaterials have been developed and tested for potential use in pharmacology. It is not our intention to cover all aspects of nanomaterials and nanomedicine. This book has four sections covering inorganic nanomaterials, organic nanomaterials, pharmaceutical properties of nanomaterials, and applications of nanomaterials in medicine. Several examples of inorganic and organic nanomaterials are provided to demonstrate how to design and develop nanomaterials for pharmacological purposes. The key pharmaceutical properties, including biocompatibility, tissue interaction, pharmaceutics, and pharmacokinetics, of nanomaterials are discussed with a focus on the safety and pharmaceutical considerations of nanomaterials in translational development. The pharmacological applications of nanomaterials are depicted in treating various human diseases, including cancer, cardiovascular diseases, immune disorders, infectious diseases, gastrointestinal disorders, bone diseases, and respiratory disorders.

Although recent developments in nanotechnology have created endless opportunities for new therapeutics to treat human diseases, we should pursue clinical use of nanomaterials with care and responsibility. The tragic story of Thorotrast, a colloidal X-ray contrast agent based on ThO_2 broadly used from the 1930s to the 1950s, or a nanomedicine in modern terms, should remind us of the potential long-term side effects of the nanomaterials that remain in the body for a long time. Thorotrast was considered a safe contrast agent for X-ray imaging with few acute side effects. Its 400-plus year half-life in the human body gave rise to liver failure and cancer in many patients who were exposed to Thorotrast, many years later. For the students and scientists who are entering the field of nanotechnology and nanomedicine, the understanding of the potential benefits and risks of nanomaterials in pharmacology will be helpful to avoid the pitfalls, to maximize the potential of nanomaterials in pharmacology, and to thrive in the field of nanomedicine.

Finally, we would like to sincerely thank all the contributors for their tremendous efforts to prepare the chapters and to share their knowledge in various aspects of nanomaterials and nanomedicine.

Cleveland, OH, USA *Zheng-Rong Lu*
Hirakata, Osaka, Japan *Shinji Sakuma*

Contents

Contributors

TAKAMI AKAGI • *Department of Applied Chemistry, Graduate School of Engineering, Osaka University, Suita, Japan; Graduate School of Frontier Bioscience, Osaka University, Suita, Japan*

MITSURU AKASHI • *Department of Applied Chemistry, Graduate School of Engineering, Osaka University, Suita, Japan; Graduate School of Frontier Bioscience, Osaka University, Suita, Japan*

HIDENORI ANDO • *Department of Pharmacokinetics and Biopharmaceutics, Subdivision of Biopharmaceutical Sciences, Institute of Biomedical Sciences, Tokushima University, Tokushima, Japan; Department of Cancer Metabolism and Therapy, Subdivision of Biopharmaceutical Sciences, Institute of Biomedical Sciences, Tokushima University, Tokushima, Japan*

KATSUHIKO ARIGA • *World Premier International (WPI) Research Center for Materials Nanoarchitectonics (MANA), National Institute for Materials Science (NIMS), Tsukuba, Japan; Core Research for Evolutional Science and Technology (CREST), Japan Science and Technology Agency (JST), Tokyo, Japan*

HIDETOSHI ARIMA • *Graduate School of Pharmaceutical Sciences, Kumamoto University, Kumamoto, Japan; Program for Leading Graduate Schools "HIGO (Health Life Science: Interdisciplinary and Glocal Oriented) Program", Kumamoto University, Kumamoto, Japan*

BARBARA BENARDO • *Department of Radiology, Perelman School of Medicine, University of Pennsylvania, Philadelphia, PA, USA*

TATIANA K. BRONICH • *Department of Pharmaceutical Sciences, College of Pharmacy, University of Nebraska Medical Center, Omaha, NE, USA; Center for Drug Delivery and Nanomedicine, College of Pharmacy, University of Nebraska Medical Center, Omaha, NE, USA*

RABEE CHEHELTANI • *Department of Radiology, Perelman School of Medicine, University of Pennsylvania, Philadelphia, PA, USA*

PETER CHHOUR • *Department of Radiology, Perelman School of Medicine, University of Pennsylvania, Philadelphia, PA, USA; Department of Bioengineering, University of Pennsylvania, Philadelphia, PA, USA*

DAVID P. CORMODE • *Department of Radiology, Perelman School of Medicine, University of Pennsylvania, Philadelphia, PA, USA; Department of Bioengineering, University of Pennsylvania, Philadelphia, PA, USA; Department of Cardiology, University of Pennsylvania, Philadelphia, PA, USA*

ANNA E. CZAPAR • *Department of Pathology, Case Western Reserve University School of Medicine and Engineering, Cleveland, OH, USA*

SWAPNIL S. DESALE • *Department of Pharmaceutical Sciences, College of Pharmacy, University of Nebraska Medical Center, Omaha, NE, USA; Center for Drug Delivery and Nanomedicine, College of Pharmacy, University of Nebraska Medical Center, Omaha, NE, USA*

YOSHIMINE FUJII • *Center for Pharmaceutical and Biomedical Analysis, Daiichi Sankyo RD Novare Co., Ltd., Tokyo, Japan*

MASAHIRO GOTO • *Department of Applied Chemistry, Graduate School of Engineering, Kyushu University, Fukuoka, Japan; Center for Future Chemistry, Kyushu University, Fukuoka, Japan*

ANIRBAN SEN GUPTA • *Department of Biomedical Engineering, Case Western Reserve University, Cleveland, OH, USA*

TAISHI HIGASHI • *Graduate School of Pharmaceutical Sciences, Kumamoto University, Kumamoto, Japan*

KAZUMA HIGASHISAKA • *Laboratory of Toxicology and Safety Science, Graduate School of Pharmaceutical Sciences, Osaka University, Suita, Osaka, Japan; Laboratory of Biopharmaceutical Research, National Institute of Biomedical Innovation, Ibaraki, Osaka, Japan*

TATSUHIRO ISHIDA • *Department of Pharmacokinetics and Biopharmaceutics, Subdivision of Biopharmaceutical Sciences, Institute of Biomedical Sciences, Tokushima University, Tokushima, Japan; Department of Cancer Metabolism and Therapy, Subdivision of Biopharmaceutical Sciences, Institute of Biomedical Sciences, Tokushima University, Tokushima, Japan*

QINGMIN JI • *World Premier International (WPI) Research Center for Materials Nanoarchitectonics (MANA), National Institute for Materials Science (NIMS), Tsukuba, Japan*

EFSTATHIOS KARATHANASIS • *Department of Radiology, Case Western Reserve University, Cleveland, OH, USA; Department of Biomedical Engineering, Case Western Reserve University, Cleveland, OH, USA*

KOHSAKU KAWAKAMI • *International Center for Materials Nanoarchitectonics, National Institute for Materials Science, Tsukuba, Ibaraki, Japan*

MOMOKO KITAOKA • *Department of Applied Chemistry, Graduate School of Engineering, Kyushu University, Fukuoka, Japan*

JIAYING LIU • *The Wallace H. Coulter Department of Biomedical Engineering, Georgia Institute of Technology and Emory University, Atlanta, GA, USA*

ZHENG-RONG LU • *Department of Biomedical Engineering, Case Western Reserve University, Cleveland, OH, USA*

KAZUO MARUYAMA • *Laboratory of Drug and Gene Delivery System Research, Faculty of Pharma-Sciences, Teikyo University, Tokyo, Japan*

SHAAMEEN MIAN • *Department of Bioengineering, University of Pennsylvania, Philadelphia, PA, USA*

KEIICHI MOTOYAMA • *Graduate School of Pharmaceutical Sciences, Kumamoto University, Kumamoto, Japan*

CHAOFENG MU • *Department of Nanomedicine, Houston Methodist Hospital Research Institute, Houston, TX, USA*

PRATAP C. NAHA • *Department of Radiology, Perelman School of Medicine, University of Pennsylvania, Philadelphia, PA, USA*

YOICHI NEGISHI • *Department of Drug Delivery and Molecular Biopharmaceutics, School of Pharmacy, Tokyo University of Pharmacy and Life Sciences, Tokyo, Japan*

MAKIYA NISHIKAWA • *Department of Biopharmaceutics and Drug Metabolism, Graduate School of Pharmaceutical Sciences, Kyoto University, Kyoto, Japan*

YUSUKE ODA • *Laboratory of Drug and Gene Delivery System Research, Faculty of Pharma-Sciences, Teikyo University, Tokyo, Japan*

HIROAKI OKADA • *Okada DDS Research Institute Inc., Tokyo, Japan*

DAIKI OMATA • *Laboratory of Drug and Gene Delivery System Research, Faculty of Pharma-Sciences, Teikyo University, Tokyo, Japan*
TETSUYA OZEKI • *Drug Delivery and Nano Pharmaceutics, Graduate School of Pharmaceutical Sciences, Nagoya City University, Nagoya, Aichi, Japan*
PALLAB PRADHAN • *The Wallace H. Coulter Department of Biomedical Engineering, The Parker H. Petit Institute for Bioengineering and Bioscience, The Georgia Tech Center for ImmunoEngineering, Georgia Institute of Technology and Emory University, Atlanta, GA, USA*
KE REN • *Department of Pharmaceutical Sciences, College of Pharmacy, University of Nebraska Medical Center, Omaha, NE, USA*
KRISHNENDU ROY • *The Wallace H. Coulter Department of Biomedical Engineering, The Parker H. Petit Institute for Bioengineering and Bioscience, The Georgia Tech Center for ImmunoEngineering, Georgia Institute of Technology and Emory University, Atlanta, GA, USA*
SHINJI SAKUMA • *Laboratory of Drug Delivery System, Faculty of Pharmaceutical Sciences, Setsunan University, Hirakata, Osaka, Japan*
HAIFA SHEN • *Department of Nanomedicine, Houston Methodist Hospital Research Institute, Houston, TX, USA*
TARO SHIMIZU • *Department of Pharmacokinetics and Biopharmaceutics, Subdivision of Biopharmaceutical Sciences, Institute of Biomedical Sciences, Tokushima University, Tokushima, Japan*
NICOLE F. STEINMETZ • *Department of Biomedical Engineering, Case Western Reserve University School of Medicine and Engineering, Cleveland, OH, USA; Department of Radiology, Case Western Reserve University School of Medicine and Engineering, Cleveland, OH, USA; Department of Materials Science and Engineering, Case Western Reserve University School of Medicine and Engineering, Cleveland, OH, USA; Department of Macromolecular Science and Engineering, Case Western Reserve University School of Medicine and Engineering, Cleveland, OH, USA*
DA SUN • *Department of Biomedical Engineering, Case Western Reserve University, Cleveland, OH, USA*
RYO SUZUKI • *Laboratory of Drug and Gene Delivery System Research, Faculty of Pharma-Sciences, Teikyo University, Tokyo, Japan; Robert M. Berne Cardiovascular Research Center, University of Virginia, Charlottesville, VA, USA*
TATSUAKI TAGAMI • *Drug Delivery and Nano Pharmaceutics, Graduate School of Pharmaceutical Sciences, Nagoya City University, Nagoya, Aichi, Japan*
MOEKO TAKI • *Drug Delivery and Nano Pharmaceutics, Graduate School of Pharmaceutical Sciences, Nagoya City University, Nagoya, Aichi, Japan*
MINGQIAN TAN • *Division of Biotechnology, Chinese Academy of Sciences, Dalian Institute of Chemical Physics, Dalian, China*
RANDALL TOY • *Department of Biomedical Engineering, Georgia Institute of Technology, Atlanta, GA, USA*
YASUO TSUTSUMI • *Laboratory of Toxicology and Safety Science, Graduate School of Pharmaceutical Sciences, Osaka University, Suita, Osaka, Japan; Laboratory of Biopharmaceutical Research, National Institute of Biomedical Innovation, Ibaraki, Osaka, Japan; The Center for Advanced Medical Engineering and Informatics, Osaka University, Suita, Osaka, Japan*

MASAMI UKAWA • *Department of Pharmacokinetics and Biopharmaceutics, Subdivision of Biopharmaceutical Sciences, Institute of Biomedical Sciences, Tokushima University, Tokushima, Japan; Department of Cancer Metabolism and Therapy, Subdivision of Biopharmaceutical Sciences, Institute of Biomedical Sciences, Tokushima University, Tokushima, Japan*

JOHAN UNGA • *Laboratory of Drug and Gene Delivery System Research, Faculty of Pharma-Sciences, Teikyo University, Tokyo, Japan*

AMITA VAIDYA • *Department of Biomedical Engineering, Case Western Reserve University, Cleveland, OH, USA*

BEIBEI WANG • *Division of Biotechnology, Chinese Academy of Sciences, Dalian Institute of Chemical Physics, Dalian, China*

DONG WANG • *Department of Pharmaceutical Sciences, College of Pharmacy, University of Nebraska Medical Center, Omaha, NE, USA*

XIN WEI • *Department of Pharmaceutical Sciences, College of Pharmacy, University of Nebraska Medical Center, Omaha, NE, USA*

XIAOHUI WU • *Department of Biomedical Engineering, Case Western Reserve University, Cleveland, OH, USA*

YASUO YOSHIOKA • *Laboratory of Toxicology and Safety Science, Graduate School of Pharmaceutical Sciences, Osaka University, Suita, Osaka, Japan; Laboratory of Biopharmaceutical Research, National Institute of Biomedical Innovation, Ibaraki, Osaka, Japan*

GUANPING YU • *Department of Biomedical Engineering, Case Western Reserve University, Cleveland, OH, USA*

JINJIN ZHANG • *Department of Pharmaceutical Sciences, College of Pharmacy, University of Nebraska Medical Center, Omaha, NE, USA; Center for Drug Delivery and Nanomedicine, College of Pharmacy, University of Nebraska Medical Center, Omaha, NE, USA*

LINGLI ZHANG • *Department of Pharmacy Practice, College of Pharmacy, University of Nebraska Medical Center, Omaha, NE, USA; West China Second University Hospital, Sichuan University, Chengdu, Sichuan, China*

Chapter 1

Synthetic Polymer-based Nanomaterials

Swapnil S. Desale, Jinjin Zhang, and Tatiana K. Bronich

Abstract

Synthetic polymers play an essential role in the development of conventional pharmaceutical formulations as well as devices for controlled drug delivery and represent the most commonly used "building blocks" for engineering of various nanomedicines. In this chapter we review several classes of synthetic polymers that are widely used for the design of drug delivery systems, synthetic methodologies to tailor their physicochemical properties, and therapeutic applications and developments.

Key words Nanomedicines, Polymers, Polymerization, Nanoparticles, Drug delivery

1 Introduction

Nanomedicine is a rapidly developing area of biomedical research that uses devices of nanoscale size to address urgent needs for effectively detecting diseases and improving drug and gene delivery. Such nanomaterial (NM)-based delivery vehicles have the ability to improve drug pharmacokinetics, biodistribution, cell- or tissue-specific targeting, and drug exposure kinetics, resulting in enhanced efficacy and improved tolerability [1–3]. The most sophisticated nanocarriers can simultaneously deliver multiple therapeutic and/or imaging agents and thus enable both diagnosis and therapy. Polymers are playing an essential role in the development of conventional pharmaceutical formulations as well as devices for controlled drug delivery and represent the most commonly used "building blocks" for engineering of the NM-based drug delivery systems. The advances in synthetic polymer chemistry led to the exceptional diversity and control over the composition, architecture and functionality of the polymers, which in turn enables the building of NM with tunable properties for various biomedical applications. This chapter first highlights several classes of synthetic polymers, which are currently the most widely used for the design of NM-based drug delivery systems. The remainder of the chapter focuses on some examples of polymeric NMs and their applications in drug and gene delivery.

Zheng-Rong Lu and Shinji Sakuma (eds.), *Nanomaterials in Pharmacology*, Methods in Pharmacology and Toxicology,
DOI 10.1007/978-1-4939-3121-7_1, © Springer Science+Business Media New York 2016

2 Synthetic Polymers

Polymers can be classified as homopolymers and copolymers based on their composition. Homopolymer is defined as the polymer containing a single type of repeating units, while copolymer is composed of two or more different monomers. Both homopolymers and copolymers have been used extensively for drug delivery applications. The development of these polymer-based drug delivery systems relies on novel polymeric architectures and appropriate synthetic methodologies to tailor their physicochemical properties.

3 Polyesters

Among all degradable polymers, aliphatic polyester-based polymeric structures are receiving special attention because of their compatibility with the natural environment and their ability to undergo hydrolytic and biological degradation [4]. Among the wide variety of aliphatic polyesters, poly(D,L-lactide-co-glycolide) (PLGA), poly(lactic acid) (PLA), poly(caprolactone) (PCL) are the most commonly used polymers for controlled drug release applications. There are two methods of the synthesis of aliphatic polyesters: polycondensation of diols and dicarboxylic acids or hydroxycarboxylic acids and ring-opening polymerization (ROP) of cyclic monomers (Scheme 1) [5, 6]. The polycondensation is hampered by drawbacks such as typically required high temperatures and long reaction times that favor side reactions, necessity of continuous water removal to achieve high conversions and high molecular weights. The polymers obtained in this process are characterized by high polydispersity. ROP yields polymer products with high molecular weight, lower polydispersity and, therefore, is a preferred route to obtain aliphatic polyesters [7, 8]. Various organometallic compounds, such as oxides, carboxylates, and alkoxides are used as effective catalysts for the controlled synthesis

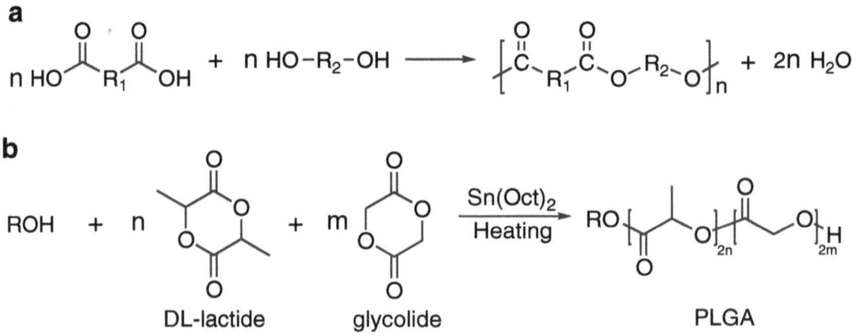

Scheme 1 (**a**) Synthesis of polyesters by polycondensation of dicarboxylic acids and diols; (**b**) synthesis of PLGA copolymer by ROP using alcohol as an initiator and stannous octoate as the catalyst

of polyesters using ROP [9]. Alternately, polyesters without toxic metallic residuals, which is an important requirement for biomedical and pharmaceutical applications, can be prepared by using enzyme-catalyzed polymerizations [10]. Unlike chemical catalysts, enzymes function under mild conditions, enable high enantioselectivity and regioselectivity, and are recyclable. Extensive research efforts have been expended in the past years to refine the ROP technique for the synthesis of the polyesters with controlled architecture and tailor-made properties. To obtain a polymer with a particular combination of desirable properties, copolymerization techniques have been extensively used. Controlling the composition, morphology, glass transition temperature, and degradation rate of the copolymers allows regulation of the drug release behavior from such matrices. Nanoparticles formulated from biodegradable polyesters are of great interest for drug delivery purposes. A wide variety of hydrophilic or hydrophobic drugs and biological macromolecules can be encapsulated into biodegradable polyesters-based nanoparticles and delivered to specific organs or cells [11]. A number of techniques are available for the formulation of polyester-based nanoparticles (or nanocapsules). The choice of a particular approach mainly depends on the physicochemical properties of the polymer (i.e., solubility and molecular weight) and the drug physicochemical properties (i.e., hydrophobicity/ hydrophilicity, sensitivity to the solvent). Currently, the most popular methods are emulsion/solvent evaporation or diffusion, double emulsion, nanoprecipitation, and the salting out procedure. The emulsion/solvent evaporation method involves the preparation of an oil-in-water emulsion, where a small quantity of water-immiscible organic solvent containing polymer and hydrophobic drug (oil phase) is emulsified in an aqueous phase containing a stabilizer [12, 13]. The most common stabilizers are hydrophilic molecules such as polyvinyl alcohol (PVA), polysorbates (TWEEN®), or sodium cholate. Stable nanoparticles are formed in the aqueous phase by organic solvent evaporation under increased temperature or reduced pressure. In the emulsion/diffusion method, the oil phase containing polymer is dissolved in a partially water-miscible solvent (e.g., ethyl acetate, propylene carbonate) [14, 15]. The addition of a certain volume of water to the oil-in-water emulsion induces a change in the equilibrium of the system and causes the partially water-miscible solvent to diffuse from the droplets into the aqueous phase. This reduces the polymer's solubility and results in particle formation. Another approach is the double-emulsion, W/O/W, method [16, 17]. The main benefit of the double-emulsion method is its ability to efficiently encapsulate hydrophilic drugs and proteins. In this approach, the drug, dissolved in water, is added to an organic solvent containing polymer, forming a water-in-oil emulsion. Then a small quantity of this initial emulsion is added to a second aqueous phase containing an emulsifier, such as PVA, to stabilize the particles. Nanoparticles are then obtained by evaporation of the organic solvent. Typically this method yields nanoparticles with larger sizes than single emulsion method with moderate drug loading and encapsulation efficiency. Nanoprecipitation (or solvent displacement) method utilizes interfacial polymer deposition to form nanoparticles [18–20]. In this simple process, polymer and a drug are dissolved in a water-miscible solvent and this solution is then added dropwise to an aqueous solution (non-solvent) with or without stabilizer. Solvent diffusion results in polymer precipitation on the interface between the aqueous phase and finely dispersed oil droplets, resulting in the formation of solid particles. Depending on the solvent choice and solvent–non-solvent ratio, this method is suitable for encapsulation of both hydrophilic and hydrophobic drugs as well as protein-based therapeutics. In general, nanoparticles of smaller sizes but with lower entrapment efficiencies are obtained through this method when compared to other methods. Finally, the salting out method is an oil-in-water emulsion comprised of a primary aqueous phase containing stabilizer and a high concentration of salt (e.g., magnesium chloride hexahydrate) and polymer dissolved in a water-miscible solvent, such as acetone or tetrahydrofuran [21]. Due to the presence of a high concentration of salt, there is no diffusion of the solvent into the aqueous phase. Fast addition of a large amount of water to this oil-in-water emulsion reduces the ionic strength and leads to the migration of the water-miscible organic solvent into the aqueous phase, inducing formation of solid particles. In this method, particles must be purified to remove residual salt and solvent prior to use. A central challenge in the development of drug-encapsulated polymeric nanoparticles is the inability to control the mixing processes required for their synthesis, which results in variable nanoparticle physicochemical properties (size, surface composition, and drug loading). To address this challenge the Langer group [22] developed a rapid and tunable mixing procedure utilizing hydrodynamic flow focusing in microchannels to control nanoprecipitation and prepare nanoparticles in a reproducible manner. The microfluidic technique allows tuning the size of the resulting particles by varying flow rates, polymer composition, molecular weight or polymer concentration in organic solution. Remarkably, higher drug encapsulation was also reported for the polymeric nanoparticles prepared through microfluidics [22]. Recently, DeSimone and colleagues have developed a unique nanofabrication process called Particle Replication In Nonwetting Templates (PRINT) [23]. Using soft-lithography techniques adopted from the semiconductor industry, PRINT enables the production of monodisperse polymeric nanoparticles with well-defined control over particle size, shape, composition, and surface chemistry, and permits the loading of a wide range of cargoes with high loading efficiency [24, 25].

4 Polyanhydrides

Polyanhydrides, polymers containing hydrolytically labile anhydride linkages in hydrophobic backbone, have been investigated for more than three decades as important biomaterials used for short-term release of drugs [26]. Polyanhydrides are characterized by their fast degradation followed by rapid erosion of material, but at the same time can be designed to release drugs that last from days to weeks by suitable choice of monomers. Numerous polymers have been synthesized in this class of material by various polymerization techniques such as melt condensation, ROP, interfacial condensation, dehydrochlorination, and dehydrative coupling agents [27]. The most convenient method of synthesizing high molecular weight polyanhydride copolymer is by the melt polycondensation of anhydride prepolymers (Scheme 2) [28, 29].

Solution polymerizations at ambient temperature are typically utilized to prepare polyanhydrides from heat-sensitive monomers and generally yield low molecular weight polymers. The degradation of polyanhydrides is a hydrolytically triggered process and depends on the uptake of water into the polymer matrix and pH of the medium. The rate of water uptake is dependent on factors such as crystallinity, polymer composition, and molecular weight. It was reported that polyanhydrides derived from monomers containing aromatic moieties degrade much slower than aliphatic polyanhydrides [30]. Thus, the degradation rate can be tuned by controlling the composition of the corresponding copolymers. They degrade in vitro as well as in vivo to the nontoxic consistent dicarboxylic acids. Importantly, the materials based on the polyanhydrides show no evidence of inflammatory reaction [31]. Polyanhydrides constitute the only class of surface eroding polymers approved for clinical trial use by the Food and Drug Administration (FDA). One of the commonly used techniques for the preparation of polyanhydride-based nanoparticles is the solvent displacement method followed by freeze or spray drying [32–34]. Another method known as an anti-solvent nanoprecipitation technique utilized by Ulery et al. [35] and others [36–38] allows fabrication of the nanoparticles with relatively uniform size and shape. In biomedical research, polyanhydride-based nanoparticles have been widely explored as a vaccine adjuvant because of their ability to induce potent immune response in a pathogen-mimicking manner without side effects [37, 39–42].

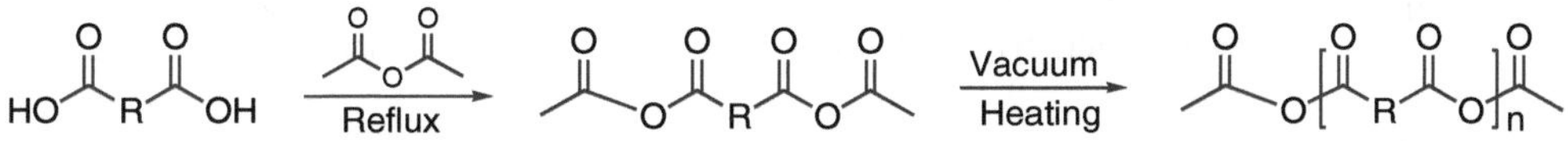

Scheme 2 Synthesis of polyanhydride prepolymer and polymer from a dicarboxylic acid

5 *N*-(2-Hydroxypropyl) Methacrylamide (HPMA) Copolymers

Among synthetic polymeric drug carriers, the water-soluble HPMA copolymers are the most studied for the last 40 years [43]. HPMA polymer–drug conjugates have been developed as nanomedicines for delivery of a number of therapeutics, including anticancer and anti-inflammatory agents [44–46]. HPMA polymers and their drug conjugates were initially synthesized by conventional free radical polymerization techniques. Recent advances in living radical polymerization methods, including atom transfer radical polymerization (ATRP) and reversible addition-fragmentation chain transfer (RAFT), allowed for the controlled synthesis of well-defined HPMA copolymers with narrow molecular weight distributions (Scheme 3) [47, 48].

HPMA copolymers have many attributes that make them ideally suited for the development as drug carriers. These polymers are biocompatible, non-immunogenic and can be tailored to the characteristics of the specific target. The molecular weight of HPMA copolymers can be adjusted to alter biodistribution, tissue localization and elimination from the body. The proper selection of the spacer between the drug and HPMA carrier (e.g., oligopeptide sequence, hydrazone bond, cis-aconityl spacer) allowed for controlled drug release within the tissue [49–52]. The HPMA copolymer conjugates containing doxorubicin were the first synthetic polymer-based therapeutics to enter clinical trials. Since then, numerous conjugates have been synthesized to contain drug or drug combinations, proteins and peptides, as well as targeting moieties and/or imaging probes. In addition, HPMA polymers were used for the modification of proteins, surface modification of biomaterials, masking and retargeting of therapeutic viruses and as macromolecular platforms for contrast agents.

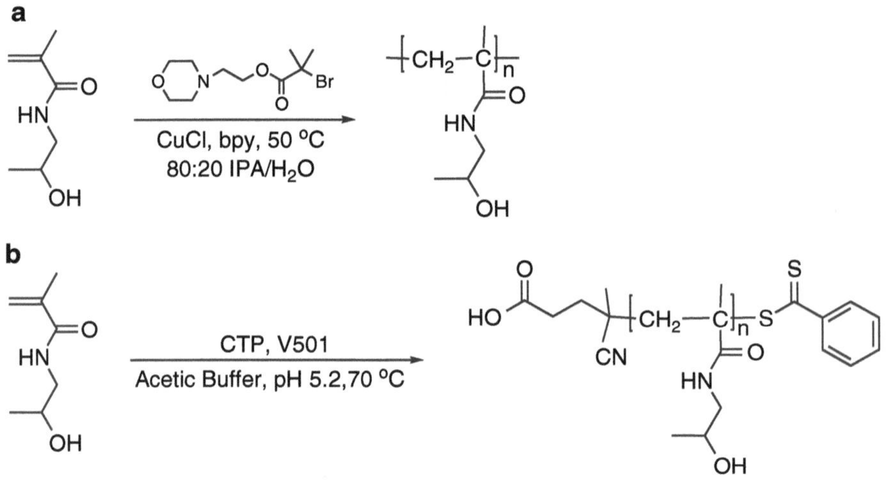

Scheme 3 Synthesis of HPMA polymer by (**a**) ATRP and (**b**) RAFT polymerization methods

6 Polyethylenimine (PEI)

PEIs are synthetic cationic polymers that have been widely employed as the most prominent polynucleotide delivery systems [53]. Depending on the linkage of the repeating ethylenimine units, PEI possesses either branched or linear topology (Scheme 4). Branched PEI is synthesized by polymerization of aziridine either in aqueous or alcoholic solutions [54–56], where the reaction is controlled by adjusting the temperature and initiator concentration, or in a rather vigorous bulk polymerization of anhydrous aziridine at a lower temperature [57]. Linear PEI has been synthesized via cationic ROP of either *N*-(2-tetrahydropyranyl)azidirine [58] or unsubstituted and 2-substituted 2-oxazolines followed by acid or base-catalyzed hydrolysis of the corresponding N-substituted polymer [59, 60].

The efficiency of PEI as transfection agent as well as its cytotoxicity is closely linked to the polymer characteristics such as molecular weight, the degree of branching, charge density and buffering capacity. Generally, the low molecular weight linear or branched PEIs have low cytotoxicity but display poor transfection efficiency. In order to solve the efficiency versus toxicity problems, cross-linked PEIs were synthesized to include biodegradable cross-links that facilitate an increase in molecular weight but then following cross-link degradation, allowing the release of lower molecular weight components to reduce cytotoxicity [61]. Alternatively, star-like PEI derivatives with high charge density have been designed; these polymers utilize low molecular weight PEIs that are conjugated to a central multivalent polymer core [62–64].

7 Amino Acid-based Polymers

Polymers based on natural L-amino acids are an attractive class of materials given their biocompatibility, controlled biodegradability, and metabolizable degradation products. Incorporation of amino

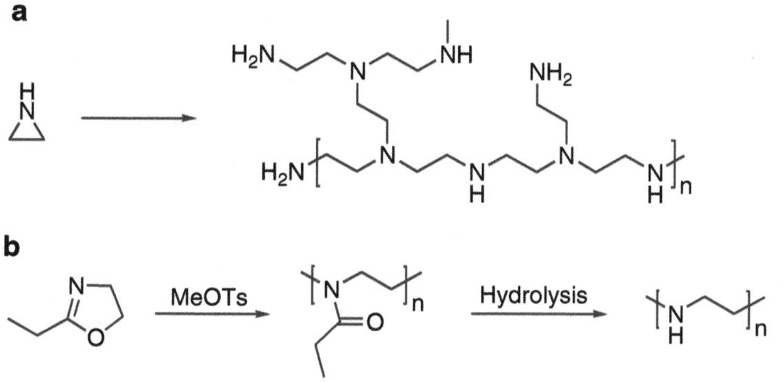

Scheme 4 Synthesis of (**a**) branched PEI by acid catalyzed polymerization of aziridine and (**b**) linear PEI by ROP of 2-ethyl-2-oxazoline

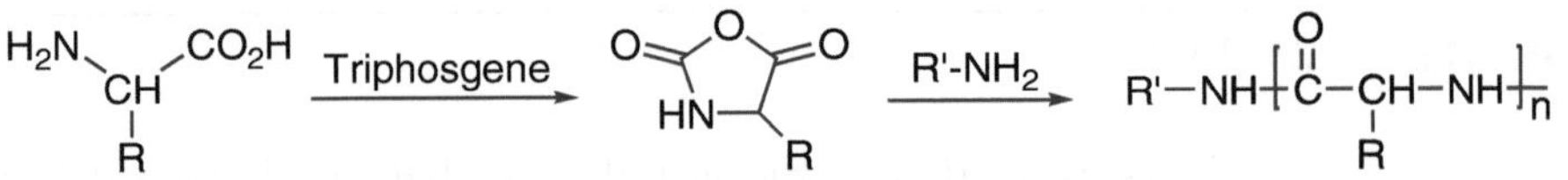

Scheme 5 Synthesis of polypeptides via α-amino acid *N*-carboxyanhydride ROP

acids as a building block into synthetic polymers not only allows for adjusting hydrophilic/hydrophobic properties of the resulting polymers and tune their degradability but also imparts chemical functionalities to facilitate further modification with bioactive molecules (e.g., drugs, imaging probes, or targeting ligands). The most common and efficient method to produce polypeptides of sufficient molecular weight is ROP of *N*-carboxyanhydrides (NCAs) [65]. NCAs are easily synthesized through a reaction between amino acids and phosgene or a phosgene derivative (e.g., triphosgene), and the polymerization is commonly initiated using amino-functional molecules (Scheme 5).

In recent years, the advances in NCA polymerizations, either using metal initiators or improved conventional initiators, allowed for the synthesis of broad range of block copolymers and side-chain functionalized polypeptides with controlled characteristics (molecular weight, sequence, composition, and molecular weight distribution) [66]. In addition, the diversity of synthetic polymer chemistries and "click" reactions offer the ability to covalently link a variety of different polymers together and prepare hybrid materials with functional macromolecular architectures and tunable physicochemical properties to meet various requirements of biomedical applications.

8 Dendrimers

Dendrimers are a unique class of polymeric materials most frequently synthesized using divergent or convergent strategies by a series of controlled polymerization reactions [67]. Divergent synthesis grows outwards from a multifunctional core molecule and comprises of two steps: first is the activation of functional surface groups, and second is the addition of branching monomer units. The process is repeated for several generations and a dendrimer is built layer after layer. While this method is successful for the production of relatively large quantities of dendrimers, problems occur from side reactions and incomplete reactions of the end groups that lead to structural defects. Convergent synthesis, on the other hand, starts at the surface and proceeds inwards before the attachment of the synthesized dendrons to the core [68]. In the convergent growth, a small number of reactive sites are functionalized in each step resulting in less number of side reactions and more precise control over molecular weight of the dendrimer.

However, convergent synthesis strategy is generally limited to the construction of lower-generation dendrimers due to steric difficulties upon attachment of the dendrons to the core molecule. In contrast to other synthetic polymers, dendrimers are nearly monodisperse in molecular weight and size. They are highly branched macromolecules of nanoscale molecular size with multiple surface group functionalities and practically perfect spherical topology in case of higher generations. Functionalization of their terminal groups provides an exceptional opportunity for the immobilization of multiple bioactive molecules and solubilizing groups in a specific and controllable manner. Alternatively, the numerous internal cavities in the dendrimer cores can be loaded with various drugs via hydrophobic interaction, hydrogen bonds or chemical conjugation. Surface modification of the dendrimer by a modification with polyethylene glycol (PEG), acetylation or esterification is often used to improve the drug loading capacity of the resulting dendrimers. It also renders them more biocompatible, less immunogenic, and less toxic, especially those decorated by free amino functionalities [69–71]. Because of these characteristics, dendrimers have been widely studied as nanoscale containers for delivery of therapeutic payloads. The flexibility to tailor both the core and surface of these systems allows optimizing the properties of drug carriers for the specific applications. Dendrimers of various structure, amphiphilicity, and architecture were explored as carriers for anticancer, antimalarial, antiviral, antitubercular, antimicrobial, and antihypertensive drugs [72]. Their application as scaffolds of prodrugs is particularly interesting [73–75]. Furthermore, several groups addressed the strategies for the synthesis of the degradable dendrimers that can achieve high accumulation and retention in diseased tissues, but allow rapid and safe elimination of nontoxic dendrimer fragments [76]. Biodegradable dendrimers are commonly prepared by inclusion of ester groups in the polymer backbone, which will be chemically hydrolyzed and/or enzymatically cleaved by esterases in physiological solutions [77]. For example, Frechet and colleagues reported efficient synthesis of robust and biodegradable PEGylated dendrimer based on a polyester–polyamide hybrid core. The architecture has been designed to avoid destructive side reactions during the synthesis while maintaining the dendrimer's degradability [78]. Polycationic dendrimers can be complexed with nucleic acids and used for gene therapy. Applications of dendrimers as protein mimics [79], biomimetic regeneration of hydroxyapatite [80], and mimicking in angiogenesis [81] has also been reported. Furthermore, dendrimers can act as "nano-drugs" themselves and their therapeutic potential has been explored against various diseases [82]. As an example, dendrimer-based nanomedicine mixed in carbomer gel (VivaGel®) is being developed as a vaginal microbicide gel to prevent the transmission of genital herpes and human immunodeficiency virus [83].

The active ingredient of this gel is a dendrimer comprising a divalent benzhydrylamine core and four generations of lysine branches capped with sulfonated naphthyl groups that impart hydrophobicity, and a high anionic charge to the dendrimer surface. Initial human trials have shown VivaGel to be safe and well-tolerated, and Phase II clinical studies for its efficacy are ongoing. Despite the promise of dendrimers-based drug delivery systems, their translation into actual therapies is challenging due to their lengthy synthesis and the need to develop nontoxic and biocompatible dendrimers.

9 Polymer Therapeutics

The term "Polymer Therapeutics" was coined by Prof. Ruth Duncan to define a family of new chemical entities that comprises a variety of complex macromolecular systems containing a water-soluble polymeric carrier covalently bound to the bioactive molecule(s). These polymeric drugs include polymer–drug and polymer–protein conjugates, polymeric micelles where drug is covalently bound to the polymer, and polyplexes (containing covalent linkers) developed as nonviral vectors for the delivery of nucleic acids [84]. Polymer is an integral and functional part of such multifunctional systems for improved drug, protein and gene delivery [30, 85, 86]. The linkers are typically sensitive to the conditions that are unique for the targeted site (e.g., an acidic environment, presence of specific enzyme), which increases the specificity of drug delivery and release. In addition, a targeting moiety may also be introduced into the conjugate to increase its therapeutic index. PEGylation has become a well-established technology for the use of proteins as drugs. When attached to a protein, peptide and more recently to an aptamers, typically via conjugation of a monomethoxylated PEG segment bearing a reactive moiety at one of the polymer termini, PEG imparts prolonged blood residency and diminished immunogenicity of the bioconjugate. The most studied polymer–drug conjugates are based on HPMA copolymer and PEG backbones and, initially, their design was focused on cancer treatments and incorporated common chemotherapeutic agents (e.g., doxorubicin, taxanes, camptothecin, or platinates) [87]. Over the years, numerous conjugates have been synthesized which contain drugs that act on the emerging targets for cancer therapy such as angiogenesis, apoptotic pathways, kinases and others. As an example, HPMA–fumagillol, the first antiangiogenic conjugate, proved to be effective at inhibiting tumor growth and exhibited a significantly better toxicity as compared to free drug [88]. It was demonstrated that HPMA copolymer–wortmannin conjugate retained the ability to inhibit type I PI3-kinase activity [89], and HPMA–geldanamycin conjugate inhibited the capacity of heat shock proteins such as HSP-90 to form complexes with client oncoproteins [90, 91]. Therapies focusing on the activation of apoptotic pathways are also promising anticancer strategies [92]. The PEGylation of curcumin, a Jab1 inhibitor, and the conjugation of Bcl2-inhibitor HA14 to HPMA, are two examples of this proapoptotic approach [93, 94]. In addition, polymer–drug conjugates were actively explored for the treatment of other diseases including infections [95], inflammation [96], rheumatoid arthritis [97] and diabetes [98]. Several preclinical studies have already illustrated the potential of conjugates in regenerative medicine, for example, for wound healing [99], ischemia [100], or osteoporosis [101]. The new concepts such as delivering drug combinations via one polymer carrier [102], exploring new polymer architectures (branched, grafted, and star polymers and dendrimers) or use of coiled-coil peptides motifs as linkers [103] are the recent developments in the field of polymer therapeutics. To address the concerns regarding the possible accumulation of the nondegradable polymers in the body, an increasing number of biodegradable polymers such as poly(glutamic acid) (PGA) [104], polyacetal Fleximer [105], poly(malic acid) [106], dextrin [107] have been investigated as platforms for the design of new polymer therapeutics. Translational research in polymer therapeutics has yielded ten marketed PEG-protein/aptamer conjugates [105, 108]. In the case of polymer–drug conjugates progression to regulatory approval has been slower. The closest to market is Opaxio™ (PGA-paclitaxel conjugate, also known as Xyotax or CT-2103) developed by Cell Therapeutics Inc. [http://www.celltherapeutics.com/opaxio], which is in advanced Phase III clinical trials. Opaxio™ sister conjugate CT-2106, PGA-camptothecin conjugate, is also in Phase II clinical trial. Promising results are emerging from a number of ongoing clinical studies involving anticancer conjugates such as ProLindac™, an HPMA copolymer DACH-platinate from Access Pharmaceuticals that has successfully completed a European Phase II clinical trial in patients with ovarian cancer [109]. PEG-irinotecan conjugate (NKTR-102) is undergoing Phase III evaluation in patients with metastatic breast cancer and is also being studied in Phase II clinical trials in ovarian and colorectal cancer [http://Nektar.com]. Mersana is commercializing XMT1001 (Fleximer®-camptothecin conjugate) as its lead candidate but has also a potent antiangiogenic conjugate XMT1107 (Fleximer®-fumagillin) in Phase I studies. Overall, the design and clinical development of new polymer therapeutics hold a significant potential of this group of NMs for targeting a wide range of the diseases.

10 Polymeric Micelles

Amphiphilic block or graft copolymers comprised of two or more chains with different hydrophobicity have been used extensively in pharmaceutical applications ranging from sustained-release technologies to gene delivery. These copolymers are known to spontaneously self-assemble in an aqueous solution into nanoscopic polymeric micelles (10–100 nm) having fairly narrow size distribution. The nature of the self-assembly process allows for significant versatility in the chemical composition of the polymeric micelles and thus permits fine tuning of the material properties, morphology and sizes. These micelles have unique core–shell architectures with hydrophobic polymer chains segregating into a micelle core surrounded by a shell of hydrophilic chains. Hydrophobic drugs can be entrapped into the micelle core non-specifically through hydrophobic interactions or specifically by chemical conjugation to the core-forming block of the copolymer via a carefully designed pH- or enzyme-sensitive linker that can be cleaved to release a drug in its active form. A variety of drugs with diverse physicochemical properties can be incorporated into the core by engineering the structure of the core-forming segment of the copolymer to attain sufficiently strong interaction with drug molecules. These polymeric micelle systems can also be used for co-delivery of two or more drugs with similar or different properties for combination therapy, or to combine multiple modalities within a single carrier [110, 111]. Hydrophilic shell serves as a stabilizing interface between the hydrophobic core and external milieu and most commonly consists of PEG chains with a molecular weight ranging from 2 to 15 kDa. In addition, shell can inhibit protein binding and opsonization during systemic administration, which allows them to remain in the circulation longer by evading the mononuclear phagocytic system. Also, modification of the shell with various ligands using different surface chemistries enables the micelle to be targeted to a specific site. A much wider range of hydrophobic blocks have been explored as drug loading cores. Examples include polyesters, polyanhydrides, poly(L-amino acids), poly(methyl methacrylate), phospholipids/long chain fatty acids, polypropylene oxide (in Pluronics/poloxamers). The choice of hydrophobic block is largely dictated by drug compatibility with the hydrophobic core (when drug is physically loaded) and the stability of the micelle. Micelles must be stable enough to retain drug cargo upon administration and remain intact long enough to accumulate in sufficient concentrations at the target site. The thermodynamic tendency for micelles to dissociate is primarily controlled by the length of the hydrophobic block while the kinetic (rate of dissociation) stability depends on many factors, including the size of a hydrophobic block, the mass ratio of hydrophilic to hydrophobic blocks, and physical state of the micelle core [112]. The incorporation of hydrophobic drugs may also further enhance micelle stability. Among the different strategies to enhance the kinetic stability of polymeric micelles, core- or shell-cross-linking have been shown to limit the premature disassembly and slow down the release of the encapsulated drug [113]. The resulting cross-linked micelles are, in essence, nanoscale single molecules that are stable upon dilution and can withstand environmental challenges and shear forces without structural deterioration. For example, Iijima et al. [114] have shown that core cross-linked micelles of PEG-b-poly(D,L-lactide) possess high stability against dilution, temperature change, and even dissolution of surfactants. Wooley and coworkers [115, 116] cross-linked the micellar corona and obtained the so-called shell-cross-linked knedel-like micelles—robust nanostructures with a permeable cross-linked shell. However, the reversible stabilization of the micellar structure will be more desirable to achieve efficient intracellular drug release and circumvent micelle accumulation in the body. To this end, the use of degradable polymer components or the introduction of reversible cross-links allowed development in situ degradable micelles [117–119]. High loading capacity and controlled drug release profile are key features for the potential drug delivery system. The loading capacity and loading efficiency of the polymeric micelles is influenced by several factors, including both structure of core-forming block and a drug, molecular characteristics of the copolymer, such as composition, molecular weight, and the solution temperature. The maximum loading level is largely influenced by the interaction between the drug and core-forming block, and stronger interactions enable saturation to be reached at a lower polymer concentration. The drug loading can also be improved by enhancing the local environment of the micelle core through the means of conjugation of small amount of drug [120] or conjugation of side chains with similar structure to the drug [121]. In addition, the location of the incorporated molecules within polymeric micelles (micelle core or the core–shell interface) determines the extent of solubilization as well as the rate of drug release [122, 123]. In general, for drugs physically incorporated in polymeric micelles, release is controlled by the rate of diffusion of the drug from the micellar core, stability of the micelles, and the rate of biodegradation of the copolymer. If the micelle is stable and the rate of polymer biodegradation is slow, the diffusion rate of the drug will be mainly determined by the compatibility between the drug and core-forming block of copolymer, amount of drug loaded, the molecular volume of drug, length of the core forming block, and physical state of the core. Moreover, external conditions such as change in pH, temperature or application of ultrasound [124] can also trigger drug release from polymeric micelles. Another important but less investigated factor that can affect different characteristics of polymeric micelles is the morphology and dimensions of micellar aggregates. Indeed, filamentous polymeric micelles ("filomicelles," also referred to as "worm micelles") with single dimensions as long as 18 μm (the diameter is ~57 nm) synthesized from amphiphilic PEG-*b*-PCL copolymer were reported to solubilize twice as much paclitaxel as spherical micelles [125].

Recently, Wooley's group [126] demonstrated that shell-cross-linked, rod-shaped micelles prepared from pH-sensitive poly(acrylic acid)-*b*-poly(p-hydroxystyrene) block copolymer exhibited a higher doxorubicin-loading capacity and rate of release compared to their spherical counterparts derived from the same copolymer precursor. Importantly, it was also demonstrated that rational design of polymeric micelles and other NMs of a given geometry (size and shape) offers an unprecedented control of their longevity in circulation and targeting to selective cellular and subcellular locations [127–129]. Further understanding of structure–activity relationships of such complex multicomponent nanomedicines is essential to determine the criteria for the successful development of polymeric micelle therapeutics. Currently several micelle formulations based on amphiphilic block copolymers are in clinical trials for treating a variety of cancers [130–133]. In addition, the first targeted micellar formulation (BIND-014) has recently reached clinical development [134].

The field of polymeric micelles was significantly advanced by employing charge-driven self-assembly of block copolymers containing water-soluble ionic and nonionic block (double hydrophilic block copolymers or block ionomers). The micellization of these copolymers can be induced by adding oppositely charged molecules such as synthetic [135, 136] or natural (DNA, proteins) [137–139] polyelectrolytes, surfactants/lipids [140, 141], or metal ions [142, 143]. These molecules form electrostatic complexes with the charged blocks of block ionomers, and prompt spontaneous segregation of the resulting complexes into micelle-like structures with electrostatically neutralized polyion cores and hydrophilic polymer shells. Ionic block lengths, charge density, and ionic strength of a solution affect the formation of stable block ionomer complexes and, therefore, control the amount of the drug that can be incorporated within the micelles [139, 144]. As an example, the metal-complex formation of ionic block copolymer, PEG-PGA, was explored to prepare polymeric micelles incorporating anticancer drug cisplatin. In preclinical studies, they exhibited remarkably prolonged blood circulation and effective accumulation in solid tumors [145]. This formulation is currently being evaluated in Phase III clinical trial as a treatment for pancreatic cancer under the name NC-6004 (Nanoplatin; NanoCarrier Co., Ltd.; Japan) [146].

Since being proposed independently by Kabanov and Kataoka [147, 148] in 1995, this approach has been widely used for developing nonviral gene delivery systems using cationic block or graft copolymers. In this case, the neutralization of positive charges on the polycation block by negatively charged DNA or siRNA leads to the formation of polyion micelles. Advanced and tunable characteristics of the cationic copolymers such as chemical structure and length of the segments, rigidity, hydrophilicity, charge density, biodegradability allow to modulate gene-delivery properties such as

DNA binding, colloidal stability of the complexes, toxicity, endosomal escape, vector unpacking, and transfection efficiency [149–151]. Similar to nucleic acid, charged proteins and peptides can be entrapped into a polyion micelle core [137, 152–154]. Recently, this strategy was successfully used for the delivery of antioxidant enzymes to the central nervous system [155–157]. There has also been a focus on the development of micellar carriers that are able to deliver both a therapeutic drug and a nucleic acid [158]. As an example, Wang and coworkers reported micelles composed of biodegradable PEG-poly(ε-caprolactone)-b-poly(2-aminoethylethylene phosphate) triblock copolymers, PEG-PCL-PPEEA, with the capacity to encapsulate hydrophobic paclitaxel into PCL core and complex siRNA against polo-like kinase 1 to the cationic PPEEA block. These micelles simultaneously delivered two payloads into the same tumor cells both in vitro and in vivo, and inhibited tumor growth in a synergistic manner following systemic administration [159].

11 Polymersomes

Polymersomes (polymeric vesicles) is another class of supramolecular assemblies formed by amphiphilic block copolymers in diluted aqueous solutions. Typically the formation of vesicular structures is favored for the copolymers with relatively low weight fraction of hydrophilic block (~20–40 %) [160]. Polymersome sizes vary from 50 nm to 10 μm depending on the chemical composition and the length of polymer blocks, the preparation method, as well as reaction conditions [161]. The copolymers of various architectures (diblock, triblock, graft, and dendritic) have been utilized as building blocks for design and preparation of polymersomes [162–165]. Nonbiodegradable poly(ethyl ethylene), poly(butadiene), poly(dimethylsiloxane), poly(propylene oxide), polystyrene as well as biodegradable PLA, PCL, and poly(trimethylene carbonate) have been used as a hydrophobic part of the block copolymers [166–171]. PEG, PGA and poly(acrylic acid) have been frequently selected as water-soluble blocks. More recently, so-called PICsomes (polyion complex vesicles) have been developed by electrostatic self-assembly of oppositely charged block- and homoionomers [172]. The key distinction between polymersomes and spherical micelles is that the former have an interior aqueous cavity surrounded by a wall that consists of entangled chains [173]. Due to the higher molecular weight of the polymers, polymersome membranes are generally thicker (8–22 nm), stronger, and hence, intrinsically more stable and less permeable than conventional liposomes. The thickness of the membrane is determined by the length of the hydrophobic block and can be tuned through fine control of the polymer chemical composition [167, 174–176]. The enhanced structural integrity and much denser hydrophilic polymer brush on the surface of the polymersomes lead to their more persistent circulation in the bloodstream [177]. Polymersomes are able to encapsulate hydrophilic, hydrophobic and amphiphilic molecules like any other vesicular structure, but their membrane tunability and superior stability are unique and undoubtedly beneficial for potential applications in drug delivery as well as medical diagnostics. Examples of drug-loaded polymersomes are increasingly broad and now include anticancer drugs, oligonucleotides, therapeutic proteins, diagnostic probes, or their combinations [178–182]. In addition, targetability of the polymersomes with various ligands attached to the surface has been demonstrated [183–187]. Recently, modulation of the membrane stability or permeability in response to specific stimulus has received a lot of attention as a strategy for controlled drug release from polymersomes. Numerous stimuli (e.g., pH, redox potential, temperature, magnetic field, light, and ultrasound) have been exploited in the design of stimuli-responsive polymersomes [188]. While these systems are still at the level of research and development, their structural versatility and improved properties in terms of stability and multifunctionality make them excellent candidates for potential biomedical applications.

12 Polymeric Nanogels

The term "nanogels" usually defines hydrogel particles of nanoscale size formed by physically or chemically cross-linked polymer networks [85]. Polymeric nanogels can be prepared by physical self-assembly of interactive polymers [189] or by cross-linking reaction of preformed polymers [190]. Nanoemulsion or microemulsion polymerization methods are often used to obtain nanogels with well-controlled sizes [191–193]. Another attractive set of synthetic techniques for preparation of nanogel particles is based on a template-assisted nanofabrication and exploit the internal water phase of liposomes [194], cross-linking of polymeric micelles [195, 196] or lithographic PRINT process [24]. Various chemical cross-linking reactions have now been developed, including photocross-linking, carbodiimide-mediated amide bond cross-linking, quaternization of amino groups, and "click" chemistry [143, 197–199]. Labile bonds are frequently introduced into nanogels during their synthesis to make them degradable and facilitate drug release. Dispersed in the water, the nanogels are highly swollen and can incorporate 30 % wt. and more of biological molecules and drugs through electrostatic, van der Waals and/or hydrophobic interactions or covalent bonding with the nanogel chains. These loading capacities are unusually high and exceed those of liposomes and polymeric micelles [85, 200]. As a result of drug loading, the nanogels collapse forming stable nanoparticles, in which biological agent becomes entrapped. Introducing dispersing hydrophilic polymers (e.g., PEG) in a nanogel structure can prevent their aggregation. During the collapse of the drug-nanogel complex hydrophilic polymer chains become exposed at the surface and form a protective layer around the nanogel. The control and versatility of polymer chemistry allows designing a broad range of drug formulations and inclusion of multiple therapeutic cargos within the same nanogel carrier [85, 196, 201]. Stimuli-responsive drug release via temperature or pH-induced volume collapse can also be very attractive for drug delivery applications. The functionalization of the nanogel surface can further facilitate their selective accumulation in the target tissue or cells [202–204]. Development of nanogels that can carry, protect, target and release therapeutic agents in spatially and temporally controlled manner is actively ongoing and their rational design can provide a platform for multiple applications.

Over the last decade, the field of polymer-based biomaterials for delivery of low molecular drugs, proteins and nucleic acids has seen exponential growth. Only selected examples were reviewed here due to the large number of contributions on this topic. Indeed, the recent advances in polymer chemistry have allowed the development of a diverse range of NMs of various sizes, shapes, surface chemistries, and targeting properties. Polymer composition also plays an essential role in function and application of such macromolecular carriers. There is growing evidence that some synthetic polymers can display biological response-modifying activity and can influence the molecular mechanism of action of a drug. Several of the polymer-based nanocarriers are already in clinical use and numerous of the others are undergoing various stages of preclinical and clinical evaluation. Although considerable progress has been made, further synthetic improvements are needed to design safe, more "intelligent" and efficient drug delivery platforms.

References

1. Brigger I, Dubernet C, Couvreur P (2002) Nanoparticles in cancer therapy and diagnosis. Adv Drug Deliv Rev 54(5):631–651
2. Lavan DA, McGuire T, Langer R (2003) Small-scale systems for in vivo drug delivery. Nat Biotechnol 21(10):1184–1191
3. Brannon-Peppas L, Blanchette JO (2012) Nanoparticle and targeted systems for cancer therapy. Adv Drug Deliv Rev 64:206–212
4. Vert M (2005) Aliphatic polyesters: great degradable polymers that cannot do everything. Biomacromolecules 6(2):538–546
5. Jérôme C, Lecomte P (2008) Recent advances in the synthesis of aliphatic polyesters by ring-opening polymerization. Adv Drug Deliv Rev 60(9):1056–1076
6. Labet M, Thielemans W (2009) Synthesis of polycaprolactone: a review. Chem Soc Rev 38(12):3484–3504
7. Lou X, Detrembleur C, Jérôme R (2003) Novel aliphatic polyesters based on functional cyclic (di) esters. Macromol Rapid Commun 24(2):161–172
8. Williams CK (2007) Synthesis of functionalized biodegradable polyesters. Chem Soc Rev 36(10):1573–1580
9. Penczek S, Cypryk M, Duda A, Kubisa P, Słomkowski S (2007) Living ring-opening polymerizations of heterocyclic monomers. Prog Polym Sci 32(2):247–282
10. Gross RA, Ganesh M, Lu W (2010) Enzyme-catalysis breathes new life into polyester

condensation polymerizations. Trends Biotechnol 28(8):435–443
11. Soppimath KS, Aminabhavi TM, Kulkarni AR, Rudzinski WE (2001) Biodegradable polymeric nanoparticles as drug delivery devices. J Control Release 70(1):1–20
12. Desgouilles S, Vauthier C, Bazile D, Vacus J, Grossiord J-L, Veillard M et al (2003) The design of nanoparticles obtained by solvent evaporation: a comprehensive study. Langmuir 19(22):9504–9510
13. Lai M-K, Tsiang R-C (2004) Encapsulating acetaminophen into poly (L-lactide) microcapsules by solvent-evaporation technique in an O/W emulsion. J Microencapsul 21(3): 307–316
14. Hariharan S, Bhardwaj V, Bala I, Sitterberg J, Bakowsky U, Kumar MR (2006) Design of estradiol loaded PLGA nanoparticulate formulations: a potential oral delivery system for hormone therapy. Pharm Res 23(1):184–195
15. Messai I, Delair T (2005) Adsorption of chitosan onto poly (D, L-lactic acid) particles: a physico-chemical investigation. Macromol Chem Phys 206(16):1665–1674
16. Keegan ME, Falcone JL, Leung TC, Saltzman WM (2004) Biodegradable microspheres with enhanced capacity for covalently bound surface ligands. Macromolecules 37(26):9779–9784
17. Zambaux M, Bonneaux F, Gref R, Maincent P, Dellacherie E, Alonso M et al (1998) Influence of experimental parameters on the characteristics of poly (lactic acid) nanoparticles prepared by a double emulsion method. J Control Release 50(1):31–40
18. Paiphansiri U, Tangboriboonrat P, Landfester K (2006) Polymeric nanocapsules containing an antiseptic agent obtained by controlled nanoprecipitation onto water-in-oil miniemulsion droplets. Macromol Biosci 6(1):33–40
19. Govender T, Stolnik S, Garnett MC, Illum L, Davis SS (1999) PLGA nanoparticles prepared by nanoprecipitation: drug loading and release studies of a water soluble drug. J Control Release 57(2):171–185
20. Jung T, Breitenbach A, Kissel T (2000) Sulfobutylated poly (vinyl alcohol)-graft-poly (lactide-co-glycolide) s facilitate the preparation of small negatively charged biodegradable nanospheres. J Control Release 67(2):157–169
21. Allémann E, Leroux J-C, Gurny R, Doelker E (1993) In vitro extended-release properties of drug-loaded poly (DL-lactic acid) nanoparticles produced by a salting-out procedure. Pharm Res 10(12):1732–1737
22. Karnik R, Gu F, Basto P, Cannizzaro C, Dean L, Kyei-Manu W et al (2008) Microfluidic platform for controlled synthesis of polymeric nanoparticles. Nano Lett 8(9):2906–2912
23. Rolland JP, Maynor BW, Euliss LE, Exner AE, Denison GM, DeSimone JM (2005) Direct fabrication and harvesting of monodisperse, shape-specific nanobiomaterials. J Am Chem Soc 127(28):10096–10100
24. Gratton SE, Pohlhaus PD, Lee J, Guo J, Cho MJ, DeSimone JM (2007) Nanofabricated particles for engineered drug therapies: a preliminary biodistribution study of PRINT™ nanoparticles. J Control Release 121(1):10–18
25. Enlow EM, Luft JC, Napier ME, DeSimone JM (2011) Potent engineered PLGA nanoparticles by virtue of exceptionally high chemotherapeutic loadings. Nano Lett 11(2):808–813
26. Chasin M, Lewis D, Langer R (1988) Polyanhydrides for controlled drug delivery. Biopharm Manufact 1:33–46
27. Kumar N, Langer RS, Domb AJ (2002) Polyanhydrides: an overview. Adv Drug Deliv Rev 54(7):889–910
28. Conix A (1966) Poly [1, 3-bis (p-carboxyphenoxy)-propane anhydride], macromolecular synthesis, vol 2. Wiley, New York, NY
29. Domb A, Langer R (1987) Polyanhydrides. I. Preparation of high molecular weight polyanhydrides. J Polym Sci A Polym Chem 25(12):3373–3386
30. Leong K, Brott B, Langer R (1985) Bioerodible polyanhydrides as drug-carrier matrices. I: Characterization, degradation, and release characteristics. J Biomed Mater Res 19(8):941–955
31. Katti D, Lakshmi S, Langer R, Laurencin C (2002) Toxicity, biodegradation and elimination of polyanhydrides. Adv Drug Deliv Rev 54(7):933–961
32. Rebouças JDS, Irache JM, Camacho AI, Esparza I, del Pozo V, Sanz ML et al (2012) Development of poly (anhydride) nanoparticles loaded with peanut proteins: the influence of preparation method on the immunogenic properties. Eur J Pharm Biopharm 82(2):241–249
33. Agüeros M, Ruiz-Gatón L, Vauthier C, Bouchemal K, Espuelas S, Ponchel G et al (2009) Combined hydroxypropyl-β-cyclodextrin and poly (anhydride) nanoparticles improve the oral permeability of paclitaxel. Eur J Pharm Sci 38(4):405–413
34. Arbos P, Campanero M, Arangoa M, Renedo M, Irache J (2003) Influence of the surface characteristics of PVM/MA nanoparticles on their bioadhesive properties. J Control Release 89(1):19–30

35. Ulery BD, Phanse Y, Sinha A, Wannemuehler MJ, Narasimhan B, Bellaire BH (2009) Polymer chemistry influences monocytic uptake of polyanhydride nanospheres. Pharm Res 26(3):683–690
36. Petersen L, Sackett C, Narasimhan B (2010) High-throughput analysis of protein stability in polyanhydride nanoparticles. Acta Biomater 6(10):3873–3881
37. Chavez-Santoscoy A, Carrillo-Conde B, Song E-H, Phanse Y, Ramer-Tait AE, Pohl NL et al. (2011) Targeted activation of antigen presenting cells with mannose-modified polyanhydride nanoparticles. Trans Soc Biomater 34
38. Haughney SL, Petersen LK, Schoofs AD, Ramer-Tait AE, King JD, Briles DE et al (2013) Retention of structure, antigenicity, and biological function of pneumococcal surface protein A (PspA) released from polyanhydride nanoparticles. Acta Biomater 9(9):8262–8271
39. Petersen LK, Ramer-Tait AE, Broderick SR, Kong C-S, Ulery BD, Rajan K et al (2011) Activation of innate immune responses in a pathogen-mimicking manner by amphiphilic polyanhydride nanoparticle adjuvants. Biomaterials 32(28):6815–6822
40. Chavez-Santoscoy AV, Roychoudhury R, Pohl NL, Wannemuehler MJ, Narasimhan B, Ramer-Tait AE (2012) Tailoring the immune response by targeting C-type lectin receptors on alveolar macrophages using "pathogen-like" amphiphilic polyanhydride nanoparticles. Biomaterials 33(18):4762–4772
41. Petersen L, Phanse Y, Ramer-Tait A, Wannemuehler M, Narasimhan B (2012) Amphiphilic polyanhydride nanoparticles stabilize Bacillus anthracis protective antigen. Mol Pharm 9(4):874–882
42. Ulery BD, Petersen LK, Phanse Y, Kong CS, Broderick SR, Kumar D et al (2011) Rational design of pathogen-mimicking amphiphilic materials as nanoadjuvants. Sci Rep 1:198
43. Kopeček J, Kopečková P (2010) HPMA copolymers: origins, early developments, present, and future. Adv Drug Deliv Rev 62(2):122–149
44. Duncan R (2006) Polymer conjugates as anticancer nanomedicines. Nat Rev Cancer 6(9):688–701
45. Kopeček J, Kopečková P, Minko T, Lu Z-R (2000) HPMA copolymer–anticancer drug conjugates: design, activity, and mechanism of action. Eur J Pharm Biopharm 50(1):61–81
46. Wang D, Miller SC, Liu X, Anderson B, Wang XS, Goldring SR (2007) Novel dexamethasone-HPMA copolymer conjugate and its potential application in treatment of rheumatoid arthritis. Arthritis Res Ther 9(1):R2
47. Teodorescu M, Matyjaszewski K (1999) Atom transfer radical polymerization of (meth) acrylamides. Macromolecules 32(15):4826–4831
48. Scales CW, Vasilieva YA, Convertine AJ, Lowe AB, McCormick CL (2005) Direct, controlled synthesis of the nonimmunogenic, hydrophilic polymer, poly (N-(2-hydroxypropyl) methacrylamide) via RAFT in aqueous media. Biomacromolecules 6(4):1846–1850
49. Duncan R, Kopeckova-Rejmanova P, Strohalm J, Hume I, Cable H, Pohl J et al (1987) Anticancer agents coupled to N-(2-hydroxypropyl) methacrylamide copolymers. I. Evaluation of daunomycin and puromycin conjugates in vitro. Br J Cancer 55(2):165
50. Šubr V, Kopeček J, Pohl J, Baudyš M, Kostka V (1988) Cleavage of oligopeptide side-chains in N-(2-hydroxypropyl) meth-acrylamide copolymers by mixtures of lysosomal enzymes. J Control Release 8(2):133–140
51. Subr V, Strohalm J, Ulbrich K, Duncan R, Hume I (1992) Polymers containing enzymatically degradable bonds, XII. Effect of spacer structure on the rate of release of daunomycin and adriamycin from poly [N-(2-hydroxypropyl)-methacrylamide] copolymer drag carriers in vitro and antitumour activity measured in vivo. J Control Release 18(2):123–132
52. Liu X-M, Quan L-D, Tian J, Alnouti Y, Fu K, Thiele GM et al (2008) Synthesis and evaluation of a well-defined HPMA copolymer–dexamethasone conjugate for effective treatment of rheumatoid arthritis. Pharm Res 25(12):2910–2919
53. Lemkine G, Demeneix B (2001) Polyethylenimines for in vivo gene delivery. Curr Opin Mol Ther 3(2):178–182
54. von Harpe A, Petersen H, Li Y, Kissel T (2000) Characterization of commercially available and synthesized polyethylenimines for gene delivery. J Control Release 69(2):309–322
55. Kunath K, von Harpe A, Fischer D, Petersen H, Bickel U, Voigt K et al (2003) Low-molecular-weight polyethylenimine as a non-viral vector for DNA delivery: comparison of physicochemical properties, transfection efficiency and in vivo distribution with high-molecular-weight polyethylenimine. J Control Release 89(1):113–125
56. Fischer D, Bieber T, Li Y, Elsässer H-P, Kissel T (1999) A novel non-viral vector for DNA delivery based on low molecular weight,

branched polyethylenimine: effect of molecular weight on transfection efficiency and cytotoxicity. Pharm Res 16(8):1273–1279

57. Dick C, Ham G (1970) Characterization of polyethylenimine. J Macromol Sci Pure Appl Chem 4(6):1301–1314
58. Weyts KF, Goethals EJ (1988) New synthesis of linear polyethyleneimine. Polym Bull 19(1):13–19
59. Saegusa T, Ikeda H, Fujii H (1972) Isomerization polymerization of 2-oxazoline. I. Preparation of unsubstituted 2-oxazoline polymer. Polym J 3(1):35–39
60. Saegusa T, Ikeda H, Fujii H (1972) Isomerization polymerization of 2-oxazoline. IV. Kinetic study of 2-methyl-2-oxazoline polymerization. Macromolecules 5(4): 359–362
61. Peng Q, Zhong Z, Zhuo R (2008) Disulfide cross-linked polyethylenimines (PEI) prepared via thiolation of low molecular weight PEI as highly efficient gene vectors. Bioconjug Chem 19(2):499–506
62. Nakayama Y, Kakei C, Ishikawa A, Zhou Y-M, Nemoto Y, Uchida K (2007) Synthesis and in vitro evaluation of novel star-shaped block copolymers (blocked star vectors) for efficient gene delivery. Bioconjug Chem 18(6):2037–2044
63. Banerjee P, Weissleder R, Bogdanov A (2006) Linear polyethyleneimine grafted to a hyperbranched poly (ethylene glycol)-like core: a copolymer for gene delivery. Bioconjug Chem 17(1):125–131
64. Namgung R, Kim J, Singha K, Kim CH, Kim WJ (2009) Synergistic effect of low cytotoxic linear polyethylenimine and multiarm polyethylene glycol: study of physicochemical properties and in vitro gene transfection. Mol Pharm 6(6):1826–1835
65. Hadjichristidis N, Iatrou H, Pitsikalis M, Sakellariou G (2009) Synthesis of well-defined polypeptide-based materials via the ring-opening polymerization of α-amino acid N-carboxyanhydrides. Chem Rev 109(11):5528–5578
66. Cheng J, Deming TJ (2012) Synthesis of polypeptides by ring-opening polymerization of α-amino acid N-carboxyanhydrides, Peptide-based materials. Springer, New York, NY, pp 1–26
67. Hodge P (1993) Polymer science branches out. Nature 362:18–19
68. Hawker CJ, Frechet JM (1990) Preparation of polymers with controlled molecular architecture. A new convergent approach to dendritic macromolecules. J Am Chem Soc 112(21):7638–7647
69. Jevprasesphant R, Penny J, Jalal R, Attwood D, McKeown N, D'emanuele A (2003) The influence of surface modification on the cytotoxicity of PAMAM dendrimers. Int J Pharm 252(1):263–266
70. Choi JS, Nam K, Park J-Y, Kim J-B, Lee J-K, Park J-S (2004) Enhanced transfection efficiency of PAMAM dendrimer by surface modification with L-arginine. J Control Release 99(3):445–456
71. Kim Y, Klutz AM, Jacobson KA (2008) Systematic investigation of polyamidoamine dendrimers surface-modified with poly (ethylene glycol) for drug delivery applications: synthesis, characterization, and evaluation of cytotoxicity. Bioconjug Chem 19(8):1660–1672
72. Kesharwani P, Jain K, Jain NK (2014) Dendrimer as nanocarrier for drug delivery. Prog Polym Sci 39(2):268–307
73. Kukowska-Latallo JF, Candido KA, Cao Z, Nigavekar SS, Majoros IJ, Thomas TP et al (2005) Nanoparticle targeting of anticancer drug improves therapeutic response in animal model of human epithelial cancer. Cancer Res 65(12):5317–5324
74. McCarthy TD, Karellas P, Henderson SA, Giannis M, O'Keefe DF, Heery G et al (2005) Dendrimers as drugs: discovery and preclinical and clinical development of dendrimer-based microbicides for HIV and STI prevention. Mol Pharm 2(4):312–318
75. Sampathkumar S-G, Yarema KJ (2005) Targeting cancer cells with dendrimers. Chem Biol 12(1):5
76. Medina SH, El-Sayed ME (2009) Dendrimers as carriers for delivery of chemotherapeutic agents. Chem Rev 109(7):3141–3157
77. Twibanire JAK, Grindley TB (2014) Polyester dendrimers: smart carriers for drug delivery. Polymers 6(1):179–213
78. van der Poll DG, Kieler-Ferguson HM, Floyd WC, Guillaudeu SJ, Jerger K, Szoka FC et al (2010) Design, synthesis, and biological evaluation of a robust, biodegradable dendrimer. Bioconjug Chem 21(4):764–773
79. Liu L, Breslow R (2003) Dendrimeric pyridoxamine enzyme mimics. J Am Chem Soc 125(40):12110–12111
80. Wu D, Yang J, Li J, Chen L, Tang B, Chen X et al (2013) Hydroxyapatite-anchored dendrimer for in situ remineralization of human tooth enamel. Biomaterials 34(21):5036–5047
81. Kasai S, Nagasawa H, Shimamura M, Uto Y, Hori H (2002) Design and synthesis of antiangiogenic/heparin-binding arginine dendrimer mimicking the surface of endostatin. Bioorg Med Chem Lett 12(6):951–954

82. Gajbhiye V, Palanirajan VK, Tekade RK, Jain NK (2009) Dendrimers as therapeutic agents: a systematic review. J Pharm Pharmacol 61(8):989–1003
83. Rupp R, Rosenthal SL, Stanberry LR (2007) VivaGel™(SPL7013 Gel): a candidate dendrimer–microbicide for the prevention of HIV and HSV infection. Int J Nanomedicine 2(4):561
84. Duncan R (2003) The dawning era of polymer therapeutics. Nat Rev Drug Discov 2(5): 347–360
85. Kabanov AV, Vinogradov SV (2009) Nanogels as pharmaceutical carriers: finite networks of infinite capabilities. Angew Chem Int Ed Engl 48(30):5418–5429
86. Vicent MJ, Duncan R (2006) Polymer conjugates: nanosized medicines for treating cancer. Trends Biotechnol 24(1):39–47
87. Vicent MJ, Ringsdorf H, Duncan R (2009) Polymer therapeutics: clinical applications and challenges for development. Adv Drug Deliv Rev 61(13):1117–1120
88. Satchi-Fainaro R, Puder M, Davies JW, Tran HT, Sampson DA, Greene AK et al (2004) Targeting angiogenesis with a conjugate of HPMA copolymer and TNP-470. Nat Med 10(3):255–261
89. Varticovski L, Lu Z-R, Mitchell K, de Aos I, Kopeček J (2001) Water-soluble HPMA copolymer–wortmannin conjugate retains phosphoinositide 3-kinase inhibitory activity in vitro and in vivo. J Control Release 74(1):275–281
90. Larson N, Ray A, Malugin A, Pike DB, Ghandehari H (2010) HPMA copolymer-aminohexylgeldanamycin conjugates targeting cell surface expressed GRP78 in prostate cancer. Pharm Res 27(12):2683–2693
91. Kasuya Y, Lu Z-R, Kopečková P, Tabibi SE, Kopeček J (2002) Influence of the structure of drug moieties on the in vitro efficacy of HPMA copolymer–geldanamycin derivative conjugates. Pharm Res 19(2):115–123
92. Vicent MJ (2007) Polymer-drug conjugates as modulators of cellular apoptosis. AAPS J 9(2):E200–E207
93. Li J, Wang Y, Yang C, Wang P, Oelschlager DK, Zheng Y et al (2009) Polyethylene glycosylated curcumin conjugate inhibits pancreatic cancer cell growth through inactivation of Jab1. Mol Pharmacol 76(1):81–90
94. Oman M, Liu J, Chen J, Durrant D, Yang H-S, He Y et al (2006) Using N-(2-hydroxypropyl) methacrylamide copolymer drug bioconjugate as a novel approach to deliver a Bcl-2-targeting compound HA14-1 in vivo. Gene Ther Mol Biol A 10:113–122
95. Vicent MJ, Cascales L, Carbajo RJ, Cortés N, Messeguer A, Pérez Payá E (2010) Nanoconjugates as intracorporeal neutralizers of bacterial endotoxins. J Control Release 142(2):277–285
96. Santamaría B, Benito-Martin A, Ucero AC, Aroeira LS, Reyero A, Vicent MJ et al (2009) A nanoconjugate Apaf-1 inhibitor protects mesothelial cells from cytokine-induced injury. PLoS One 4(8):e6634
97. Liu X-M, Quan L-D, Tian J, Laquer FC, Ciborowski P, Wang D (2010) Syntheses of click PEG–dexamethasone conjugates for the treatment of rheumatoid arthritis. Biomacromolecules 11(10):2621–2628
98. Ikumi Y, Kida T, Sakuma S, Yamashita S, Akashi M (2008) Polymer–phloridzin conjugates as an anti-diabetic drug that Inhibits glucose absorption through the Na+/glucose cotransporter (SGLT1) in the small intestine. J Control Release 125(1):42–49
99. Shaunak S, Thomas S, Gianasi E, Godwin A, Jones E, Teo I et al (2004) Polyvalent dendrimer glucosamine conjugates prevent scar tissue formation. Nat Biotechnol 22(8):977–984
100. Mondragon L, Orzaez M, Sanclimens G, Moure A, Arminan A, Sepulveda P et al (2008) Modulation of cellular apoptosis with apoptotic protease-activating factor 1 (Apaf-1) inhibitors. J Med Chem 51(3):521–529
101. Pan H, Sima M, Kopečková P, Wu K, Gao S et al (2008) Biodistribution and pharmacokinetic studies of bone-targeting N-(2-hydroxypropyl) methacrylamide copolymer–alendronate conjugates. Mol Pharm 5(4):548–558
102. Greco F, Vicent MJ (2009) Combination therapy: opportunities and challenges for polymer–drug conjugates as anticancer nanomedicines. Adv Drug Deliv Rev 61(13):1203–1213
103. Deacon SP, Apostolovic B, Carbajo RJ, Schott A-K, Beck K, Vicent MJ et al (2010) Polymer coiled-coil conjugates: potential for development as a new class of therapeutic "molecular switch". Biomacromolecules 12(1):19–27
104. Chipman SD, Oldham FB, Pezzoni G, Singer JW (2006) Biological and clinical characterization of paclitaxel poliglumex (PPX, CT-2103), a macromolecular polymer–drug conjugate. Int J Nanomedicine 1(4):375
105. Sausville E, Garbo L, Weiss G, Shkolny D, Yurkovetskiy A, Bethune C et al (2010) Phase I study of XMT-1001 given IV every 3 weeks to patients with advanced solid tumors. J Clin Oncol 28:13121
106. Lee B-S, Fujita M, Khazenzon NM, Wawrowsky KA, Wachsmann-Hogiu S, Farkas

DL et al (2006) Polycefin, a new prototype of a multifunctional nanoconjugate based on poly (β-L-malic acid) for drug delivery. Bioconjug Chem 17(2):317–326
107. Hreczuk-Hirst D, Chicco D, German L, Duncan R (2001) Dextrins as potential carriers for drug targeting: tailored rates of dextrin degradation by introduction of pendant groups. Int J Pharm 230(1):57–66
108. Becker R, Dembek C, White LA, Garrison LP (2012) The cost offsets and cost-effectiveness associated with pegylated drugs: a review of the literature. Expert Rev Pharmacoecon Outcomes Res 12:775
109. Duncan R, Vicent MJ (2010) Do HPMA copolymer conjugates have a future as clinically useful nanomedicines? A critical overview of current status and future opportunities. Adv Drug Deliv Rev 62(2):272–282
110. Godsey ME, Suryaprakash S, Leong KW (2013) Materials innovation for co-delivery of diverse therapeutic cargos. RSC Adv 3(47):24794–24811
111. Zhu L, Perche F, Wang T, Torchilin VP (2014) Matrix metalloproteinase 2-sensitive multifunctional polymeric micelles for tumor-specific co-delivery of siRNA and hydrophobic drugs. Biomaterials 35(13):4213–4222
112. Allen C, Maysinger D, Eisenberg A (1999) Nano-engineering block copolymer aggregates for drug delivery. Colloids Surf B Biointerfaces 16(1):3–27
113. O'Reilly RK, Hawker CJ, Wooley KL (2006) Cross-linked block copolymer micelles: functional nanostructures of great potential and versatility. Chem Soc Rev 35(11):1068–1083
114. Iijima M, Nagasaki Y, Okada T, Kato M, Kataoka K (1999) Core-polymerized reactive micelles from heterotelechelic amphiphilic block copolymers. Macromolecules 32(4): 1140–1146
115. Thurmond KB, Kowalewski T, Wooley KL (1996) Water-soluble knedel-like structures: the preparation of shell-cross-linked small particles. J Am Chem Soc 118(30):7239–7240
116. Elsabahy M, Wooley KL (2012) Strategies toward well-defined polymer nanoparticles inspired by nature: chemistry versus versatility. J Polym Sci A Polym Chem 50(10): 1869–1880
117. Li Y, Lokitz BS, Armes SP, McCormick CL (2006) Synthesis of reversible shell cross-linked micelles for controlled release of bioactive agents. Macromolecules 39(8): 2726–2728
118. Kim JO, Sahay G, Kabanov AV, Bronich TK (2010) Polymeric micelles with ionic cores containing biodegradable cross-links for delivery of chemotherapeutic agents. Biomacromolecules 11(4):919–926
119. Li YL, Zhu L, Liu Z, Cheng R, Meng F, Cui JH et al (2009) Reversibly stabilized multifunctional dextran nanoparticles efficiently deliver doxorubicin into the nuclei of cancer cells. Angew Chem Int Ed Engl 48(52): 9914–9918
120. Nakanishi T, Fukushima S, Okamoto K, Suzuki M, Matsumura Y, Yokoyama M et al (2001) Development of the polymer micelle carrier system for doxorubicin. J Control Release 74(1):295–302
121. Adams ML, Kwon GS (2003) Relative aggregation state and hemolytic activity of amphotericin B encapsulated by poly (ethylene oxide)- block–poly (N-hexyl-l-aspartamide)-acyl conjugate micelles: effects of acyl chain length. J Control Release 87(1):23–32
122. Teng Y, Morrison M, Munk P, Webber S, Procházka K (1998) Release kinetics studies of aromatic molecules into water from block polymer micelles. Macromolecules 31(11):3578–3587
123. Choucair A, Eisenberg A (2003) Interfacial solubilization of model amphiphilic molecules in block copolymer micelles. J Am Chem Soc 125(39):11993–12000
124. Husseini GA, Christensen DA, Rapoport NY, Pitt WG (2002) Ultrasonic release of doxorubicin from Pluronic P105 micelles stabilized with an interpenetrating network of N,N-diethylacrylamide. J Control Release 83(2):303–305
125. Cai S, Vijayan K, Cheng D, Lima EM, Discher DE (2007) Micelles of different morphologies—advantages of worm-like filomicelles of PEO-PCL in paclitaxel delivery. Pharm Res 24(11):2099–2109
126. Lee NS, Lin LY, Neumann WL, Freskos JN, Karwa A, Shieh JJ et al (2011) Influence of nanostructure morphology on host capacity and kinetics of guest release. Small 7(14):1998–2003
127. Geng Y, Dalhaimer P, Cai S, Tsai R, Tewari M, Minko T et al (2007) Shape effects of filaments versus spherical particles in flow and drug delivery. Nat Nanotechnol 2(4): 249–255
128. Simone EA, Dziubla TD, Muzykantov VR (2008) Polymeric carriers: role of geometry in drug delivery. Expert Opin Drug Deliv 5:1283
129. Zhang K, Fang H, Chen Z, Taylor J-SA, Wooley KL (2008) Shape effects of nanoparticles conjugated with cell-penetrating peptides (HIV Tat PTD) on CHO cell uptake. Bioconjug Chem 19(9):1880–1887

130. Valle JW, Armstrong A, Newman C, Alakhov V, Pietrzynski G, Brewer J et al (2011) A phase 2 study of SP1049C, doxorubicin in P-glycoprotein-targeting pluronics, in patients with advanced adenocarcinoma of the esophagus and gastroesophageal junction. Invest New Drugs 29(5):1029–1037
131. Kim T-Y, Kim D-W, Chung J-Y, Shin SG, Kim S-C, Heo DS et al (2004) Phase I and pharmacokinetic study of Genexol-PM, a cremophor-free, polymeric micelle-formulated paclitaxel, in patients with advanced malignancies. Clin Cancer Res 10(11):3708–3716
132. Hamaguchi T, Matsumura Y, Suzuki M, Shimizu K, Goda R, Nakamura I et al (2005) NK105, a paclitaxel-incorporating micellar nanoparticle formulation, can extend in vivo antitumour activity and reduce the neurotoxicity of paclitaxel. Br J Cancer 92(7):1240–1246
133. Chin K, Kato K, Yoshikawa T, Yamaguchi K, Esaki T, Tsuji Y et al (2010) Phase II study of NK105, a paclitaxel-incorporating micellar nanoparticle as second-line treatment for advanced or recurrent gastric cancer. J Clin Oncol 28(15S):4041
134. Hrkach J, Von Hoff D, Ali MM, Andrianova E, Auer J, Campbell T et al (2012) Preclinical development and clinical translation of a PSMA-targeted docetaxel nanoparticle with a differentiated pharmacological profile. Sci Transl Med 4(128):128ra39
135. Kabanov AV, Bronich TK, Kabanov VA, Yu K, Eisenberg A (1996) Soluble stoichiometric complexes from poly (N-ethyl-4-vinylpyridinium) cations and poly (ethylene oxide)-block-polymethacrylate anions. Macromolecules 29(21):6797–6802
136. Harada A, Nakanishi K, Ichimura S, Kojima C, Kono K (2009) Spontaneous formation of narrowly-distributed self-assembly from polyamidoamine dendron-poly (L-lysine) block copolymers through helix-coil transition of poly (L-lysine) block. J Polym Sci A Polym Chem 47(4):1217–1223
137. Batrakova EV, Li S, Reynolds AD, Mosley RL, Bronich TK, Kabanov AV et al (2007) A macrophage-nanozyme delivery system for Parkinson's disease. Bioconjug Chem 18(5):1498–1506
138. Kishimura A, Koide A, Osada K, Yamasaki Y, Kataoka K (2007) Encapsulation of myoglobin in PEGylated polyion complex vesicles made from a pair of oppositely charged block ionomers: a physiologically available oxygen carrier. Angew Chem Int Ed Engl 46(32):6085–6088
139. Kakizawa Y, Kataoka K (2002) Block copolymer micelles for delivery of gene and related compounds. Adv Drug Deliv Rev 54(2):203–222
140. Bronich TK, Kabanov AV, Kabanov VA, Yu K, Eisenberg A (1997) Soluble complexes from poly (ethylene oxide)-block-polymethacrylate anions and N-alkylpyridinium cations. Macromolecules 30(12):3519–3525
141. Kabanov AV, Bronich T, Kabanov V, Yu K, Eisenberg A (1998) Spontaneous formation of vesicles from complexes of block ionomers and surfactants. J Am Chem Soc 120(38):9941–9942
142. Yokoyama M, Okano T, Sakurai Y, Suwa S, Kataoka K (1996) Introduction of cisplatin into polymeric micelle. J Control Release 39(2):351–356
143. Bronich TK, Keifer PA, Shlyakhtenko LS, Kabanov AV (2005) Polymer micelle with cross-linked ionic core. J Am Chem Soc 127(23):8236–8237
144. Kabanov AV, Kabanov VA (1998) Interpolyelectrolyte and block ionomer complexes for gene delivery: physico-chemical aspects. Adv Drug Deliv Rev 30(1):49–60
145. Nishiyama N, Okazaki S, Cabral H, Miyamoto M, Kato Y, Sugiyama Y et al (2003) Novel cisplatin-incorporated polymeric micelles can eradicate solid tumors in mice. Cancer Res 63(24):8977–8983
146. Heinemann V, Quietzsch D, Gieseler F, Gonnermann M, Schönekäs H, Rost A et al (2006) Randomized phase III trial of gemcitabine plus cisplatin compared with gemcitabine alone in advanced pancreatic cancer. J Clin Oncol 24(24):3946–3952
147. Kabanov AV, Vinogradov SV, Suzdaltseva YG, Alakhov VY (1995) Water-soluble block polycations as carriers for oligonucleotide delivery. Bioconjug Chem 6(6):639–643
148. Harada A, Kataoka K (1995) Formation of polyion complex micelles in an aqueous milieu from a pair of oppositely-charged block copolymers with poly (ethylene glycol) segments. Macromolecules 28(15):5294–5299
149. Miyata K, Nishiyama N, Kataoka K (2012) Rational design of smart supramolecular assemblies for gene delivery: chemical challenges in the creation of artificial viruses. Chem Soc Rev 41(7):2562–2574
150. Itaka K, Yamauchi K, Harada A, Nakamura K, Kawaguchi H, Kataoka K (2003) Polyion complex micelles from plasmid DNA and poly (ethylene glycol)–poly (l-lysine) block copolymer as serum-tolerable polyplex system: physicochemical properties of micelles relevant to gene transfection efficiency. Biomaterials 24(24):4495–4506

151. Katayose S, Kataoka K (1997) Water-soluble polyion complex associates of DNA and poly (ethylene glycol)-poly (L-lysine) block copolymer. Bioconjug Chem 8(5):702–707
152. Harada A, Kataoka K (2001) Pronounced activity of enzymes through the incorporation into the core of polyion complex micelles made from charged block copolymers. J Control Release 72(1):85–91
153. Yuan X, Harada A, Yamasaki Y, Kataoka K (2005) Stabilization of lysozyme-incorporated polyion complex micelles by the ω-end derivatization of poly (ethylene glycol)-poly (α, β-aspartic acid) block copolymers with hydrophobic groups. Langmuir 21(7):2668–2674
154. Zhang J, Mulvenon A, Makarov E, Wagoner J, Knibbe J, Kim JO et al (2013) Antiviral peptide nanocomplexes as a potential therapeutic modality for HIV/HCV co-infection. Biomaterials 34(15):3846–3857
155. Klyachko NL, Manickam DS, Brynskikh AM, Uglanova SV, Li S, Higginbotham SM et al (2012) Cross-linked antioxidant nanozymes for improved delivery to CNS. Nanomedicine (Lond) 8(1):119–129
156. Manickam DS, Brynskikh AM, Kopanic JL, Sorgen PL, Klyachko NL, Batrakova EV et al (2012) Well-defined cross-linked antioxidant nanozymes for treatment of ischemic brain injury. J Control Release 162(3):636–645
157. Savalia K, Manickam DS, Rosenbaugh EG, Tian J, Ahmad TM, Kabanov AV et al (2014) Neuronal uptake of nanoformulated superoxide dismutase and attenuation of angiotensin II-dependent hypertension following central administration. Free Radic Biol Med 73:299
158. Jhaveri AM, Torchilin VP (2014) Multifunctional polymeric micelles for delivery of drugs and siRNA. Front Pharmacol 5:77
159. Sun T-M, Du J-Z, Yao Y-D, Mao C-Q, Dou S, Huang S-Y et al (2011) Simultaneous delivery of siRNA and paclitaxel via a "two-in-one" micelleplex promotes synergistic tumor suppression. ACS Nano 5(2):1483–1494
160. Lee JCM, Bermudez H, Discher BM, Sheehan MA, Won YY, Bates FS et al (2001) Preparation, stability, and in vitro performance of vesicles made with diblock copolymers. Biotechnol Bioeng 73(2):135–145
161. Yu G-e, Eisenberg A (1998) Multiple morphologies formed from an amphiphilic ABC triblock copolymer in solution. Macromolecules 31(16):5546–5549
162. Jain JP, Kumar N (2010) Self assembly of amphiphilic (PEG) 3-PLA copolymer as polymersomes: preparation, characterization, and their evaluation as drug carrier. Biomacromolecules 11(4):1027–1035
163. Ayen WY, Chintankumar B, Jain JP, Kumar N (2011) Effect of PEG chain length and hydrophilic weight fraction on polymersomes prepared from branched (PEG) 3-PLA co-polymers. Polym Adv Technol 22(1):158–165
164. Zheng C, Qiu L, Zhu K (2009) Novel polymersomes based on amphiphilic graft polyphosphazenes and their encapsulation of water-soluble anti-cancer drug. Polymer 50(5):1173–1177
165. del Barrio J, Oriol L, Sánchez C, Serrano JL, Di Cicco A, Keller P et al (2010) Self-assembly of linear–dendritic diblock copolymers: from nanofibers to polymersomes. J Am Chem Soc 132(11):3762–3769
166. Schillén K, Bryskhe K, Mel'Nikova YS (1999) Vesicles formed from a poly (ethylene oxide)-poly (propylene oxide)-poly (ethylene oxide) triblock copolymer in dilute aqueous solution. Macromolecules 32(20):6885–6888
167. Discher BM, Won Y-Y, Ege DS, Lee JC, Bates FS, Discher DE et al (1999) Polymersomes: tough vesicles made from diblock copolymers. Science 284(5417):1143–1146
168. Kukula H, Schlaad H, Antonietti M, Förster S (2002) The formation of polymer vesicles or "Peptosomes" by polybutadiene-b lock-poly (l-glutamate) s in dilute aqueous solution. J Am Chem Soc 124(8):1658–1663
169. Ding J, Liu G (1997) Polyisoprene-block-poly (2-cinnamoylethyl methacrylate) vesicles and their aggregates. Macromolecules 30(3):655–657
170. Nardin C, Hirt T, Leukel J, Meier W (2000) Polymerized ABA triblock copolymer vesicles. Langmuir 16(3):1035–1041
171. Meng F, Engbers GH, Feijen J (2005) Biodegradable polymersomes as a basis for artificial cells: encapsulation, release and targeting. J Control Release 101(1):187–198
172. Chuanoi S, Kishimura A, Dong W-F, Anraku Y, Yamasaki Y, Kataoka K (2013) Structural factors directing nanosized polyion complex vesicles (Nano-PICsomes) to form a pair of block aniomer/homo catiomers: studies on the aniomer segment length and the catiomer side-chain structure. Polym J 46:130
173. Battaglia G, Ryan AJ (2005) Bilayers and interdigitation in block copolymer vesicles. J Am Chem Soc 127(24):8757–8764
174. Meng F, Hiemstra C, Engbers GH, Feijen J (2003) Biodegradable polymersomes. Macromolecules 36(9):3004–3006
175. Dimova R, Seifert U, Pouligny B, Förster S, Döbereiner H-G (2002) Hyperviscous diblock copolymer vesicles. Eur J Phys E 7(3):241–250

176. Nardin C, Widmer J, Winterhalter M, Meier W (2001) Amphiphilic block copolymer nanocontainers as bioreactors. Eur J Phys E 4(4):403–410
177. Lee JS, Ankone M, Pieters E, Schiffelers RM, Hennink WE, Feijen J (2011) Circulation kinetics and biodistribution of dual-labeled polymersomes with modulated surface charge in tumor-bearing mice: comparison with stealth liposomes. J Control Release 155(2):282–288
178. Ghoroghchian PP, Li G, Levine DH, Davis KP, Bates FS, Hammer DA et al (2006) Bioresorbable vesicles formed through spontaneous self-assembly of amphiphilic poly (ethylene oxide)-block-polycaprolactone. Macromolecules 39(5):1673–1675
179. Ahmed F, Pakunlu RI, Brannan A, Bates F, Minko T, Discher DE (2006) Biodegradable polymersomes loaded with both paclitaxel and doxorubicin permeate and shrink tumors, inducing apoptosis in proportion to accumulated drug. J Control Release 116(2):150–158
180. Kim Y, Tewari M, Pajerowski JD, Cai S, Sen S, Williams J et al (2009) Polymersome delivery of siRNA and antisense oligonucleotides. J Control Release 134(2):132–140
181. Chen W, Meng F, Cheng R, Zhong Z (2010) pH-Sensitive degradable polymersomes for triggered release of anticancer drugs: a comparative study with micelles. J Control Release 142(1):40–46
182. Hickey RJ, Koski J, Meng X, Riggleman RA, Zhang P, Park S-J (2014) Size-controlled self-assembly of superparamagnetic polymersomes. ACS Nano 8(1):495–502
183. Pangburn TO, Georgiou K, Bates FS, Kokkoli E (2012) Targeted polymersome delivery of siRNA induces cell death of breast cancer cells dependent upon Orai3 protein expression. Langmuir 28(35):12816–12830
184. Lin JJ, Ghoroghchian PP, Zhang Y, Hammer DA (2006) Adhesion of antibody-functionalized polymersomes. Langmuir 22(9):3975–3979
185. Kim B-S, Yang W-Y, Ryu J-H, Yoo Y-S, Lee M (2005) Carbohydrate-coated nanocapsules from amphiphilic rod–coil molecule: binding to bacterial type 1 pili. Chem Commun 15:2035–2037
186. Yang X, Grailer JJ, Rowland IJ, Javadi A, Hurley SA, Matson VZ et al (2010) Multifunctional stable and pH-responsive polymer vesicles formed by heterofunctional triblock copolymer for targeted anticancer drug delivery and ultrasensitive MR imaging. ACS Nano 4(11):6805–6817
187. Brož P, Benito SM, Saw C, Burger P, Heider H, Pfisterer M et al (2005) Cell targeting by a generic receptor-targeted polymer nanocontainer platform. J Control Release 102(2):475–488
188. Lee JS, Feijen J (2012) Polymersomes for drug delivery: design, formation and characterization. J Control Release 161(2):473–483
189. Sasaki Y, Akiyoshi K (2012) Self-assembled nanogel engineering for advanced biomedical technology. Chem Lett 41(3):202–208
190. Vinogradov SV, Bronich TK, Kabanov AV (2002) Nanosized cationic hydrogels for drug delivery: preparation, properties and interactions with cells. Adv Drug Deliv Rev 54(1):135–147
191. McAllister K, Sazani P, Adam M, Cho MJ, Rubinstein M, Samulski RJ et al (2002) Polymeric nanogels produced via inverse microemulsion polymerization as potential gene and antisense delivery agents. J Am Chem Soc 124(51):15198–15207
192. Oh JK, Tang C, Gao H, Tsarevsky NV, Matyjaszewski K (2006) Inverse miniemulsion ATRP: a new method for synthesis and functionalization of well-defined water-soluble/cross-linked polymeric particles. J Am Chem Soc 128(16):5578–5584
193. Murthy N, Xu M, Schuck S, Kunisawa J, Shastri N, Fréchet JM (2003) A macromolecular delivery vehicle for protein-based vaccines: acid-degradable protein-loaded microgels. Proc Natl Acad Sci U S A 100(9):4995–5000
194. Murphy EA, Majeti BK, Mukthavaram R, Acevedo LM, Barnes LA, Cheresh DA (2011) Targeted nanogels: a versatile platform for drug delivery to tumors. Mol Cancer Ther 10(6):972–982
195. Turner JL, Wooley KL (2004) Nanoscale cage-like structures derived from polyisoprene-containing shell cross-linked nanoparticle templates. Nano Lett 4(4):683–688
196. Desale SS, Cohen SM, Zhao Y, Kabanov AV, Bronich TK (2013) Biodegradable hybrid polymer micelles for combination drug therapy in ovarian cancer. J Control Release 171(3):339–348
197. Wooley K, Remsen E (1998) Amphiphilic core–shell nanospheres obtained by intramicellar shell crosslinking of polymer micelles with poly (ethylene oxide) linkers. Chem Commun 13:1415–1416
198. Bütün V, Lowe A, Billingham N, Armes S (1999) Synthesis of zwitterionic shell cross-

linked micelles. J Am Chem Soc 121(17): 4288–4289

199. Zhang J, Zhou Y, Zhu Z, Ge Z, Liu S (2008) Polyion complex micelles possessing thermo-responsive coronas and their covalent core stabilization via "click" chemistry. Macromolecules 41(4):1444–1454

200. Torchilin VP (2012) Multifunctional nano-carriers. Adv Drug Deliv Rev 64:302–315

201. Kim JO, Kabanov AV, Bronich TK (2009) Polymer micelles with cross-linked polyanion core for delivery of a cationic drug doxorubicin. J Control Release 138(3):197–204

202. Vinogradov SV, Batrakova EV, Kabanov AV (2004) Nanogels for oligonucleotide delivery to the brain. Bioconjug Chem 15(1):50–60

203. Nukolova NV, Oberoi HS, Cohen SM, Kabanov AV, Bronich TK (2011) Folate-decorated nanogels for targeted therapy of ovarian cancer. Biomaterials 32(23):5417–5426

204. Nukolova NV, Oberoi HS, Zhao Y, Chekhonin VP, Kabanov AV, Bronich TK (2013) LHRH-targeted nanogels as a delivery system for cisplatin to ovarian cancer. Mol Pharm 10(10):3913–3921

Chapter 2

Cyclodextrin-Based Drug Carriers for Low Molecular Weight Drugs, Proteins, and Nucleic Acids

Taishi Higashi, Keiichi Motoyama, and Hidetoshi Arima

Abstract

Currently, active pharmaceutical ingredients (APIs) have diversified from low molecular weight compounds to proteins, gene, or oligonucleotides, and the advanced drug delivery systems are required to determine the optimum pharmaceutical formulations. In this context, a large number of oligo-/polysaccharide-based nanomaterials such as cellulose, dextran, chitosan/chitin, mannan, hyaluronic acid, and sacran are utilized as advanced drug carriers for the various drugs. On the other hand, cyclodextrins (CyDs) have mainly been used as pharmaceutical excipients for low molecular weight drugs to improve their solubility, stability, taste, bioavailability, etc. However, the use of CyDs as drug carriers for proteins and nucleic acids is limited because of their weak interactions. Of note, CyD-based drug carriers combined with various functional materials such as ligands, polymers, nanosphere, microsphere, liposome, and micelle have recently been developed for low molecular weight drugs, proteins, or nucleic acids. In the present chapter, we review recent oligo-/polysaccharide- and CyD-based drug carriers for various drugs.

Key words Saccharide, Cyclodextrin, Drug delivery system, Low molecular weight drugs, Proteins, Nucleic acids, Folic acid, Polypseudorotaxane, Polyethylene glycol, Dendrimer

1 Introduction

Recently, active pharmaceutical ingredients (APIs) have been extending from low molecular weight compounds to proteins or nucleic acids. As a result, advanced pharmaceutical techniques are required to develop the drugs including proteins or nucleic acids. For instance, improvements of solubility, stability, and/or blood retention are required to develop protein drugs [1]. In the case of nucleic acids, improvements of their transfer efficiencies to target tissues and cells are necessary [2]. To achieve these techniques, various biomaterials such as polymers, sugars, liposome, micelle, and nanosphere are utilized [3–7].

Oligo-/polysaccharides are promising biomaterials possessing the multifunctions and high safety and used as targeting ligands, pharmaceutical excipients, gelatinizers, etc. in the pharmaceutical

Zheng-Rong Lu and Shinji Sakuma (eds.), *Nanomaterials in Pharmacology*, Methods in Pharmacology and Toxicology, DOI 10.1007/978-1-4939-3121-7_2, © Springer Science+Business Media New York 2016

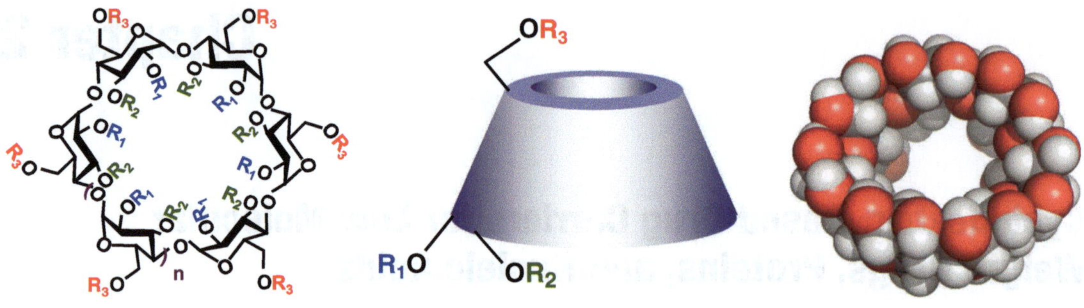

n=1, α-CyDs ; n=2, β-CyDs ; n=3, γ-CyDs.

Cylodextrin derivative	R_1	R_2	R_3
Methyl-cyclodextrin (M-CyD)	R_1, R_2, R_3 = H or CH_3		
2,6-Di-*O*-methyl-3-*O*-acetyl-cyclodextrin (DMA-CyD)	CH_3	$COCH_3$	CH_3
2-Hydroxypropyl-cyclodextrin (HP-CyD)	R_1, R_2, R_3 = H or $CH_2CH(OH)CH_3$		
6-*O*-Glucuronylglucosyl-cyclodextrin (GUG-CyD)	H	H	H or glucuronylglucose

Fig. 1 Structures of CyDs and their derivatives

fields. For example, oligo-/polysaccharides including mannose or fucose and galactose are utilized as targeting ligands for Kupffer cell and hepatocyte, respectively [8, 9]. Also, cellulose and its derivatives are useful excipients to prepare the tablets [10]. Sucrose, trehalose, sorbitol, and some oligo-/polysaccharides are used as stabilizers for protein drugs [11, 12]. Alginate, carrageenan, gellan gum, xanthan gum, etc. form hydrogels encapsulating the drugs and are utilized as controlled release carriers for various drugs [13]. Thus, oligo-/polysaccharides have been fundamental biomaterials in the pharmaceutical fields.

Cyclodextrins (CyDs) are cyclic oligosaccharides composed of six (α-CyD), seven (β-CyD), and eight (γ-CyD) glucopyranose units, containing a hydrophobic central cavity and hydrophilic outer surface (Fig. 1) [14]. CyDs are known to form inclusion complexes with a variety of guest molecules in solution and in a solid state, and the solubilization of lipophilic drugs by CyDs has been widely utilized in the pharmaceutical fields [15, 16]. In the cell biology fields, CyDs at higher concentration induce hemolysis and decrease the integrity of the mucosal epithelial cells and extract cholesterol, phospholipids, and proteins from biological membranes, which are useful for investigating the function of caveolae, lipid rafts, and cholesterol transporter [17]. However, the interactions between CyDs and proteins or nucleic acids are negligible, resulting in a limitation to utilize CyDs as drug carriers for these drugs.

Recently, oligo-/polysaccharide- and CyD-based drug carriers combined with various functional materials such as ligands, polymers, nanosphere, microsphere, liposome, and micelle are developed for low molecular weight drugs, proteins, or nucleic acids [18–22].

In this chapter, we introduce a number of recent oligo-/polysaccharide- and CyD-based drug carriers for various drugs. Especially, we focus on CyD-based multifunctional drug carriers in this review.

2 Oligo-/Polysaccharide-Based Drug Carriers

Recently, a large number of oligo-/polysaccharide-based drug carriers combined with various functional materials are developed and utilized for low molecular weight compounds to proteins or nucleic acids. Song et al. prepared sucrose- and maltose-modified liposomes encapsulating doxorubicin (DOX) [23]. Both sugar-modified liposomes enhanced the cellular uptake of DOX via lectin-mediated endocytosis and showed high antitumor activity in vitro. Ishii et al. prepared oligomannose-coated liposome [24]. This liposome had the potentials as a delivery carrier and an adjuvant of antigens to dendritic cells. In addition, Higuchi et al. demonstrated the utility of fucosylated cationic liposome as a Kupffer cell-selective delivery carrier for NF-κB decoy [25]. The NF-κB decoy complex with fucosylated cationic liposome could be useful for treatment of cytokine-related liver disease.

Oligo-/polysaccharides have also been used as sustained release drug carriers for various drugs. For example, chitosan is utilized as controlled release carriers for insulin, streptomycin, bovine serum albumin, etc. [26]. Chitosan is a cationic biodegradable polysaccharide and is one of the most widely used biopolymers in drug delivery system (DDS). Interestingly, chitosan is also used as antimicrobial, wound healing, hypocholesterolemic, and antiulcer agents [26]. Meanwhile, dextran is used as sustained release drug carriers for antibiotics, tacrolimus, imaging agents, etc. [27]. For example, the conjugation with dextran provides prolonged blood half-life and passive targeting ability to various drugs such as proteins and antitumor drugs [27]. In addition, Tokatlian et al. prepared porous hydrogels consisting of hyaluronic acid which is one of the anionic polysaccharides and demonstrated their utility as nonviral DNA carriers [28]. Furthermore, Chen et al. reported that diisocyanate/Pluronic F127/hyaluronic acid hydrogel provides sustained and thermo-responsive release of DOX and shows potent antitumor effect in vitro [29].

Recently, Okajima et al. extracted supergiant ampholytic sugar chains from the Japanese indigenous cyanobacterium *Aphanothece sacrum* and named it sacran [30]. Sacran consists of glucose, galactose, mannose, xylose, rhamnose, fucose, galacturonic acid, glucuronic acid, alanine, galactosamine, and muramic acid. Surprisingly, molecular weight of sacran is markedly high (>20 MDa) and sacran forms film and hydrogel. More recently, Motoyama et al. utilized sacran as sustained release drug carriers [31]. Sacran formed hydrogels in the presence of various charged drugs such as 4-biphenyl acetic acid, prednisolone, and chlorpheniramine maleate. In addition, the sacran hydrogels prolonged the release of the drugs, and the release could be controlled by the concentration of aluminum chloride as a cross-linker. Thus, sacran has the potentials for novel sustained release drug carriers.

3 Cyclodextrin-Based Drug Carriers for Low Molecular Weight Drugs

Currently, a large number of low molecular weight drugs are used in the clinical field, although trend of APIs has shifted to proteins and nucleic acids. So far, CyDs have been utilized as pharmaceutical excipients to improve solubility, stability, bioavailability, etc. of low molecular weight drugs. Recently, CyD-based supramolecular compounds are developed as drug carriers for low molecular weight drugs. For instance, Namgung et al. developed a novel drug carrier formed by multivalent host-guest interactions between a polymer/CyD conjugate and a polymer/paclitaxel conjugate [32]. This multivalent host-guest interaction between CyD and paclitaxel provided the formation of stable nanoparticle, and this nano-assembly delivered paclitaxel into the targeted cancer cells and released the drug via a degradation of ester linkages between paclitaxel and the polymer backbone, resulting in significant antitumor activity in a mouse tumor model. Salmaso et al. prepared the β-CyD conjugate with folic acid through a polyethylene glycol (PEG) spacer [33–35]. β-CyD moiety in this conjugate included rhodamine-B, and the resulting complex was incorporated into KB cells, a folate receptor-α (FR-α)-overexpressing human epidermal carcinoma cell line, but not into MCF7 cells, a non-FR-α-expressing human lung carcinoma cell line [33–35]. Zhang et al. prepared the folic acid/PEG-β-CyD conjugate through a click chemistry strategy [36]. This conjugate formed nanoparticle with 5-fluorouracil in aqueous solution and provided selective uptake of the drug through FR-α-mediated endocytosis.

Recently, Okamatsu et al. developed folic acid-appended β-CyDs possessing one or two caproic acids between folic acid and a β-CyD molecule as a spacer (Fol-cap1-β-CyD or Fol-cap2-β-CyD) and evaluated them as novel tumor targeting carriers for antitumor drugs [37, 38]. In these conjugates, the β-CyD moiety works as a reservoir of antitumor drugs, and spacer provides strong host-guest interaction. Actually, both Fol-cap1-β-CyD and Fol-cap2-β-CyD formed stable inclusion complexes with DOX at pH 7.3 with high stability constants ($>10^6$ M^{-1}). In addition, Fol-cap-β-CyDs increased cellular uptake of DOX in KB cells. Interestingly, stability constants of Fol-cap-β-CyDs and DOX markedly decreased at pH 6.8, implying the drug release in the lysosome (Fig. 2). Also, Fol-cap-β-CyDs increased cytotoxic activities of DOX, vinblastine, and paclitaxel in KB cells, but not in A549 cells, a FR-α-negative

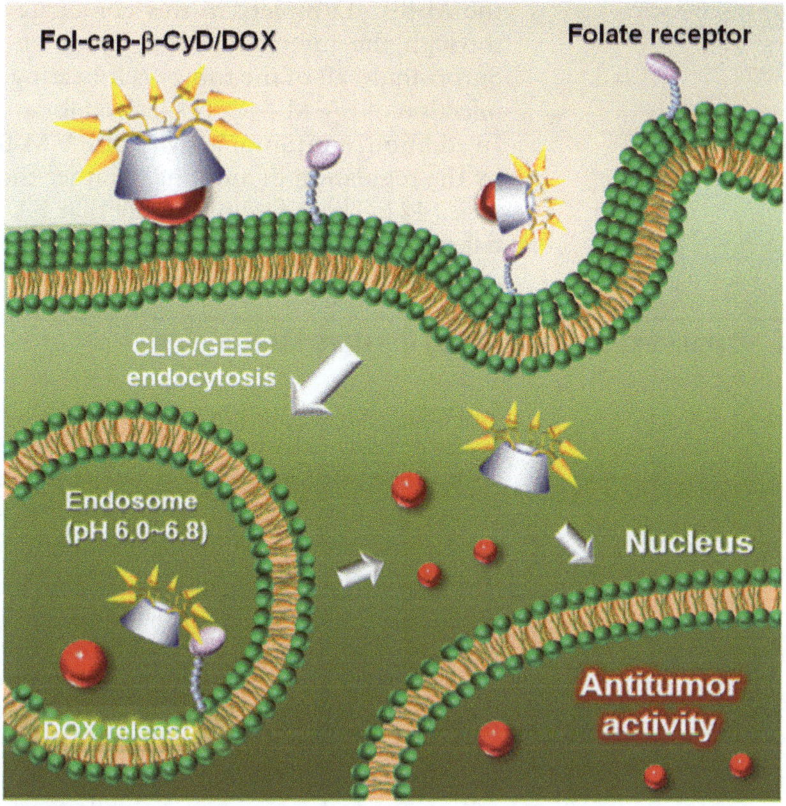

Fig. 2 Proposed mechanism for antitumor effect of DOX complexes with Fol-cap-β-CyDs

human lung adenocarcinoma epithelial cell line. Furthermore, the complexes of DOX with Fol-cap-β-CyDs showed significant antitumor activity, not only after the intratumoral administration but also after the intravenous administration to mice subcutaneously inoculated colon-26 cells, a FR-α-positive mouse colon adenocarcinoma cell line. Thus, Fol-cap-β-CyDs could be useful as promising antitumor drug carriers.

Motoyama et al. developed folate-appended methyl-β-CyD (FA-M-β-CyD) as a novel antitumor drug carrier [39, 40]. The M-β-CyD moiety in the conjugates formed stable inclusion complexes with DOX and paclitaxel. In addition, FA-M-β-CyD increased antitumor activity of DOX and paclitaxel in KB cells, but not 5-fluorouracil. Moreover, FA-M-β-CyD/DOX complex showed markedly high antitumor activity compared to DOX alone and M-β-CyD/DOX complex in vivo. These results suggest the potentials of FA-M-β-CyD as tumor-selective carriers for antitumor drugs.

Meanwhile, Onodera et al. reported that FA-M-β-CyD shows excellent antitumor activity by itself after an intratumoral or intravenous injection to colon-26 cell-bearing mice [41]. In this case, the M-β-CyD moiety in this conjugate shows antitumor activity through the interaction with lipids on the cellular membranes. Surprisingly, all of the tumor cell-bearing mice after an intravenous injection of FA-M-β-CyD survived for at least more than 140 days. In addition, antitumor activity of FA-M-β-CyD could be mediated by the regulation of autophagy rather than the induction of apoptosis [42]. These findings imply that FA-M-β-CyD has the potential as a novel anticancer agent.

4 Cyclodextrin-Based Drug Carriers for Proteins

Currently, a large number of protein drugs are used in the pharmaceutical fields. However, low stability, low proteolytic resistance, immunogenicity, and short circulating half-life of the proteins often hinder the development of protein drugs. In addition, controlled release systems of proteins are also required to achieve the optimum treatments. Therefore, various methods such as additions of pharmaceutical excipients, PEGylation techniques, and point mutations are applied to improve the properties of protein drugs [1].

PEGylation technology has been widely used to improve therapeutic efficacies of protein drugs [43]. For example, when PEG is covalently attached to a protein, it transfers many of the polymer's favorable characteristics to the resulting conjugate, i.e., a number of benefits such as increased circulating half-life, enhanced proteolytic resistance, reduced antigenicity and immunogenicity, reduced aggregation, and improved bioavailability. However, the activities of proteins are lost by PEGylation because of a steric hindrance formed by PEG chains.

Most recently, Arima and colleagues developed self-assembly PEGylation retaining the activity (SPRA) technology via a host-guest interaction between β-CyD and adamantane, i.e., the inclusion complexation of adamantane/insulin conjugate and PEGylated β-CyD (Fig. 3) (unpublished data). This supramolecular PEGylated insulin could dissociate a PEG chain from the assembly, resulting in the prolonged hypoglycemic effect without loss of the activity.

CyDs can also form inclusion complexes with linear polymers such as PEG. Harada et al. first reported the supramolecular assemblies of PEG and α-CyD, namely, polypseudorotaxane, in which a number of the cyclic molecules are spontaneously threaded onto the polymer chain [44, 45]. On the other hand, γ-CyD forms the polypseudorotaxane with double-stranded PEG [46]. These polypseudorotaxanes are less soluble in water, although CyDs in the polypseudorotaxanes can be dethreaded from the polymer chain by dilution. When both ends of the polymer chains in polypseudorotaxanes are covalently capped with bulky molecules, CyDs are trapped in and cannot be dethreaded from the assembly, giving the so-called polyrotaxane [47].

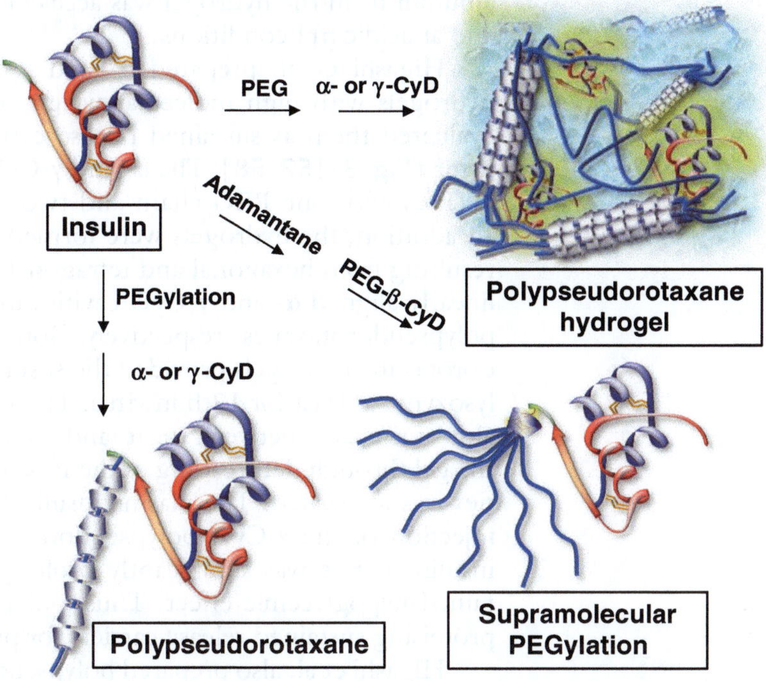

Fig. 3 CyD-based controlled release systems for insulin introduced in this review

Recently, drug carriers utilizing polyrotaxanes or polypseudorotaxanes have been developed for protein drugs. Li et al. reported the sustained release system for macromolecular drugs using polypseudorotaxane hydrogels consisting of α-CyD and high molecular weight PEGs (M.W. 8000–100,000) [48]. Both components spontaneously formed polypseudorotaxane hydrogels possessing the thixotropic property. In addition, the hydrogels showed the sustained release profiles of FITC-dextran, a model compound, at least for 130 h in vitro. Also, the polypseudorotaxane hydrogels consisting of CyDs and PEG-poly[(R)-3-hydroxybutyrate]-PEG triblock copolymer or PEG-b-poly ε-caprolactone diblock copolymer were also used as drug carriers [49–53]. Zhao et al. prepared biodegradable polypseudorotaxane hydrogel consisting of α-CyD and PEG-b-poly ε-caprolactone-grafted chitooligosaccharide [54]. This hydrogel provided the sustained release of bovine serum albumin at least for 140 h in vitro. Polypseudorotaxane hydrogel consisting of PEG-appended heparin and α-CyD was also used as a sustained drug release carrier [55]. α-CyD and poly(PEG methyl ether methacrylate)-co-poly[2-(dimethylamino) ether methacrylate] formed a polypseudorotaxane hydrogel [56]. The structure of this hydrogel could be disrupted by an increase in temperature and a decrease in pH, resulting from dethreading of α-CyD from PEG chains and ionization of dimethylamino groups in the axile molecule, respectively. Moreover, the release of bovine serum albumin from the hydrogel was accelerated at higher temperature and at acidic pH conditions.

Higashi et al. prepared α- and γ-CyD polypseudorotaxane hydrogels with high molecular weight PEG (M.W. 20,000) and evaluated them as sustained release carriers for insulin and lysozyme (Fig. 3) [57, 58]. The α- and γ-CyDs formed polypseudorotaxanes with one PEG chain and two PEG chains, respectively. In addition, the hydrogels were formed by physical cross-linking, resulting from hexagonal and tetragonal columnar channels of the linearly aligned α- and γ-CyD cavities in the crystal phases of the polypseudorotaxanes, respectively. Both α- and γ-CyD polypseudorotaxane hydrogels provided the sustained release of insulin and lysozyme at least for 12 h in vitro. These release mechanisms were almost the same between the α- and γ-CyD systems, and erosion of the gel through dethreading of the PEG chains from the CyD cavities was associated. The plasma insulin level after a subcutaneous injection of the γ-CyD polypseudorotaxane hydrogel containing insulin to rats was significantly prolonged, resulting in the sustained hypoglycemic effect. Thus, polypseudorotaxanes could be promising sustained release carriers for protein drugs.

Higashi et al. also prepared polypseudorotaxanes of PEGylated insulin and PEGylated lysozyme with α- and γ-CyDs (Fig. 3) [59–62]. α- and γ-CyDs formed polypseudorotaxanes with both PEGylated proteins by including one PEG chain and two PEG chains, respectively. The release of PEGylated proteins from the polypseudorotaxanes was prolonged and could be controlled by concentration of CyDs in the medium or a degree of substitution of PEG. Importantly, the conformation and enzymatic activity of the PEGylated proteins were negligibly changed before and after the release from the polypseudorotaxanes. Moreover, γ-CyD polypseudorotaxane with PEGylated insulin markedly sustained the plasma insulin level and the hypoglycemic effect after a subcutaneous administration to rats. To the best of our knowledge, this is the first report describing the successful sustained drug release system based on the polyrotaxane or polypseudorotaxane in vivo. These findings suggest the potentials of polypseudorotaxanes as sustained release systems for PEGylated protein drugs.

5 Cyclodextrin-Based Drug Carriers for Nucleic Acids

Gene therapy is emerging as a potential strategy for the treatment of genetic diseases, cancers, cardiovascular diseases, and infectious diseases [2]. In addition, RNA interference (RNAi) induced by small interfering RNA (siRNA) is a highly efficient regulatory process that causes posttranscriptional gene silencing in most eukaryotic cells, and it represents a promising new approach for producing gene-specific inhibition and knockouts, producing transgenic animal models, and designing new therapeutics [63]. Likewise, vector-based short-hairpin RNAs (shRNAs) expression systems have been developed in order to prolong the RNAi effect [64]. Currently, these nucleic acids are expected as promising drugs. However, the lack of effective technique to deliver these nucleic acids into the diseased organs and cells hampers the development of the drugs including gene, siRNA, shRNA, etc. [65, 66].

Recently, numerous CyD-appended polymers have been developed and utilized as gene and oligonucleotide carriers [67], e.g., β-CyD-appended polypropylenimine dendrimer [68], polyethylenimine (PEI) conjugate with 2-hydroxypropyl-β-CyD (HP-β-CyD) or HP-γ-CyD [69], cationic polyrotaxanes [70–72], biocleavable polyrotaxane [73, 74], cationic amphiphilic β-CyD [75, 76], and PEI conjugate with HP-β-CyD and folic acid [77]. Davis and colleagues have developed nanoparticles consisting of cationic β-CyD-polymer and adamantine-PEG or adamantine-PEG-transferrin for gene [78, 79], DNAzyme [80], and siRNA [81, 82] delivery. Importantly, this carrier provided evidence of inducing an RNAi mechanism of action in a human from the delivered siRNA [83].

Arima and colleagues have developed polyamidoamine Starburst™ dendrimer (dendrimers) conjugates with CyDs (Fig. 4) and utilized them as gene and oligonucleotide carriers [84–86]. Firstly, Arima et al. prepared dendrimer (generation 2 (G2)) conjugates with α-, β-, and γ-CyDs and named them α-, β-, and γ-CDEs (G2), respectively [87]. Of these CDEs, luciferase gene transfer activity of α-CDE (G2) was approximately 100 times higher than that of dendrimer (G2), resulting from the cooperative influence of the endosomal disrupting effect of α-CyD and the proton sponge effect of dendrimer in the α-CDE (G2) molecule. Next, Kihara et al. investigated the optimum generation of dendrimer and degree of substitution (DS) of α-CyD in the α-CDE molecule [88]. As a result, α-CDE (G3, DS 2) showed the highest transfection efficiency with low cytotoxicity. Importantly, α-CDE (G3, DS 2) showed higher in vivo gene transfer activity than dendrimer in the spleen, liver, and kidney with negligible changes in blood chemistry data such as lactate dehydrogenase (LDH), aspartate aminotransferase (AST), alanine aminotransferase (ALT), blood urea nitrogen (BUN), and creatinine (CRE) [89].

Tsutsumi et al. examined the utility of α-CDE (G3, DS 2) as a siRNA carrier [90, 91]. α-CDE (G3, DS 2) showed superior transfection efficiency to dendrimer or commercially available transfection reagents not only in the cotransfection system, i.e., the ternary complex of luciferase reporter plasmids (pGL3), siRNA, and a carrier (pGL3/siRNA/carrier), but also in the binary system. Tsutsumi et al. also demonstrated the potentials of α-CDE (G3, DS 2) as a novel carrier for shRNA as well as siRNA [92].

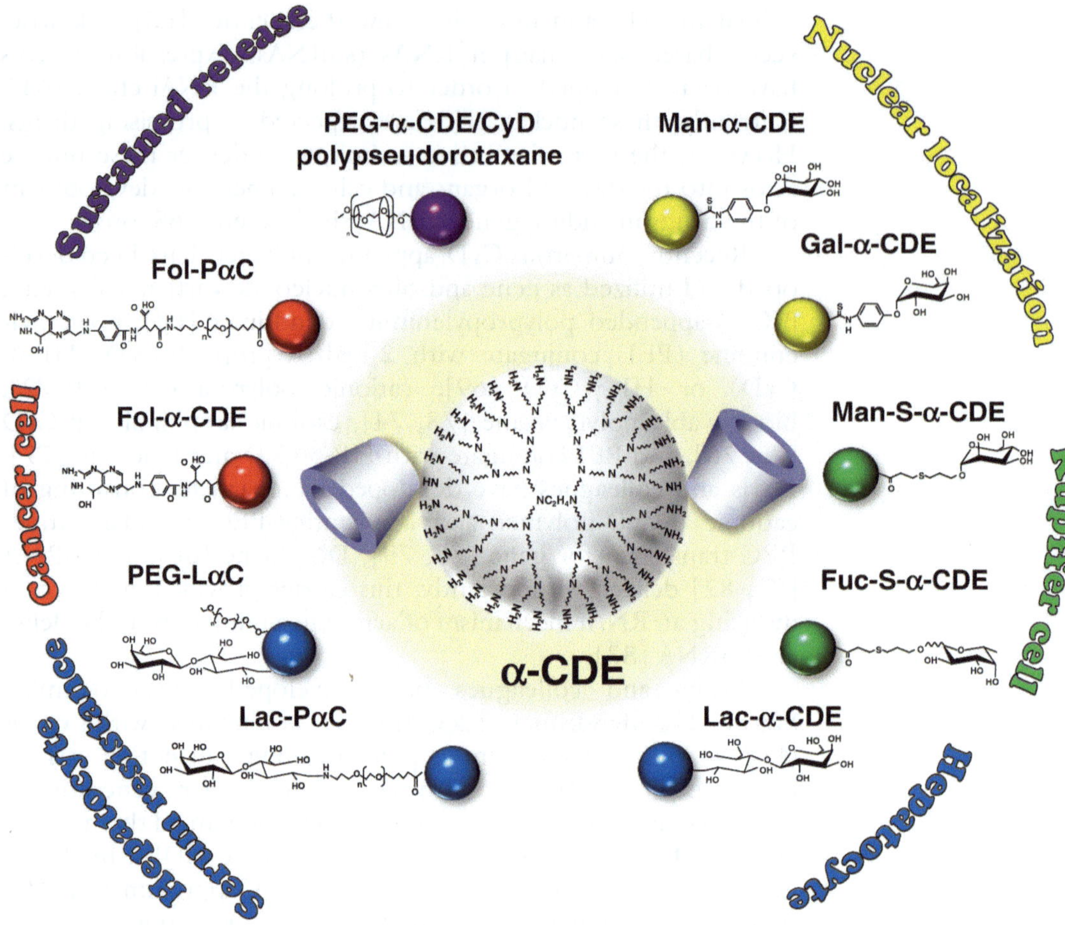

Fig. 4 Structures of various α-CDEs modified with functional molecules

Recently, Anno et al. developed novel dendrimer (G2) conjugate with 6-*O*-α-(4-*O*-α-D-glucuronyl)-D-glucosyl-β-CyD (GUG-β-CyD) and named it GUG-β-CDE (G2) [93]. GUG-β-CDE (G2, DS 1.8) showed higher gene transfer activity than α-CDE (G2, DS 1.2) and β-CDE (G2, DS 1.3) in vitro and in vivo, probably due to its efficient endosomal escape and suitable plasmid DNA (pDNA) release from the polyplex [94, 95]. More recently, Anno et al. demonstrated the utility of GUG-β-CDE (G2, DS 1.8) as a siRNA carrier [96]. The polyplex of GUG-β-CDE (G2, DS 1.8) and a target siRNA against transthyretin (TTR) mRNA (siTTR) showed much higher RNAi effect than that with α-CDE (G2, DS 1.1) or β-CDE (G2, DS 1.3) with negligible cytotoxicity. Thus, GUG-β-CDE has a great potential for novel polymeric pDNA and siRNA carriers as well as α-CDE.

Currently, various targeting ligand-appended α-CDEs are developed by Arima and colleagues. To develop mannose receptor-mediated gene transfer carriers, Wada et al. prepared mannose-modified α-CDEs via an α-D-mannopyranosylphenyl group as a spacer (Man-α-CDEs (G2, G3), Fig. 4) [97, 98]. Man-α-CDEs showed high gene transfer activity, compared to α-CDEs in NR8383 cells, a mannose receptor-positive rat pulmonary alveolar macrophage cell line. However, Man-α-CDEs also showed high gene transfer activity in MDCK, a mannose receptor-negative canine kidney cell line; NIH3T3, a mannose receptor-negative mouse embryo fibroblast cell line; and A549 cells, a mannose receptor-negative human lung adenocarcinoma epithelial cell line, suggesting the mannose receptor-independent gene transfer activity of Man-α-CDEs. Through the detailed investigation, the mechanisms for the cell-nonspecific high gene transfer activity of Man-α-CDEs may be due to (1) protection of pDNA against methylation through DNA methyltransferases, (2) high serum resistance, and (3) high nuclear localization ability.

Most recently, Arima and colleagues newly prepared α-D-mannopyranosylpropylthiopropyonylated α-CDEs (G2) (Man-S-α-CDEs (G2), Fig. 4) (unpublished data). Importantly, Man-S-α-CDE (G2) had mannose receptor-dependent high gene transfer activity in NR8383 cells and JAWSII cells, a mannose receptor-positive immature mice dendritic cell line, but did not in colon-26 cells, a mannose receptor-negative colon adenocarcinoma cell line.

To prepare Kupffer cell-selective decoy DNA carrier, Akao et al. prepared α-D-fucopyranosylpropylthiopropynylated α-CDE (G2) (Fuc-S-α-CDE (G2), Fig. 4) [99]. Fuc-S-α-CDE (G2)/NF-κB decoy complex markedly suppressed nitric oxide and tumor necrosis factor-α (TNF-α) production from lipopolysaccharide (LPS)-simulated NR8383 cells, a fucose receptor-positive cell line, resulting from adequate physicochemical properties and fucose receptor-mediated cellular uptake. The intravenous administration of NF-κB decoy complex with Fuc-S-α-CDE (G2) extended the survival of LPS-induced fulminant hepatitis model mice. In addition, the complex highly accumulated in the liver, and this accumulation was inhibited by the pretreatment with $GdCl_3$, a specific inhibitor of Kupffer cell uptake. Furthermore, the serum AST, ALT, and TNF-α levels in LPS-induced fulminant hepatitis model mice were decreased by the intravenous administration of NF-κB decoy complex with Fuc-S-α-CDE (G2), compared with naked NF-κB decoy alone. Thus, Fuc-S-α-CDE (G2) is useful as a novel Kupffer cell-selective NF-κB decoy carrier for the treatment of LPS-induced fulminant hepatitis in mice.

To develop the hepatocyte-selective gene transfer carrier, Wada et al. prepared galactose-appended α-CDE having an α-D-galactopyranosylphenyl group as a spacer (Gal-α-CDE (G2), Fig. 4) [100]. Unfortunately, Gal-α-CDE (G2) did not show hepatocyte-specific gene transfer activity, although it showed high gene transfer activity compared to α-CDE (G2) in HepG2 cells, an asialoglycoprotein receptor (ASGPR)-positive human hepatocellular carcinoma cell line. Therefore, Arima and colleagues newly prepared lactose-modified α-CDEs (Lac-α-CDEs) possessing glucose moiety as a spacer between galactose and dendrimer molecules (Fig. 4) [101, 102]. Lac-α-CDE (G2) showed hepatocyte-specific gene transfer activity in HepG2 cells. Importantly, in vivo gene transfer activity of Lac-α-CDE (G2) was much higher than that of α-CDE (G2) or jetPEI™-Hepatocyte in the liver.

Transthyretin (TTR)-related familial amyloidotic polyneuropathy (FAP), which is induced by amyloidogenic TTR, is an autosomal dominant form of fatal hereditary amyloidosis characterized by systemic accumulation of amyloid fibrils in peripheral nerves and other organs. To evaluate the utility of Lac-α-CDE (G3) as a siRNA carrier for treatment of FAP, Hayashi et al. investigated the RNAi effect of siTTR complexes with Lac-α-CDE (G3) in vitro and in vivo [103, 104]. siRNA complex with Lac-α-CDE (G3) showed the high RNAi effect, compared to that with jetPEI™-Hepatocyte in HepG2 cells. In addition, Lac-α-CDE (G3)/siRNA complex significantly decreased *TTR* mRNA expression in the liver, suggesting the potential of Lac-α-CDE (G3) as a hepatocyte-selective siRNA carrier for treatment of FAP. Furthermore, to improve in vivo RNAi transfer activity of Lac-α-CDE (G3), Hayashi et al. also prepared two PEG-appended Lac-α-CDEs (G3), i.e., PEG-grafted Lac-α-CDE (G3) (PEG-LαC (G3), Fig. 4) and PEGylated lactose-grafted α-CDE (Lac-PαC (G3), Fig. 4) (unpublished data). Both siRNA complexes with PEG-LαC (G3) and Lac-PαC (G3) showed the superior serum resistance to that with Lac-α-CDE (G3). Moreover, siTTR complex with PEG-LαC (G3) showed significant RNAi effect in the liver at a lower dose (5 mg/kg of siRNA) rather than that with Lac-α-CDE (G3) (9 mg/kg of siRNA), suggesting the potential of PEG-LαC (G3) as a siRNA carrier for treatment of FAP. Additionally, PEG-LαC (G3) was also found to be useful as a gene transfer carrier [105].

To develop a cancer cell-specific gene transfer carrier, Arima et al. prepared folate-appended α-CDE (G3) (Fol-α-CDEs (G3)) and folate-PEG-appended α-CDE (G3) (Fol-PαC (G3), Fig. 4) [106]. Fol-PαC (G3) showed significantly higher gene transfer activity than α-CDE (G3) in KB cells, FR-α-negative cells, but not in A549 cells, FR-α-negative cells. Meanwhile, the activity of Fol-α-CDE (G3) was lower than that of α-CDE (G3) in KB cells, probably due to low interaction between folate moieties in the Fol-α-CDE (G3) molecule and FR-α. Hence, Fol-PαC (G3) could be useful as a cancer cell-selective gene transfer carrier.

Arima et al. also examined the utility of Fol-PαC (G3) as a siRNA carrier [107]. siRNA complex with Fol-PαC (G3) showed the high RNAi effect with negligible cytotoxicity in KB cells. Moreover, the siRNA complex with Fol-PαC (G3) tended to show the in vivo RNAi effects after the intravenous administration in tumor cell-bearing mice. However, the RNAi effect of the complex was not satisfactory. Most recently, to improve in vivo siRNA transfer activity of Fol-PαC, Arima and colleagues newly prepared Fol-PαC (G4). Actually, siRNA complex with Fol-PαC (G4) showed noteworthy serum resistance, providing the significant RNAi effect in vivo after the intravenous administration in tumor cell-bearing mice (unpublished data). Currently, the utility of Fol-PαC (G4) as siRNA transfer carrier for treatment of cancer is examined using anticancer siRNA.

To develop the novel sustained release system for gene, Motoyama et al. prepared polypseudorotaxanes of PEGylated dendrimer (G2) or PEGylated α-CDE (G2) (PEG-α-CDE, (G2)) with CyDs (Fig. 4) [108, 109]. The pDNA complexes with PEGylated dendrimer (G2) and PEG-α-CDE (G2) formed insoluble precipitates with α-CyD and γ-CyDs, but not with β-CyD. Importantly, the CyD polypseudorotaxanes prolonged a release of pDNA and provided sustained gene transfer activity after the intramuscular administration to mice at least for 14 days. Thus, CyD polypseudorotaxane with PEG-α-CDE (G2) has potential as sustained release system for DNA.

6 Conclusion

CyDs have mainly used as pharmaceutical excipients for low molecular weight drugs to improve their solubility, stability, taste, bioavailability, etc. so far. As we introduced in this review, CyDs are recently used to achieve targeting for low molecular weight drugs through the functionalization with ligands. In addition, a large number of CyD-based supramolecules are developed for proteins and nucleic acids. Interestingly, these drugs are loaded in CyD-based drug carriers through different mechanism. For example, low molecular weight drugs such as DOX are directly included in the β-CyD moiety of folic acid-appended β-CyDs. Proteins are incorporated into the pores of polypseudorotaxane hydrogels. In the case of gene and oligonucleotides, the nucleic acids are encapsulated in the nanoparticles including CyD-based carriers through their electrostatic interaction. Of note, CyDs are also expected as novel and safe API candidates for intractable diseases such as cancer [41, 42, 110, 111], Niemann-Pick disease type C [112–116], FAP [117], Alzheimer disease [118, 119], and LPS-induced fulminant hepatitis [120, 121], even though the detail was left out in this review. Finally, we expect that more CyDs and CyD-based supramolecules are used in the clinical field on the horizon.

References

1. Frokjaer S, Otzen DE (2005) Protein drug stability: a formulation challenge. Nat Rev Drug Discov 4:298–306
2. Pfeifer A, Verma IM (2001) Gene therapy: promises and problems. Annu Rev Genomics Hum Genet 2:177–211
3. Ali M, Brocchini S (2006) Synthetic approaches to uniform polymers. Adv Drug Deliv Rev 58:1671–1687
4. Alvarez-Lorenzo C, Blanco-Fernandez B, Puga AM, Concheiro A (2013) Crosslinked ionic polysaccharides for stimuli-sensitive drug delivery. Adv Drug Deliv Rev 65:1148–1171
5. Torchilin VP (2005) Recent advances with liposomes as pharmaceutical carriers. Nat Rev Drug Discov 4:145–160
6. Cabral H, Nishiyama N, Kataoka K (2011) Supramolecular nanodevices: from design validation to theranostic nanomedicine. Acc Chem Res 44:999–1008
7. Petros RA, DeSimone JM (2010) Strategies in the design of nanoparticles for therapeutic applications. Nat Rev Drug Discov 9:615–627
8. Barratt G, Tenu JP, Yapo A, Petit JF (1986) Preparation and characterisation of liposomes containing mannosylated phospholipids capable of targeting drugs to macrophages. Biochim Biophys Acta 862:153–164
9. Huang H, Sakurai F, Higuchi Y, Kawakami S, Hashida M, Kawabata K, Mizuguchi H (2009) Suppressive effects of sugar-modified cationic liposome/NF-κB decoy complexes on adenovirus vector-induced innate immune responses. J Control Release 133:139–145
10. Thoorens G, Krier F, Leclercq B, Carlin B, Evrard B (2014) Microcrystalline cellulose, a direct compression binder in a quality by design environment-a review. Int J Pharm 473:64–72
11. Chang L, Shepherd D, Sun J, Ouellette D, Grant KL, Tang XC, Pikal MJ (2005) Mechanism of protein stabilization by sugars during freeze-drying and storage: native structure preservation, specific interaction, and/or immobilization in a glassy matrix? J Pharm Sci 94:1427–1444
12. Crowe JH, Crowe LM, Carpenter JF, Aurell Wistrom C (1987) Stabilization of dry phospholipid bilayers and proteins by sugars. Biochem J 242:1–10
13. Jana S, Gandhi A, Sen KK, Basu SK (2011) Natural polymers and their application in drug delivery and biomedical field. J PharmaSciTech 1:16–27
14. Szejtli J (1994) Medicinal applications of cyclodextrins. Med Res Rev 14:353–386
15. Uekama K, Hirayama F, Irie T (1998) Cyclodextrin drug carrier systems. Chem Rev 98:2045–2076
16. Davis ME, Brewster ME (2004) Cyclodextrin-based pharmaceutics: past, present and future. Nat Rev Drug Discov 3:1023–1035
17. Irie T, Uekama K (1997) Pharmaceutical applications of cyclodextrins. III. Toxicological issues and safety evaluation. J Pharm Sci 86:147–162
18. Kang Y, Guo K, Li BJ, Zhang S (2014) Nanoassemblies driven by cyclodextrin-based inclusion complexation. Chem Commun 50:11083–11092
19. Zhang J, Ma PX (2013) Cyclodextrin-based supramolecular systems for drug delivery: recent progress and future perspective. Adv Drug Deliv Rev 65:1215–1233
20. Li J, Loh XJ (2008) Cyclodextrin-based supramolecular architectures: syntheses, structures, and applications for drug and gene delivery. Adv Drug Deliv Rev 60:1000–1017
21. Chen J, Lu WL, Gu W, Lu SS, Chen ZP, Cai BC, Yang XX (2014) Drug-in-cyclodextrin-in-liposomes: a promising delivery system for hydrophobic drugs. Expert Opin Drug Deliv 11:565–577
22. Challa R, Ahuja A, Ali J, Khar RK (2005) Cyclodextrins in drug delivery: an updated review. AAPS PharmSciTech 6:E329–E357
23. Song CK, Jung SH, Kim DD, Jeong KS, Shin BC, Seong H (2009) Disaccharide-modified liposomes and their *in vitro* intracellular uptake. Int J Pharm 380:161–169
24. Ishii M, Kato C, Hakamata A, Kojima N (2011) Targeting with oligomannose-coated liposomes promotes maturation and splenic trafficking of dendritic cells in the peritoneal cavity. Int Immunopharmacol 11:164–171
25. Higuchi Y, Kawakami S, Yamashita F, Hashida M (2007) The potential role of fucosylated cationic liposome/NFκB decoy complexes in the treatment of cytokine-related liver disease. Biomaterials 28:532–539
26. Chaudhury A, Das S (2011) Recent advancement of chitosan-based nanoparticles for oral controlled delivery of insulin and other therapeutic agents. AAPS PharmSciTech 12:10–20
27. Mehvar R (2000) Dextrans for targeted and sustained delivery of therapeutic and imaging agents. J Control Release 69:1–25
28. Tokatlian T, Cam C, Segura T (2014) Non-viral DNA delivery from porous hyaluronic

acid hydrogels in mice. Biomaterials 35: 825–835
29. Chen YY, Wu HC, Sun JS, Dong GC, Wang TW (2013) Injectable and thermoresponsive self-assembled nanocomposite hydrogel for long-term anticancer drug delivery. Langmuir 29:3721–3729
30. Okajima MK, Bamba T, Kaneso Y, Hirata K, Fukusai E, Kajiyama S, Kaneko T (2008) Supergiant ampholytic sugar chains with imbalanced charge ratio form saline ultra-absorbent hydrogels. Macromolecules 41: 4061–4064
31. Motoyama K, Tanida Y, Hata K, Hayashi T, Higashi T, Ishitsuka Y, Kondo Y, Irie T, Kaneko S, Arima H (2014) Potential use of a megamolecular polysaccharide sacran as a hydrogel-based sustained release system. Chem Pharm Bull 62:636–641
32. Namgung R, Lee MY, Kim J, Jang Y, Lee BH, Kim IS, Sokkar P, Rhee YM, Hoffman AS, Kim WJ (2014) Poly-cyclodextrin and poly-paclitaxel nano-assembly for anticancer therapy. Nat Commun 5:3702
33. Salmaso S, Bersani S, Semenzato A, Caliceti P (2007) New cyclodextrin bioconjugates for active tumour targeting. J Drug Target 15: 379–390
34. Salmaso S, Semenzato A, Caliceti P, Hoebeke J, Sonvico F, Dubernet C, Couvreur P (2004) Specific antitumor targetable β-cyclodextrin-poly(ethylene glycol)-folic acid drug delivery bioconjugate. Bioconjug Chem 15: 997–1004
35. Caliceti P, Salmaso S, Semenzato A, Carofiglio T, Fornasier R, Fermeglia M, Ferrone M, Pricl S (2003) Synthesis and physicochemical characterization of folate-cyclodextrin bio-conjugate for active drug delivery. Bioconjug Chem 14:899–908
36. Zhang H, Cai Z, Sun Y, Yu F, Chen Y, Sun B (2012) Folate-conjugated β-cyclodextrin from click chemistry strategy and for tumor-targeted drug delivery. J Biomed Mater Res A 100:2441–2449
37. Okamatsu A, Motoyama K, Onodera R, Higashi T, Koshigoe T, Shimada Y, Hattori K, Takeuchi T, Arima H (2013) Folate-appended β-cyclodextrin as a promising tumor targeting carrier for antitumor drugs *in vitro* and *in vivo*. Bioconjug Chem 24:724–733
38. Okamatsu A, Motoyama K, Onodera R, Higashi T, Koshigoe T, Shimada Y, Hattori K, Takeuchi T, Arima H (2013) Design and evaluation of folate-appended α-, β-, and γ-cyclodextrins having a caproic acid as a tumor selective antitumor drug carrier *in vitro* and *in vivo*. Biomacromolecules 14:4420–4428
39. Onodera R, Motoyama K, Arima H (2011) Design and evaluation of folate-appended methyl-β-cyclodextrin as a new antitumor agent. J Incl Phenom Macrocycl Chem 70:321–326
40. Motoyama K, Onodera R, Okamatsu A, Higashi T, Kariya R, Okada S, Arima H (2014) Potential use of the complex of doxorubicin with folate-conjugated methyl-β-cyclodextrin for tumor-selective cancer chemotherapy. J Drug Target 22:211–219
41. Onodera R, Motoyama K, Okamatsu A, Higashi T, Arima H (2013) Potential use of folate-appended methyl-β-cyclodextrin as an anticancer agent. Sci Rep 3:1104
42. Onodera R, Motoyama K, Tanaka N, Ohyama A, Okamatsu A, Higashi T, Kariya R, Okada S, Arima H (2014) Involvement of autophagy in antitumor activity of folate-appended methyl-β-cyclodextrin. Sci Rep 4:4417
43. Harris JM, Chess RB (2003) Effect of pegylation on pharmaceuticals. Nat Rev Drug Discov 2:214–221
44. Harada A, Kamachi M (1990) Complex formation between poly(ethylene glycol) and α-cyclodextrin. Macromolecules 23: 2821–2823
45. Harada A, Li J, Kamachi M (1993) Preparation and properties of inclusion complexes of poly(ethylene glycol) with α-cyclodextrin. Macromolecules 26:5698–5703
46. Harada A, Li J, Kamachi M (1994) Double-stranded inclusion complexes of cyclodextrin threaded on poly(ethylene glycol). Nature 370:126–128
47. Harada A, Li J, Kamachi M (1992) The molecular necklace: a rotaxane containing many threaded α-cyclodextrins. Nature 356:325–327
48. Li J, Ni X, Leong KW (2003) Injectable drug-delivery systems based on supramolecular hydrogels formed by poly(ethylene oxide)s and α-cyclodextrin. J Biomed Mater Res A 65:196–202
49. Li J, Li X, Ni X, Wang X, Li H, Leong KW (2006) Self-assembled supramolecular hydrogels formed by biodegradable PEO-PHB-PEO triblock copolymers and α-cyclodextrin for controlled drug delivery. Biomaterials 27:4132–4140
50. Li JJ, Zhao F, Li J (2011) Supramolecular polymers based on cyclodextrins for drug and gene delivery. Adv Biochem Eng Biotechnol 125:207–249
51. Li J (2009) Cyclodextrin inclusion polymers forming hydrogels. Adv Polym Sci 222: 79–113

52. Li JJ, Zhao F, Li J (2011) Polyrotaxanes for applications in life science and biotechnology. Appl Microbiol Biotechnol 90:427–443
53. Li X, Li J (2008) Supramolecular hydrogels based on inclusion complexation between poly(ethylene oxide)-b-poly(ε-caprolactone) diblock copolymer and α-cyclodextrin and their controlled release property. J Biomed Mater Res A 86:1055–1061
54. Zhao S, Lee J, Xu W (2009) Supramolecular hydrogels formed from biodegradable ternary COS-g-PCL-b-MPEG copolymer with α-cyclodextrin and their drug release. Carbohydr Res 344:2201–2208
55. Ma D, Tu K, Zhang LM (2010) Bioactive supramolecular hydrogel with controlled dual drug release characteristics. Biomacromolecules 11:2204–2212
56. Ren L, He L, Sun T, Dong X, Chen Y, Huang J, Wang C (2009) Dual-responsive supramolecular hydrogels from water-soluble PEG-grafted copolymers and cyclodextrin. Macromol Biosci 9:902–910
57. Abu Hashim II, Higashi T, Anno T, Motoyama K, Abd-ElGawad AE, El-Shabouri MH, Borg TM, Arima H (2010) Potential use of γ-cyclodextrin polypseudorotaxane hydrogels as an injectable sustained release system for insulin. Int J Pharm 392:83–91
58. Higashi T, Tajima A, Motoyama K, Arima H (2012) Cyclodextrin/poly(ethylene glycol) polypseudorotaxane hydrogels as a promising sustained-release system for lysozyme. J Pharm Sci 101:2891–2899
59. Higashi T, Hirayama F, Arima H, Uekama K (2007) Polypseudorotaxanes of pegylated insulin with cyclodextrins: application to sustained release system. Bioorg Med Chem Lett 17:1871–1874
60. Higashi T, Hirayama F, Misumi S, Arima H, Uekama K (2008) Design and evaluation of polypseudorotaxanes of pegylated insulin with cyclodextrins as sustained release system. Biomaterials 29:3866–3871
61. Higashi T, Hirayama F, Misumi S, Motoyama K, Arima H, Uekama K (2009) Polypseudorotaxane formation of randomly-pegylated insulin with cyclodextrins: slow release and resistance to enzymatic degradation. Chem Pharm Bull 57:541–544
62. Higashi T, Hirayama F, Yamashita S, Misumi S, Arima H, Uekama K (2009) Slow-release system of pegylated lysozyme utilizing formation of polypseudorotaxanes with cyclodextrins. Int J Pharm 374:26–32
63. Wang J, Lu Z, Wientjes MG, Au JLS (2010) Delivery of siRNA therapeutics: barriers and carriers. AAPS J 12:492–503
64. Rao DD, Vorhies JS, Senzer N, Nemunaitis J (2009) siRNA vs. shRNA: similarities and differences. Adv Drug Deliv Rev 61:746–759
65. Blau HM, Springer ML (1995) Gene therapy - a novel form of drug delivery. N Engl J Med 333:1204–1207
66. Grimm D (2009) Small silencing RNAs: state-of-the-art. Adv Drug Deliv Rev 61:672–703
67. Hu QD, Tang GP, Chu PK (2014) Cyclodextrin-based host-guest supramolecular nanoparticles for delivery: from design to applications. Acc Chem Res 47:2017–2025
68. Zhang W, Chen Z, Song X, Si J, Tang G (2008) Low generation polypropylenimine dendrimer graft β-cyclodextrin: an efficient vector for gene delivery system. Technol Cancer Res Treat 7:103–108
69. Huang H, Tang G, Wang Q, Li D, Shen F, Zhou J, Yu H (2006) Two novel non-viral gene delivery vectors: low molecular weight polyethylenimine cross-linked by (2-hydroxypropyl)-β-cyclodextrin or (2-hydroxypropyl)-γ-cyclodextrin. Chem Commun 42:2382–2384
70. Yang C, Wang X, Li H, Goh SH, Li J (2007) Synthesis and characterization of polyrotaxanes consisting of cationic α-cyclodextrins threaded on poly[(ethylene oxide)-ran-(propylene oxide)] as gene carriers. Biomacromolecules 8:3365–3374
71. Zhou Y, Wang H, Wang C, Li Y, Lu W, Chen S, Luo J, Jiang Y, Chen J (2012) Receptor-mediated, tumor-targeted gene delivery using folate-terminated polyrotaxanes. Mol Pharm 9:1067–1076
72. Huang H, Cao D, Qin L, Tian S, Liang Y, Pan S, Feng M (2014) Dilution-stable PAMAM G1-grafted polyrotaxane supermolecules deliver gene into cells through a caveolae-dependent pathway. Mol Pharm 11:2323–2333
73. Ooya T, Choi HS, Yamashita A, Yui N, Sugaya Y, Kano A, Maruyama A, Akita H, Ito R, Kogure K, Harashima H (2006) Biocleavable polyrotaxane-plasmid DNA polyplex for enhanced gene delivery. J Am Chem Soc 128:3852–3853
74. Tamura A, Yui N (2013) Cellular internalization and gene silencing of siRNA polyplexes by cytocleavable cationic polyrotaxanes with tailored rigid backbones. Biomaterials 34:2480–2491
75. Diaz-Moscoso A, Guilloteau N, Bienvenu C, Mendez-Ardoy A, Blanco JL, Benito JM, Le Gourrierec L, Di Giorgio C, Vierling P, Defaye J, Mellet CO, Fernandez JM (2011) Mannosyl-coated nanocomplexes from amphiphilic cyclodextrins and pDNA for site-

specific gene delivery. Biomaterials 32: 7263–7273

76. Diaz-Moscoso A, Vercauteren D, Rejman J, Benito JM, Ortiz Mellet C, De Smedt SC, Fernandez JM (2010) Insights in cellular uptake mechanisms of pDNA-polycationic amphiphilic cyclodextrin nanoparticles (CDplexes). J Control Release 143:318–325
77. Li JM, Wang YY, Zhang W, Su H, Ji LN, Mao ZW (2013) Low-weight polyethylenimine cross-linked 2-hydroxypopyl-β-cyclodextrin and folic acid as an efficient and nontoxic siRNA carrier for gene silencing and tumor inhibition by VEGF siRNA. Int J Nanomedicine 8:2101–2117
78. Gonzalez H, Hwang SJ, Davis ME (1999) New class of polymers for the delivery of macromolecular therapeutics. Bioconjug Chem 10:1068–1074
79. Pun SH, Davis ME (2002) Development of a nonviral gene delivery vehicle for systemic application. Bioconjug Chem 13:630–639
80. Pun SH, Tack F, Bellocq NC, Cheng J, Grubbs BH, Jensen GS, Davis ME, Brewster M, Janicot M, Janssens B, Floren W, Bakker A (2004) Targeted delivery of RNA-cleaving DNA enzyme (DNAzyme) to tumor tissue by transferrin-modified, cyclodextrin-based particles. Cancer Biol Ther 3:641–650
81. Davis ME (2009) The first targeted delivery of siRNA in humans via a self-assembling, cyclodextrin polymer-based nanoparticle: from concept to clinic. Mol Pharm 6:659–668
82. Heidel JD, Yu Z, Liu JY, Rele SM, Liang Y, Zeidan RK, Kornbrust DJ, Davis ME (2007) Administration in non-human primates of escalating intravenous doses of targeted nanoparticles containing ribonucleotide reductase subunit M2 siRNA. Proc Natl Acad Sci U S A 104:5715–5721
83. Davis ME, Zuckerman JE, Choi CH, Seligson D, Tolcher A, Alabi CA, Yen Y, Heidel JD, Ribas A (2010) Evidence of RNAi in humans from systemically administered siRNA via targeted nanoparticles. Nature 464:1067–1070
84. Arima H, Motoyama K, Higashi T (2012) Polyamidoamine dendrimer conjugates with cyclodextrins as novel carriers for DNA, shRNA and siRNA. Pharmaceutics 4:130–148
85. Arima H, Motoyama K, Higashi T (2011) Potential use of polyamidoamine dendrimer conjugates with cyclodextrins as novel carriers for siRNA. Pharmaceuticals (Basel) 5:61–78
86. Arima H, Motoyama K, Higashi T (2013) Sugar-appended polyamidoamine dendrimer conjugates with cyclodextrins as cell-specific non-viral vectors. Adv Drug Deliv Rev 65: 1204–1214
87. Arima H, Kihara F, Hirayama F, Uekama K (2001) Enhancement of gene expression by polyamidoamine dendrimer conjugates with α-, β- and γ-cyclodextrins. Bioconjug Chem 12:476–484
88. Kihara F, Arima H, Tsutsumi T, Hirayama F, Uekama K (2002) Effects of structure of polyamidoamine dendrimer on gene transfer efficiency of the dendrimer conjugate with α-cyclodextrin. Bioconjug Chem 13:1211–1219
89. Kihara F, Arima H, Tsutsumi T, Hirayama F, Uekama K (2003) *In vitro* and *in vivo* gene transfer by an optimized α-cyclodextrin conjugate with polyamidoamine dendrimer. Bioconjug Chem 14:342–350
90. Tsutsumi T, Hirayama F, Uekama K, Arima H (2007) Evaluation of polyamidoamine dendrimer/α-cyclodextrin conjugate (generation 3, G3) as a novel carrier for small interfering RNA (siRNA). J Control Release 119:349–359
91. Arima H, Tsutsumi T, Yoshimatsu A, Ikeda H, Motoyama K, Higashi T, Hirayama F, Uekama K (2011) Inhibitory effect of siRNA complexes with polyamidoamine dendrimer/α-cyclodextrin conjugate (generation 3, G3) on endogenous gene expression. Eur J Pharm Sci 44:375–384
92. Tsutsumi T, Hirayama F, Uekama K, Arima H (2008) Potential use of polyamidoamine dendrimer/α-cyclodextrin conjugate (generation 3, G3) as a novel carrier for short hairpin RNA-expressing plasmid DNA. J Pharm Sci 97:3022–3034
93. Anno T, Motoyama K, Higashi T, Hirayama F, Uekama K, Arima H (2011) Preparation and evaluation of polyamidoamine dendrimer (G2)/branched-β-cyclodextrin conjugate as a novel gene transfer carrier. J Incl Phenom Macrocycl Chem 70:339–344
94. Anno T, Higashi T, Motoyama K, Hirayama F, Uekama K, Arima H (2012) Potential use of glucuronylglucosyl-β-cyclodextrin/dendrimer conjugate (G2) as a DNA carrier *in vitro* and *in vivo*. J Drug Target 20:272–280
95. Anno T, Higashi T, Motoyama K, Hirayama F, Uekama K, Arima H (2012) Possible enhancing mechanisms for gene transfer activity of glucuronylglucosyl-β-cyclodextrin/dendrimer conjugate. Int J Pharm 426:239–247
96. Anno T, Higashi T, Hayashi Y, Motoyama K, Jono H, Ando Y, Arima H (2014) Potential use of glucuronylglucosyl-β-cyclodextrin/dendrimer conjugate (G2) as a siRNA carrier

for the treatment of familial amyloidotic polyneuropathy. J Drug Target 22:883–890
97. Wada K, Arima H, Tsutsumi T, Chihara Y, Hattori K, Hirayama F, Uekama K (2005) Improvement of gene delivery mediated by mannosylated dendrimer/α-cyclodextrin conjugates. J Control Release 104:397–413
98. Arima H, Chihara Y, Arizono M, Yamashita S, Wada K, Hirayama F, Uekama K (2006) Enhancement of gene transfer activity mediated by mannosylated dendrimer/α-cyclodextrin conjugate (generation 3, G3). J Control Release 116:64–74
99. Akao C, Tanaka T, Onodera R, Ohyama A, Sato N, Motoyama K, Higashi T, Arima H (2014) Potential use of fucose-appended dendrimer/α-cyclodextrin conjugates as NF-κB decoy carriers for the treatment of lipopolysaccharide-induced fulminant hepatitis in mice. J Control Release 193:35–41
100. Wada K, Arima H, Tsutsumi T, Hirayama F, Uekama K (2005) Enhancing effects of galactosylated dendrimer/α-cyclodextrin conjugates on gene transfer efficiency. Biol Pharm Bull 28:500–505
101. Arima H, Yamashita S, Mori Y, Hayashi Y, Motoyama K, Hattori K, Takeuchi T, Jono H, Ando Y, Hirayama F, Uekama K (2010) *In vitro* and *in vivo* gene delivery mediated by lactosylated dendrimer/α-cyclodextrin conjugates (G2) into hepatocytes. J Control Release 146:106–117
102. Motoyama K, Mori Y, Yamashita S, Hayashi Y, Jono H, Ando Y, Hirayama F, Uekama K, Arima H (2011) *In vitro* gene delivery mediated by lactosylated dendrimer (generation 3, G3)/α-cyclodextrin conjugates into hepatocytes. J Incl Phenom Macrocycl Chem 70:333–338
103. Hayashi Y, Mori Y, Yamashita S, Motoyama K, Higashi T, Jono H, Ando Y, Arima H (2012) Potential use of lactosylated dendrimer (G3)/α-cyclodextrin conjugates as hepatocyte-specific siRNA carriers for the treatment of familial amyloidotic polyneuropathy. Mol Pharm 9:1645–1653
104. Hayashi Y, Mori Y, Higashi T, Motoyama K, Jono H, Sah DW, Ando Y, Arima H (2012) Systemic delivery of transthyretin siRNA mediated by lactosylated dendrimer/α-cyclodextrin conjugates into hepatocyte for familial amyloidotic polyneuropathy therapy. Amyloid 19:47–49
105. Hayashi Y, Higashi T, Motoyama K, Mori Y, Jono H, Ando Y, Arima H (2013) Design and evaluation of polyamidoamine dendrimer conjugate with PEG, α-cyclodextrin and lactose as a novel hepatocyte-selective gene carrier *in vitro* and *in vivo*. J Drug Target 21:487–496
106. Arima H, Arizono M, Higashi T, Yoshimatsu A, Ikeda H, Motoyama K, Hattori K, Takeuchi T, Hirayama F, Uekama K (2012) Potential use of folate-polyethylene glycol (PEG)-appended dendrimer (G3) conjugate with α-cyclodextrin as DNA carriers to tumor cells. Cancer Gene Ther 19:358–366
107. Arima H, Yoshimatsu A, Ikeda H, Ohyama A, Motoyama K, Higashi T, Tsuchiya A, Niidome T, Katayama Y, Hattori K, Takeuchi T (2012) Folate-PEG-appended dendrimer conjugate with α-cyclodextrin as a novel cancer cell-selective siRNA delivery carrier. Mol Pharm 9:2591–2604
108. Motoyama K, Hayashida K, Arima H (2011) Potential use of polypseudorotaxanes of pegylated polyamidoamine dendrimer with cyclodextrins as novel sustained release systems for DNA. Chem Pharm Bull 59:476–479
109. Motoyama K, Hayashida K, Higashi T, Arima H (2012) Polypseudorotaxanes of pegylated α-cyclodextrin/polyamidoamine dendrimer conjugate with cyclodextrins as a sustained release system for DNA. Bioorg Med Chem 20:1425–1433
110. Grosse PY, Bressolle F, Pinguet F (1998) Antiproliferative effect of methyl-β-cyclodextrin *in vitro* and in human tumour xenografted athymic nude mice. Br J Cancer 78:1165–1169
111. Onodera R, Motoyama K, Okamatsu A, Higashi T, Kariya R, Okada S, Arima H (2013) Involvement of cholesterol depletion from lipid rafts in apoptosis induced by methyl-β-cyclodextrin. Int J Pharm 452: 116–123
112. Camargo F, Erickson RP, Garver WS, Hossain GS, Carbone PN, Heidenreich RA, Blanchard J (2001) Cyclodextrins in the treatment of a mouse model of Niemann-Pick C disease. Life Sci 70:131–142
113. Liu B, Turley SD, Burns DK, Miller AM, Repa JJ, Dietschy JM (2009) Reversal of defective lysosomal transport in NPC disease ameliorates liver dysfunction and neurodegeneration in the npc1$^{-/-}$ mouse. Proc Natl Acad Sci U S A 106:2377–2382
114. Tamura A, Yui N (2014) Lysosomal-specific cholesterol reduction by biocleavable polyrotaxanes for ameliorating Niemann-Pick type C disease. Sci Rep 4:4356
115. Mondjinou YA, McCauliff LA, Kulkarni A, Paul L, Hyun SH, Zhang Z, Wu Z, Wirth M, Storch J, Thompson DH (2013) Synthesis of 2-hydroxypropyl-β-cyclodextrin/pluronic-based polyrotaxanes via heterogeneous reaction

as potential Niemann-Pick type C therapeutics. Biomacromolecules 14:4189–4197

116. Matsuo M, Togawa M, Hirabaru K, Mochinaga S, Narita A, Adachi M, Egashira M, Irie T, Ohno K (2013) Effects of cyclodextrin in two patients with Niemann-Pick Type C disease. Mol Genet Metab 108:76–81
117. Jono H, Anno T, Motoyama K, Misumi Y, Tasaki M, Oshima T, Mori Y, Mizuguchi M, Ueda M, Shono M, Obayashi K, Arima H, Ando Y (2011) Cyclodextrin, a novel therapeutic tool for suppressing amyloidogenic transthyretin misfolding in transthyretin-related amyloidosis. Biochem J 437:35–42
118. Camilleri P, Haskins NJ, Howlett DR (1994) β-Cyclodextrin interacts with the Alzheimer amyloid β-A4 peptide. FEBS Lett 341: 256–258
119. Yao J, Ho D, Calingasan NY, Pipalia NH, Lin MT, Beal MF (2012) Neuroprotection by cyclodextrin in cell and mouse models of Alzheimer disease. J Exp Med 209: 2501–2513
120. Motoyama K, Arima H, Nishimoto Y, Miyake K, Hirayama F, Uekama K (2005) Involvement of CD14 in the inhibitory effects of dimethyl-α-cyclodextrin on lipopolysaccharide signaling in macrophages. FEBS Lett 579:1707–1714
121. Arima H, Motoyama K, Matsukawa A, Nishimoto Y, Hirayama F, Uekama K (2005) Inhibitory effects of dimethylacetyl-β-cyclodextrin on lipopolysaccharide-induced macrophage activation and endotoxin shock in mice. Biochem Pharmacol 70: 1506–1517

Chapter 3

Development of Dendrimer-Based Nanomaterials for Diagnostic and Therapeutic Applications

Beibei Wang, Zheng-Rong Lu, and Mingqian Tan

Abstract

Dendrimer-based nanomaterials are a promising generation of nanoagents for diagnostic and therapeutic applications. The present chapter initially describes dendrimers history, architectures, synthesis strategies, and main types. Then the physicochemical characteristics of dendrimers are discussed in detail. Numerous designs and applications of dendrimer-based nanomaterials in biological systems are then reviewed. This chapter focuses on their applications on drug or gene delivery devices. Besides, biocompatibility of dendrimer-based nanomaterials is also highlighted, such as in vitro and in vivo toxicity, as well as immunogenicity and biopermeability.

Key words Dendrimer-based materials, Drug delivery, Gene delivery, Biocompatibility

1 Introduction

Dendrimers are defined as synthetic polymers characterized by a highly branched architecture, three dimensional shape, monodispersity, and nanometric size range. In synthetic organic chemistry, dendritic structures are originated from a special type of molecules named "cascade" polymers, firstly reported by Vögtle et al. [1] at the end of the 1970s. During the period of 1970–1990, development of polymer science together with synthetic organic chemistry gave rise to larger dendritic structures [1–5]. These hyper-branched molecules were named "dendrimers," which is derived from the Greek term dendron, meaning "tree" or "branch" [6]. In literature, they are also commonly named as "Cascade molecules," "Arborols," "Dendritic molecules"; or as "nanometric architectures" due to their nanoscopic size [7–9].

In comparison with linear polymers, dendrimers have highly branched architecture with precisely tailored surface groups. A dendrimer molecule is generally constituted of three domains: a core, branches and diverse surface groups. A core, the center of dendrimer, is generally an atom or a molecule presenting two or

Zheng-Rong Lu and Shinji Sakuma (eds.), *Nanomaterials in Pharmacology*, Methods in Pharmacology and Toxicology, DOI 10.1007/978-1-4939-3121-7_3, © Springer Science+Business Media New York 2016

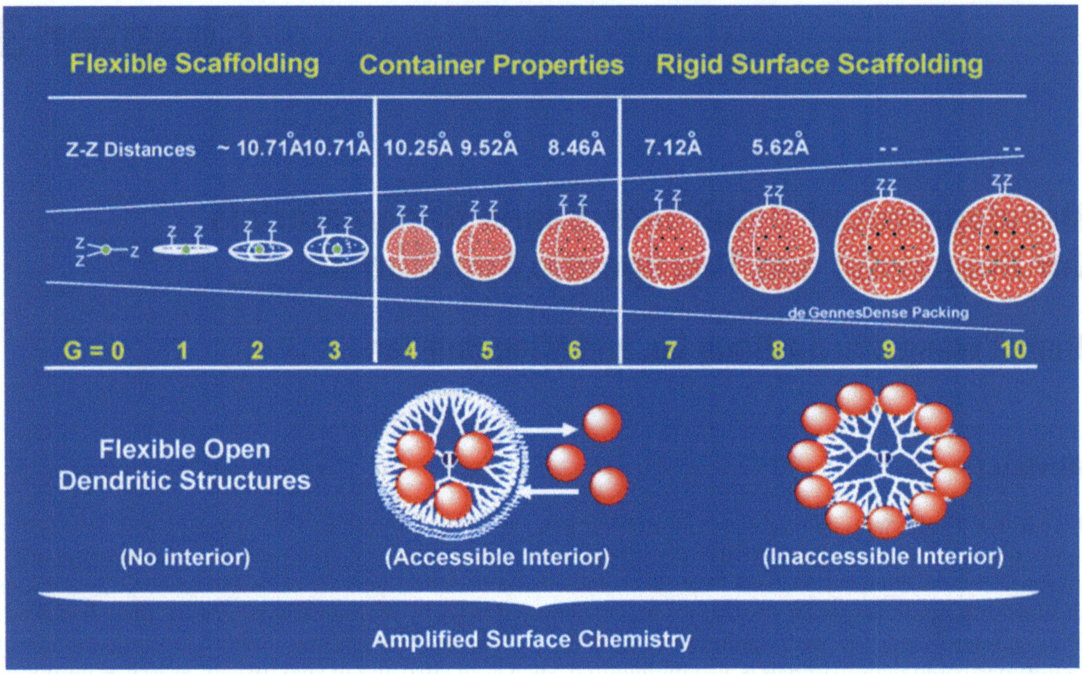

Fig. 1 Periodic properties of PAMAM dendrimers generations G = 0–10 depicting the distances between surface charges (Z–Z), including the "de Gennes dense packing," the generation-dependent size and shape of dendrimers, and their "nanoscale-container" and "nano-scaffolding" properties [12]

more identical chemical function groups. Due to no cascade point, the core is sometimes called generation "zero" (G0). Branches, which radiate from the core, are formed by repeat units with at least one junction. The repetitions present a series of concentric layers which are denoted as "generations" (G). There are generally diverse terminal functional groups on the surface of dendrimer architecture. When there are carboxylate as surface groups, the intermediate molecules are called dendrimers of half generation, e.g., G1.5 or G2.5 [10, 11].

The size of the globular dendrimer macromolecule grows with the added generation. Take polyamides and amines dendrimer (PAMAMs) for an example, the diameter of this core–shell molecule increase linearly, approximately at rate of 1 nm per generation, while the surface groups amplify exponentially (Fig. 1) [12]. On a molecular level, dendrimers are nano-sized macromolecules with the dendritic branching resulting globular structures, generally with a small "volume." Small dendrimers have open structure indicated by model simulation, while larger dendrimers (G > 3) have a compact structure. They usually show a spherical or cylinder shape which is depended on the extension of the core. When a functional unit is embedded within a large dendrimer, its accessibility and the diverse local environments may have significant effect on the dendrimer properties [13].

Besides PAMAM dendrimer, polypropylene imines (PPI), and Fréchet-type poly(ester-acrylate/amine) (PEA) are also common dendrimers reported in literature [14–20]. A variety of new dendritic structures are also emerging such as dendrimers based on calixarene or carbohydrate [21, 22] core structures, polylysine nanoglobules [23–26] or core containing "third period" elements such as silicon or phosphorus [27].

This chapter focuses on the design, synthesis, characterization of dendritic nanomaterials and their pharmacological applications, such as the delivery function for imaging agents, drugs or genes in antibacterial, antiviral and antitumor treatment. The biocompatibility, immunogenicity, and biopermeability of the dendritic nanomaterials are also discussed.

1.1 Synthesis of Dendrimer

The synthesis of dendrimer mainly includes two major strategies: [10] (1) the divergent method, in which a dendron grows radially from the core site, and branching units successively attached to another in a radial, branch-upon-branch scheme according to certain rules and principles; (2) the convergent method, in which the skeleton is constructed stepwise starting from the end groups towards inside to form a dendron, and the dendrimer is finally yielded by reaction of several dendrons with a multifunctional core [28].

Divergent strategy is commonly used in dendrimer synthesis due to its major advantages, such as easily attached reagents, rapid progressing, exponential growth, and the feasibility of preparing large dendrimers. However, purification of the dendrimer by divergent strategy is complicated. The product is easily contaminated by various deletion compounds, which have very similar molecular weight, polarity, charge, hydrophilicity, etc. as the desired product. Moreover, it is a big challenge to synthesize a higher generation architecture due to the steric resistance. This may result in significant defects on the surface. For example, it is very difficult to synthesize a G5 nanoglobules from our experience and the dendrimer must be very pure in every generation to avoid surface defection in higher generation macromolecules.

Different from the divergent strategy, the convergent method possesses merits such as good monodispersity, the convenience of conjugating various types of dendritic units to one core. Notably, the convergent method has the advantage of easier purification because the accessory substances differ much from the aiming structure, in parameters such as the molecular weight, polarity, and charge. The researchers can easily separate the desired product by many available separation techniques. Still, the synthesis could be restricted by steric constraints during the process of synthesize the large dendritic units with the central core.

Both convergent and divergent approaches have pros and cons, and one should choose proper synthesis strategy according to the designed structure and generation of the final product. Carbohydrates with repeated units and spacers are usually applied as building blocks for dendritic structures, which provide resulting dendrimers with versatile characters. The significant improvements for this purpose are the introductions of "Lego" and "click" chemistries. The "lego" chemistry is based on versatile functionalized core and branched monomers, and has been applied for preparing phosphorous dendrimers [29]. Among the various "click" reactions, the copper-catalyzed azide-alkyne cycloaddition (Cu-AAC) is the most useful one. 2.0 and 3.0 G triazole dendrimers were successfully synthesized using this reaction with mild and simple reaction conditions, pure product and excellent synthetic yield [29, 30]. Another successful try for quick and reliable construction of dendrimers is double exponential growth. It allows the preparation of monomers from a single small molecule for both divergent and convergent growth. The resultant two medium compounds are then reacted to give rise to an orthogonally protected trimer. This growth process can be repeated. The biggest advantage of this approach is applicability to either divergent or convergent strategy [10].

1.2 Physicochemical Properties and Characterizations of Dendrimers

Dendritic nanomaterials with unique physicochemical properties such as mono-dispersed, three-dimensional and highly branched macromolecules with multivalency, large amount of end terminal peripheral groups and interior cavities, and host–guest interactions properties, are of great interest in pharmacological applications. They are widely used as nanocarriers for anticancer drug, imaging agents, gene because of their ability to cross cell membranes and avoid the premature clearance from the body.

The most distinguishing feature of dendritic nanomaterials is the multivalency, which has been shown to lead to a strongly increased activity compared to the corresponding monomeric interaction. With multimeric system, the binding affinity of dendritic nanomaterials is enhanced largely as compared with the monomeric system. This is usually referred to as the dendritic effect, which is able to increase specificity of a given reaction. The versatile functionalities of the dendritic nanomaterials could serve as an excellent platform for the attachment of targeting moieties, solubility modifiers, imaging nanotags, and stealth molecules which could decrease the interaction with macromolecules from the body defense system (Fig. 2). For example, folic acid and fluorescein modified dendrimers are able to specifically bind with folate receptor on the surface of a variety of cancer cells. Moreover, the multivalency with three-dimensional structure is generally useful for attaching targeting moieties, signaling groups, drugs, or biocompatibility groups, leading to a multifunctional system in an all-in-one platform. The hydrophobic and hydrophilic performance can be easily adjudged by attaching different dendritic unit for a given purpose.

The characterization of the dendritic nanomaterials can be performed with general analytical techniques, such as

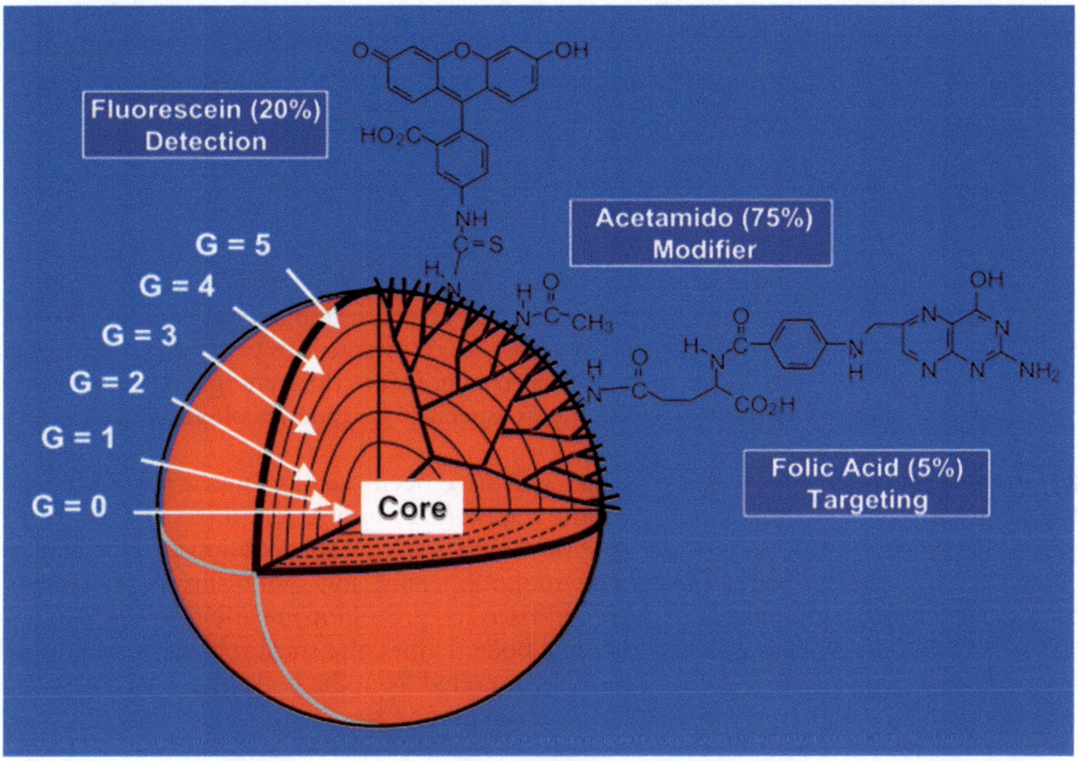

Fig. 2 Schematic presentation of dendrimers as nano-scaffold for the attachment of cell-specific ligands, modifiers, and fluorescence tags

matrix-assisted laser desorption/ionization time of flight (MALDI-TOF) mass spectrometry, gel permeation chromatography (GPC), nuclear magnetic resonance (NMR) spectrometry, ultraviolet–visible spectroscopy or ultraviolet–visible (UV–Vis) spectrophotometry, high performance liquid chromatography (HPLC), transmission electron microscope (TEM), circular dichroism, X-ray diffraction, electrophoresis, intrinsic viscosity, and Fourier transform infrared spectroscopy (FTIR) [11].

1.3 Dendrimer Nanocomposites

Dendritic nanomaterials also includes nanocomposites, which are hybrid nanoparticles formed by guest atoms or small clusters after dispersion and immobilization in dendritic polymer matrices. Dendrimers have also been linked to different carriers for different pharmaceutical and biomedical purposes. The conjugates or complexes of dendrimers with different novel carriers such as liposomes, carbon nanotubes (CNTs), and nanoparticles have resulted in more extra functions [10]. For example, Shi, Wang et al. had demonstrated that dendrimer-entrapped gold nanoparticles (Au DENPs) can be surface-modified with acetyl and hydroxyl groups, thus the toxicity of Au can be significantly reduced [31]. Buczkowski, A. et al. [32] characterized the formation of complexes between PAMAM-NH_2 G4 dendrimer and L-α-tryptophan and L-α-tyrosine in water. Their data indicated a reversible character of the formed complexes. They have a great potential in biomedical applications because of their controlled composition, predetermined size, shape, and versatile surface functionalities [33].

2 Pharmacological Applications

Owing to the exclusive monodispersity, nanometric size range, multivalency, large number of end terminal peripheral groups and interior cavities, and host–guest interactions properties, dendrimers are applied as appropriate host for different guest molecules in broad application fields especially for pharmacological uses (Fig. 3).

2.1 Dendrimer Nanomaterials as Imaging Agents

2.1.1 CT Imaging

Dendritic nanomaterials have been used as nanocarriers for attaching computed tomography (CT) iodinated contrast media, which can provide relatively high iodine concentrations, high stability, near or complete monodispersity, low osmolality, high aqueous solubility, controlled viscosity, great biocompatibility, and complete elimination from the body. Unlike the small molecular weight CT agents that are rapidly excreted from the body, the macromolecular

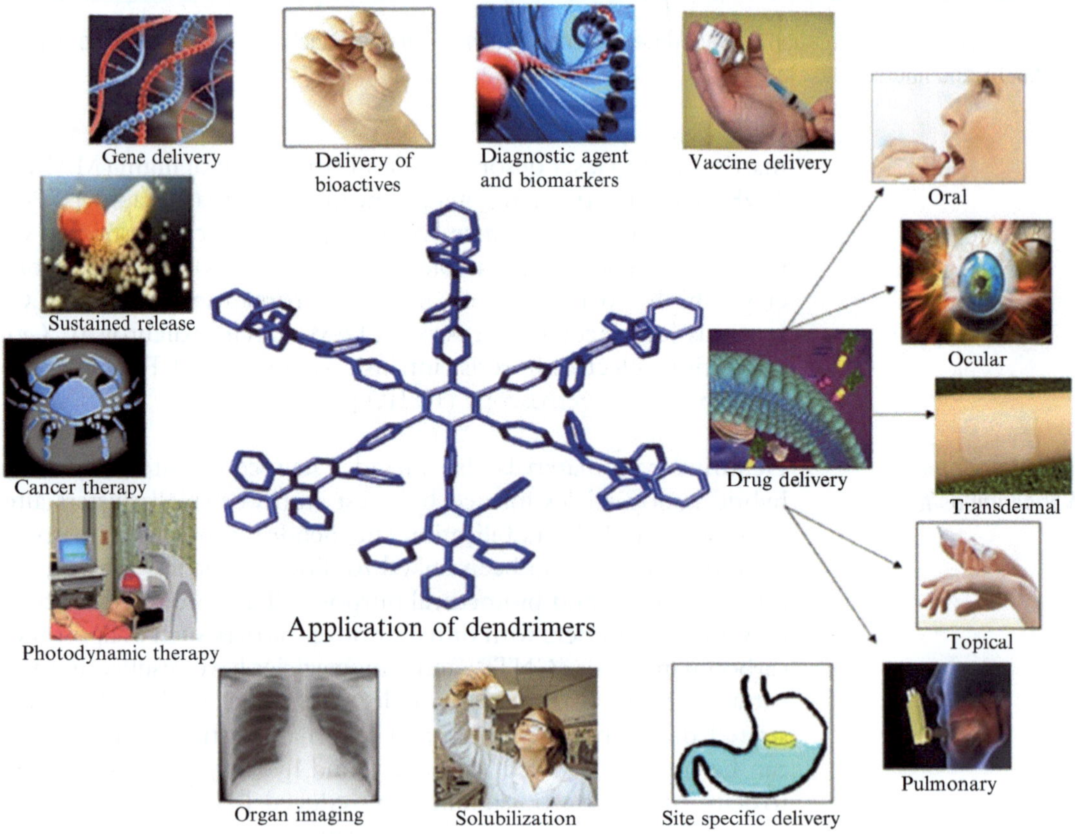

Fig. 3 Overview of dendrimers applications [10]

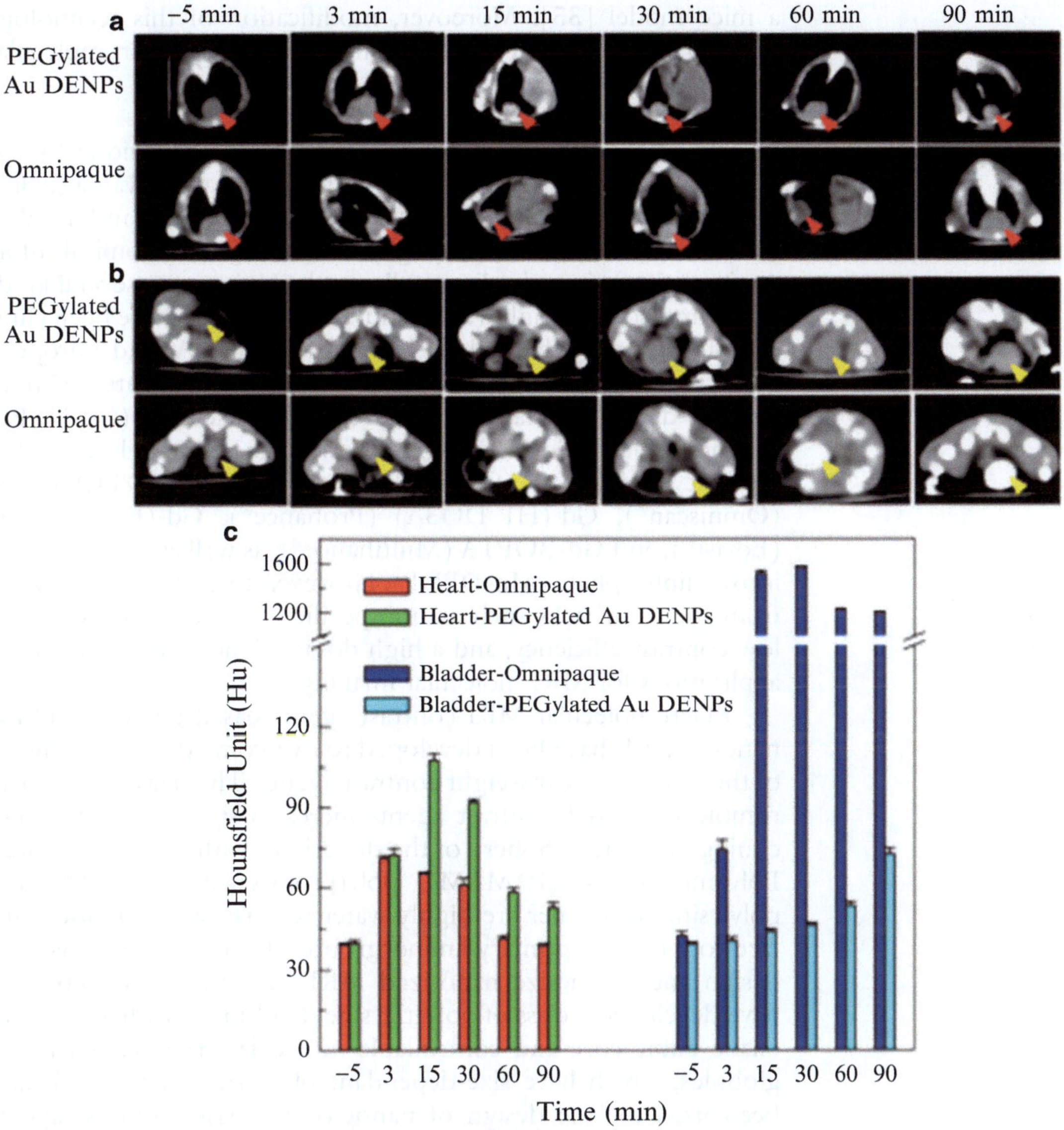

Fig. 4 CT images of the mouse heart (**a**) and bladder (**b**) before and after intravenous injection of PEGylated Au DENPs and Omnipaque, respectively. The *red* and *yellow arrow heads* indicate the heart and bladder area, respectively. (**c**) The corresponding CT value of the heart and bladder at different time points post-injection. Reprinted from reference [35]

dendrimer CT agents can significantly prolong intravascular half life and improve the pharmacokinetics property [12]. Polyethylene glycol (PEG) is usually used to further improve the biocompatibility and decrease the immunogenicity [34]. For example, dendrimer-entrapped gold nanoparticles (Au DENPs) were prepared by using low-generation dendrimers modified by PEG doped with gold nanoparticles, which possess desirable stability, cytocompatibility, and X-ray attenuation properties. As shown in Fig. 4, the prepared Au DENPs enable efficient CT imaging of the heart and tumor in a mice model [35]. Moreover, modification of this technology with targeting moieties will amplify its applications in molecular imaging [31].

2.1.2 MRI Imaging

As one of the prominent noninvasive imaging techniques, magnetic resonance imaging (MRI) has shown unique advantages like high spatial resolution, non-ionizing radiation source, and the ability to extract, simultaneously, physiological and anatomical information of soft tissue in disease diagnosis. Up to now, several kinds of low molecular weight (MW) Gd(III) complexes have been clinically approved by the Federal Drug Agency (FDA) and European Medicines Agency (EMEA) as MRI contrast agents, such as Gd(III)-diethylenetriaminepentaacetic acid (Gd-DTPA, Magnevist®), Gd(III)-1,4,7,10-tetra(carboxymethyl)-1,4,7,10-teraazacyclododecane (Gd-DOTA, Dotarem®), Gd-(DTPA-BMA) (Omniscan®), Gd-(HP-DO3A) (Prohance®), Gd-(EOB-DTPA) (Eovist®), and Gd-BOPTA (Multihance®), as well as Mn(II) dipyridoxal diphosphate (Mn-DPDP). However, these agents still suffer from the drawbacks such as nonspecificity, rapid renal excretion, low contrast efficiency, and a high dosage. These are against their applications for MRI molecular imaging.

Macromolecular MRI contrast agents based on the dendritic nanomaterials have been developed to overcome the shortcomings of the low molecular weight contrast agents. The relaxivity of macromolecular MRI contrast agents increases significantly through conjugating the periphery of the dendrimer with Gd(III) chelates. Polyamidoamine (PAMAM), poly(propyleneimine) (PPI) and polylysine dendrimer are highly water soluble, with a unique surface topology of primary amino groups. They have been used to design and synthesize nanosized MRI contrast agents [36]. We have developed a class of poly-L-lysine dendrimers with a silsesquioxane cubic core and controllable molecular sizes named nanoglobules, which have size-dependant pharmacokinetics and have been used for the design of nanoglobular MRI contrast agents [23–26, 37]. For molecular MRI, the local concentration of receptors is generally too low to reach detectable concentrations of monovalent target-specific contrast agent, while binding multiple MRI labels to the targeting unit may compensate for insufficient accumulation. In our previous work (Fig. 5), the targeting peptides can be directly conjugated on the surface of nanoglobules for tumor-specific extracellular matrix recognition, resulting in significant contrast enhancement in MR cancer molecular imaging [24]. The nanoglobular agents of lower generation (<4) can be readily excreted from the body with reduced tissue retention. Future challenges in the field of macromolecular MRI contrast agents include the rational design and facile synthesis of multifunctional target-specific nanostructures by the combination of target moiety and multiple MRI tags onto a single scaffold. In addition, the synthesis

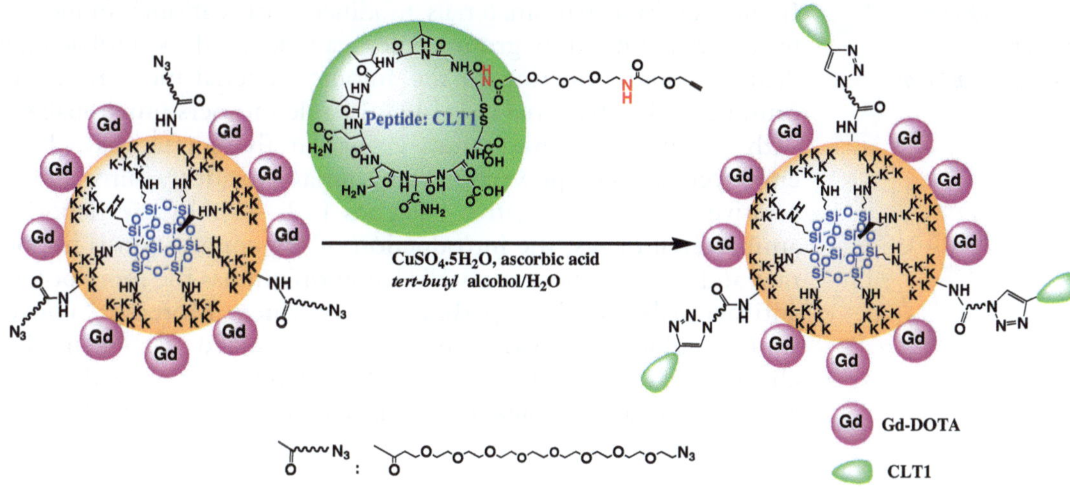

Fig. 5 Schematic illustration of nanoglobular MRI contrast agents for tumor targeted molecular imaging. Image is adapted with permission from reference [25] Copyright (2010) American Chemical Society

of bimodality agents with MRI and PET of optical imaging unit on a single scaffold is a challenge too for the use of advantages of different imaging techniques [38].

2.1.3 Fluorescent Probes

The first synthesis method of a dendrimer emitting blue fluorescence was described by Staneva, Bosch et al. [39]. The PAMAM dendrimer from first generation was modified with eight 4-*N*, *N*-dimethylaminoethyloxy-1, 8-naphthalimide in the dendrimer periphery. The sensor ability of this dendrimer to metal cations (Ag^{2+}, Co^{2+}, Pb^{2+}, Zn^{2+}, Ni^{2+}, Cu^{2+}, and Fe^{3+}) was examined and revealed that it can be used as a sensitive detector for the cations investigated. The fluorescence intensity of the dendrimer has also been investigated as a pH function of the environment, showing potential for detecting protons.

2.2 Dendrimer-Based Nano-drugs

2.2.1 Dendrimer Nanomaterials as Antiviral Drugs

By mimicking the features of anionic cell surfaces, dendritic nanomaterials can be designed as antiviral drugs by attaching sulfonate residues or sialic acid residues on their surface. Through the competing with the cellular surface for binding of virus, the anionic nanomaterials can reduce the risk of the possibility of cell-virus infection. For instance, Starpharma et al. has employed a polylysine dendrimer conjugated naphthalene disulfonate units as the active pharmaceutical ingredient in Viva Gel, a topical vaginal microbicide for HIV prevention, to prevent the virus from infecting cells through attaching to receptors located on the viral coat of HIV-1 [40]. Viva Gel has entered phase II clinical trials in humans and the dendrimer drug can not only act as an inhibitor at early stage virus/cell adsorption, but also hinder viral replication process through interfering with the reverse transcriptase and/or integrase enzymes at later stages [41].

2.2.2 Dendrimer Nanomaterials as Antibacterial Drugs

If the dendritic nanomaterials modified with cationic amines or tetraalkyl ammonium groups, they can be used as antibacterial drugs through adhering to the anionic bacterial membrane and causing further bacterial lysis [42]. PPI dendrimers functionalized with tertiary alkyl ammonium groups at the surface have been employed as very powerful antibacterial biocides against gram-positive and gram-negative bacterias [43, 44]. In the dendritic antibacterial drugs, the introduction of the counter ion is important and the cationic tertiary alkyl ammonium has the more potent antibacterials over the hyperbranched polymers. Moreover, a novel water-soluble PAMAM dendrimer-quaternized carboxymethyl chitosan was prepared via EDC/NHS chemistry, displayed higher antibacterial activity against gram-negative bacteria Escherichia coli (*E. coli*) [45].

2.2.3 Dendrimer Nanomaterials as Antitumor Drugs

The research using dendritic nanomaterials as platform for the development of antitumor drugs has drawn great attention because of the promising antitumor effect with increased drug loading, reduced hemolytic toxicity, and prolonged drug release. Some antitumor drugs including chemotherapeutic and photodynamic therapy (PDT) drugs have been conjugated onto the dendritic nanomaterials. Ly et al. [46] prepared a pegylated PAMAM dendrimer loaded with fluorouracil for the treatment of breast tumor cells MCF-7. The antitumor drugs showed a slow release profile of the drug and an antiproliferative activity against MCF-7 cells as compared to its pegylated counterpart. In vivo tumor xenograft study demonstrated that the 5-FU encapsulated pegylated dendrimer exhibited a significant decrement in volume of the tumor. Tao et al. [47] reported a novel PDT drug-carrier system with the third-generation PAMAM dendrimer grafted to the surface of porous hollow silica nanoparticles modified with gluconic acid. This nanostructure with the size of 100–200 nm and pore structures was then loaded with aluminum phthalocyanine tetrasulfonate to generate singlet oxygen under visible light excitation. Cellular PTD experiments revealed that the dendrimer-based antitumor drugs exhibited a good biocompatibility with lower toxicity and a greater killing efficacy against MCF-7 tumor cells as compared with free photosensitizer.

2.2.4 Dendrimer Nanomaterials in Vaccines

Since small molecular weight substances has low immunogenicity to generate immunogenic reaction, dendritic nanomaterials are also can be used as immunogenic carriers through the increasing the molecular weight of the substance to produce human vaccine. Dendritic nanomaterials are well defined, reproducible immunogens with multivalency for the attachment of antigenic substances. For example, Daftarian et al. [48] reported a new platform using G5 PAMAM dendrimer conjugated with class II-targeting peptides for effective and selective delivery of DNA to antigen-presenting cells.

The immune stimulatory potency is largely enhanced by the dendritic platform in a transfected murine. In vivo study of subcutaneous administration of DNA–peptide–dendrimer complexes transfected dendritic cells in the draining lymph nodes exhibited a promoted generation of high affinity T cells, and elicited rejection of established tumors. Skwarczynski et al. [49] described a self-assembled dendritic nanostructure consisting of a polyacrylate core and an antigen peptides of the minimal B-cell epitope (J14, KQAEDKVKASREAKKQVEKALEQLEDKVK). The nanostructure was about 20 nm diameter in water with less toxic core and exhibited a high affinity for self-assembly into nanoparticles. The peptide alone had no native secondary helical conformation and produced little or no immunogenicity, while peptide conjugated nanostructures were able to induce high levels of systemic J14-specific IgG antibody. Taken together, the dendritic nanomaterials may have great potential as a platform for the producing antibody after proper attaching epitope on their surface.

2.3 Dendrimer Nanomaterials in Gene Delivery

Unique properties of dendrimers such as tailored architecture and diverse multivalent surface groups make these dendritic nanomaterials highly potential to be applied as delivery vectors for therapeutic genes. The relationship between dendrimer structure and the morphology and physicochemistry of the delivery nucleic acid complexes plays an important role in the rational design of dendrimer carriers. The first successful attempt of employing dendritic nanomaterials for transfection purposes was reported by Haensler and Szoka in 1993 using PAMAM dendrimers as a platform [50]. The self-assembling process between dendrimers and genes is based on electrostatic interactions of the surface amine groups of dendrimer and nucleic acids. The binding ability increases along with increasing generation of the dendrimer [51]. A dendrimer-like polymer (e.g., Superfect®) has become a popular commercial product for gene vectors [52]. The application of dendrimer nanomaterials in gene delivery for cancer gene therapy has attracted much attention recently. For example, Santander-Ortega et al. [53] reported DAB-AM16 dendrimer DNA delivery system contained a substantial proportion of free polymer to inhibit tumor growth. DAB-AM16 is a dendritic polymer with a globular structure, consisting of poly(propylene imine) branches that emerge from a diaminobutane core. They found that the electrolytes and proteins present in physiological media play a crucial role to reduce the toxicity associated with their cationic groups. Wang et al. recently reported the synthesis of fluorinated dendrimers for use as gene vectors, which were able to achieve excellent gene transfection efficacy in several tumor cell lines (higher than 90 % in HEK293 and HeLa cells) at extremely low N/P ratios. Compared with several commercial transfection reagents such as Lipofectamine 2000 and SuperFect, the fluorinated dendritic vectors showed superior efficacy and biocompatibility with enhanced cellular uptake of the dendrimer/DNA polyplexes and facilitating their endosomal escape. In a word, the concept of utilizing dendritic architectures for gene-delivery purposes is a promising approach to create well-defined, efficient, and less toxic nonviral gene vectors. More research on the relationships between structure and activity will stimulate the design of more active gene vectors and hopefully be suitable for prospective clinical development.

3 Principles for Application in Biological Systems

The major constraints to the biological applications of dendritic nanomaterials include hemolytic toxicity, immunogenicity, RES uptake, stability, hydrophobicity, and drug leakage [10]. In order to successfully apply in vivo, besides being nontoxic, dendrimer-based nanomaterials have to be non-immunogenic as well if not applied as vaccines. They also are required to be able to cross bio-barriers and reach to the targeting tissues or cells [6].

3.1 In Vitro Toxicity

Toxicity of dendrimer-based nanomaterials is strongly influenced by the properties of their terminal groups. Dendrimers with negatively charged or neutral groups on the surface are generally nontoxic, while positively charged ones causing varying degrees of toxicity, especially species with polycationic groups are easy to cause cell lysis by destabilizing cell membranes. The exact mechanism of this phenomenon has not yet been fully revealed [54].

Comparative cytotoxicity studies on different cell-lines showed that PAMAM dendrimers are less toxic than the lysine based dendrimer [50]. The PAMAM dendrimers has shown generation-dependent cytotoxicity. The higher generation dendrimers show increased cytotoxicity, which is in accordance with general studies that polymers with larger molecular size present more cytotoxicity [55, 56]. Besides, heme toxicity studies conclude that the same dendrimer has hemolytic effect on rat blood cells which also increases with larger generation [57]. Myotoxicity studies on rodent muscles isolated from male Sprague Dawley rats revealed that the G4-PAMAM dendrimer was more myotoxic, comparing with cationic liposomes and proteins [58]. In summary, amino-terminated dendrimers are generally cytotoxic because of their globular shapes and less flexible structures [57], but still show lower toxicity comparing to more flexible linear macromolecules with amino groups. Another factor related to the cytotoxicity is the substitution degree on the amine functionality. The primary amines usually show more toxicity than the secondary or tertiary species [56, 59].

3.2 In Vivo Toxicity

So far not many systematic study results on the in vivo toxicity of dendrimer-based nanomaterials are available. Initially the general observation was carried out after the G5-PAMAM dendrimers were injected into mice even at the high concentration of 10 mg/kg, where they all show nontoxicity, no matter the dendrimer surface are unmodified or modified [60, 61]. In further studies they injected the unmodified amino-terminated PAMAM dendrimers together with ovalbumin into mice, where no any significant toxicity except slight adjuvant activity were found [62]. Similar results were found on new hydroxy- or methoxy-terminated dendrimers [63]. Due to their nontoxic performance in vivo, these new dendritic structures are expected to be very promising in the pharmaceutical applications [63].

3.3 Immunogenicity

Besides nontoxic, when applied in animal or human body except as vaccines, dendrimer-based nanomaterials are also required to be nonimmunogenic. An early systematic study on amino-terminated PAMAM dendrimers revealed no to very weak immunogenicity from generation 3 to 7 [60]. In later studies, however, these dendrimers showed some immunogenicity. Polyethylene glycol (PEG) chains can be introduced to modify these dendrimers to reduce immunogenicity [64], which can be explained by PEG chains increasing the hydrophilicity with low disturbing effect to the biological environment. On the opposite, to create highly immunogenic compounds such as vaccines, the surface of dendrimers can be grafted with antigens or T-cell helper epitopes to enhance this effect.

3.4 Biopermeability

In order to successfully use dendrimer nanomaterials in different levels of biological systems, their biopermeability has also to be taken into serious consideration. Dendrimers complexed with DNA can greatly improve the biopermeability on a microscopic level. Compared to free dendrimer, the dendrimer–DNA adducts can enter the cell nucleus with less resistance while fewer cytotoxicity. To further increase the transfection ability, several approaches have been developed [65, 66]. The transfection efficiency of the PAMAM dendrimer–DNA complex can be enhanced by addition of a certain amount of sulfonated β-cyclodextrins (β-CD's), due to the altered DNA–dendrimer surface charge from ionic binding between the anionic sulfonate moieties of the β-CD and the cationic amino-terminated dendrimer [67]. PEG was also applied to modify the dendrimer surface, which can increase the transfection effect of polylysine dendrimers [68]. However, many studies generally reveal that the globular shape of dendrimer architecture doesn't show advantages in gene delivery, which is in accordance with an earlier study result that the "fragmented" dendrimers had a much better transfection efficacy compared to the globular "complete" molecule [69].

Biopermeability on a macroscopic level of dendrimer-based nanomaterials also has to be taken into serious consideration. The amino-terminated PAMAM dendrimers were studied in vivo for their abilities to cross the microvascular endothelium. It was found that the extravasation time increases with increasing molecular weight and generation [70]. Research on the transepithelial transport of G0-G4 PAMAM dendrimers in Madin-Darby canine kidney cells revealed the G4 dendrimer present the best permeability, and there was no linear relationship between the generation number and permeability [55, 70]. However, studies on the para-cellular transepithelial transport in a Caco-2 cell monolayer concluded the amino-terminated PAMAM dendrimers with smaller generation presented better permeability than the species with larger generation. Another in vitro study in an everted rat intestinal sac system revealed that the negatively charged PAMAM dendrimers could rapidly cross into the intestine of rats. Compared to other polymeric systems, these faster transferred dendrimers suggested they could be used as oral delivery device [71]. After modified with lipid chains, polylysine dendrimers showed poorer uptake ability through the intestine of rats compared with the popular delivery devices such as polystyrene latex system [72].

4 Conclusion

Dendrimers are extremely well tailored, highly branched globular polymers with "volumes." As described, a variety of dendrimer-based nanomaterials have already found wide use in biological systems such as imaging agents, drug candidates, and also have widely used as carriers for drugs, genes, vaccine antigens and so on. Dendrimers endow these devices better membrane permeability, and furthermore, targeting function by specific host–guest interactions. New approaches for synthesizing and modifying dendrimers are expected to enable specific tailoring of volume size, binding motifs, surface charge density, which will make it possible to well control the sophistication of current drugs and nanocarrier agents. Meanwhile, more and more dendrimer derivated nanocomposites are merging, creating totally new types of nanocarrier or specific devices for treating human diseases. All the results from in vitro and vivo studies show dendrimer-based nanomaterials well biocompatible. Although the obstacles in the fields of delivery efficiency, targeting ability and suitability to match with specific clinical situations still remain significant, the dendrimer-based nanomaterials still present great potential to be applied in biological environments.

Acknowledgment

This work was supported by the National Nature Science Foundation of China (91227126), National Special Fund for Key Scientific Instrument and Equipment Development (2013YQ17046307) and the Nature Science Foundation of Liaoning Province, China (2013020177).

References

1. Buhleier E, Wehner W, Vogtle F (1978) Cascade-chain-like and nonskid-chain-like syntheses of molecular cavity topologies. Synthesis-Stuttgart 2:155–158
2. Tomalia DA, Baker H, Dewald J, Hall M, Kallos G, Martin S, Roeck J, Ryder J, Smith P (1985) A new class of polymers: starburst-dendritic macromolecules. Polym J 17:117–132
3. Tomalia DA, Baker H, Dewald J, Hall M, Kallos G, Martin S, Roeck J, Ryder J, Smith P (1986) Dendritic macromolecules: synthesis of starburst dendrimers. Macromolecules 19:2466–2468
4. Newkome GR, Yao Z, Baker GR, Gupta VK (1985) Micelles. Part 1. Cascade molecules: a new approach to micelles. A [27]-arborol. J Org Chem 50:2003–2004
5. Newkome GR, Yao Z, Baker GR, Gupta VK, Russo PS, Saunders MJ (1986) Chemistry of micelles series. Part 2. Cascade molecules. Synthesis and characterization of a benzene [9] 3-arborol. J Am Chem Soc 108:849–850
6. Boas U, Heegaard PM (2004) Dendrimers in drug research. Chem Soc Rev 33:43–63
7. Twyman LJ, King AS, Martin IK (2002) Catalysis inside dendrimers. Chem Soc Rev 31:69–82
8. Gillies ER, Frechet JM (2005) Dendrimers and dendritic polymers in drug delivery. Drug Discov Today 10:35–43
9. Eichman JD, Bielinska AU, Kukowska-Latallo JF, Baker JR Jr (2000) The use of PAMAM dendrimers in the efficient transfer of genetic material into cells. Pharm Sci Technolo Today 3:232–245
10. Kesharwani P, Jain K, Jain NK (2014) Dendrimer as nanocarrier for drug delivery. Prog Polym Sci 39:268–307
11. Caminade AM, Laurent R, Majoral JP (2005) Characterization of dendrimers. Adv Drug Deliv Rev 57:2130–2146
12. Svenson S, Tomalia DA (2005) Dendrimers in biomedical applications--reflections on the field. Adv Drug Deliv Rev 57:2106–2129
13. Zhao F, Li W (2011) Dendrimer/inorganic nanomaterial composites: tailoring preparation, properties, functions, and applications of inorganic nanomaterials with dendritic architectures. Sci China Chem 54:286–301
14. Wang SH, Shi X, Van Antwerp M, Cao Z, Swanson SD, Bi X, Baker JR (2007) Dendrimer-functionalized iron oxide nanoparticles for specific targeting and imaging of cancer cells. Adv Funct Mater 17:3043–3050
15. Kobayashi H, Kawamoto S, Saga T, Sato N, Hiraga A, Ishimori T, Akita Y, Mamede MH, Konishi J, Togashi K (2001) Novel liver macromolecular MR contrast agent with a polypropylenimine diaminobutyl dendrimer core: comparison to the vascular MR contrast agent with the polyamidoamine dendrimer core. Magn Reson Med 46:795–802
16. Kobayashi H, Kawamoto S, Jo S-K, Bryant HL, Brechbiel MW, Star RA (2003) Macromolecular MRI contrast agents with small dendrimers: pharmacokinetic differences between sizes and cores. Bioconjug Chem 14:388–394
17. Kitchens KM, El-Sayed ME, Ghandehari H (2005) Transepithelial and endothelial transport of poly (amidoamine) dendrimers. Adv Drug Deliv Rev 57:2163–2176
18. Gupta R, Mehra NK, Jain NK (2014) Development and characterization of sulfasalazine loaded fucosylated PPI dendrimer for the treatment of cytokine-induced liver damage. Eur J Pharm Biopharm 86:449–458
19. Bunz UH (2005) Synthesis and structure of PAEs, poly (arylene etynylene)s. Springer, Berlin, pp 1–52
20. Swanson DR, Huang B, Abdelhady HG, Tomalia DA (2007) Unique steric and geometry induced stoichiometries observed in the divergent synthesis of poly(ester-acrylate/amine) (PEA) dendrimers. New J Chem 31:1368–1378
21. Turnbull WB, Stoddart JF (2002) Design and synthesis of glycodendrimers. Rev Mol Biotechnol 90:231–255
22. Roy R, Kim JM (1999) Amphiphilic p-tert-butylcalix [4] arene scaffolds containing exposed carbohydrate dendrons. Angew Chem Int Ed 38:369–372
23. Tan MQ, Burden-Gulley SM, Li W, Wu XM, Lindner D, Brady-Kalnay SM, Gulani V, Lu ZR (2012) MR molecular imaging of prostate cancer with a peptide-targeted contrast agent in a mouse orthotopic prostate cancer model. Pharm Res 29:953–960
24. Tan MQ, Wu XM, Jeong EK, Chen QJ, Lu ZR (2010) Peptide-targeted nanoglobular Gd-DOTA monoamide conjugates for magnetic resonance cancer molecular imaging. Biomacromolecules 11:754–761
25. Tan MQ, Wu XM, Jeong EK, Chen QJ, Parker DL, Lu ZR (2010) An effective targeted nanoglobular manganese(II) chelate conjugate for magnetic resonance molecular imaging of tumor extracellular matrix. Mol Pharm 7:936–943

26. Tan MQ, Ye Z, Jeong EK, Wu XM, Parker DL, Lu ZR (2011) Synthesis and evaluation of nanoglobular macrocyclic Mn(II) chelate conjugates as non-gadolinium(III) MRI contrast agents. Bioconjug Chem 22:931–937
27. Majoral J-P, Caminade A-M (1999) Dendrimers containing heteroatoms (si, p, B, ge, or bi). Chem Rev 99:845–880
28. Fischer M, Vögtle F (1999) Dendrimers: from design to application—a progress report. Angew Chem Int Ed 38:884–905
29. Pourianazar NT, Mutlu P, Gunduz U (2014) Bioapplications of poly(amidoamine) (PAMAM) dendrimers in nanomedicine. J Nanopart Res 16:2342
30. Sebestik J, Niederhafner P, Jezek J (2011) Peptide and glycopeptide dendrimers and analogous dendrimeric structures and their biomedical applications. Amino Acids 40:301–370
31. Shi X, Wang S, Meshinchi S, Van Antwerp ME, Bi X, Lee I, Baker JR Jr (2007) Dendrimer-entrapped gold nanoparticles as a platform for cancer-cell targeting and imaging. Small 3:1245–1252
32. Buczkowski A, Urbaniak P, Belica S, Sekowski S, Bryszewska M, Palecz B (2014) Formation of complexes between PAMAM-NH2 G4 dendrimer and L-alpha-tryptophan and L-alpha-tyrosine in water. Spectrochim Acta Part A 128:647–652
33. Wolinsky JB, Grinstaff MW (2008) Therapeutic and diagnostic applications of dendrimers for cancer treatment. Adv Drug Deliv Rev 60:1037–1055
34. Fu Y, Nitecki DE, Maltby D, Simon GH, Berejnoi K, Raatschen H-J, Yeh BM, Shames DM, Brasch RC (2006) Dendritic iodinated contrast agents with PEG-cores for CT imaging: synthesis and preliminary characterization. Bioconjug Chem 17:1043–1056
35. Liu H, Wang H, Xu Y, Shen M, Zhao J, Zhang G, Shi X (2014) Synthesis of PEGylated low generation dendrimer-entrapped gold nanoparticles for CT imaging applications. Nanoscale 6:4521–4526
36. Kobayashi H, Brechbiel MW (2004) Dendrimer-based nanosized MRI contrast agents. Curr Pharm Biotechnol 5:539–549
37. Tan MQ, Ye Z, Lindner D, Brady-Kalnay SM, Lu ZR (2014) Synthesis and evaluation of a targeted nanoglobular dual-modal imaging agent for MR imaging and image-guided surgery of prostate cancer. Pharm Res 31:1469–1476
38. Langereis S, Dirksen A, Hackeng TM, van Genderen MHP, Meijer EW (2007) Dendrimers and magnetic resonance imaging. New J Chem 31:1152
39. Staneva D, Bosch P, Asiri AM, Taib LA, Grabchev I (2014) Studying pH dependence of the photophysical properties of a blue emitting fluorescent PAMAM dendrimer and evaluation of its sensor potential. Dyes Pigm 105:114–120
40. Peng J, Wu Z, Qi X, Chen Y, Li X (2013) Dendrimers as potential therapeutic tools in HIV inhibition. Molecules 18:7912–7929
41. Wrobel D, Kolanowska K, Gajek A, Gomez-Ramirez R, de la Mata J, Pedziwiatr-Werbicka E, Klajnert B, Waczulikova I, Bryszewska M (2014) Interaction of cationic carbosilane dendrimers and their complexes with siRNA with erythrocytes and red blood cell ghosts. Biochim Biophys Acta 1838:882–889
42. Castonguay A, Ladd E, van de Ven TG, Kakkar A (2012) Dendrimers as bactericides. New J Chem 36:199–204
43. Balogh L, Swanson DR, Tomalia DA, Hagnauer GL, McManus AT (2001) Dendrimer-silver complexes and nanocomposites as antimicrobial agents. Nano Lett 1:18–21
44. Chen CZ, Cooper SL (2002) Interactions between dendrimer biocides and bacterial membranes. Biomaterials 23:3359–3368
45. Wen Y, Tan ZL, Sun F, Sheng L, Zhang XY, Yao FL (2012) Synthesis and characterization of quaternized carboxymethyl chitosan/poly(amidoamine) dendrimer core-shell nanoparticles. Mater Sci Eng C-Mater 32:2026–2036
46. Ly TU, Tran NQ, Thi KDH, Phan KN, Truong HN, Nguyen CK (2013) Pegylated dendrimer and its effect in fluorouracil loading and release for enhancing antitumor activity. J Biomed Nanotechnol 9:213–220
47. Tao X, Yang YJ, Liu S, Zheng YZ, Fu J, Chen JF (2013) Poly(amidoamine) dendrimer-grafted porous hollow silica nanoparticles for enhanced intracellular photodynamic therapy. Acta Biomater 9:6431–6438
48. Daftarian P, Kaifer AE, Li W, Blomberg BB, Frasca D, Roth F, Chowdhury R, Berg EA, Fishman JB, Al Sayegh HA, Blackwelder P, Inverardi L, Perez VL, Lemmon V, Serafini P (2011) Peptide-conjugated PAMAM dendrimer as a universal DNA vaccine platform to target antigen-presenting cells. Cancer Res 71:7452–7462
49. Skwarczynski M, Zaman M, Urbani CN, Lin IC, Jia ZF, Batzloff MR, Good MF, Monteiro MF, Toth I (2010) Polyacrylate dendrimer nanoparticles: a self-adjuvanting vaccine delivery system. Angew Chem Int Ed 49:5742–5745
50. Haensler J, Szoka FC Jr (1993) Polyamidoamine cascade polymers mediate efficient transfection

of cells in culture. Bioconjug Chem 4: 372–379
51. Chen W, Turro NJ, Tomalia DA (2000) Using ethidium bromide to probe the interactions between DNA and dendrimers. Langmuir 16:15–19
52. Tschiche A, Malhotra S, Haag R (2014) Nonviral gene delivery with dendritic self-assembling architectures. Nanomedicine UK 9: 667–693
53. Santander-Ortega MJ, de la Fuente M, Lozano MV, Tsui ML, Bolton K, Uchegbu IF, Schatzlein AG (2014) Optimisation of synthetic vector systems for cancer gene therapy—the role of the excess of cationic dendrimer under physiological conditions. Curr Top Med Chem 14:1172–1181
54. Rittner K, Benavente A, Bompard-Sorlet A, Heitz F, Divita G, Brasseur R, Jacobs E (2002) New basic membrane-destabilizing peptides for plasmid-based gene delivery in vitro and in vivo. Mol Ther 5:104–114
55. El-Sayed M, Ginski M, Rhodes C, Ghandehari H (2002) Transepithelial transport of poly (amidoamine) dendrimers across Caco-2 cell monolayers. J Control Release 81:355–365
56. Fischer D, Li Y, Ahlemeyer B, Krieglstein J, Kissel T (2003) In vitro cytotoxicity testing of polycations: influence of polymer structure on cell viability and hemolysis. Biomaterials 24: 1121–1131
57. Malik N, Wiwattanapatapee R, Klopsch R, Lorenz K, Frey H, Weener J, Meijer E, Paulus W, Duncan R (2000) Dendrimers: relationship between structure and biocompatibility in vitro, and preliminary studies on the biodistribution of 125I-labelled polyamidoamine dendrimers in vivo. J Control Release 65:133–148
58. Brazeau GA, Attia S, Poxon S, Hughes JA (1998) In vitro myotoxicity of selected cationic macromolecules used in non-viral gene delivery. Pharm Res 15:680–684
59. Ferruti P, Knobloch S, Ranucci E, Gianasi E, Duncan R (1997) A novel chemical modification of poly-L-lysine reducing toxicity while preserving cationic properties. Proc Int Symp Control Rel Bioact Mater 24:45–46
60. Roberts JC, Bhalgat MK, Zera RT (1996) Preliminary biological evaluation of polyamidoamine (PAMAM) Starburst dendrimers. J Biomed Mater Res 30:53–65
61. Bourne N, Stanberry L, Kern E, Holan G, Matthews B, Bernstein D (2000) Dendrimers, a new class of candidate topical microbicides with activity against herpes simplex virus infection. Antimicrob Agents Chemother 44: 2471–2474
62. Rajananthanan P, Attard GS, Sheikh NA, Morrow WJW (1999) Evaluation of novel aggregate structures as adjuvants: composition, toxicity studies and humoral responses. Vaccine 17:715–730
63. Ihre HR, Padilla De Jesús OL, Szoka FC, Fréchet JM (2002) Polyester dendritic systems for drug delivery applications: design, synthesis, and characterization. Bioconjug Chem 13:443–452
64. Kobayashi H, Kawamoto S, Saga T, Sato N, Hiraga A, Ishimori T, Konishi J, Togashi K, Brechbiel MW (2001) Positive effects of polyethylene glycol conjugation to generation-4 polyamidoamine dendrimers as macromolecular MR contrast agents. Magn Reson Med 46:781–788
65. Shah DS, Sakthivel T, Toth I, Florence AT, Wilderspin AF (2000) DNA transfection and transfected cell viability using amphipathic asymmetric dendrimers. Int J Pharm 208: 41–48
66. Wimmer N, Marano RJ, Kearns PS, Rakoczy EP, Toth I (2002) Syntheses of polycationic dendrimers on lipophilic peptide core for complexation and transport of oligonucleotides. Bioorg Med Chem Lett 12:2635–2637
67. Roessler BJ, Bielinska AU, Janczak K, Lee I, Baker JR Jr (2001) Substituted β-cyclodextrins interact with PAMAM dendrimer–DNA complexes and modify transfection efficiency. Biochem Biophys Res Commun 283: 124–129
68. Männistö M, Vanderkerken S, Toncheva V, Elomaa M, Ruponen M, Schacht E, Urtti A (2002) Structure–activity relationships of poly (l-lysines): effects of pegylation and molecular shape on physicochemical and biological properties in gene delivery. J Control Release 83:169–182
69. Tang MX, Redemann CT, Szoka FC (1996) In vitro gene delivery by degraded polyamidoamine dendrimers. Bioconjug Chem 7:703–714
70. Tajarobi F, El-Sayed M, Rege B, Polli J, Ghandehari H (2001) Transport of poly amidoamine dendrimers across Madin–Darby canine kidney cells. Int J Pharm 215:263–267
71. Wiwattanapatapee R, Carreño-Gómez B, Malik N, Duncan R (2000) Anionic PAMAM dendrimers rapidly cross adult rat intestine in vitro: a potential oral delivery system? Pharm Res 17:991–998
72. Florence A, Sakthivel T, Toth I (2000) Oral uptake and translocation of a polylysine dendrimer with a lipid surface. J Control Release 65:253–259

Chapter 4

Paving the Way Toward Translational Application of Virus-Based Nanoparticles (VNPs): Preclinical Evaluation of Their Biological Fates

Anna E. Czapar and Nicole F. Steinmetz

Abstract

Plant based viral nanoparticles (VNPs) are an attractive platform for a variety of biomedical applications including tissue-specific imaging and drug delivery. As with any novel biomaterial, thorough in vivo evaluation is required to assess safety profiles and pave the way for potential clinical application. In this chapter we discuss protocols for study of the immune response, pharmacokinetics, biodistribution, as well as blood and tissue compatibility of VNPs.

Key words Plant virus, Cowpea mosaic virus, Potato virus X, Tobacco mosaic virus, Immune response, Pharmacokinetics, Biodistribution, Biocompatibility, Imaging, Drug delivery

1 Virus-Based Nanoparticles in Preclinical Development and Testing

Nanoparticles have an increasingly expanding range of potential medical applications including tissue-specific drug delivery, image contrast enhancement for diagnosis and prognosis, and immune modulation, including vaccine development. There are many classes of nanomaterials in preclinical development and clinical testing; one such class of nanomaterials is the proteinaceous, virus-based nanoparticles (VNPs) from bacteriophages, animal viruses, and plant viruses. VNPs offer several advantages over synthetic nanoparticles: They can be produced in large quantities in a relatively short period of time via fermentation, tissue culture, or molecular farming in plants; since virus production is genetically encoded each progeny particle formed is highly monodisperse; viral structures are known to atomic resolution and can be tailored to incorporate tissue-specific ligands, contrast agents, or therapeutic agents through synthetic or chemical biology methods with spatial control (Fig. 1). The variety of capsid shapes and the combination of genetic control and available surface chemistries allows

Zheng-Rong Lu and Shinji Sakuma (eds.), *Nanomaterials in Pharmacology*, Methods in Pharmacology and Toxicology, DOI 10.1007/978-1-4939-3121-7_4, © Springer Science+Business Media New York 2016

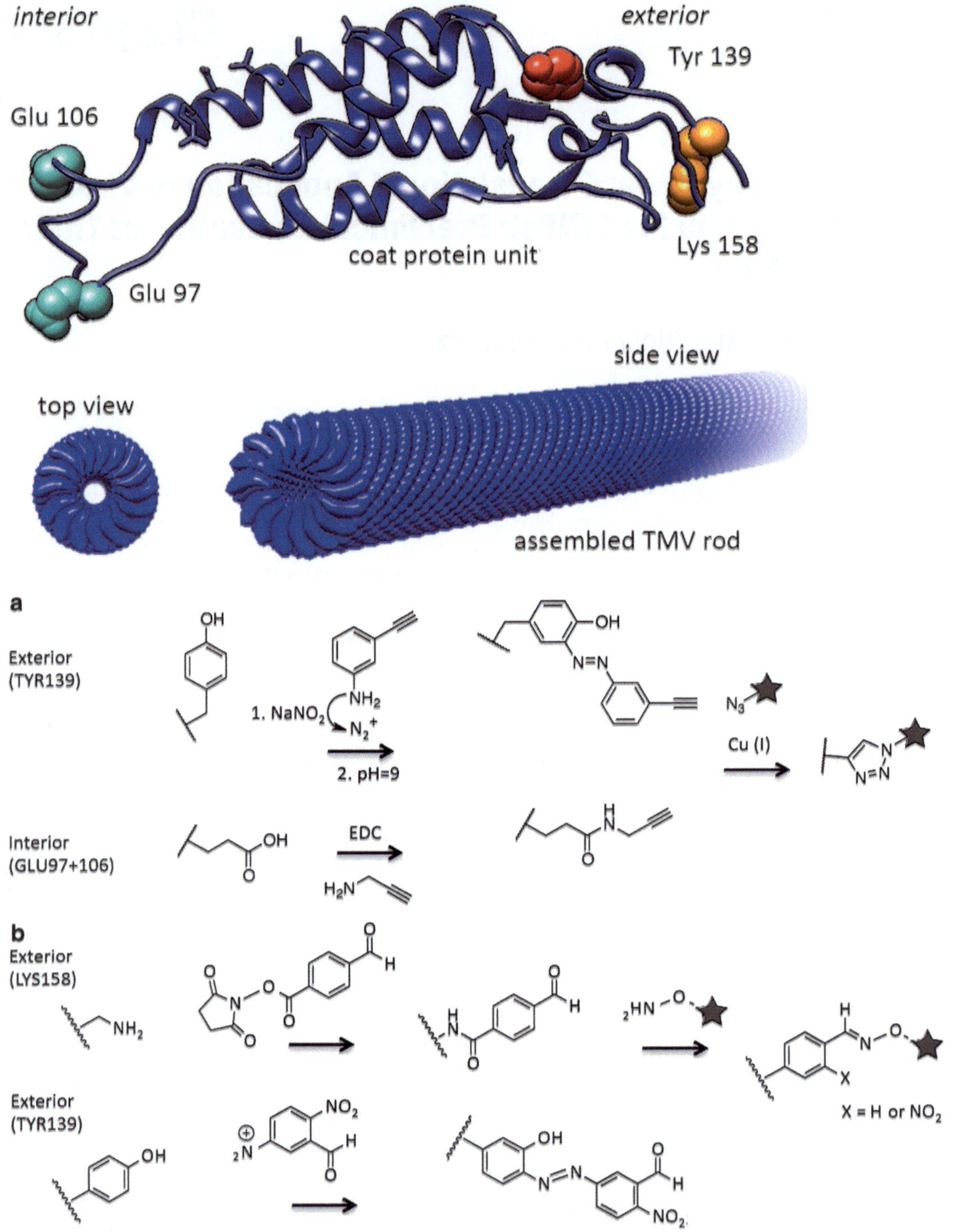

Fig. 1 *Left panel*: TMV and its coat protein; highlighting Glutamic acids on the interior surface and Tyrosine and Lysine residue on the exterior surface. TMV measures 300 × 18 nm with a 4 nm-wide interior channel. *Right panel*: Typical bioconjugation schemes for chemical modification of Glutamic acids, Tyrosine side chains, or Lysine residues on the TMV coat protein

for the synthesis of diverse particle libraries useful for a wide range of applications [1–3].

Another advantage for in vivo medical applications is that the protein-based carriers are biodegradable and removed from cells and tissues through the cellular machinery. This is in stark contrast to some synthetic materials, which may persist in the body for extended periods [4–7]. An additional advantage of plant viruses and bacteriophages, as opposed to mammalian viruses, is that plant viruses do not infect or replicate in humans, and therefore are unlikely to produce downstream signal transduction events or pathogenic effects [2].

A potential disadvantage of bacterial and plant produced protein carriers is that these materials are generally immunogenic. However, it is important to acknowledge that immunogenicity is a translational challenge to be addressed for many systems, including synthetic nanoparticles; in fact, the production of carrier-specific antibodies has been reported for various inorganic and synthetic systems [8–13]. The key questions to be addressed are whether the immune responses are part of the natural clearance mechanisms or whether this poses potential adverse effects. Generally it is accepted that the immunogenic properties of nanoparticles, protein-based carriers [14, 15] as well as plant viruses [16] can be attenuated by stealth polymer coating, for example using polyethylene glycol (PEG) [15, 17–20]. The hydrophilic PEG shield decreases serum protein adsorption, which in turn decreases clearance by the macrophagocytic system (MPS) and deposition in non-target cells and organs, such as components of the immune system.

While nanoparticles, including VNPs, may provide intriguing opportunities as next-generation medicines for diagnostic and therapeutic applications, understanding the biological response of any nanomaterials is imperative to developing nanotechnology that may have clinical utility. In recent years, our laboratory has focused on gaining a fundamental understanding on the in vivo fate of plant virus-based carriers for nanomedical applications [21–23]. This chapter describes methods for the propagation of plant-derived VNPs and evaluation of their immune interactions, biodistribution, and pharmacokinetics; methods for in vitro and in vivo testing are described. While we focus this chapter is on VNPs, many of the protocols described could be applied for preclinical testing of other types of nano-based contrast agents or therapeutics.

2 Methods Presented in This Chapter

We recently published detailed experimental procedures for the propagation of tobacco mosaic virus (TMV, [24]), cowpea mosaic virus (CPMV, [25]), and potato virus X (PVX, [26]).

Protocols for chemical and genetic modification of these virus-based nanocarriers as well their characterization is also described in these chapters; therefore we would like to refer the reader to these publications with regard to VNP propagation, purification, modification, and characterization. In the following sections we will describe protocols for determining VNP–immune interactions, their blood compatibility, pharmacokinetics, and biodistribution. Studies involve macrophage and dendritic cell coculture with VNPs to examine differential immune cell uptake, cytokine expression, and inflammasome response. Blood sampling from mice pre- and post-dosing with VNPs is described to determine antibody titers, while naïve blood samples are used to assess the levels of hemolysis, coagulation, and complement activation upon VNP administration. Finally, we will report several methods to evaluate pharmacokinetics and biodistribution including optical methods, elemental analysis, or genetic profiling (it should be noted that radiolabeling is a suitable alternative, but since our lab does not utilize radiochemistry, these methods will not be further discussed in this chapter; the reader is referred to the following publications [9, 27]).

3 Nanomaterial-Target and Non-target Cell Interactions

In concert with in vivo animal studies, in vitro assays should be considered: target and non-target cell interactions can be studied using tissue culture methods in conjunction with confocal microscopy or flow cytometry [28, 29]. For example, cancer target cell uptake of RGD-modified VNPs targeted to tumor-associated integrin receptors can be evaluated by comparison with non-targeted VNPs or in competition binding assays using a molar excess of the free targeting ligands [28]. Further, interactions with cells of the immune system should be considered, including mouse or human macrophage cell lines and bone marrow-derived dendritic cells (BMDC) [30]. Phagocytic uptake versus target cell uptake should be studied side-by-side comparing different surface chemistries, i.e., targeting ligands (e.g., RGD) and polymer shields (e.g., PEG). An increased target cell uptake and decreased immune cell uptake of VNPs could indicate decreased MPS clearance in vivo, resulting in increased delivery to target tissues. Nevertheless, while in vitro testing is expected to provide insights into the in vivo fates, only in vivo studies can provide detailed information on biodistribution and clearance (see below).

In addition to measuring VNP–cell interactions, cytokine signaling should be evaluated, as it will provide more detailed insights into potential adverse effects such as onset of acute or chronic inflammation. A good initial evaluation is to examine production of TNF-α, IL-6, and IL-1β. TNF-α and IL-6 are mediators of the acute and chronic phases of the inflammatory response; both are good indicators of potential immune reactions and adverse responses to nanoparticle administration [6]. IL-1β is an important mediator of inflammation, neutrophil and macrophage recruitment, and the febrile response. Production of IL-1β is associated with the inflammasome, a caspase-activating complex found in macrophages and monocytes that is active during infection, cell damage, and stress [31]. Increased production of IL-1β has been observed with administration of several formulations of synthetic nanoparticles [6, 32–34]. Although IL-1β production upon VNP–cell interaction has not been reported yet, it might be critical to establish whether or not IL-1β signaling occurs when cargo-loaded VNPs are in use.

3.1 Protocols for (Virus-Based) Nanoparticle In Vitro Cell Uptake and Signaling

3.1.1 Flow Cytometry to Evaluate Immune Cell Uptake

To evaluate cell uptake in immune cells, mouse or human macrophage cell lines as well as bone-marrow derived dendritic cells should be used. Here, we describe a protocol that is similar to that described in Ref. [35]; a sample result is shown in Fig. 2.

1. Grow RAW264.7 (ATTC) to confluency, wash three times with PBS, and collect using enzyme-free Hank's based Cell Dissociation Buffer. It should be noted that RAW 264.7 cells are highly susceptible to genetic drift, therefore they should be used from an early passage number. Add cells to 96-well v-bottom plates (1×10^6 cells/200 μL/well) and incubate with 10,000 or 100,000 TMV particles/cell, in triplicate for either 20 min or 2 h at 37 °C and 5 % CO_2. The VNPs should be added in 0.1 M potassium phosphate buffer pH 7.0 (1 mg/mL) with or with cargo (e.g., drug) and/or surface modification (e.g., PEG).
2. In parallel, bone marrow-derived dendritic cells (BMDCs) should be studied. BMDCs can be isolated using techniques previously described (ref. [36]), cells should be used 7–10 days post-isolation. For cell uptake studies, collect BMDC from plates using Lidocaine–EDTA (40 mg/mL Lidocaine, 10 mM EDTA in PBS, pH 7.4), add to 96-well v-bottom plates (1×10^6 cells/200 μL/well) and incubate for 2 h with 10,000 particles/cell and 5 % CO_2.
3. Following incubation with (virus-based) nanoparticles, cells should be washed twice in FACS buffer and fixed in 2 % (v/v) paraformaldehyde in FACS buffer for 10 min at room temperature (FACS buffer: 1 mM EDTA, 25 mM HEPES (Fisher Scientific), 1 % (v/v) FBS (Atlanta Biologicals) in PBS (Fisher Scientific), pH 7.0). Then wash cells twice after fixation, resuspend in 400 μL FACS buffer, and store at 4 °C until analysis.
4. Analyze cells using a BD LSRII Flow Cytometer and record 10,000 gated events. Analyze data using FlowJo 8.6.3 software. A sample result is shown in Fig. 2. Here PEGylated and native potato virus X (PVX)-based nanoparticle formulations were compared. Cell uptake data indicate that PEG shielding is effective to reduce PVX nanoparticle–immune cell interactions. It should be noted that, while flow cytometry provides

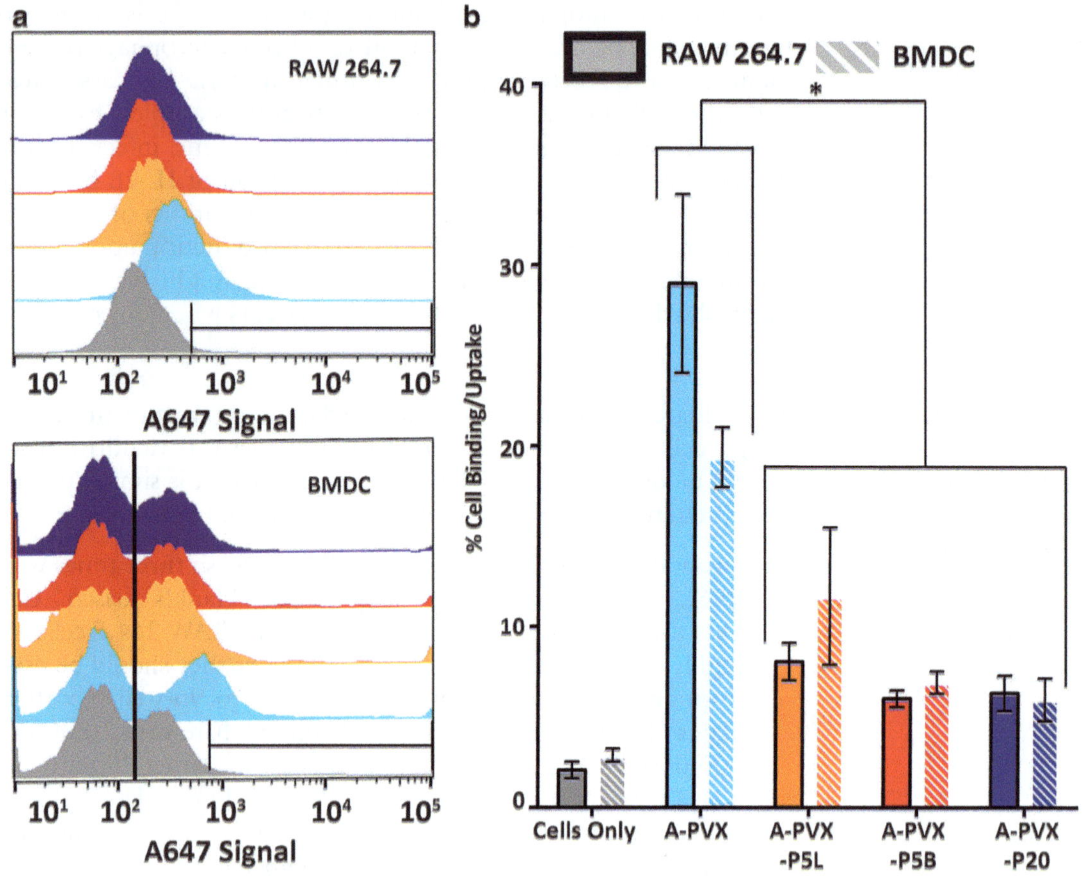

Fig. 2 A-PVX-PEG–cell interactions measured by flow cytometry. A-PVX-PEG formulations were incubated with RAW264.7 and BMDC at a concentration of 10,000 particles/cell for 2 h. (**a**) Histograms of A647 signal versus count for A-PVX-PEG particles in RAW264.7 (*top*) and BMDC (*bottom*). *Gray*=cells only, *light blue*=A-PVX, *orange*=A-PVX-P5L, *red*=A-PVX-P5B, *purple*=A-PVX-P20. Any counts within the indicated gate represent positive cells. At least 10,000 events were considered; all studies were done in triplicate and data were analyzed using FlowJo software. (**b**) Statistical analysis and quantitative data showing percent cell uptake of A-PVX-PEG particles in RAW264.7 or BMDC. *$p<0.05$. Data are reproduced from Ref. [35]

quantitative data on nanoparticle–cell interactions, flow cytometry does not indicate whether cell binding or cell uptake occurred; to investigate this further confocal microscopy is recommended.

3.1.2 Cytokine Activation Assessment Using BMDC

These protocols are similar to those described in Ref. [35]. While there is a library of cytokines that may be produced upon (plant virus) nanoparticle–cell interactions, a good starting point is to assay for the inflammatory cytokines TNFα, IL-6, and IL-1β.

TNFα and IL-6 Production

1. Seed BMDC onto treated plates at a concentration of 1×10^6 cells/mL and allow growth in complete high glucose DMEM for 7 days. Before the start of the assay, centrifuge plates at $400\times g$ for 5 min. Aspirate culture medium and add fresh com-

plete high glucose DMEM. Add VNPs in 0.1 M potassium phosphate buffer pH 7.0 (1 mg/mL) with or with cargo (e.g., drug) and/or surface modification (e.g., PEG), to the cells at a concentration of 100,000 particles/cell for 6 or 24 h.

2. Collect media by centrifugation and analyze for TNFα and IL-6 using ELISA kits. IL-6 activation should be analyzed following 6-h treatment with cytochalasin D. Add cytochalasin D (10 μg/mL final concentration) 10 min prior to addition of nanoparticles. Lipopolysaccharide (LPS) (30 ng/mL final concentration), Pam3Cys (200 ng/mL final concentration), and PolyI:C (25 μg/mL final concentration) can be used as positive controls with untreated media as a negative control. All methods should be performed as described by the manufacturer's instructions. Determine concentration of cytokine for each sample using a standard curve based on TNFα and IL-6 of known concentration supplied with each kit.

IL-1β Production

1. Grow BMDC for 8 days following the protocol described in TNFα and IL-6 production protocol above. Divide BMDC into two groups and treat one group with LPS for 4 h prior to addition of VNP formulations to increase the total concentration of IL-1β present in the cell culture. Treat both groups with VNP stimuli at a concentration of 100,000 particles/cell for 6 h. Use alum (480 μg/mL final concentration), LPS (1 μg/mL final concentration), Nigericin (10 μM final concentration), and untreated media as controls for both groups. It should be noted that pretreatment with LPS causes IL-1β baseline concentration to increase allowing for a more measureable difference in between nanoparticle formulations which may have only a small difference in inflammasome activation.
2. Collect media as described above and analyze for IL-1β using mouse IL-1β/ILF2 DuoSet ELISA kit (R&D Systems). All methods should be performed as described by the manufacturer's instructions. Determine concentration of IL-1β for each sample using a standard curve of IL-1β of known concentration supplied with the kit.

4 Assays to Evaluate Nanoparticle–Blood Compatibility Through Study of Coagulation and Hemolysis

Evaluation of blood compatibility is important because for imaging and drug delivery administration of the nano-formulation is often via intravital injection. Two assays should be considered: Coagulation, measured with rotational thromboelastometry and hemolysis, measured using absorbance [37]. Coagulation tests should take into consideration both the speed of clot formation and the total clot thickness. An increase or decrease in the speed of clot formation would indicate that VNPs are activating or inactivating platelets or factors in the clotting cascade. An increase or decrease in clot thickness, however, would indicate an increased or decreased nanoparticle–fibrin(ogen) and nanoparticle–platelet interaction. Changes in either parameter could make patients susceptible to cardiovascular events or bleeding disorders [21].

While the mechanism of nanoparticle-induced hemolysis is unclear and has been attributed both to immune and non-immune mediated causes, determining the effects of any nanoparticle system on hemolysis is important for evaluating safety. We reported that hemolysis has not been observed using TMV-based nanoparticles [21]. It should, however, be noted that the VNPs under investigation in this study did not contain any surface lysine side chains; and other groups reported that multivalent amine groups can induce red blood cell (RBC) lysis in a dose-dependent manner [37]. Therefore it would be critical to evaluate other VNP systems, for example, cowpea mosaic virus (CPMV) or potato virus X (PVX), both of which display multivalent surface lysines, 300 in the case of 30 nm-sized icosahedral CPMV [38], or 1270 in the case of 515 × 13 nm-sized PVX [39]. Hemolysis can be monitored by measuring the concentration of free hemoglobin in a blood sample as hemoglobin is released when cells are lysed. Free hemoglobin can be detected at a wavelength of 540 nm [35].

4.1 Protocols for Evaluation of Blood Compatibility

This protocol is similar to those described in Refs. [21, 35, 40], an example data set is shown in Fig. 3. Here TMVnanoparticles were studies; the formulations did not induce blood lysis or clotting.

4.1.1 Hemolysis Assay

1. Within 1 h of collection, centrifuge pooled whole blood from healthy Balb/c mice (Charles River) at 500 × *g* for 10 min. Remove the supernatant and replace with calcium/magnesium-free DPBS (HyClone) to reach previous volume. Repeat centrifugation two more times at 1000 × *g* for 10 min. Count RBCs and dilute to 1×10^9 cells/mL (~1:10 dilution) in DPBS.
2. Mix 50 μL of RBCs with 50 μL VNP samples (5 mg/mL) and incubate in 37 °C water bath for 1 h. VNPs should be added in of 7000–8000 particles/RBC; this represents roughly 1000 times the concentration in murine blood following injection. DPBS should be used as a negative control as it should cause little or no hemolysis and 1 % (v/v) Triton X-100 should be used as a positive control.
3. Centrifuge the solution for 10 min at 1000 × *g* to remove intact RBCs. Measure the absorbance of the resulting supernatant at 540 nm for hemoglobin content. Calculate the percent hemolysis by dividing the absorbance at 540 nm of each sample by the absorbance measured for 1 % Triton X-100.

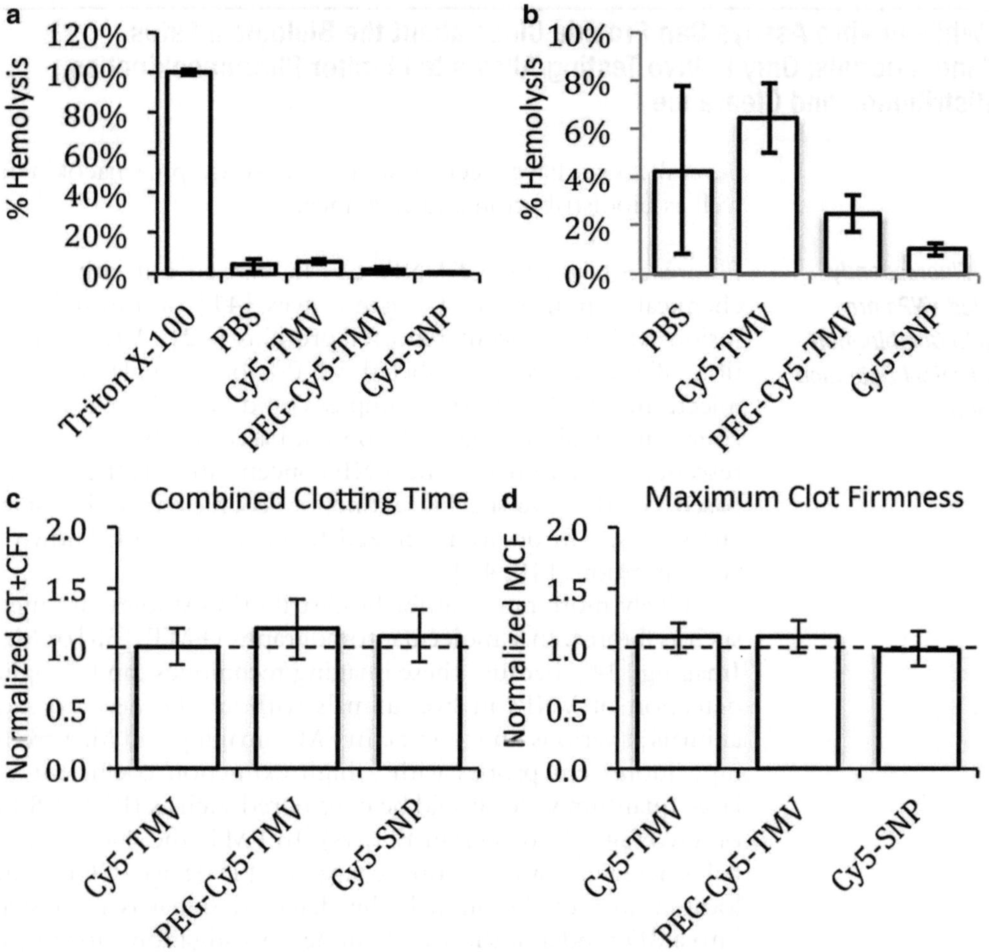

Fig. 3 Blood biocompatibility assays. (**a**) Red blood cell (RBC) hemolysis assay. (**b**) Zoomed in RBC hemolysis assay showing Cy5-TMV, PEG-Cy5-TMV, and Cy5-SNP do not lyse RBCs. (**c**) Effect of Cy5-TMV, PEG-Cy5-TMV, and Cy5-SNP on clotting (normalized to saline control), measured in rotational thromboelastometry (ROTEM). There were no significant changes in the combined clotting time (CT + CFT) and maximum clot firmness (MCF) compared to the saline control (*dotted line*). Error bars represent S.D. This figure is reproduced from Ref. [21]

4.1.2 Coagulation Assay

This protocol is similar to that described in Ref. [21], an example data set is shown in Fig. 3.

1. Add sodium citrate to pooled whole blood collected from healthy Balb/c mice to a concentration of 3.8 % (v/v). Using a Gamma ROTEM measure coagulability with the company's non-activated (NATEM) test in the presence of either saline or VNP formulations (20 μL, 5 mg/mL). Samples from each mouse should be normalized to a saline control.
2. Consider outcomes including the clotting time (CT), clot formation time (CFT), and the maximum clot firmness (MCF). Perform statistical analysis using a one-way ANOVA of the not normalized data with a Dunnett's comparison test between the treatment groups and the saline control.

5 While In Vitro Assays Can Provide Clues about the Biological Fates of Nanomaterials; Only In Vivo Testing Allows to Monitor Pharmacokinetics, Biodistribution and Clearance

Several assays have been described to study pharmacokinetics as well as biodistribution and clearance.

5.1 Fluorescently Labeled VNPs are Used in Combination with Optical Detection Methods

Fluorescent labeling of VNPs can be carried out either through chemical conjugation of organic dyes [41] or through genetic fusion with fluorescent reporter proteins [42]. After administration of the fluorescent-labeled VNPs, for example, via tail vein injection, blood and tissue samples could be collected over a time course and analyzed for VNP content based on absorbance or fluorescence measurement. The VNP concentration is then calculated based on the dye-specific extinction coefficient and a standard curve of serum or homogenized tissue spiked with known VNP concentrations [40, 43].

Likely more practical for biodistribution studies, are methods such as fluorescence molecular tomography (FMT) [35] or Maestro Imaging [44], because these imaging techniques can be applied to detection of VNPs in live animals without the need to sacrifice animals at various time points. In FMT imaging and Maestro imaging, fluorescent probes with a high extinction coefficient with a large quantum yield should be considered such as IRDye® 800 CW or VivoTag-S 750 (Perkin Elmers). In FMT, the fluorescence signal is detected using multiple charge couple device (CCD) cameras located around the animal; the detected signal is reconstructed into a 3D model of the sample under investigation allowing analysis of whole animals or select regions of interest [45]. Maestro is similar in some respects to FMT but is used more commonly ex vivo as it is detects fluorescence only in a 2D plane and thus is less descriptive of 3D structures and distribution [46].

5.1.1 Protocols for Evaluation of In Vivo Pharmacokinetics and Biodistribution Profiles Using Fluorescently Labeled VNPs

Pharmacokinetics of Fluorescently Labeled VNPs

This protocol is similar to that described in Ref. [35]; sample data are shown in Fig. 4 [23].

1. For any study involving fluorescent read outs, animals should be maintained on an alfalfa-free diet for 2 weeks prior to administration to reduce tissue autofluorescence.
2. Administer fluorescently labeled VNPs via the tail vein injection. Collect 200 μL blood into heparin-collected tubes using retro-orbital bleeding. Time course studies should be conducted at time points up to 36 h.
3. Isolate serum by centrifuging at 14,500 × *g* for 10 min. Read fluorescence using microplate reader and correlate the fluorescence reading to a standard curve normalized for each particle, use this standard curve to determine the amount of particle at

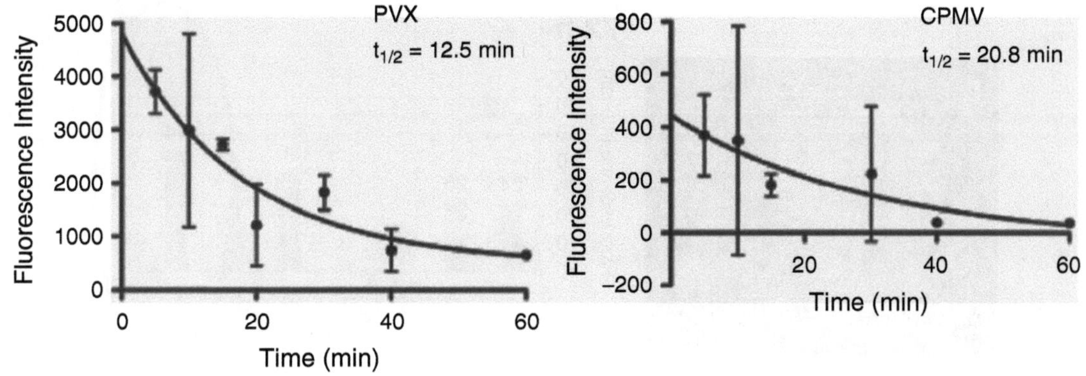

Fig. 4 Plasma clearance of A647-labeled, PEGylated PVX and CPMV. Pharmacokinetics were evaluated using healthy Balb/c mice. Blood was collected over a 60 min time period, plasma extracted, and the fluorescence intensity measured. This figure is reproduced from Ref. [22]

each time point. Determine percent of injected dose using the fluorescence reading of the amount of nanoparticles per 50 μL of serum from each time point.

Fluorescence to Determine VNP Biodistribution Ex Vivo Using a Plate Reader

This protocol is similar to that described in Ref. [21] or [40].

1. Inject Balb/c mice with fluorescently labeled VNPs at a dose of 10 mg/kg body weight in 100 μL sterile, endotoxin-free PBS. As a control, inject a mouse with 100 μL sterile, endotoxin-free PBS without nanoparticles. This control will be referred to as sham-inoculated.
2. Euthanize animals and remove the following tissues and snap freeze in liquid nitrogen, weigh, and store at −20 °C: spleen, kidney, liver, lung, stomach, duodenum, jejunum, ileum, lymph nodes, and brains. Homogenize isolated tissues in PBS (100 mg organ/mL PBS) and centrifuge at 7500 × *g* for 10 min at 4 °C to precipitate cell debris.
3. Use a fluorescence plate reader to measure the fluorescence intensity (λ_{Ex} 600 nm and λ_{Em} 665 nm if using Cy5 dye).
4. Add a known amount of labeled VNPs to tissue supernatants of the sham-inoculated control to determine the tissue-specific dye excitation and emission for each tissue. Take five separate scans of each tissue supernatant sample, subtract the tissue specific emission of the sham-inoculated control sample as background, and average the adjusted emissions. Use measured emission to calculate total concentration of VNPs.

Biodistribution of Fluorescently Labeled VNPs Via FMT Imaging In Vivo

This protocol is similar to that described in Ref. [35].

1. As with other fluorescent studies, mice should be maintained on alfalfa-free diet (Teklad) to reduce tissue autofluorescence. Inject 100 μg fluorescently labeled VNPs in 100 μL sterile PBS via the tail vein.

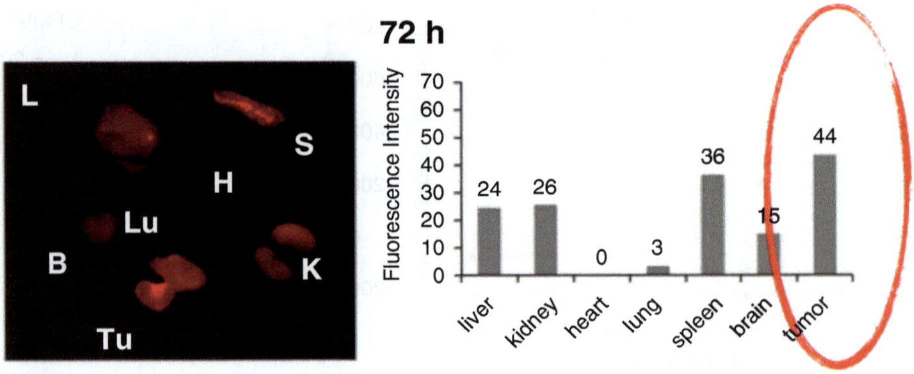

Fig. 5 Biodistribution of A647-labeled, PEGylated PVX 72 h post intravenous administration into the tail vein of nude mice with HT-29 tumor xenografts. Maestro imaging (*left*) was used to quantify the amount of PVX deposited per tissue. This figure is reproduced from Ref. [22]

2. Anesthetize mice with inhaled O_2/isoflurane (1–3 % isoflurane) prior to imaging; animals should be kept under anesthesia during the procedure. Using a FMT in vivo imaging system (FMT 2500 quantitative tomography in vivo imaging system (Perkin-Elmer)) take measurements prior to injection (0 min), and 30 min, 1 h, 2 h, 4 h, 6 h, 8 h, 24 h, 32 h, and 52 h post-administration. For each image, regions choose a region of interest (ROI) for the whole body, liver, spleen, and bladder.
3. Calculate the fluorescence intensity using the normalized total fluorescence within each ROI. The concentration of VNPs per ROI can be estimated based on a standard curve of VNPs at known concentration in phantom tissue (buffer or agarose plugs) and taking into account the number of dyes per VNP.

Biodistribution of Fluorescently Labeled TMV Via Maestro Imaging Ex Vivo

This protocol is similar to that described in Ref. [22] or [23]; Fig. 5 shows a typical result.

1. As with other fluorescent studies, mice should be maintained on alfalfa-free diet (Teklad) to reduce tissue autofluorescence. Inject fluorescently labeled VNPs (10 mg/kg body-weight) via the tail vein. Animals should be euthanized at 24 and 72 h and tissues collected. For a study of biodistribution, healthy animals, such as Balb/c mice, 8–14 weeks old (Charles River) could be used. Alternatively, tumor homing can be investigated using orthotopic 4T1 mammary tumor xenografts in 8-week-old female Balb/c mice, as described in Ref. [23].
2. Image the livers, spleen, and tumors using the Maestro imaging system (Maestro™ Imaging System (Perkin Elmer)) with yellow excitation and emission filters (if using A647 dye) with a 800 ms exposure time. Analyze fluorescence intensity using Maestro software tool and normalize for number of dyes per VNP. It should be noted that tissues should ideally be imaged immediately following harvest when still fresh, but can be frozen and thawed prior to imaging.

5.2 Metal Ion-Labeled VNPs Are Used in Combination with Inductively Coupled Plasma Mass Spectrometry (ICP-MS) or Optical Emission Spectroscopy (ICP-OES)

Techniques that allow to determine the concentration of metal-loaded, e.g., Gd(DOTA)-conjugated VNPs [47, 48] or other metal-containing nanoparticles, such as gold nanoparticles [49] with part-per-billion accuracy while not being limited to potential bleaching or quenching as observed with some organic fluorophores. ICP-MS/OES utilizes high-energy argon gas plasma to energize elemental components into ions, which are then separated and detected by MS or OES. Much like fluorescence detection using a plate reader, ICP-MS/OES is limited to quantitative tissue and blood analysis ex vivo [21, 50].

5.2.1 Protocols for Determination of the Biodistribution of Metal Ion-Labeled VNPs via Inductively Coupled Plasma-Optical Emission Spectrometry

This protocol is similar to that described in Ref. [47]; and these methods can be used to determine biodistribution as well as pharmacokinetics.

1. Inject 100 μg of Gd or Tb labeled VNPs in 100 μL PBS into Balb/c mice via the tail vein. VNPs can be labeled with metal ions either through complexation of the metal ions with the nucleic acids, e.g., CPMV particles can be labeled with Gd^{3+} or Tb^{3+} ions either by binding to nucleoprotein sites on the interior of the particle; or by covalent attachment of a Gd(DOTA) derivative to the external surface of the capsid by the CuAAC reaction, as described in Ref. [47].
2. Euthanize mice and collect organs at least 30 min following injection. Freeze-dry organs in liquid nitrogen and digest with in nitric acid at a concentration of 20 % (v/v) for 18–24 h. Insoluble materials that cannot be digested should be filtered out of the solution.
3. Using a Varian VISTA AX CCD simultaneous spectrometer, construct calibration plots for Gd or Tb in the concentration range of 0–1000 ppb. Inject all samples with 10 ppm yttrium chloride internal standard to normalize differences in nebulization between samples. Measure the concentration of Gd and Tb in each sample and use this value to calculate the concentration of VNPs in each tissue sample by using the amount of Gd and Tb per VNP.

5.3 Detection and Quantification of VNPs Can Also Be Carried out Making Use of the Encapsidated RNA Components of the Viruses Itself

Since many plant viruses are single-stranded RNA viruses, reverse transcription polymerase chain reaction (RT-PCR) in combination with sequencing and/or quantitative PCR methods can be used to measure the concentration of intact viral nanoparticles in blood samples and digested tissues [40]. This method is useful for measuring the concentration of intact viruses but cannot measure virus-like nanoparticles that do not contain viral RNA. Additionally, this method may not give useful information about the cargo of viral nanoparticles delivered.

5.3.1 Protocol for RT-PCR for Detection of TMV

This protocol is similar to that described in Ref. [51].

1. Inject Balb/c mice with TMVnanoparticles (300 μg in 100 μL sterile PBS) via the tail vein. As a control 100 μL sterile PBS without TMV particles should be injected. Euthanize animals, remove the following tissues and snap freeze in liquid nitrogen, weigh, and store at −20 °C: spleen, kidney, liver, lung, stomach, duodenum, jejunum, ileum, lymph nodes, and brains.
2. Add 1 mL trizol reagent per 50–100 mg frozen tissues, homogenize with a handheld homogenizer, and incubate at room temperature for 8 min. Centrifuge samples for 10 min at 10,000 × *g* and transfer supernatant to a fresh tube. Add 0.2 M chloroform per 1 mL trizol reagent and incubate at room temperature for 8 min. Centrifuge samples for 5 min at 14,000 × *g* at 4 °C for 8 min and transfer the aqueous phase to a fresh tube.
3. To precipitate the RNA, add 0.5 mL isopropanol per 1 mL TRI and incubate for 5 min at room temperature. Centrifuge the samples at for 10 additional minutes at 14,000 rpm at 4 °C; a pellet of RNA should be visible. Wash the pellet by adding 1 mL 70 % (v/v) ethanol per 1 mL TRI. Centrifuge the sample for 5 min at 14,000 rpm at 4 °C and allow the pellet to air-dry. Resuspend the RNA pellet in 40 μL RNAse-free water and incubate at 50–60 °C for 10 min. Determine the concentration and A_{260}/A_{280} ratio using photometrical measurement.
4. Synthesize cDNA using MMLV-RT and downstream TMV RNA CPr (see below for the oligonucleotide sequences). Mix the CPr primer (60 pmol) with 1 μg of each tissue RNA and heat to 70 °C for 5 min. Following the incubation, add: 20 units of RNAsin; 4 mM each of dATP, dTTP, dCTP, and dGTP; 60 pmol each of the upstream (CPf) and downstream primer (CPr); 0.5 units of Taq polymerase; 1.5 mM Taq polymerase buffer containing Mg; and purified water. Perform 30 cycles consisting of 1 min denaturation at 95 °C, 1 min annealing at 55 °C, and 1 min extension at 72 °C. This should result in a 270 bp PCR product.

   This method required the use of VNP-specific oligonucleotides, for example for TMV the following primer pairs (from Integrated DNA Technologies) could be used:

   TMV CP2-r: 5′-ACCGTTGCGTCGTCTACTCT-3′

   TMV CP2-f: 5′-CAAGCTCGAACTGTCGTTCA-3′
5. Analyze PCR products on a 0.8 % agarose gel alongside a 1-kb ladder and visualize with ethidium bromide. Spot densitometry can also be used to quantitatively compare to control. Note that RT-PCR is a highly sensitive method; it was shown to be capable of detecting as few as ten copies as CPMV.

5.4 PET Imaging and Other Radiolabels

Positron emission tomography (PET) uses radionuclides, isotopes with a short half-life (minutes to hours) which emit positrons, particles with a charge opposite that of an electron; collisions between positrons and electrons in the tissues causes photon emission that can be detected and used to construct an image. Recently, fluorine-18 has been used to label the interior of the bacteriophage MS2 (mtMS2), providing information about the biodistribution of mtMS2 in vivo [27]. In addition to PET imaging using live subjects; tissues could also be detected and analyzed ex vivo using a gamma well detector; this could be helpful when accumulation of the nanoparticles in tissues is low and below the in vivo detection threshold. Other radiolabeling options include iodine-125, a radioactive compound easily detected in excised tissues [9]. While there are significant differences between these labels, they share several advantages over fluorescence labeling, including no risk of photoquenching or photobleaching. A disadvantage of use of radiolabels is the potential difficulty associated with handling and disposal. For protocols the reader is referred to the references discussed herein.

6 Antibody Titers, Antibody Recognition, and Complement Activation

Determining antibody titers is an important milestone to gain insights into the immunogenic properties of (viral) drug delivery vehicles and contrast agents. Antibody titers and antibody recognition may provide critical implications on whether repeated administrations of the proposed formulation are possible. A nanoparticle that induces high antibody titers may be cleared rapidly upon repeat administration, therefore resulting in an altered longitudinal pharmacokinetic profile and reduced tissue targeting properties. Enzyme-linked immunosorbent assay (ELISA) is the standard method to determine the titers and subtypes of carrier and cargo-specific antibodies produced upon single or repeat VNP administration. Similarly, sandwich ELISAs are useful to determine whether antibodies produced recognize and neutralize the VNPs; for example, while antibodies against PEGylated stealth VNPs may still be raised (at lower titers compared to non-PEGylated VNPs [16]), the antibodies may not recognize the PEGylated VNP version [35], and therefore may not interfere with the pharmacokinetics and pharmacodynamics.

In the context of immune modulation, activation of the complement system is another potential indicator of immune activation. Complement activation refers to a cascade of biochemical reactions leading to activation of proteins that bolster cell and humoral immunity. An increase in complement activation can increase MPS clearance and non-target deposition, therefore resulting in reduced VNP circulation time and therefore reducing potential interactions with the target cells and tissues. Additionally,

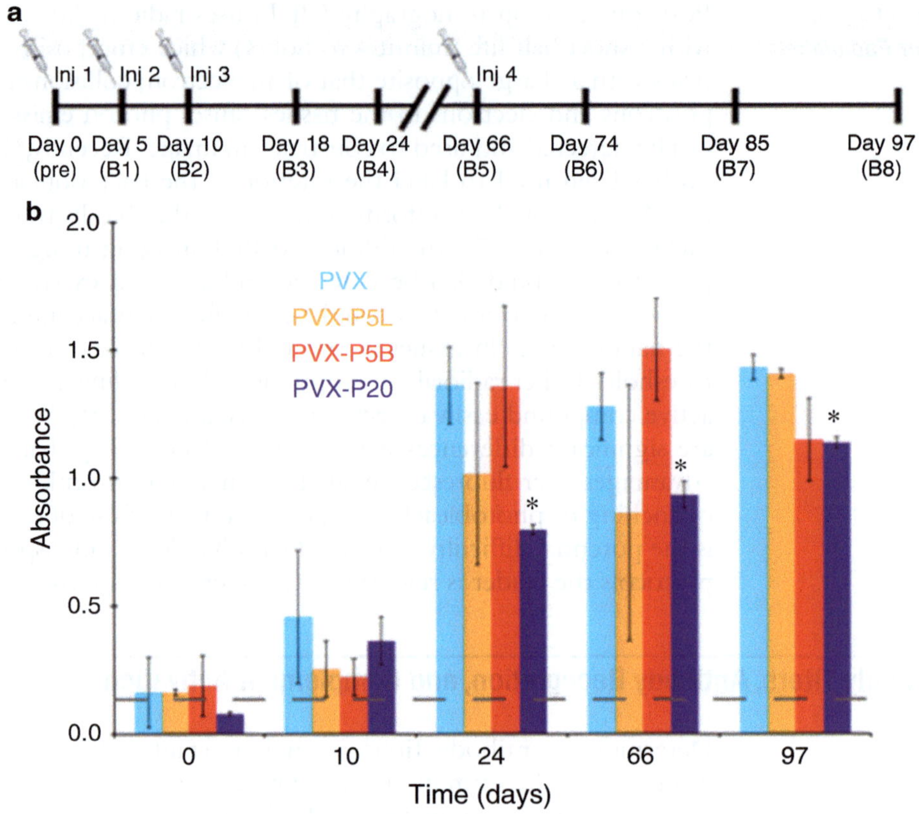

Fig. 6 Anti-PVX IgG titers and reactivity. (**a**) Timeline of treatment schedule; time points of PVX administration and blood collection are indicated. (**b**) Anti-PVX IgG titers of sera from mice treated with PVX, PVX-P5L, PVX-P5B, and PVX-P20. All data were analyzed using Excel software and Student's *t*-test *$p < 0.05$; Ab = antibody; AP = alkaline phosphatase. Data are reproduced from Ref. [35]

activation of complement is responsible for hypersensitivity and anaphylaxis, potentially life-threatening conditions. Protein C3 is a major component of the complement system that circulates in an inactive form and is activated by conversion to a small fragment (C3a) and a large fragment (C3b). By determining the relative concentrations of the inactive C3 to the active C3b, nanoparticle-induced activation of complement can be assessed [37, 52]. For screening purposes, these assays could be conducted using blood samples ex vivo.

6.1 Protocols for Determining Immune Responses

6.1.1 Determining Antibody Titer Using Enzyme Linked Immunosorbent Assay (ELISA)

This protocol is similar to that described in Ref. [35], a representative data set is shown in Fig. 6. Generally foreign proteins, such as plant or bacterially produced proteins can elicit an immune response and lead to production of antibodies. Therefore it is important to determine the antibody titers (this section). For repeat administration, it is also critical to evaluate whether the produced antibodies may neutralize the formulation (see Sect. 6.1.2). Shielding techniques, such as coating of the protein-based formulations with polymers (e.g., PEG) can be used to overcome antibody recognition and also reduce clearance by mononuclear phagocytic cells (see Fig. 2).

1. Inject healthy male Balb/c mice via tail vein with VNP formulations containing 100 μg in 100 μL sterile PBS; the schedule and administration route should mimic the schedule used in the desired applications; e.g., weekly injections for chemotherapy delivery or less frequent when imaging applications are proposed. A group injected with the protein ovalbumin should be used as a control.
2. Collect blood via retro-orbital bleeding using heparin-coated tubes on days 0 (pre-bleed), 5, 10, 18, 24, 66, 74, 85, and 97. Isolate serum by centrifuging samples at 10,000 × *g* for 10 min and analyzed using enzyme-linked immunosorbent assay (ELISA). Note, on days on which both injections and blood draws were performed, that blood draws should be performed first.
3. Coat 96-well plate with 10 μg/well of either VNP or ovalbumin in coating buffer and incubate overnight at 4 °C. Following coating, block wells using 200 μL/well blocking buffer at 37 °C for 1 h. After blocking, add 100 μL of sera at various dilutions in blocking buffer and incubate at 37 °C for 2 h. After serum incubation, add 100 μL of alkaline phosphatase-labeled goat anti-mouse IgG and incubate for 1 h at 37 °C. Stop reaction using 100 μL of 2 M NaOH. Read absorbance at 405 nm using a microplate reader.

6.1.2 Sandwich ELISA to Determine Whether Antibodies Produced Are Neutralizing

This protocol is similar to that described in Ref. [35].

1. Perform VNP administration and blood sample collections as in previous protocol.
2. Coat 96-well immuno plates overnight at 4 °C with a rabbit anti-VNP antibodies in coating buffer.
3. After coating, block wells with blocking buffer for 1 h at 37 °C.
4. Following blocking, add 5 μg of various VNP formulations in 150 μL incubation buffer and incubate for 1 h at 37 °C.
5. After incubation with VNP particles, 150 μL of sera were added at a dilution of 1:25,000 in incubation buffer and incubated for 1 h at 37 °C.
6. Develop wells by adding 100 μL of 1-step PNPP substrate for 10 min at 4 °C.
7. Stop the reaction by adding 100 μL of 2 M NaOH.
8. Read absorbance at 405 nm using a microplate reader (Tecan).

6.1.3 Complement Activation in Mouse or Human Blood Samples

This protocol is similar to that described in Ref. [52].

1. Obtain blood from healthy Balb/c mice or donor and centrifuge at 500 × *g* for 10 min. Save the serum contained within the supernatant.

2. Prepare veronal-buffered saline (VBS) containing 0.15 mM Ca^{2+} and 0.5 mM Mg^{2+} ions (VBS^{2+}) and VBS containing 40 nM EDTA (VBS–EDTA).
3. Incubate VNPs or other nanoparticle suspensions (200 μL) under gentle agitation at 37 °C with 100 μL collected serum and 100 μL of VBS^{2+}. Use VBS–EDTA as a negative control of complement activation. Serum should also be incubated with only VBS^{2+} to determine the base complement activation under these experimental conditions. Use sephadex® G 25 superfine incubated in serum diluted in VBS^{2+} as a positive control of complement activation.
4. Following incubation, use electrophoresis on a 1 % agarose gel to electrofocus 5 μL of each sample. Agarose gel plates should contain a polyclonal antibody to human C3. Stain films with Coomassie blue to identify C3 and C3b.
5. Measure the height of the peaks shown on the immunoelectrophoretic plate. Activation of complement can be expressed as a ratio of the peak height of C3b detected and the height of C3.

7 Summary and Future Prospects

As for any new nanotechnology, risks, benefits, and biologic interactions must be carefully evaluated. In order to best understand the risks and benefits of nanotechnology, it is necessary to study many aspects of immune and other physiologic responses. Advanced understanding of the mechanisms of the body's response will allow for better prediction of how nanoparticle composition and characteristics will induce responses. A complete understanding of the in vivo fates of nanotechnologies will enable tailoring their properties to advance the technology development. In the future, improved imaging modalities may allow for better quantitative evaluation of nanoparticle trafficking. At the same time, innovative shielding, camouflage, and targeting strategies will enable to navigate the physiological barriers to home to the desired tissue, cell, or molecular target.

Acknowledgements

This work was supported by the following grants from the National Science Foundation (NSF): CMMI NM 1333651 (VNP nanomanufacturing) and NSF CHEM MSN 1306447 (VNP polymer hybrids), American Heart Association grant AHA14GRNT19890005 (VNP-based materials in cardiovascular research), Susan G. Komen Grant CCT14298962 (VNP research targeting breast cancer), and Mt. Sinai Foundation and Case Western Reserve University start-up funds to N.F.S. A.E.C. was supported in part by NIH grant T32 GM007250 and TL1 TR000441. The authors thank Amy M. Wen for helpful discussion.

References

1. Liu Z, Qiao J, Niu Z, Wang Q (2012) Natural supramolecular building blocks: from virus coat proteins to viral nanoparticles. Chem Soc Rev 41(18):6178–6194
2. Steinmetz NF (2010) Viral nanoparticles as platforms for next-generation therapeutics and imaging devices. Nanomedicine 6(5):634–641
3. Venter PA, Dirksen A, Thomas D, Manchester M, Dawson PE, Schneemann A (2011) Multivalent display of proteins on viral nanoparticles using molecular recognition and chemical ligation strategies. Biomacromolecules 12(6):2293–2301
4. Semmler-Behnke M, Kreyling WG, Lipka J, Fertsch S, Wenk A, Takenaka S, Schmid G, Brandau W (2008) Biodistribution of 1.4- and 18-nm gold particles in rats. Small 4(12): 2108–2111
5. Tarn D, Ashley CE, Xue M, Carnes EC, Zink JI, Brinker CJ (2013) Mesoporous silica nanoparticle nanocarriers: biofunctionality and biocompatibility. Acc Chem Res 46:792–801
6. Jaganathan H, Godin B (2012) Biocompatibility assessment of Si-based nano- and micro-particles. Adv Drug Deliv Rev 64(15): 1800–1819
7. Liu Y, Zhao Y, Sun B, Chen C (2012) Understanding the toxicity of carbon nanotubes. Acc Chem Res. doi:10.1021/ar300028m
8. Baiu DC, Brazel CS, Bao Y, Otto M (2013) Interactions of iron oxide nanoparticles with the immune system: challenges and opportunities for their use in nano-oncology. Curr Pharm Des 19(37):6606–6621
9. Kaiser CR, Flenniken ML, Gillitzer E, Harmsen AL, Harmsen AG, Jutila MA, Douglas T, Young MJ (2007) Biodistribution studies of protein cage nanoparticles demonstrate broad tissue distribution and rapid clearance in vivo. Int J Nanomedicine 2(4):715–733
10. Meng J, Yang M, Jia F, Xu Z, Kong H, Xu H (2011) Immune responses of BALB/c mice to subcutaneously injected multi-walled carbon nanotubes. Nanotoxicology 5(4):583–591
11. Raja KS, Wang Q, Gonzalez MJ, Manchester M, Johnson JE, Finn MG (2003) Hybrid virus-polymer materials. 1. Synthesis and properties of PEG-decorated cowpea mosaic virus. Biomacromolecules 4(3):472–476
12. Semple SC, Harasym TO, Clow KA, Ansell SM, Klimuk SK, Hope MJ (2005) Immunogenicity and rapid blood clearance of liposomes containing polyethylene glycol-lipid conjugates and nucleic Acid. J Pharmacol Exp Ther 312(3):1020–1026
13. Shimizu T, Ishida T, Kiwada H (2013) Transport of PEGylated liposomes from the splenic marginal zone to the follicle in the induction phase of the accelerated blood clearance phenomenon. Immunobiology 218(5): 725–732
14. Jokerst JV, Lobovkina T, Zare RN, Gambhir SS (2011) Nanoparticle PEGylation for imaging and therapy. Nanomedicine (Lond) 6(4): 715–728
15. Veronese FM, Pasut G (2005) PEGylation, successful approach to drug delivery. Drug Discov Today 10(21):1451–1458
16. Raja KS, Wang Q, Gonzalez MJ, Manchester M, Johnson JE, Finn MG (2003) Hybrid virus-polymer materials. 1. Synthesis and properties of PEG-decorated cowpea mosaic virus. Biomacromolecules 3:472–476
17. Harris JM, Chess RB (2003) Effect of pegylation on pharmaceuticals. Nat Rev Drug Discov 2(3):214–221
18. Jokerst JV, Lobovkina T, Zare RN, Gambhir SS (2011) Nanoparticle PEGylation for imaging and therapy. Nanomedicine 6(4):715–728
19. Roberts MJ, Bentley MD, Harris JM (2002) Chemistry for peptide and protein PEGylation. Adv Drug Deliv Rev 54(4):459–476
20. Wattendorf U, Merkle HP (2008) PEGylation as a tool for the biomedical engineering of surface modified microparticles. J Pharm Sci
21. Bruckman MA, Randolph LN, VanMeter A, Hern S, Shoffstall AJ, Taurog RE, Steinmetz NF (2014) Biodistribution, pharmacokinetics, and blood compatibility of native and PEGylated tobacco mosaic virus nano-rods and -spheres in mice. Virology 449:163–173
22. Shukla S, Ablack AL, Wen AM, Lee KL, Lewis JD, Steinmetz NF (2013) Increased tumor homing and tissue penetration of the filamentous plant viral nanoparticle Potato virus X. Mol Pharm 10(1):33–42
23. Shukla S, Wen AM, Ayat NR, Commandeur U, Gopalkrishnan R, Broome AM, Lozada KW,

Keri RA, Steinmetz NF (2014) Biodistribution and clearance of a filamentous plant virus in healthy and tumor-bearing mice. Nanomedicine (Lond) 9(2):221–235

24. Bruckman MA, Steinmetz NF (2014) Chemical modification of the inner and outer surfaces of Tobacco Mosaic Virus (TMV). Methods Mol Biol 1108:173–185
25. Cho CF, Shukla S, Simpson EJ, Steinmetz NF, Luyt LG, Lewis JD (2014) Molecular targeted viral nanoparticles as tools for imaging cancer. Methods Mol Biol 1108:211–230
26. Lee KL, Uhde-Holzem K, Fischer R, Commandeur U, Steinmetz NF (2014) Genetic engineering and chemical conjugation of potato virus X. Methods Mol Biol 1108:3–21
27. Hooker JM, O'Neil JP, Romanini DW, Taylor SE, Francis MB (2008) Genome-free viral capsids as carriers for positron emission tomography radiolabels. Mol Imaging Biol 10(4):182–191
28. Hovlid ML, Steinmetz NF, Laufer B, Lau JL, Kuzelka J, Wang Q, Hyypia T, Nemerow GR, Kessler H, Manchester M, Finn MG (2012) Guiding plant virus particles to integrin-displaying cells. Nanoscale 4(12):3698–3705
29. Plummer EM, Thomas D, Destito G, Shriver LP, Manchester M (2012) Interaction of cowpea mosaic virus nanoparticles with surface vimentin and inflammatory cells in atherosclerotic lesions. Nanomedicine (Lond) 7(6):877–888
30. Agrawal A, Manchester M (2012) Differential uptake of chemically modified cowpea mosaic virus nanoparticles in macrophage subpopulations present in inflammatory and tumor microenvironments. Biomacromolecules 13(10):3320–3326
31. Martinon F, Burns K, Tschopp J (2002) The inflammasome: a molecular platform triggering activation of inflammatory caspases and processing of proIL-beta. Mol Cell 10(2):417–426
32. Kusaka T, Nakayama M, Nakamura K, Ishimiya M, Furusawa E, Ogasawara K (2014) Effect of silica particle size on macrophage inflammatory responses. PLoS One 9(3):e92634
33. Yang M, Flavin K, Kopf I, Radics G, Hearnden CH, McManus GJ, Moran B, Villalta-Cerdas A, Echegoyen LA, Giordani S, Lavelle EC (2013) Functionalization of carbon nanoparticles modulates inflammatory cell recruitment and NLRP3 inflammasome activation. Small 9(24):4194–4206
34. Schanen BC, Das S, Reilly CM, Warren WL, Self WT, Seal S, Drake DR III (2013) Immunomodulation and T helper TH(1)/TH(2) response polarization by CeO(2) and TiO(2) nanoparticles. PLoS One 8(5):e62816
35. Lee KL, Shukla S, Wu M, Ayat NR, El Sanadi CE, Wen AM, Edelbrock JF, Pokorski JK, Commandeur U, Dubyak GR, Steinmetz NF (2014) Stealth filaments: polymer chain length and conformation affect the in vivo fate of PEGylated potato virus X. Acta Biomater 19:166–79
36. Stoll S, Delon J, Brotz TM, Germain RN (2002) Dynamic imaging of T cell-dendritic cell interactions in lymph nodes. Science 296(5574):1873–1876
37. Dobrovolskaia MA, Aggarwal P, Hall JB, McNeil SE (2008) Preclinical studies to understand nanoparticle interaction with the immune system and its potential effects on nanoparticle biodistribution. Mol Pharm 5(4):487–495
38. Chatterji A, Ochoa W, Paine M, Ratna BR, Johnson JE, Lin T (2004) New addresses on an addressable virus nanoblock: uniquely reactive Lys residues on cowpea mosaic virus. Chem Biol 11(6):855–863
39. Steinmetz NF, Mertens ME, Taurog RE, Johnson JE, Commandeur U, Fischer R, Manchester M (2010) Potato virus X as a novel platform for potential biomedical applications. Nano Lett 10(1):305–312
40. Rae CS, Khor IW, Wang Q, Destito G, Gonzalez MJ, Singh P, Thomas DM, Estrada MN, Powell E, Finn MG, Manchester M (2005) Systemic trafficking of plant virus nanoparticles in mice via the oral route. Virology 343(2):224–235
41. Lewis JD, Destito G, Zijlstra A, Gonzalez MJ, Quigley JP, Manchester M, Stuhlmann H (2006) Viral nanoparticles as tools for intravital vascular imaging. Nat Med 12(3):354–360
42. Shukla S, Dickmeis C, Nagarajan AS, Fischer R, Commandeur U, Steinmetz NF (2014) Molecular farming of fluorescent virus-based nanoparticles for optical imaging in plants, human cells and mouse models. Biomater Sci 2:784–797
43. Knudsen KB, Northeved H, Gjetting T, Permin A, Andresen TL, Wegener KM, Lam HR, Lykkesfeldt J (2014) Biodistribution of rhodamine B fluorescence-labeled cationic nanoparticles in rats. J Nanopart Res 16(2):2221
44. Kumar R, Roy I, Ohulchanskky TY, Vathy LA, Bergey EJ, Sajjad M, Prasad PN (2010) In vivo biodistribution and clearance studies using multimodal organically modified silica nanoparticles. ACS Nano 4(2):699–708
45. Bai J, Xu Z (2013) Fluorescence molecular tomography. In: Tian J (ed) Molecular imaging: fundamentals and applications. Zhejiang University Press, Hangzhou China, pp 185–216
46. Halig LV, Wang D, Wang AY, Chen ZG, Fei B (2013) Biodistribution study of nanoparticle

encapsulated photodynamic therapy drugs using multispectral imaging. Proc SPIE Int Soc Opt Eng 8672

47. Singh P, Prasuhn D, Yeh RM, Destito G, Rae CS, Osborn K, Finn MG, Manchester M (2007) Bio-distribution, toxicity and pathology of cowpea mosaic virus nanoparticles in vivo. J Control Release 120(1–2): 41–50
48. Prasuhn DE Jr, Singh P, Strable E, Brown S, Manchester M, Finn MG (2008) Plasma clearance of bacteriophage Qbeta particles as a function of surface charge. J Am Chem Soc 130(4):1328–34
49. Stern ST, Hall JB, Yu LL, Wood LJ, Paciotti GF, Tamarkin L, Long SE, McNeil SE (2010) Translational considerations for cancer nanomedicine. J Control Release 146(2):164–174
50. Chan S, Gerson B, Reitz RE, Sadjadi SA (1998) Technical and clinical aspects of spectrometric analysis of trace elements in clinical samples. Clin Lab Med 18(4):615–629
51. Mertens ME (2009) Rod-shaped viral nanoparticles as building blocks for biomedical applications. In: Molekulare biotechnologie. RWTH Aachen University, Aachen Germany, p 98
52. Bertholon I, Vauthier C, Labarre D (2006) Complement activation by core-shell poly(isobutylcyanoacrylate)-polysaccharide nanoparticles: influences of surface morphology, length, and type of polysaccharide. Pharm Res 23(6):1313–1323

Chapter 5

Gold Nanoparticles for Biomedical Applications: Synthesis and In Vitro Evaluation

Peter Chhour, Pratap C. Naha, Rabee Cheheltani, Barbara Benardo, Shaameen Mian, and David P. Cormode

Abstract

Gold nanoparticles can be synthesized in a wide range of sizes and shapes. They can be coated with molecules, polymers, or phospholipids that yield solubility and stability in biological fluids. Gold is inert and is generally regarded as biocompatible. Depending on their shape and structure, gold nanoparticles can have a number of remarkable properties, such as strong and tunable attenuation of light, fluorescence, conversion of light to heat, and attenuation of X-rays. Due to these properties, gold nanoparticles have a wide range of biomedical applications. They have been used as contrast agents for fluorescence, optical, photoacoustic, and X-ray imaging. They can function as drug or gene delivery vectors. They can also play roles in photothermal or radiosensitization treatment regimens. We herein present methods to synthesize, coat, and purify spherical gold nanoparticles that are 15–100 nm in diameter. We describe protocols to characterize these gold nanoparticles with dynamic light scattering, transmission electron microscopy, inductively coupled plasma-optical emission spectroscopy (ICP-OES) and for computed tomography contrast generation. Last, we detail methods to assess nanoparticle uptake by cells, effect on cell viability, and effect on cell function.

Key words Gold nanoparticles, Nanomedicine, Characterization, Electron microscopy computed tomography, Cell uptake, Cell viability, Cytokine expression

1 Introduction

There has been tremendous interest in the use of nanoparticles in medicine for over two decades [1]. Nanoparticles can have a number of advantages over small molecule agents such as long circulation half-lives, enhanced accumulation in diseased tissue, efficient targeting, high payloads and can easily be made multifunctional (i.e., can deliver multiple drugs, contrast agents, or combinations of the two) [2]. Furthermore, nanoparticles can sometimes have properties that are unavailable in small molecules, such as the superparamagnetism of iron oxides, which generates strong contrast for magnetic resonance imaging [3, 4]. Nanoparticles have

Zheng-Rong Lu and Shinji Sakuma (eds.), *Nanomaterials in Pharmacology*, Methods in Pharmacology and Toxicology, DOI 10.1007/978-1-4939-3121-7_5, © Springer Science+Business Media New York 2016

therefore been used for drug delivery, gene transfection, vaccination, as contrast agents and in numerous other applications [5, 6]. Many nanoparticles are now in clinical use, with Doxil, a doxorubicin loaded liposome anticancer drug, and Feridex, a dextran-coated iron oxide nanoparticle MRI contrast agent, among the first to be approved [7].

Gold nanoparticles (AuNP) have been used by humanity for more than 2000 years. For example, the Lycurgus cup, a decorative goblet, is colored using gold nanoparticles and was made in the fifth to fourth century BC [8]. Medical applications have been proposed for gold nanoparticles for centuries [9], but it is not until the last decade or so that informed, scientific work has been done to study their biomedical effects [10, 11]. Gold nanoparticles have a number of unusual properties that are valuable in biomedical applications [12]. They absorb light very strongly and their absorption maxima can be tuned from the visible to the near infrared (a region where tissue absorbs weakly and is therefore useful for biomedical applications) [13]. Certain gold nanoparticle types, such as nanorods, are fluorescent in this region, yielding applications in optical imaging [14]. Gold nanoparticles are also efficient at converting absorbed light into heat and transmitting that heat to the surroundings. These features have led to applications in photothermal therapy and photoacoustic imaging [15–17]. Gold nanoparticles enhance the Raman spectra of molecules close to their surface by orders of magnitude, which has led to a technique known as surface enhanced Raman spectroscopy (SERS) imaging [18, 19]. Furthermore, they have been used as vectors to deliver drugs or nucleic acid [20–23]. Last, gold attenuates high energy photons such as X-rays strongly, so gold nanoparticles have found use as contrast agents in X-ray based imaging techniques such as computed tomography (CT) [7, 24], as well as adjuvants for radiotherapy [25, 26]. Gold nanoshells are undergoing clinical trials in both head and neck cancer [27] and coronary artery disease [28, 29] for tissue ablation. A phase I clinical trial has been completed by Aurimmune using TNFα bound to gold nanoparticles in patients with advanced solid organ tumors and reported no adverse effects [30]. These trials indicate the safety of gold nanoparticles in humans and a path to eventual clinical use.

To facilitate these and other applications, synthetic routes to a range of morphologies and sizes have been developed. Gold nanoparticles have been synthesized as spheres, rods, cages, shells, stars, cubes, plates, and other shapes [31–36]. Gold nanospheres and nanorods, for example, can be controllably synthesized to be from tens to hundreds of nanometers in size [37–39]. Once gold cores have been synthesized, additional steps typically have to be taken to coat them with molecules, polymers or lipids that yield aqueous solubility and biocompatibility [40, 41]. As alluded to above, the shape and size of gold nanoparticles highly influences their properties. For example, the aspect ratio of gold nanorods affects the wavelength of their peak absorption and emission maxima and therefore affects their properties for photothermal therapy or fluorescence imaging. Hence, methods to carefully characterize the products of gold nanoparticle syntheses are very important, in order to establish structure–function relationships and to understand how changes in synthetic conditions can alter structure. In addition, it is important to study how these nanoparticles interact with cells. In the case of nanoparticles designed as contrast agents, the goal would be to have minimal impact on cells. In the case of therapeutics, the goal would be to avoid adverse affects on normal cells, but to destroy pathological cells. In addition, thorough evidence of biocompatibility and efficacy for the nanoparticle's purpose is needed before proceeding to in vivo experiments. For all these reasons, understanding the interactions of gold nanoparticles with cells in culture is crucial.

In this chapter, we provide example syntheses of gold nanoparticles and describe their characterization, evaluation for an example biomedical application (CT) and several assessments of their biocompatibility in vitro. Specifically, we describe a synthesis of 15 nm gold nanoparticles, coating with polyethylene glycol molecules to render them biocompatible and their purification so that they are ready for use in biomedical applications. We also describe routes to gold nanoparticles of core sizes between 15 and 100 nm. We describe the characterization of these nanoparticles with transmission electron microscopy (TEM), dynamic light scattering (DLS), zeta potential measurements, and inductively coupled plasma optical emission spectrometry (ICP-OES). We also describe how to determine the CT contrast generation properties of the nanoparticles. Methods to determine the amount of gold nanoparticles taken up in cells in vitro are outlined. Several methods to assess the effect of gold nanoparticles on cell viability, cell cytoskeleton, and cytokine production are detailed. Figure 1 outlines the developmental process of going from gold nanoparticle synthesis and characterization to biomedical evaluation.

2 Materials

2.1 Synthesis and Purification of Gold Nanoparticles

Gold(III) chloride trihydrate, sodium citrate dihydrate and hydroquinone (all Sigma-Aldrich) are typically used for the synthesis of 15–100 nm gold cores. Polyethylene glycol (PEG) thiol ligands (Creative PEGWorks) with a molecular weight of 2 kDa and various distal chemical groups are used to cap the gold nanoparticles.

2.2 Determining Nanoparticle Uptake

Dulbecco's modified eagle's medium (DMEM) supplemented with 10 % fetal bovine serum and 1 % penicillin/streptomycin (10,000 units/mL, 10,000 μg/mL) is typically used to culture

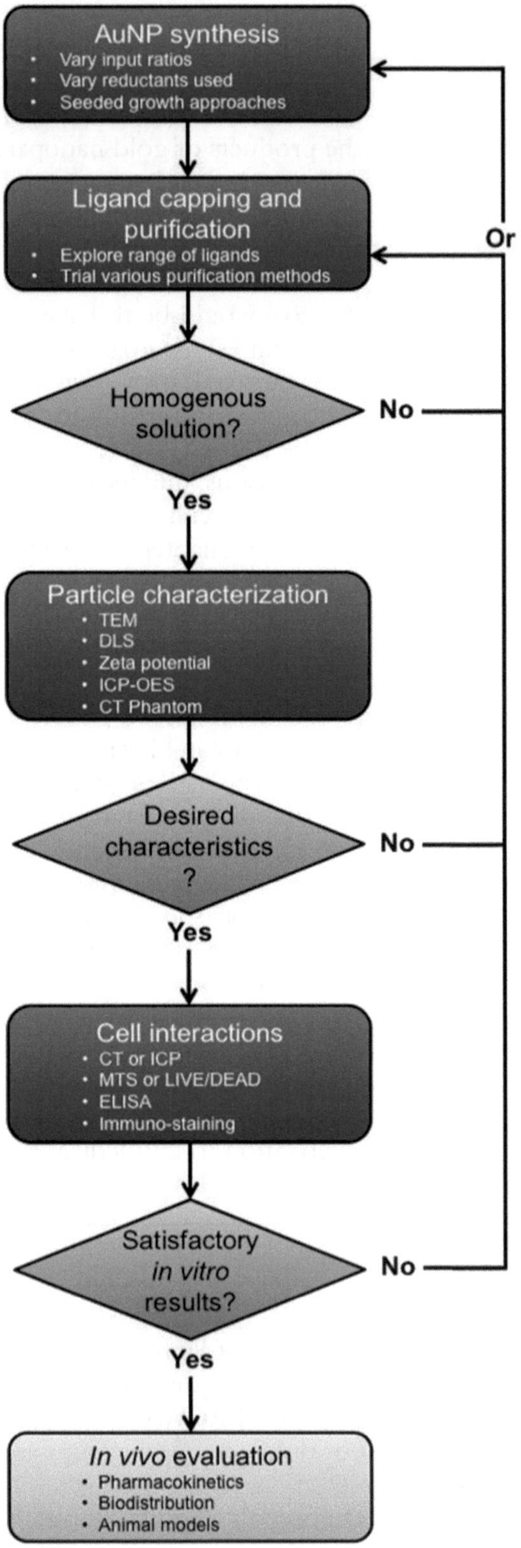

Fig. 1 Flowchart for gold nanoparticle synthesis and characterization

cells on plastic. Dulbecco's phosphate buffered saline (DPBS) is used for washing. Aqua regia is made in a 3:1 ratio of hydrochloric acid and nitric acid (**Note 1**). 4 % paraformaldehyde (PFA) diluted in DPBS is used as a fixative.

2.3 MTS Assay to Determine Cell Viability

An MTS assay kit from Promega Corp is used. This assay kit contains solutions of MTS and an electron coupling reagent (phenazine methosulfate; PMS). These solutions are combined upon receipt, aliquoted and frozen.

2.4 LIVE/DEAD Assay to Determine Cell Viability

The LIVE/DEAD® Viability/Cytotoxicity Kit for mammalian cells (Life Technologies) is used for cell toxicity evaluation. A stock solution of 3.2 mM Hoechst 33342 is used to stain nuclei (Life Technologies). Staining cocktail is made fresh before each experiment from 2 μL of stock Hoechst solution, 4 μL of stock ethidium homodimer-1 solution and 1 μL of stock Calcein AM in 2 mL of DPBS. Staining cocktail contains a final concentration of 2 μM Calcein AM, 4 μM ethidium homodimer-1, and 3.2 μM Hoechst 33342.

2.5 Evaluating Nanoparticle Effect on Cytokine Expression

Lipopolysaccharides from *E. coli* (LPS, Sigma-Aldrich, L6529) are used to stimulate cytokine release. ELISA kits (Life Technologies) are used for cytokine quantification.

3 Methods

3.1 Synthesis and Purification of Gold Nanoparticles

3.1.1 Synthesis of 15 nm Spherical Gold Cores

There are many methods used to synthesize gold nanoparticles in a range of shapes and sizes [12]. One of the most commonly used methods is that of Turkevich, where a boiling solution of gold(III) chloride trihydrate is reduced with sodium citrate in water [31]. The citrate ions also act as capping agents, coating the surface of the resulting nanoparticles (for biological applications, the citrate ions have to be substituted with ligands that provide stability in saline solutions, see later for example methods). A typical synthesis based on the Turkevich method produces 15 nm gold cores, although larger sizes can be accessed with this method by reducing the amount of sodium citrate added [38]. Smaller gold nanoparticles (1–5 nm) can be synthesized by use of sodium borohydride in addition to sodium citrate [42].

Another classic method for the synthesis of gold nanoparticles is the Brust method [43]. In this approach, gold chloride is transferred from water to toluene or another hydrophobic solvent using a phase transfer reagent. A capping ligand such as dodecanethiol is added, before sodium borohydride is added to form the nanoparticles. The resulting gold nanoparticles are 1–5 nm in size, depending on the amount of ligand used—the less ligand, the larger the cores produced [44]. As these AuNP are capped with dodecanethiol or ligands like it, they are therefore hydrophobic. For use in biological applications they need to be rendered soluble in saline solutions. Approaches to this include ligand substitution, coating with amphiphiles or embedding in a matrix such as PLGA or an oil [40, 45–47]. Gold nanoparticles can be synthesized via this method on the gram scale and are robustly stable. However transfer to aqueous media can be cumbersome and only small sized cores can be made.

As mentioned above, many other gold nanoparticles morphologies can be made, such as rods, cages, shells, stars and so forth [31–36]. Rods can be made from gold seeds that are extended by use of a growth solution and cetyl trimethylammonium bromide (CTAB) [37]. CTAB preferentially binds to the (100) facets of the gold seed, resulting in deposition predominantly on one axis. Cages and shells are often made by deposition of gold onto a template [13]. For example, shells can be made by deposition of gold onto silica spheres [34]. Gold seeds are incubated with the silica and attach to the silica surface. These seeds act as nucleation points for a gold growth solution, resulting in shell formation [48]. In some cases the template is removed by chemical processes that leave the gold undisturbed (in which case it is known as a sacrificial template). The Xia group have used silver cubes as such templates, which results in gold nanocages, via the use of iron(III) nitrate or ammonia etchants [49]. Gold nanostars have been synthesized under a number of conditions. For example, Kumar et al. reported the synthesis of gold nanostars via the addition of gold chloride and poly(vinylpyrrolidone) (PVP) to 15 nm, PVP-coated gold seeds [50]. The reader is encouraged to consult the references for more detail on the synthesis of gold nanoparticles of unusual morphology.

A synthesis of 15 nm gold cores based on the Turkevich method is described here. 98 mg of gold(III) chloride trihydrate is dissolved in 250 mL of deionized (DI) water and brought to a boil. 285 mg of sodium citrate dehydrate dissolved in 25 mL DI water is added. Upon the addition of sodium citrate, the yellow solution should turn colorless, then black, followed by deep red. The solution should be allowed to reflux for 15 min and then allowed to cool to room temperature. If the glassware/stirrer is not well-cleaned, the solution may turn black, but not change color to red. In this case, the gold nanoparticles will aggregate at the bottom of the flask and cannot be redispersed. Rinsing the glassware with aqua regia prior to the reaction will thoroughly clean the glassware and prevent aggregation.

3.1.2 Capping and Purification

Gold nanoparticles must be stable in biological media to be useful in biomedical applications [40]. Stability is needed in vivo in particular, so that the nanoparticles can circulate and reach their target tissues. Citrate-coated gold nanoparticles, for example, will immediately aggregate and precipitate when added to biological media. Polyethylene glycol (PEG) coatings provide AuNP with stealth properties, i.e., they are stable, circulate well in blood, and evade the immune system [41]. These coatings also provide excellent solubility in biological media and have good biocompatibility. As an example, we present below the capping of 15 nm gold cores with PEG-thiol ligands. The thiol groups attach to the gold surface, and PEG provides a highly stable coating for the gold nanoparticles [41]. Coated gold nanoparticles are purified before use in biological experiments to ensure that results such as effects on cell viability are due to the gold nanoparticles, as opposed to free ligands in solution. For example, there was concern that gold nanorods produced significant toxicity, but it was found that the toxicity in fact arose from residual CTAB from their synthesis [51]. Similar approaches could be taken with many thiol ligands, although the stability that they confer in biological media needs to be individually tested. This can be done by dispersing the coated gold nanoparticles in a medium such as DPBS or cell culture media and recording the absorbance of the gold nanoparticles in the medium over time. Unstable gold nanoparticles will typically form a black precipitate in a short period of time.

In the method presented below, purification is achieved by exploiting the high density of the gold nanoparticles compared to the molecules and ions used in the synthesis. Therefore the gold nanoparticles will sink to the bottom of the tube under centrifugation. The supernatant is removed and the nanoparticles redispersed in fresh solution. This is repeated several times in order to produce a highly purified agent. There are various alternative approaches to achieve this same goal. One variation of the above approach is to centrifuge the agent on a density gradient made from potassium bromide or sucrose. Such as approach is particularly valuable when there is only a small difference in density between the product and by-products, such as the loading of low density lipoprotein with 3 nm gold nanoparticles [47]. In addition, the larger size of gold nanoparticles can be exploited through the use of molecular weight cut-off (MWCO) centrifugal concentrator tubes (e.g., 10,000 MWCO), where the impurities flow through the filter into the waste compartment and the nanoparticles are retained in the upper chamber [52]. In a related approach, MWCO diafiltration columns connected to a pump and reservoirs of fresh buffer can be used [53]. Precipitation with a solvent in which the gold nanoparticles are insoluble and then washing with solvents in which the impurities are soluble is used in the Brust method [43].

A method for capping with a methoxy-PEG thiol and purification with a floor centrifuge of 15 nm, spherical AuNP synthesized in Sect. 3.1.1 is described below. The radial centrifugal force (rcf) and times given here are optimized for this core size and coating.

The rcf and time needed to isolate the gold cores will vary depending on the formulation and will need to be determined empirically. In addition, in our experience, the time and rcf needed to pull down AuNP will vary between centrifuge models.

1. Dissolve 25 mg of the PEG-thiol ligand in 1 mL of deionized water.
2. Add 1 mL of the 25 mg/mL PEG-thiol solution to each 250 mL gold nanoparticle batch (*see* Sec. 3.1.1) for a final concentration of 0.048 mM.
3. Leave the solution to incubate at room temperature for 24 h.
4. Split the resulting solution evenly into eight 50 mL high-speed centrifuge tubes (~32 mL in each tube) and spin the solution down in a centrifuge at 14,500 rcf for 120 min.
5. Discard the supernatant. Collect the pellets into 1 mL Eppendorf tubes and centrifuge at 17,000 rcf for 45 min.
6. Discard the supernatant. Collect the pellets into a single tube and resuspend them in 1 mL of deionized water.
7. Pass the resulting solution through a 450 nm millipore filter to sterilize and remove any aggregates.

3.1.3 Seeded Growth Synthesis of Large Gold Cores

Gold cores larger than 15 nm can be synthesized via the Turkevich method, by simply decreasing the amount of citrate added to the gold nanoparticles, as reported by Frens [38]. However, in our experience, these nanoparticles are faceted, heterogeneous in shape and vary in size. Nanoparticles that are more homogenous in size and shape (Fig. 2) can be formed via a seeded growth approach [39], as described below. As was mentioned in Sect. 3.1.1, synthesis of seeds and subsequent growth on the seeds is a commonly used method to access AuNP shapes and sizes that are difficult to obtain from a direct synthesis method. In this case, relatively small gold cores (i.e., 15 nm) can be made in a homogenous fashion, therefore use of a growth solution allows access to homogenous larger core sizes. The growth solution uses gold chloride with weak reducing agents, i.e., hydroquinone and sodium citrate. At room temperature, these agents are not strong enough to cause the nucleation of new gold cores, but can cause gold ions to deposit onto existing gold cores, therefore the product is simply larger gold cores than the seeds used. Large AuNP can be stored in ambient environment without degradation. Particles may sink to the bottom of the flask but can be homogenously redistributed by vortexing.

1. Synthesize a 15 nm gold core stock solution as per the method of Turkevich described above (*see* Sect. 3.1.1). Centrifuge as per Sect. 3.1.2 and resuspend in deionized (DI) water at a concentration of 250 μg/mL. Do not add additional capping ligands.
2. Dissolve 30 mg of gold(III) chloride trihydrate in 3 mL of deionized water to create a 1 % solution.

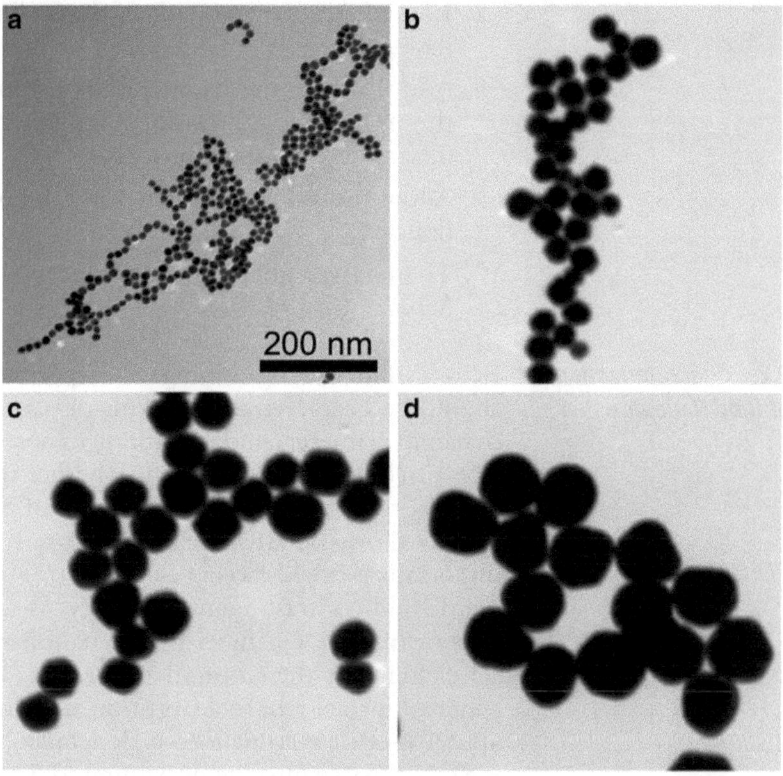

Fig. 2 Transmission electron microscopy of gold nanoparticles. (**a**) 15 nm gold "seed" nanocrystals. (**b–d**) Larger gold nanocrystals (30, 80, and 100 nm) grown from the seeds. Scale the same in **a–d**

3. Dissolve 113 mg of hydroquinone in 3 mL of deionized water to create a 0.34 M solution (**Note 2**).
4. Add 290 mL of DI water to a 500 mL Erlenmeyer flask with a stir bar and set on a stir plate at 300 rpm.
5. Add 3 mL of the gold(III) chloride solution to the flask.
6. Depending on the size of the gold core desired, add one of the following volumes of 15 nm gold cores synthesized as above to the flask:

Volume of 15 nm gold cores (μL)	Resulting particle size (nm)
12,000	30
3000	45
2250	60
810	80
450	100

7. Immediately add 660 μL of the sodium citrate solution to the flask.
8. Add 3 mL of the hydroquinone solution to the flask and stir the solution vigorously. A rapid color change should be observed during this process.
9. Allow the solution to stir for 1 h to ensure the reaction has finished.
10. These larger gold cores can be capped and purified as in Sect. 3.1.2.

3.2 Characterization of Gold Nanoparticles

Before undertaking biological experiments, gold nanoparticles should be characterized in terms of particle size (core and hydrodynamic diameter) and quantitative measurement of gold content. The aim of this is to determine whether the AuNP meet the design criteria, to allow the impact of size and morphology to be probed and to allow the effect of AuNP dose to be studied. This is very important as these factors can have tremendous impacts on therapeutic and contrast agent efficiency, as well as affecting uptake in cells or tumors. Changes in gold nanoparticle shape result in drastic changes in their optical properties. For example, 5 nm gold spheres normally have adsorption maxima at about 520 nm. The absorbance of gold nanorods depends on their aspect ratio, but it is easily tunable into the near-infrared, i.e., 650–900 nm, the wavelengths where tissue absorbs least [37]. Light-based therapeutic and imaging techniques such as photothermal ablation or photoacoustics typically use lasers whose wavelengths are in the near infrared for this reason. In addition, gold nanostars produce strong enhancement of Raman spectra at the tips of their points, thereby producing strong contrast in SERS based imaging [50]. Therefore, careful determination of structure and shape is crucial to producing nanoparticles of the desired properties.

AuNP can be characterized using dynamic light scattering (DLS) to measure their hydrodynamic diameter and transmission electron microscopy (TEM) to determine their core diameter [41]. Nanoparticle surface charge can be determined using zeta potential measurements. Inductively coupled plasma optical emission spectrometry (ICP-OES) is one of the best techniques to determine gold concentration [26]. Other methods are sometimes used to characterize AuNP, such as scanning electron microscopy (provides information on surface morphology and size), high-resolution TEM (provides information on the crystallinity of the material), X-ray powder diffraction (used to determine crystal structures), selected area electron diffraction (SAED—also used to determine crystal structures), energy-dispersive X-ray spectroscopy (EDS—used to determine elemental composition in an electron microscopy field of view) and so forth, although the crystal structure of elemental gold does not frequently vary based on the synthesis method. However DLS, zeta potential, TEM and ICP-OES are the most commonly used characterization methods.

3.2.1 Dynamic Light Scattering

Hydrodynamic diameter measurement using DLS is one of the most frequently used methods to determine nanoparticle size. The results derived from DLS can be challenging to interpret as gold nanoparticles used in nanomedicine are composed of at least two phases, i.e., the gold core and the coating, which have different refractive indices. DLS principally observes the scatter of light from particles that results from the gold core, coating, and adsorbed water molecules around the particle. Therefore, DLS size measurements are typically larger than TEM core measurements. Furthermore, the complex shapes of gold nanoparticles can confound accurate data determination—the determination of an average diameter for a rod or a plate conveys limited information, often presenting a bimodal distribution of particle size [54]. Nevertheless, DLS can give a reasonable estimate of total size, especially for spheres. It is also interesting to determine the size of the nanoparticles in cell culture media, to simulate the size found in biological settings. In addition DLS measurements taken over time, both from stored samples and samples in cell culture media, can inform on sample stability. However, measuring particles in serum may induce artifacts due to protein aggregates that occur in some serum samples. Additionally, as small amounts of particulates such as dust in the solution can yield erroneous results, it is important to filter samples prior to measurements. The protocol for the measurement of hydrodynamic diameters of AuNP using Zetasizer Nano ZS-90 (Malvern Instrument, Malvern, UK) is described below. Take 20 μL of AuNP from a stock (ca. 5 mg/mL) and dilute with 2 mL of a solvent such as DI water or PBS. This solution should be filtered into a clear-sided cuvette and a Zetasizer (Nano ZS-90, Malvern Instrument, Malvern, UK) or similar instrument to determine the hydrodynamic diameter. The solvent chosen for DLS measurements is important, as the measurement will vary depending on the solvent used. Normally a saline solution such as PBS is used. Filtering the sample prior to measurement is important, as small amounts of particulates such as dust in the solution can yield erroneous results.

3.2.2 Zeta Potential

Zeta potential measurements determine the surface charge of nanoparticles. Zeta potential can frequently be measured using the same devices used to measure DLS, using modified cells, but samples are prepared in the same way. Zeta potential measurements help to predict the properties of nanoparticles in biological media. Highly positively charged nanoparticles will likely aggregate in serum, have short circulation half-lives and be rapidly phagocytosed by cells of the reticuloendothelial system, such as macrophages [55]. Nanoparticles whose surface charge is close to neutral or negatively charged are more likely to be stable in serum and avoid phagocytosis [55].

3.2.3 Transmission Electron Microscopy

TEM can be used to determine nanoparticle size and shape. The most frequently used method of sample preparation is to simply drop the sample onto the grid and allow it to dry. The sample is then imaged using conventional TEM. This method is frequently sufficient to analyze the sample. However, for complex structures, more advanced approaches may be additionally informative. For example, air-dried samples can be imaged with TEM tomography, where the grid is rotated and the sample imaged from many angles. These images are then computationally processed to create three dimensional images of nanoparticles. This can be very useful to determine the structure of complex assemblies, such as when gold nanocrystals are embedded in polymer matrices [56]. In addition, cryo-electron microscopy is an approach where a small volume of the sample is flash-frozen, sectioned and imaged at low temperatures. This has the advantage that the sample is viewed in a native state, although the procedure is more complicated and the nature of the sample can limit the magnification used, as the beam can damage the sample. Depending on the model and configuration of the electron microscope, some of the additional characterization methods mentioned in Sect. 3.2 may be available, such as EDS or SAED.

Transmission electron microscopy of AuNP using a JEOL 1010 microscope is described below. Example images are displayed in Fig. 2. Dilute 5 μL of AuNP from stock (~5 mg/mL) with 500 μL of filtered DI water (final concentration ~50 μg/mL). 10 μL of this AuNP suspension is dropped onto a carbon-coated copper grid (FCF-200-Cu, Electron Microscopy Sciences, PA, USA) and allowed to dry. The prepared grid is gently placed on the TEM sample holder and inserted into the electron microscope. Images are acquired of the AuNP. Image J software (NIH, USA) can be used to analyze their core diameters.

3.2.4 ICP-OES

Knowledge of gold concentration, as determined by ICP-OES, allows precise dosing of AuNP for in vivo and in vitro experiments. ICP-OES is typically sensitive enough for characterizing samples. If the gold nanoparticles are diluted, e.g., after incubation with cells or injection into animals, the sensitivity of ICP-OES may not be good enough to determine concentrations. In these cases, more sensitive methods such as ICP-mass spectrometry (ICP-MS) may be needed. The measurement of the gold concentration in a AuNP formulation using ICP-OES (Spectro Genesis ICP) is described below.

1. Take 5, 10 and 25 μL of AuNP from stock and add to three separate 15 mL falcon tubes.
2. Add 1 mL of aqua regia (3:1 ratio of concentrated hydrochloric to nitric acid) to each tube to dissolve the AuNP (**Note 1**).

3. Make the final volume of each sample to 5 mL by adding DI water.
4. Dilute a gold analytical standard in the range from 0 to 50 ppm (e.g., 0, 0.5, 1, 5, 10, 25, and 50 ppm) with DI water. Gold analytical standards can be purchased from Fisher Scientific (Pittsburgh, USA).
5. Analyze the standards on the ICP-OES instrument, then proceed to the samples.
6. The results obtained from the ICP-OES are then multiplied by their respective dilution factors for each sample.
7. Average the three samples to obtain the final concentration of gold in the AuNP formulation.

3.2.5 CT Contrast Generation Evaluation

CT contrast generation (attenuation rate) is a key characteristic of CT contrast agent performance [57]. It can help predict the concentrations needed to detect signal in the blood or tissues in vivo. A phantom containing the samples is formed, this is scanned and the images are analyzed ("phantom" is a medical imaging term for an object designed to be scanned to allow contrast to be analyzed). With an eye towards translation to patients, clinical CT scanners should be used, as in the method described below. If preclinical experiments are planned, the attenuation rate can be determined with preclinical scanners also, using a smaller phantom. Tissues attenuate low energy X-rays more than high energy X-rays, an effect known as beam hardening. Therefore it is important to evaluate CT contrast with the samples submerged in a water, to simulate beam hardening. The phantom described above simulates the contrast in an abdomen, where there is little bone. Slabs of calcium phosphate can be added to the phantom to simulate conditions in the chest or other regions of the body where there is a lot of bone. For preclinical scanners, phantoms of varying sizes can be used to simulate beam hardening in mice, rats or other animals. The X-ray energies and image acquisition approach are different in clinical and preclinical scanners [58], necessitating separate CT contrast determination. When reporting the attenuation rate of a formulation, the scanner model and X-ray energies used should be reported.

1. Dilute the gold nanoparticle solution with PBS to a range of concentrations such as 5, 10, 20, 30, 40, 50, 70, and 100 mM. Pipette 1 mL of each sample into a 1.5 mL centrifuge tube. Wrap each tube with Parafilm to seal it. Make three tubes for each concentration.
2. Place each tube in the same four-way rack. Wrap the rack with Parafilm to hold the tubes in the rack.
3. Place an empty rack and then the rack containing samples into a plastic container of similar width to a human chest. Tape the racks down to the bottom of container. Fill the container with

water to a height of 21 cm to complete the phantom. The empty rack is used to raise the rack containing samples to the center of the container.

4. Scan the phantom with a clinical CT scanner, such as a Siemens Definition DS. An abdomen scan can be used. Scan with 80, 100, 120 and 140 kV. Export the data to a USB drive or a DVD.
5. Load the data into OsiriX or similar image analysis software. Analyze the data by placing an ROI on three slices for each tube and recording the attenuation values. Ensure that the ROI used is always the same size and placed in the same area of each tube.
6. Average the values for each tube and then make averages for each concentration. Plot attenuation versus concentration. The slope of the line is the attenuation rate.

3.3 Interactions of Nanoparticles with Cells

3.3.1 Determining Nanoparticle Uptake

Quantifying the cellular uptake of gold nanoparticles is an important parameter for many biomedical applications. In vitro quantification can demonstrate whether targeted AuNP are taken up by their desired cell type or whether "stealthy" AuNP avoid cell uptake, for example [59]. In cases where gold nanoparticles are being used for therapy, studying uptake will be informative as to whether a therapeutic effect is expected—if there is minimal gold nanoparticle uptake, little therapeutic effect should be expected. Studies have shown that gold nanoparticle's size can play a significant role in the interaction between particles and cells. Some reports have shown a parabolic relationship between the size of gold nanoparticles and cellular uptake, suggesting an ideal size for uptake [60, 61]. Chithrani et al. evaluated gold nanoparticles of the same shape and coating but with varied sizes and found 50 nm diameter particles to have the highest cellular uptake in HeLa cells [62]. While these results demonstrate significant size dependence for cellular uptake, a variety of factors including gold dosing, gold nanoparticle coating and cell type undoubtedly contribute to the overall cellular uptake [63]. Therefore the optimal size for highest uptake (or conversely for lowest uptake) will need to be determined for each nanoparticle on an individual basis.

Nanoparticle uptake can be determined through direct and indirect methods. Here, we describe a direct quantification method using ICP-OES and an indirect method utilizing the X-ray attenuation properties of AuNP with CT. For the latter, the X-ray attenuation from gold nanoparticles is linearly correlated to the amount of gold present in the sample. ICP-OES is more sensitive than CT for determining gold nanoparticle uptake. However, CT is higher throughput (dozens of pellets can be imaged in a single scan) and substantial gold nanoparticle uptake will be apparent in CT. These two techniques will quantify total uptake. It can also be interesting to study the sub-cellular localization of gold nanoparticles. This can be done by the electron microscopy methods described in Sect. 3.2.2. Cells can be prepared for TEM using the same approach as for CT, except 2.5 % glutaraldehyde is used for fixation. Electron microscopy pathology labs will then be able to prepare the cells for TEM using standard methods used for tissue.

1. Culture cells into 6-well plates at 2 M cells/well. Allow cells to equilibrate overnight at 37 °C, 5 % CO_2 (**Note 3**).
2. Remove the cell culture media. Prepare AuNP at desired concentration in cell culture media. Add 1 mL of AuNP treatment into each well. Incubate at 37 °C, 5 % CO_2 for the desired treatment time (**Note 4**).
3. Remove the cell culture media in each well and gently wash wells two times with DPBS.
4. Detach cells from wells using a scraper or trypsin–EDTA. Collect cells in 1.5 mL Eppendorf tubes and centrifuge at 300 rcf for 5 min to form cell pellets. These pellets can either be analyzed with ICP-OES (**step 5**) or CT (**step 6**).
5. For ICP-OES quantification:
   (a) Remove the supernatant and disperse cell pellet with 1 mL of aqua regia. Allow approximately for 20–30 min for digestion.
   (b) Centrifuge samples at 300 rcf for 5 min to pellet cellular debris. Collect supernatant and place in 15 mL falcon tubes.
   (c) Dilute samples with DI H_2O to 5 mL of total volume.
   (d) Evaluate gold concentration of samples using ICP-OES system such as the Spectro-Genesis, as detailed in Sect. 3.2.3.
   (e) Using these results and total treated dose, AuNP uptake % can be evaluated.
6. For CT attenuation quantification:
   (a) Remove the supernatant from pellets formed in **steps 1–4** and disperse them with 200 μL of 4 % PFA.
   (b) Transfer fixed cell solution into 250 μL tubes and allow the cells to settle overnight.
   (c) Arrange tubes in rack and wrap with Parafilm.
   (d) Scan the samples with a clinical scanner such as the Siemens Definition DS.
   (e) Load images into an image analysis software package such as OsiriX. Draw ROIs in each cell pellet on three slices, recording attenuation values. Attenuation values can be used as an indirect measure of gold uptake in each sample. *See* Fig. 3 for example data.

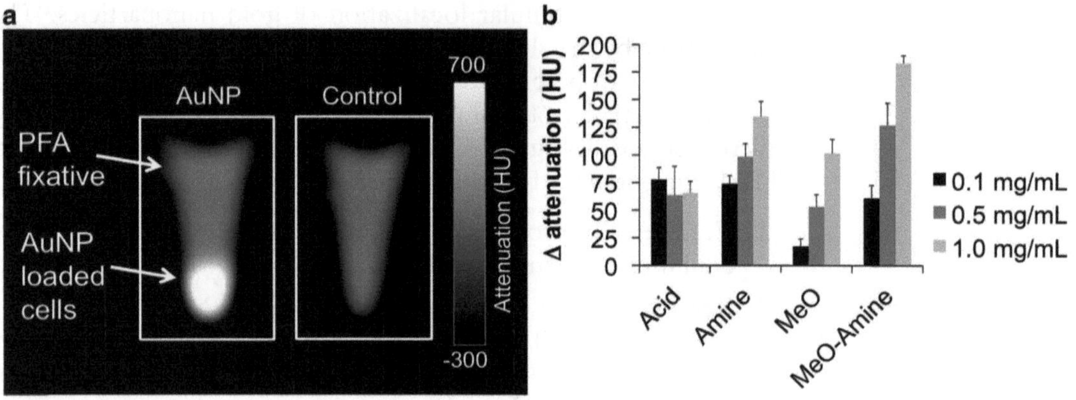

Fig. 3 (**a**) CT images of cell pellets. (**b**) Results of analysis of CT images of pellets of cells that had been incubated with 15 nm AuNP coated with PEG ligands with the named groups at their distal ends. MeO = methoxy. MeO-Amine denotes AuNP coated with a 1:1 mixture of those ligands

3.3.2 MTS Assay to Determine Cell Viability

While gold nanoparticles are frequently found to be biocompatible, certain physical characteristics and coatings may affect the cytotoxicity of the gold nanoparticles. Groups have studied the cytotoxicity of gold nanorods as compared to gold nanospheres in multiple cell types and found a shape dependent interaction between nanomaterials and cells [64–66]. For example, Schaeublin et al. showed that gold nanorods coated with PEG still caused toxicity to keratinocytes in a dose dependent manner whereas spherical nanoparticles did not cause toxicity [67]. Cytotoxicity can also be affected by gold nanoparticle core size and capping ligands used to coat gold nanoparticles. Characteristics such as charge, hydrophobicity, and polarity of the coating have been found to affect biocompatibility [68, 69]. Furthermore, nanoparticle size was shown to influence cellular interactions and cytotoxicity [70, 71]. The MTS assay is a colorimetric method for determining the number of viable cells. Cells bioreduce the tetrazolium compound [3-(4,5-dimethylthiazol-2-yl)-5-(3-carboxymethoxyphenyl)-2-(4-sulfophenyl)-2H-tetrazolium, inner salt; MTS] into a formazan product that is soluble in cell culture medium. The absorbance of formazan at 490 nm can be measured directly from the 96-well plates and is directly related to the number of living cells in culture. It should be noted that this assay is useful for instances where the cell uptake of the nanoparticle agent is low. When a significant uptake of the nanoparticles agent by cells is observed, the color of the agent in the cells can affect the accuracy of the measured absorbance. In these cases, the LIVE/DEAD assay can be used as an alternative for measuring cell viability in vitro (*see* below). These two assays are measures of cell viability. Various other effects of nanoparticles can be studied also. We have described how to measure effects on cytokine production and cell area below. Additional assays include alamar blue (viability), MTT (viability), carboxy-H2DCFDA (reactive oxygen species), thiobarbituric acid reactive substances (oxidative stress), alkaline comet (DNA damage), YO-PRO-1/ propidium iodide (apoptosis), and activating transcription factor 6 (unfolded protein response) among many others [72, 73].

1. Culture cells into a 96-well plate overnight at 37 °C, 5 % CO_2. The optimum number of cells per well depends on the cell type, cell growth rate, and the treatment time. For most cell types and treatment times of less than 24 h, 5–10 k cells seeded/well produces a signal in the linear range of the assay.
2. Remove the media and add 100 μL per well of fresh cell culture media containing gold nanoparticles diluted to the desired dose. Use at least 6 wells/condition including untreated wells as controls.
3. Incubate at 37 °C, 5 % CO_2 for the desired treatment time.
4. Dilute combined MTS/PMS solution with cell culture media in a 1:5 ratio.
5. Remove the gold nanoparticle solution and gently wash the wells with DPBS.
6. Pipet 120 μL of MTS/PMS in cell culture media into each well of the plate.
7. Incubate the plate for 1–4 h at 37 °C in a humidified, 5 % CO_2 atmosphere.
8. Record the absorbance at 490 nm using a plate reader.

3.3.3 LIVE/DEAD Assay to Determine Cell Viability

The cytotoxic effects of AuNP are an important consideration for any biomedical application. Gold has been shown to remain inert in biological systems, however various coatings of gold nanoparticles may alter the cytotoxicity of the particles. Therefore it is important to understand how a particular AuNP formulation may affect the viability of different cells. AuNP can quench fluorescent signal or increase the absorbance in a system. As many cell viability assays rely these readouts, erroneous results may be found when cells significantly take up AuNP. Here we present a method that directly quantifies cell viability by staining and counting cells. This method has the advantage of giving results in a binary fashion, with cells either stained as viable or as dying rather than depending on signal intensity. The number of cells to seed per dish will vary depending on cell type. Typically, ~50 % confluency at the end of the treatment should be the aim. If the cells are too confluent, difficulties may arise with the use of automated counting software.

1. Culture cells into glass bottom culture dishes at 75 k cells/dish for overnight at 37 °C, and 5 % CO_2.
2. Remove the cell culture media. Prepare AuNP at desired concentration(s) in cell culture media. Add 300 μL of AuNP treatment into each dish. Incubate at 37 °C, 5 % CO_2 for the

desired treatment time. Untreated cells should be used as controls (**Note 4**).

3. Remove cell culture media from each dish and gently wash twice with DPBS.
4. Place 300 μL of staining cocktail into each dish. Incubate each dish at 37 °C, 5 % CO_2 for 20 min.
5. Using a fluorescent microscope, 10× images are taken in each well using separate excitation filters for DAPI, FITC, and Texas red or similar filters. DAPI filter will excite Hoechst stain indicating total cells in the field of view. FITC filter will excite the Calcein AM stain indicating living cells. Texas red filter will excite the ethidium homodimer-1 stain indicating dead cells (**Note 5**).
6. Use image processing software (e.g., MATLAB or ImageJ) to count the number of cells in each image for each filter. Viability % can be calculated by dividing the number of living cells by total cells (**Note 6**).

3.3.4 Evaluating Nanoparticle Effect on Cytokine Expression

Many cell types release cytokines as a part of their ordinary function, or will do so under inflammatory stimuli. Therefore measurement of cytokine expression can be a subtler marker of adverse effect on the cells than viability measurements. Here we describe a method to quantify the tumor necrosis factor–α (TNF-α) release from monocyte cells (RAW 264.7) stimulated with lipopolysaccharides (LPS) using a sandwich ELISA kit. The release of this cytokine upon stimulation with LPS is a hallmark of monocyte function. If gold nanoparticles do not affect its release, that indicates minimal impact on the cells.

Generation of Samples

1. Culture cells into a 96-well plate at 15 k cells/well overnight at 37 °C, 5 % CO_2.
2. Remove the cell culture media. Prepare AuNP at desired concentration(s) in cell culture media. Add 100 μL of AuNP treatment into each well and incubate at 37 °C, 5 % CO_2 for the desired treatment time. Untreated cells should be used as controls (**Note 4**).
3. Remove cell culture media in each well and gently wash wells two times with DPBS.
4. Replace 100 μL of cell culture media in each well supplemented with 100 ng/mL of LPS and incubate at 37 °C, 5 % CO_2 for 3 h.
5. Collect cell culture media and use fresh for ELISA or store at −80 °C.
6. Count cells from each well using a hemocytometer.

*ELISA for TNF-α (**Note** 7)*

1. Dilute TNF-α standard stock in concentrations of 1000, 500, 250, 125, 62.5, 31.2, 15.6 and 0 pg/mL.
2. Using a 96-well plate pre-coated with anti-TNF-α, add 100 μL of standard into wells used for standard measurement. Run in duplicates.
3. Dilute previously generated media samples 1:4 in standard diluent buffer from kit. Add 100 μL of diluted samples in pre-coated wells. Run in duplicates.
4. Add 50 μL of biotin-labeled anti-TNF-α into each well. Cover plate and incubate at room temperature for 90 min.
5. Wash wells four times with diluted wash buffer from kit (**Note 8**).
6. Add 100 μL of diluted Streptavidin-HRP from kit into each well. Cover plate and incubate at room temperature for 30 min.
7. Wash wells four times with diluted wash buffer from kit.
8. Add 100 μL of stabilized chromogen to each well. Wells will become blue. Cover plate and incubate at room temperature for 20 min in the dark (**Note 9**).
9. Add 100 μL of stop solution from kit to each well. Wells will become yellow.
10. Read absorbance at 450 nm using a plate reader.
11. Generate standard curve using standard measurements. Calculate concentrations of TNF-α in samples by using the linear regression from the standard curve. Account for 1:4 dilution of samples. Concentrations can be normalized by the number of cells counted in each well.

3.3.5 Effect of AuNP on Cell Cytoskeleton

Cell cytoskeleton components such as actin and tubulin create a filamentous intracellular structure which is responsible for maintaining cell shape, providing mechanical strength, facilitating intracellular transport and playing a major role in chromosome separation during cell division. It has been reported that deformation of the cell cytoskeleton network can occur upon exposure to AuNP. This effect can be related to the exposure dose, particle size, exposure time [63, 70, 74] or shape of the nanoparticles [74, 75]. A common method to visualize actin in the cell is staining with phalloidin conjugated to a fluorophore. Phalloidin binds between F-actin subunits, which allow for visualization of the distribution of actin within the cell. Similarly, tubulin can be visualized with immunocytochemistry using antibodies against tubulin. The protocol for determining the effect of AuNP on BJ5ta (human fibroblast) cell cytoskeleton is described below with staining for both actin and tubulin [76].

1. Maintain the BJ5ta cells in a culture medium containing four parts of Dulbecco's Modified Eagle's Medium (DMEM), one part of Medium 199, 10 % fetal bovine serum (Gibco) and 0.01 mg/mL of hygromycin B (Sigma-Aldrich).
2. Transfer 50 k cells to a 35 mm glass bottom petri dish (In Vitro Scientific, USA) and incubate the cells at 37 °C in a 5 % CO_2 humidified incubator for 24 h.
3. Wash the cell monolayer with sterile PBS and then incubate with AuNP at desired concentration(s) for required exposure time points (such as 1, 4, 6, or 24 h).
4. After incubation for a given time point/concentration, remove the cell culture media and wash the cell monolayer twice with sterile DPBS.
5. Fix the cells by adding 400 μL of 4 % paraformaldehyde (Electron Microscopy Sciences, PA, USA) to the petri dish and incubate for 20 min at room temperature.
6. Wash the cells twice with DPBS and then incubate the cells with 400 μL of 0.1 % Triton™ X-100 (Sigma-Aldrich) for 4 min at room temperature.
7. Wash the cells twice with DPBS and then block the cells by adding 800 μL of blocking buffer (1 % bovine serum albumin in DPBS) for 30 min at room temperature.
8. After blocking, incubate the cells with a primary antibody against α-tubulin (1/150 dilution with blocking buffer, ab80779, abcam, Cambridge UK) for 2 h at room temperature.
9. Wash the cells three times with blocking buffer. Incubate cells with secondary AF-488 conjugated goat anti-mouse antibody (one drop in 500 μL of blocking buffer, Life Technologies, Grand Island, NY, USA) and AF-546 conjugated phalloidin (1/300 dilution, Life Technologies) for 1 h at room temperature.
10. Wash the cells three times with DPBS and add two drops of Prolong gold antifade reagent with DAPI (Life Technologies).
11. Image the cells using a fluorescence microscope, such as a Nikon Eclipse (Nikon Instruments Inc, Melville, NY, USA) equipped with a mercury bulb as the light source. DAPI, FITC, and Tx-Red excitation filters can be used for DAPI, tubulin, and actin, respectively.
12. Acquire fluorescence images of cells at 20× magnification and the images can be merged using NIS-Elements microscope imaging software (Nikon Instruments Inc).
13. Measure the cell areas using image J software.

4 Notes

1. Undiluted aqua regia (3:1 HCl–HNO_3) can be difficult to handle. Diluting with four parts deionized water (3:1:4 HCl–HNO_3–DI H_2O) makes it easier to handle.
2. Hydroquinone solutions should be made just before use and stored in light-proof, tightly closed containers. Do not expose to heat.
3. The number of cells to seed per well will vary depending on cell type. 90 % confluency after 24 h should be the aim in order to generate a substantial pellet that can be visualized with CT.
4. Prepare media with AuNP before adding to wells. When adding AuNP to cells, pipette gently onto along the walls of the well and not directly onto the cells.
5. Typically, four different fields of the same plate are acquired from each dish. Each field has an image from each corresponding filter (DAPI, FITC, Texas red). Values are averaged across the four fields for a better representation of the dish.
6. The Calcein AM stains all of the cytoplasm, and therefore cells close together can be incorrectly counted as one cell by automated software. Living cells can be alternatively calculated using the total number of cells (Hoechst 33342) and dead cells (Ethidium Homodimer-1).
7. Depending on the cytokine, the directions may vary in terms of incubation temperature and times.
8. Washing steps must be thorough. Fill each well with wash buffer and soak for 15–30 s. After removing wash buffer, invert plate and tap against flat surface to remove remaining solution out of wells.
9. Suggested incubation time depends on expected TNF-α concentration in samples. Incubating too long will saturate signal. Trial and error may be needed to determine acceptable incubation times.

Acknowledgements

This work was supported by R00 EB012165 (D.P.C.), T32 HL007954 (P.C.), and the W. W. Smith Charitable Trust. We also thank the University of Pennsylvania for start-up funding.

References

1. Kim BYS, Rutka JT, Chan WCW (2010) Nanomedicine. N Engl J Med 363(25):2434–2443
2. Briley-Saebo KC, Geninatti Crich S, Cormode DP, Barazza A, Mulder WJM, Chen W, Giovenzana GB, Fisher EA, Aime S, Fayad ZA (2009) High-relaxivity gadolinium-modified high-density lipoproteins as magnetic resonance imaging contrast agents. J Phys Chem B 113:6283–6289
3. Corot C, Robert P, Idee J-M, Port M (2006) Recent advances in iron oxide nanocrystal technology for medical imaging. Adv Drug Deliv Rev 58:1471–1504
4. Yigit MV, Moore A, Medarova Z (2012) Magnetic nanoparticles for cancer diagnosis and therapy. Pharm Res 29(5):1180–1188
5. Chacko AM, Hood ED, Zern BJ, Muzykantov VR (2011) Targeted nanocarriers for imaging and therapy of vascular inflammation. Curr Opin Colloid Interface Sci 16(3):215–227
6. Cheng ZL, Al Zaki A, Hui JZ, Muzykantov VR, Tsourkas A (2012) Multifunctional nanoparticles: cost versus benefit of adding targeting and imaging capabilities. Science 338(6109):903–910
7. Cormode DP, Naha P, Fayad ZA (2014) Nanoparticle contrast agents for computed tomography: a focus on micelles. Contrast Media Mol Imaging 9(1):37–52
8. Daniel M-C, Astruc D (2004) Gold nanoparticles: assembly, supramolecular chemistry, quantum-size-related properties, and applications toward biology, catalysis, and nanotechnology. Chem Rev 104:293–346
9. Antonie F (1616) Panacea aurea-auro potabile. John Legatt, London
10. Thakor AS, Jokerst J, Zavaleta C, Massoud TF, Gambhir SS (2011) Gold nanoparticles: a revival in precious metal administration to patients. Nano Lett 11:4029–4036
11. Dreaden E, Alkilany A, Huang X, Murphy C, El-Sayed M (2011) The golden age: gold nanoparticles for biomedicine. Chem Soc Rev 41:2740–2779
12. Mieszawska AJ, Mulder WJM, Fayad ZA, Cormode DP (2013) Multifunctional gold nanoparticles for diagnosis and therapy of disease. Mol Pharm 10(4):831–847
13. Li N, Zhao P, Astruc D (2014) Anisotropic gold nanoparticles: synthesis, properties, applications, and toxicity. Angew Chem Int Ed Engl 53:1756–1789
14. Durr NJ, Larson T, Smith DK, Korgel BA, Sokolov K, Ben-Yakar A (2007) Two-photon luminescence imaging of cancer cells using molecularly targeted gold nanorods. Nano Lett 7(4):941–945
15. Wang B, Yantsen E, Larson T, Karpiouk AB, Sethuraman S, Su JL, Sokolov K, Emelianov SY (2009) Plasmonic intravascular photoacoustic imaging for detection of macrophages in atherosclerotic plaques. Nano Lett 9(6):2212–2217
16. von Maltzahn G, Park JH, Agrawal A, Bandaru NK, Das SK, Sailor MJ, Bhatia SN (2009) Computationally guided photothermal tumor therapy using long-circulating gold nanorod antennas. Cancer Res 69(9):3892–3900
17. Agarwal A, Huang SW, O'Donnell M, Day KC, Day M, Kotov N, Ashkenazi S (2007) Targeted gold nanorod contrast agent for prostate cancer detection by photoacoustic imaging. J Appl Phys 102(6):064701
18. Kircher MF, de la Zerda A, Jokerst JV, Zavaleta CL, Kempen PJ, Mittra E, Pitter K, Huang R, Campos C, Habte F, Sinclair R, Brennan CW, Mellinghoff IK, Holland EC, Gambhir SS (2012) A brain tumor molecular imaging strategy using a new triple-modality MRI-photoacoustic-Raman nanoparticle. Nat Med 18(5):829–834
19. Qian X, Peng X-H, Ansari DO, Yin-Goen Q, Chen GZ, Shin DM, Yang L, Young AN, Wang MD, Nie S (2008) In vivo tumor targeting and spectroscopic detection with surface-enhanced Raman nanoparticle tags. Nat Biotechnol 26(1):83–90
20. Shan Y, Luo T, Peng C, Sheng R, Cao A, Cao X, Shen M, Guo R, Tomas H, Shi X (2012) Gene delivery using dendrimer-entrapped gold nanoparticles as nonviral vectors. Biomaterials 33(10):3025–3035
21. Pearson S, Scarano W, Stenzel MH (2012) Micelles based on gold-glycopolymer complexes as new chemotherapy drug delivery agents. Chem Commun 48(39):4695–4697
22. Kong WH, Bae KH, Jo SD, Kim JS, Park TG (2012) Cationic lipid-coated gold nanoparticles as efficient and non-cytotoxic intracellular siRNA delivery vehicles. Pharm Res 29(2):362–374
23. Mieszawska AJ, Kim Y, Gianella A, van Rooy I, Priem B, Labarre MP, Ozcan C, Cormode DP, Petrov A, Langer R, Farokhzad OC, Fayad ZA, Mulder WJ (2013) Synthesis of polymer-lipid nanoparticles for image-guided delivery of dual modality therapy. Bioconjug Chem 24(9):1429–1434
24. Hainfeld JF, Slatkin DN, Focella TM, Smilowitz HM (2006) Gold nanoparticles: a

new X-ray contrast agent. Br J Radiol 79:248–253

25. Liu CJ, Wang CH, Chen ST, Chen HH, Leng WH, Chien CC, Wang CL, Kempson IM, Hwu Y, Lai TC, Hsiao M, Yang CS, Chen YJ, Margaritondo G (2010) Enhancement of cell radiation sensitivity by pegylated gold nanoparticles. Phys Med Biol 55(4):931–945
26. Al Zaki A, Joh D, Cheng ZL, De Barros ALB, Kao G, Dorsey J, Tsourkas A (2014) Gold-loaded polymeric micelles for computed tomography-guided radiation therapy treatment and radiosensitization. ACS Nano 8(1): 104–112
27. Pilot Study of AuroLase(tm) Therapy in Refractory and/or Recurrent Tumors of the Head and Neck (Clinical trial identifier: NCT00848042). http://www.clinicaltrials-gov/ct2/show/NCT00848042
28. Plasmonic Nanophotothermic Therapy of Atherosclerosis (NANOM) (Clinical trial identifier: NCT01270139). http://www.clinical-trialsgov/ct2/show/NCT01270139
29. Plasmonic Photothermal and Stem Cell Therapy of Atherosclerosis Versus Biodegradable Stenting (NANOM2) (Clinical trial identifier: NCT01436123). http://www clinicaltrialsgov/ct2/show/NCT01436123
30. Libutti SK, Paciotti GF, Byrnes AA, Alexander HR, Gannon WE, Walker M, Seidel GD, Yuldasheva N, Tamarkin L (2010) Phase I and pharmacokinetic studies of CYT-6091, a novel PEGylated colloidal gold-rhTNF nanomedicine. Clin Cancer Res 16(24):6139–6149
31. Turkevich J, Stevenson PC, Hillier J (1951) A study of the nucleation and growth processes in the synthesis of colloidal gold. Discuss Faraday Soc 11:55–75
32. Jana NR, Gearheart L, Murphy CJ (2001) Wet chemical synthesis of high aspect ratio cylindrical gold nanorods. J Phys Chem B 105(19):4065–4067
33. Skrabalak SE, Chen J, Sun Y, Lu X, Au L, Cobley CM, Xia Y (2008) Gold nanocages: synthesis, properties, and applications. Acc Chem Res 41(12):1587–1595
34. Park J, Estrada A, Sharp K, Sang K, Schwartz JA, Smith DK, Coleman C, Payne JD, Korgel BA, Dunn AK, Tunnell JW (2008) Two-photon-induced photoluminescence imaging of tumors using near-infrared excited gold nanoshells. Opt Express 16(3):1590–1599
35. Yuan H, Khoury CG, Hwang H, Wilson CM, Grant GA, Vo-Dinh T (2012) Gold nanostars: surfactant-free synthesis, 3D modelling, and two-photon photoluminescence imaging. Nanotechnology 23(7):075102
36. Liu B, Xie J, Lee JY, Ting YP, Chen JP (2005) Optimization of high-yield biological synthesis of single-crystalline gold nanoplates. J Phys Chem B 109(32):15256–15263
37. Murphy CJ, Sau TK, Gole AM, Orendorff CJ, Gao J, Gou L, Hunyadi SE, Li T (2005) Anisotropic metal nanoparticles: synthesis, assembly, and optical applications. J Phys Chem B 109:13857–13870
38. Frens G (1973) Controlled nucleation for regulation of particle size in monodisperse gold suspensions. Nat Phys Sci 241(105):20–22
39. Perrault SD, Chan WCW (2009) Synthesis and surface modification of highly monodispersed, spherical gold nanoparticles of 50–200 nm. J Am Chem Soc 131(47):17042–17043
40. Cormode DP, Sanchez-Gaytan BL, Mieszawska AJ, Fayad ZA, Mulder WJ (2013) Inorganic nanocrystals as contrast agents in MRI: synthesis, coating and introducing multifunctionality. NMR Biomed 26(7):766–780
41. Cai QY, Kim SH, Choi KS, Kim SY, Byun SJ, Kim KW, Park SH, Juhng SK, Yoon KH (2007) Colloidal gold nanoparticles as a blood-pool contrast agent for x-ray computed tomography in mice. Invest Radiol 42(12):797–806
42. Patil V, Malvankar RB, Sastry M (1999) Role of particle size in individual and competitive diffusion of carboxylic acid derivatized colloidal gold particles in thermally evaporated fatty amine films. Langmuir 15:8197–8206
43. Brust M, Walker M, Bethell D, Schiffrin DJ, Whyman R (1994) Synthesis of thiol-derivatised gold nanoparticles in a two-phase liquid–liquid system. Chem Commun 801–802
44. Hostetler MJ, Wingate JE, Zhong CJ, Harris JE, Vachet RW, Clark MR, Londono JD, Green SJ, Stokes JJ, Wignall GD, Glish GL, Porter MD, Evans ND, Murray RW (1998) Alkanethiolate gold cluster molecules with core diameters from 1.5 to 5.2 nm: core and monolayer properties as a function of core size. Langmuir 14:17–30
45. Cormode DP, Skajaa T, van Schooneveld MM, Koole R, Jarzyna P, Lobatto ME, Calcagno C, Barazza A, Gordon RE, Zanzonico P, Fisher EA, Fayad ZA, Mulder WJM (2008) Nanocrystal core high-density lipoproteins: a multimodal molecular imaging contrast agent platform. Nano Lett 8(11):3715–3723
46. Mieszawska AJ, Gianella A, Cormode DP, Zhao Y, Meijerink A, Langer R, Farokhzad OC, Fayad ZA, Mulder WJM (2012) Engineering of lipid-coated PLGA nanoparticles with a tunable payload of diagnostically active nanocrystals for medical imaging. Chem Commun 48:5835–5837

47. Allijn IE, Leong W, Tang J, Gianella A, Mieszawska AJ, Fay F, Ma G, Russell S, Callo CB, Gordon RE, Korkmaz E, Post JA, Zhao Y, Gerritsen HC, Storm G, Thran A, Proksa R, Daerr H, Fuster V, Fisher EA, Fayad ZA, Mulder WJ, Cormode DP (2013) Gold nanocrystal labeling allows low density lipoprotein imaging from the subcellular to macroscopic level. ACS Nano 7(11):9761–9770
48. Pham T, Jackson JB, Halas NJ, Lee TR (2002) Preparation and characterization of gold nanoshells coated with self-assembled monolayers. Langmuir 18(12):4915–4920
49. Lu XM, Au L, McLellan J, Li ZY, Marquez M, Xia YN (2007) Fabrication of cubic nanocages and nanoframes by dealloying Au/Ag alloy nanoboxes with an aqueous etchant based on Fe(NO3)(3) or NH4OH. Nano Lett 7(6): 1764–1769
50. Kumar PS, Pastoriza-Santos I, Rodriguez-Gonzalez B, Garcia de Abajo FJ, Liz-Marzan LM (2008) High-yield synthesis and optical response of gold nanostars. Nanotechnology 19(1):015606
51. Alkilany AM, Nagaria PK, Hexel CR, Shaw TJ, Murphy CJ, Wyatt MD (2009) Cellular uptake and cytotoxicity of gold nanorods: molecular origin of cytotoxicity and surface effects. Small 5(6):701–708
52. Cormode DP, Roessl E, Thran A, Skajaa T, Gordon RE, Schlomka JP, Fuster V, Fisher EA, Mulder WJM, Proksa R, Fayad ZA (2010) Atherosclerotic plaque composition: analysis with multicolor CT and targeted gold nanoparticles. Radiology 256(3):774–782
53. Naha P, Al-Zaki A, Hecht ER, Chorny M, Chhour P, Blankemeyer E, Yates DM, Witschey WRT, Litt HI, Tsourkas A, Cormode DP (2014) Dextran coated bismuth-iron oxide nanohybrid contrast agents for computed tomography and magnetic resonance imaging. J Mater Chem B Mater Biol Med 2(46): 8239–8248
54. Liu H, Pierre-Pierre N, Huo Q (2012) Dynamic light scattering for gold nanorod size characterization and study of nanorod-protein interactions. Gold Bull 45:187–195
55. Zahr AS, Davis CA, Pishko MV (2006) Macrophage uptake of core-shell nanoparticles surface modified with poly(ethylene glycol). Langmuir 22:8178–8185
56. Chhour P, Gallo N, Re C, Williams D, Al-Zaki A, Nichol JL, Tian Z, Paik T, Naha PC, Allcock HR, Murray CB, Tsourkas A, Cormode DP (2014) Nano-disco balls: control over surface versus core loading of diagnostically active nanocrystals into polymer nanoparticles. ACS Nano 8(9):9143–9153
57. Galper MW, Saung MT, Fuster V, Roessl E, Thran A, Proksa R, Fayad ZA, Cormode DP (2012) Effect of computed tomography scanning parameters on gold nanoparticle and iodine contrast. Invest Radiol 47(8):475–481
58. Jackson PA, Rahman WNWA, Wong CJ, Ackerly T, Geso M (2010) Potential dependent superiority of gold nanoparticles in comparison to iodinated contrast agents. Eur J Radiol 75(1):104–109
59. Albanese A, Tang PS, Chan WC (2012) The effect of nanoparticle size, shape, and surface chemistry on biological systems. Annu Rev Biomed Eng 14:1–16
60. Jiang W, Kim BY, Rutka JT, Chan WC (2008) Nanoparticle-mediated cellular response is size-dependent. Nat Nanotechnol 3(3):145–150
61. Ma X, Wu Y, Jin S, Tian Y, Zhang X, Zhao Y, Yu L, Liang XJ (2011) Gold nanoparticles induce autophagosome accumulation through size-dependent nanoparticle uptake and lysosome impairment. ACS Nano 5(11):8629–8639
62. Chithrani BD, Ghazani AA, Chan WC (2006) Determining the size and shape dependence of gold nanoparticle uptake into mammalian cells. Nano Lett 6(4):662–668
63. Soenen SJ, Manshian B, Montenegro JM, Amin F, Meermann B, Thiron T, Cornelissen M, Vanhaecke F, Doak S, Parak WJ, De Smedt S, Braeckmans K (2012) Cytotoxic effects of gold nanoparticles: a multiparametric study. ACS Nano 6(7):5767–5783
64. Alkilany AM, Murphy CJ (2010) Toxicity and cellular uptake of gold nanoparticles: what we have learned so far? J Nanopart Res 12(7):2313–2333
65. Connor EE, Mwamuka J, Gole A, Murphy CJ, Wyatt MD (2005) Gold nanoparticles are taken up by human cells but do not cause acute cytotoxicity. Small 1(3):325–327
66. Chuang SM, Lee YH, Liang RY, Roam GD, Zeng ZM, Tu HF, Wang SK, Chueh PJ (2013) Extensive evaluations of the cytotoxic effects of gold nanoparticles. Biochim Biophys Acta 1830(10):4960–4973
67. Schaeublin NM, Braydich-Stolle LK, Maurer EI, Park K, MacCuspie RI, Afrooz AR, Vaia RA, Saleh NB, Hussain SM (2012) Does shape matter? Bioeffects of gold nanomaterials in a human skin cell model. Langmuir 28(6):3248–3258
68. Goodman CM, McCusker CD, Yilmaz T, Rotello VM (2004) Toxicity of gold nanoparticles functionalized with cationic and anionic side chains. Bioconjug Chem 15(4):897–900
69. Cai H, Yao P (2014) Gold nanoparticles with different amino acid surfaces: serum albumin

adsorption, intracellular uptake and cytotoxicity. Colloids Surf B Biointerfaces 123:900–906

70. Coradeghini R, Gioria S, Garcia CP, Nativo P, Franchini F, Gilliland D, Ponti J, Rossi F (2013) Size-dependent toxicity and cell interaction mechanisms of gold nanoparticles on mouse fibroblasts. Toxicol Lett 217(3):205–216
71. Pan Y, Neuss S, Leifert A, Fischler M, Wen F, Simon U, Schmid G, Brandau W, Jahnen-Dechent W (2007) Size-dependent cytotoxicity of gold nanoparticles. Small 3(11):1941–1949
72. Naha PC, Bhattacharya K, Tenuta T, Dawson KA, Lynch I, Gracia A, Lyng FM, Byrne HJ (2010) Intracellular localisation, geno- and cytotoxic response of polyN-isopropylacrylamide (PNIPAM) nanoparticles to human keratinocyte (HaCaT) and colon cells (SW 480). Toxicol Lett 198(2):134–143
73. Naha PC, Davoren M, Lyng FM, Byrne HJ (2010) Reactive oxygen species (ROS) induced cytokine production and cytotoxicity of PAMAM dendrimers in J774A.1 cells. Toxicol Appl Pharmacol 246(1–2):91–99
74. Wu YL, Putcha N, Ng KW, Leong DT, Lim CT, Loo SC, Chen X (2013) Biophysical responses upon the interaction of nanomaterials with cellular interfaces. Acc Chem Res 46(3):782–791
75. Huang X, Teng X, Chen D, Tang F, He J (2010) The effect of the shape of mesoporous silica nanoparticles on cellular uptake and cell function. Biomaterials 31(3):438–448
76. Naha P, Chhour P, Cormode DP (2015) Systematic in vitro toxicological screening of gold nanoparticles designed for nanomedicine applications. Toxicology In Vitro, 29: 1445–1453

Chapter 6

Paramagnetic Nanoparticles

Randall Toy and Efstathios Karathanasis

Abstract

Paramagnetic nanoparticles have many applications for cancer diagnosis and therapy. More importantly, advances in nanoparticle engineering enable performance enhancements over molecular paramagnetic agents. A variety of paramagnetic materials and production methods enable the selection of nanoparticle size, shape, and surface chemistry, which are all important design parameters that determine a nanoparticle's in vivo behavior, diagnostic accuracy using magnetic resonance imaging, and therapeutic efficacy. In this chapter, we evaluate design rules that can be used in the manufacturing of a paramagnetic nanoparticle for a specific biomedical application. Moreover, we introduce ways in which paramagnetic nanoparticles may be used for targeted magnetic resonance imaging, for multimodal imaging, and as drivers for tumor therapy by hyperthermia and triggered drug release.

Key words Nanoparticles, Gadolinium, Iron oxide, Manganese, Targeting, Magnetic resonance imaging, Hyperthermia

1 Paramagnetic Nanoparticles in Medicine

Paramagnetism is a type of magnetism in which atoms with one or more unpaired electrons are attracted by an externally applied magnetic field. The application of the magnetic field causes the induction of a magnetic moment, which reverts back to the ground state upon removal of the field. This return of magnetization is termed "relaxation" and occurs at rates dependent on the paramagnetism of the material. Magnetic relaxation is described by the T1 and T2 relaxation time parameters, where T1 relaxation is the return of the longitudinal magnetization to the equilibrium state and T2 relaxation is the return of transverse magnetization to the equilibrium state. When the applied magnetic field strength is held constant, the T1 and T2 relaxation times are distinct for different tissue types. Moreover, diseased tissues often have distinct T1 and T2 values from healthy tissue. The targeted delivery of paramagnetic agents to diseased tissue can lengthen or shorten these relaxation times, which generates contrast enhancement that

Zheng-Rong Lu and Shinji Sakuma (eds.), *Nanomaterials in Pharmacology*, Methods in Pharmacology and Toxicology, DOI 10.1007/978-1-4939-3121-7_6, © Springer Science+Business Media New York 2016

further improves the ease in which abnormalities can be identified. In addition, paramagnetic agents facilitate contrast-enhanced vascular imaging, which may useful for the identification of angiogenic tumors or blood vessels that are developing atherosclerotic plaques.

Recent advances have resulted in the development of paramagnetic nanoparticles for various medical applications (Fig. 1). What are the advantages of employing a paramagnetic nanoparticle over a paramagnetic agent based on small molecules? Nanoparticles are capable of loading high amounts of molecular paramagnetic agents, which increases their overall contrast sensitivity. Through decoration of the nanoparticle surface with targeting ligands, paramagnetic nanoparticles can also be delivered directly to the targeting site due to enhanced multivalent targeting avidity. In addition, nanoparticles tend to have improved pharmacokinetics over molecular agents, which is due to their filtration through hepatic and splenic mechanisms but not through renal mechanisms. The subsequent extension in half-life increases the chances that a paramagnetic contrast agent can reach its target. Nanoparticles can also be designed to specifically deliver their payload at the target site. Their structure may incorporate pH, enzyme, or ultrasound sensitive elements that could be used to either unmask molecular contrast agents or release a therapeutic payload [1]. Most importantly, nanoparticles have the capability of shielding the body from the toxicity of some contrast agents (e.g., gadolinium), which is essential for their in vivo use.

More importantly, there is incredible flexibility with a nanoparticle's physical design, which enhances both its magnetic susceptibility and its ability to successfully reach its target. It has been well established that the size and shape of a nanoparticle influences its magnetic relaxivity, which must be considered in the rational design of magnetic resonance (MR) contrast agents. In general, larger nanoparticles exhibit a higher magnetic relaxivity, which corresponds to higher sensitivity as a contrast agent. In addition, nanoparticles of oblate shape tend to exhibit a higher magnetic

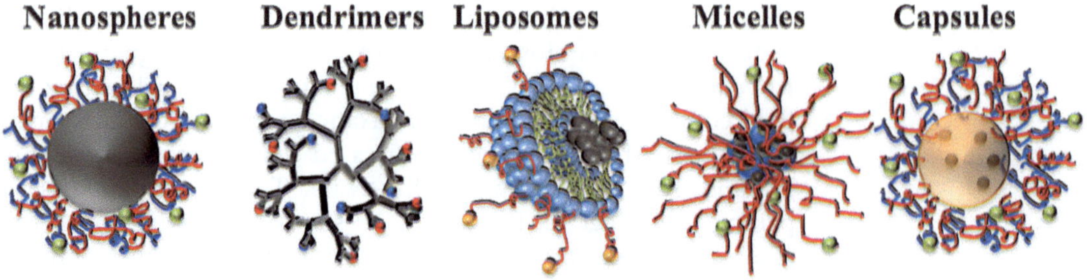

Fig. 1 Common platforms for paramagnetic nanoparticles. Contrast agents may be developed as discrete crystalline geometries (spheres, rods, cubes, etc.), or incorporated into a variety of nanoparticle platforms, such as being entrapped in dendrimers, liposomes, or micelles, or loaded into capsules

relaxivity than spherical nanoparticles. While the size and shape of a nanoparticle critically affect its response to a magnetic field, it is also an important consideration for nanoparticle delivery to a target site. In fact, extensive research has shown that the size and shape of a nanoparticle influences its pharmacology, both in terms of its circulation half-life and ability to interact with its target site. The reticuloendothelial system (RES), which consists of the liver and spleen, phagocytoses and processes nanoparticles at different rates depending on the particle size and shape. A nanoparticle's size and shape also affects its ability to escape the blood flow and marginate towards the blood vessel wall. For maximized interactions with the vascular endothelium, it is essential to design nanoparticles that are highly capable of margination. At the target site, a nanoparticle's size, shape, and surface characteristics all affect its ability to bind to a cell and undergo endocytosis mechanisms.

With these considerations in mind, this chapter seeks to illustrate the processes and materials required to produce paramagnetic nanoparticles with high diagnostic and therapeutic potential. Most importantly, we will demonstrate how the geometric and surface properties of a paramagnetic nanoparticle influence its ability to successfully reach the target site. More specifically, the relationships between nanoparticle size and shape and nanoparticle pharmacokinetics and pharmacodynamics will be explored. Ultimately, we will discuss the implications of these design criteria on paramagnetic nanoparticles produced for site-specific MR imaging and tumor therapy. Therapeutic applications of specific focus are tumor ablation via nanoparticle induced hyperthermia and triggered drug release through the magnetically induced mechanical disruption of nanoparticle composites that carry chemotherapy.

2 Classes of Paramagnetic Nanoparticles

2.1 Paramagnetic Nanoparticle T1 Contrast Agents

Lanthanide metals (e.g., gadolinium (Gd)) exhibit extremely favorable paramagnetic properties due to their high number of unpaired valence electrons. Consequently, lanthanide metals are excellent T1 shortening agents, which allow for the bright detection of small lesions. Unfortunately, a limitation of lanthanide metals is their high toxicity in free form. Chelation of the lanthanide ions decreases their toxicity while maintaining high magnetic susceptibility, which enables their use as MR imaging contrast agents. The size and loading capacity of nanoparticles enable the delivery of high amounts of lanthanide ions to the target, which allows for high detection sensitivity. For example, dendrimers have been extensively investigated as vehicles for the transport of gadolinium—the primary advantage of the dendrimer is its slow rotational dynamics, which enhances relaxivity [2]. The dendrimer's superior relaxivity is further enhanced by the functionality of its highly branched structure, which enables the conjugation of up to hundreds of gadolinium molecules per carrier. In addition, the dendrimer's size provides with extended circulation half-life, which further boosts its strength as a contrast agent. Due to these features, dendrimers have been exploited for use as blood pool and molecular MRI contrast agents [3]. One limitation of dendrimers is that the Gd payload is restricted by the number of conjugation sites available on the dendrimer. To tackle this limitation, one strategy is to synthesize nanoclusters of Gd-conjugated dendrimer [4]. Unfortunately, the clinical utility of such nanoclusters may be limited due to safety related to nephrogenic systemic fibrosis. Further advancements lead to biodegradable nanoclusters, which were based on polydisulfide linkages between the individual dendrimers to facilitate renal excretion (Fig. 2) [5]. For example, such biodegradable nanoclusters displayed a blood circulation half-life of >1.6 h in mice and generated significant contrast enhancement in the abdominal aorta for as long as 4 h. As a result of thiol–disulfide exchange, the nanoclusters were degraded and rapidly excreted via renal filtration, resulting in minimal Gd tissue retention.

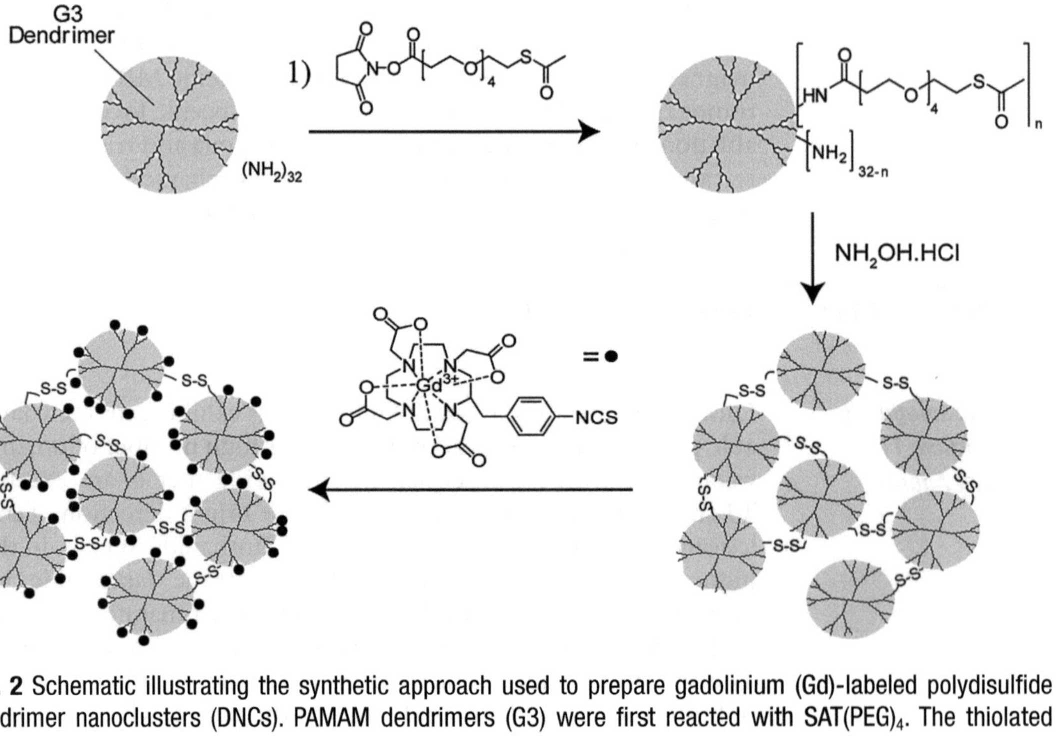

Fig. 2 Schematic illustrating the synthetic approach used to prepare gadolinium (Gd)-labeled polydisulfide dendrimer nanoclusters (DNCs). PAMAM dendrimers (G3) were first reacted with $SAT(PEG)_4$. The thiolated dendrimers were then suspended in an alkaline buffer for deprotection and to initiate the formation of polydisulfide DNCs. Once DNCs with a desirable hydrodynamic diameter were formed, free thiols were quenched with maleimide and the remaining amines were functionalized with $[Gd\text{-}C\text{-}DOTA]^{-1}$. Reproduced with permission from reference [5]

Another class of nanoparticles frequently used as T1 contrast agent is the PEGylated liposome, which provides the flexibility of conjugating Gd-chelates on their surface [6] or encapsulating a very large Gd payload in their interior aqueous core [7, 8]. Between the encapsulated and surface Gd, one should consider that the T1 relaxivity of the Gd-encapsulating liposome exhibits an upper limit due to limited proton exchange between the interior and exterior of liposomes because of the liposomal bilayer [8]. Not surprisingly, liposomes with surface Gd can generate equal or higher T1 relaxivities compared to conventional contrast agents. However, similar to dendrimers, the number of sites for Gd-chelate conjugation on the liposome is limited. Conjugation of Gd cannot exceed about 25 % of the number of surface lipid molecules due to destabilization of the liposomal membrane [6]. While this presents an upper limit to the T1 relaxivity, further improvements can be achieved by using very short chains of PEG on the liposomal surface to conjugate [9]. To further increase the T1 relaxivity of liposomes, recent efforts integrated both surface and encapsulated Gd into the same liposome resulting in a nanoparticle-based T1 relaxivity of 35,000 $(\text{mM s})^{-1}$, which is approximately 10^4 times higher than that of free Gd-chelate [10]. Overall, in addition to the prolonged blood residence time, the ability of PEGylated liposomes to escape blood circulation only in regions of leaky blood vessel provides a contrast agent that can be used as a marker of abnormal vascular permeability to detect compromised, diseased vasculature. Furthermore, it can also be used as an "exclusive" intravascular blood pool agent for interrogation of structural abnormalities of blood vessels.

Manganese nanoparticles have also recently been used in place of gadolinium nanoparticles [11]. One of the problems with Gd is its tendency to increase the incidence of nephrogenic systemic fibrosis in patients with renal disease or a recent liver transplantation. Manganese has been evaluated as an alternative T1 contrast agent for that reason. For instance, manganese has been encapsulated into doxorubicin liposomes in order to noninvasively monitor drug delivery [12]. This metal, however, also has its disadvantages, which include reduced water accessibility that leads to decreased relaxivity and a very high cardiotoxicity. Appropriate surfactants must be applied to reduce cardiotoxicity and to improve pharmacokinetics of the agent.

2.2 Superparamagnetic Iron Oxide (SPIO) Nanoparticles

Iron oxide nanoparticles are commonly used as T2-shortening contrast agents, which results in the production of dark contrast at the target site. In addition, they have been used in therapeutic applications, such as tumor ablation by hyperthermia. The magnetic properties of the contrast agent depend largely on the alloy used, which is often either maghemite or magnetite. There are two different categories of methods of production. One method of production involves the mixture of the iron oxide alloy with an acid and oleate to produce a sol gel. The size of the nanoparticles depends on the pH of the reaction mixture and the ratio of Fe(III) to Fe(II). The second method of production is the top-down fabrication method, in which nanoparticles are produced from a template or with an etching methodology [13]. An advantage of a top-down fabrication method is the high flexibility in which nanoparticles of different shapes can be produced. In addition, nanoparticles of a more defined size range can be manufactured with a top-down fabrication approach.

While iron oxide nanoparticles are easily manufactured using organic phase methods, it is often difficult to disperse them into aqueous media without aggregation. This is due to the fact that the nanocrystals are often highly hydrophobic. Therefore, a polymeric coating must be added to the nanoparticles to maintain size and allow for aqueous stability. A beneficial side effect is that polymeric coatings can also improve the circulation half-life of the nanoparticle in vivo. One common approach to modify iron oxide nanoparticles involves the use of oxysilanes, which interact with the nanoparticle surface through hydrogen bonds and provide a scaffolding for subsequent functionalization [14, 15]. These silanes can be modified with hydrophilic polymers to increase biocompatibility or functional groups to specifically add targeting moieties. Common hydrophilic surface coatings include polyethylene glycol (PEG), polyethylenimine (PEI), and chitosan. Conjugations can easily be completed through either *N*-hydroxysuccinimide (NHS) esterification or click chemistries.

In addition to the size of the iron oxide nanoparticles, the T2 relaxivity also depends on the shape and structure of the nanoparticle. It has been reported that iron oxide nanoworms display increased magnetic relaxivity in MRI compared to spheres due to enhanced orientation of the magnetic moments of the different iron oxide cores [16, 17]. Besides the effect of shape, previous studies have reported that clustering of iron oxide cores also significantly increases T2 relaxivity [18, 19]. For example, the T2 relaxivity of a chain-like nanoparticle composed of three iron oxide nanoparticles was 2.25-fold higher than that of its constituting spheres [20].

3 Designing Paramagnetic Nanoparticles for Improved In Vivo Performance

So far, we have listed a variety of materials and described a set of methods that can be used to produce paramagnetic nanoparticles. These nanoparticles have a range of applications, which include use as blood pool contrast agents, targeted contrast agents for tumor detection, and a means to destroy tumor tissue through hyperthermia or the controlled delivery of chemotherapy. Depending on the application, different pharmacokinetics and biodistribution profiles may be desired. Ideally, a blood pool agent should exhibit sufficiently long blood residence times, but be quickly cleared shortly thereafter to minimize the risk of undesired side effects. On the other hand, the requirements for a targeted contrast agent or therapeutic agent are different. For these purposes, one would want to maximize the half-life of the nanoparticle to increase the probability that the nanoparticle will reach its desired target. Extended blood circulation time endows the nanoparticle with more opportunities to escape the blood flow, move towards the vessel wall, and either bind to targeted receptors on the vascular bed or extravasate into the interstitial tissue at sites with leaky vasculature. Fortunately, the versatility of nanoparticle engineering, which allows for the production of nanoparticles of different geometries and surface chemistries, enables the precise tailoring of pharmacokinetics for the desired medical application. In particular, the effect of nanoparticle size, shape, and surface chemistry has been studied with respect to the nanoparticle's ability to highlight vasculature, identify disease sites, and impart a therapeutic effect to a disease region. In this section, we will discuss how these parameters play a role in guiding both the transport and uptake of a paramagnetic nanoparticle at the region of interest.

3.1 Effect of Nanoparticle Size on Pharmacology and Tumor Targeting

Nanoparticle size was one of the first parameters to be studied in relation to pharmacokinetics and biodistribution. Early nanoparticle research identified that the size of a liposome has a significant effect on its in vivo performance. Generally, because of their size that is greater than 5 nm, nanoparticles are not excreted through renal clearance mechanisms [21]. Instead, nanoparticles of sizes greater than 5 nm are cleared either through the liver or the spleen [22]. The exact size of the nanoparticle has direct consequences on its pharmacokinetics. For example, in the case of PEGylated liposomes, when the nanoparticle size is greater than 100 nm, a significant increase in hepatic and splenic macrophage uptake is observed. These same studies established that a size range of 60–100 nm is optimal to maximize blood circulation time [23–25]. For the design of paramagnetic nanoparticle blood pool contrast agents, sole consideration of the nanoparticle's pharmacokinetics is sufficient. The half-life should be sufficiently long to allow for MR imaging, but not of excessive duration to minimize the risk of side effects. In the design of targeted paramagnetic nanoparticle contrast agents to disease sites, however, it is also important to consider the effect of nanoparticle size on margination (i.e., ability of the nanoparticle to escape the blood flow and travel to the vessel wall), binding, and cellular uptake. The nanoparticle must be designed to maximize the probability that each of these processes will occur. In a study evaluating the margination of nanoparticles in a size range of 65–130 nm, it was determined that smaller nanoparticles are more likely to marginate to the blood vessel wall [26]. This observation can be explained through an understanding of the convective transport processes that govern the movement of a nanoparticle. Larger nanoparticles have a higher convective transport component, which influences them to follow the trajectory of the blood flow. As a result, fewer large nanoparticles have the opportunity to travel to wall of the blood vessel. Smaller nanoparticles, on the contrary, have a higher diffusive transport component. Thus, their transport is less influenced by the blood flow, which enables them to move radially throughout the blood vessel and interact with the vascular endothelium. At the same time, it is imperative not to choose a size, which is too small. A 30-nm liposome, for example, was observed to accumulate less in a tumor than a 100 nm liposome. Increased accumulation of the 30 nm liposome through targeting of a locally overexpressed receptor suggests that smaller liposomes are susceptible to washout by diffusive transport [27]. On the other hand, higher cellular uptake has been observed of larger nanoparticles. One explanation for this observation is that large ligand-functionalized nanoparticles have higher binding strength than small ligand-functionalized nanoparticles [28]. Therefore, there most likely exists an "optimal" size for a nanoparticle based on the conditions of the targeted microenvironment.

3.2 Effect of Nanoparticle Shape on Distribution and Tumor Targeting

Another way to alter the pharmacokinetics and targeting efficacy of a paramagnetic nanoparticle is to modify its shape. Incorporating an asymmetric shape results in decreased macrophage uptake, which thereby improves the nanoparticle's pharmacokinetics [29]. While the energy to phagocytose a spherical nanoparticle will be the same regardless of orientation, the energy required to phagocytose an asymmetric nanoparticle will differ depending on the angular orientation of the nanoparticle. For instance, more energy is required to phagocytose a rod shaped nanoparticle when its long axis is parallel to the cell membrane than when its short axis is parallel to the cell membrane. These energy calculations correspond well with in vivo assessments of cellular uptake and organ biodistribution, where rod-shaped nanoparticles are phagocytosed two times less when the aspect ratio is increased from 1.5 to 5 [30, 31]. Differences in nanoparticle uptake have also been observed between nanoparticles of different asymmetric shapes, including discoids, hemispheres, and ellipsoids [32]. Given the high degrees of freedom in which nanoparticle shape can be adjusted, more investigation can be done to identify the shape, which maximizes nanoparticle pharmacokinetics.

As discussed earlier, margination is a critical phenomenon that must be taken into consideration in the design of targeted paramagnetic nanoparticles (Fig. 3). Indeed, shape is a design parameter that significantly influences nanoparticle margination in blood vessels.

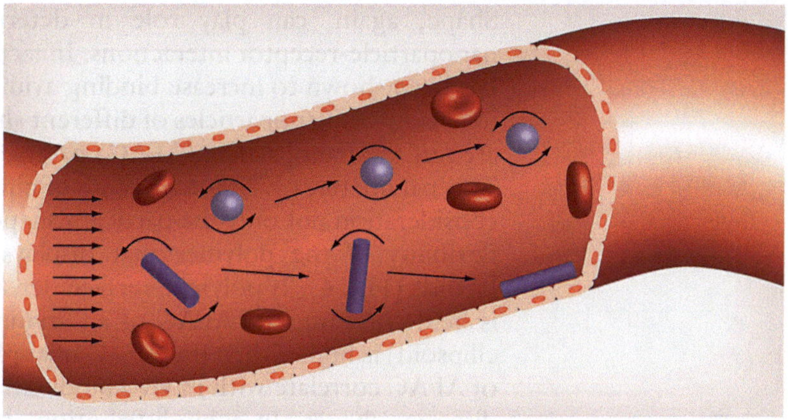

Fig. 3 Margination of flowing nanoparticles in microcirculation. The symmetry of a spherical nanoparticle results in its tendency to remain in the blood flow. Variable drag forces and torques which act on an oblate shaped nanoparticle, however, enable oscillatory movement within a blood vessel that increases meaningful interactions with the blood vessel wall. Reproduced with permission from reference [33]

Hydrodynamic forces affect both a nanoparticle's translational and rotational motion in different ways depending on the particle shape. Symmetric nanoparticles, such as spheres, have the same distribution of forces acting on them in all angular orientations. Because the distribution of hydrodynamic forces is equal, a symmetric nanoparticle will maintain a steady trajectory down the center of a blood vessel. In contrast, the drag forces and torques which act on asymmetric nanoparticles, such as rods or disks, will vary depending on the particle's angular orientation [34]. The end effect is a tumbling motion by such an asymmetric particle, which initiates an oscillatory trajectory that enables vessel wall interactions [35, 36]. Experimentally, it has been confirmed that three distinct classes of nanoparticles of different shapes—discoidal (aspect ratio (AR): 0.5), hemispherical, and ellipsoidal (AR: 0.5)—display increased margination behavior in comparison to spheres. Additionally, rod shaped particles have been observed to marginate seven times more than a spherical particle in a straight microchannel at a physiological flow rate (50 μL/min) [26]. Considering both pharmacokinetics and margination, it is suggested that asymmetry may improve the performance of long circulating blood pool paramagnetic iron oxide contrast agents.

For a targeted paramagnetic nanoparticle, however, margination is only the first necessary step that must occur. Once a targeted nanoparticle reaches the blood vessel wall, it must be able to bind to overexpressed receptors at the target site with high avidity. After the targeted nanoparticle forms ligand–receptor complexes, the cell must be able to internalize it with reasonable efficiency.

Shape, again, can play role in determining the strength of nanoparticle-receptor interactions. In fact, nanoparticle asymmetry has been shown to increase binding avidity. To compare the binding avidity of nanoparticles of different shapes, the active fractional area of the nanoparticle (AFAC) parameter was established [37]. This parameter, which is a measure of binding efficiency, takes into consideration not only the particle's shape, but also the length and flexibility of the polymer that displays the particle's targeting ligands (Fig. 4). If polymer surface density, length, and flexibility is held constant, the AFAC of an asymmetric particle (e.g., rod, ellipsoid) is higher than the AFAC of a sphere. Indeed, calculations of AFAC correlate with in vivo biodistribution of nanoparticles of different shapes. In a biodistribution study comparing antibody targeted nanorods with antibody targeted nanospheres, the targeted nanorods localized in the lungs seven times more than their targeted spherical counterparts [38]. Unfortunately, the nanoparticle shape, which imparts the highest binding avidity does not necessarily have the highest rate of uptake. Use of an oblong shape, as described earlier, leads to a decrease in phagocytosis by macrophages; this improves the pharmacokinetic profile of the nanoparticle. Under the same principle, active transport of oblong shaped nanoparticles at the target site is also decreased. When the nanoparticle's aspect ratio is very high, particle wrapping and

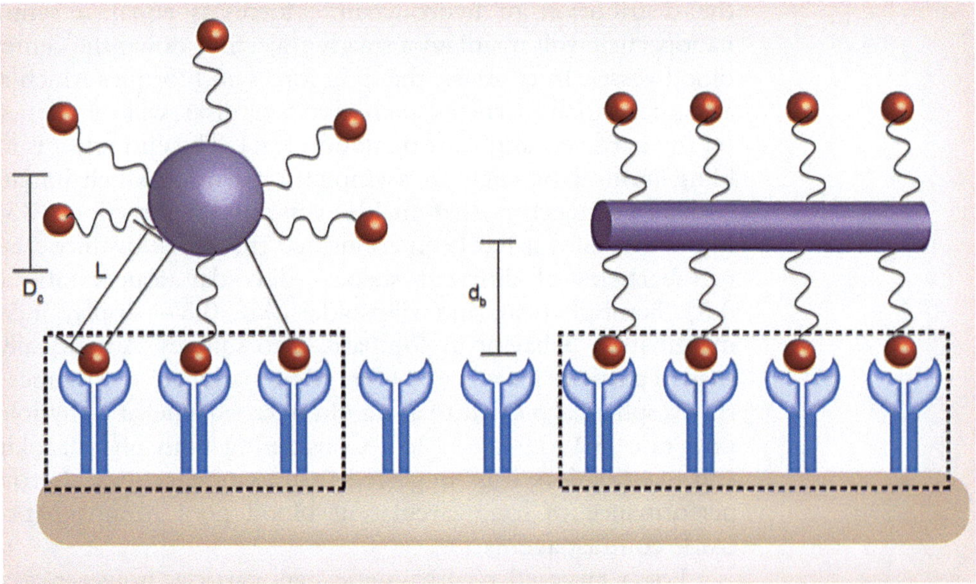

Fig. 4 Effect of shape on nanoparticle binding avidity. Shape, ligand length, and polymer flexibility all play a role in the active fractional area of a nano-carrier (AFAC). For a sphere, the AFAC is defined as $(L - d_B)/D_C$, where L is the length of the ligand, d_b is the binding distance between the nanoparticle and the receptor, and D_c is the diameter of the nano-carrier. For particles with equal surface area, the ligand length, binding distance, and shape affects AFAC. Reproduced with permission from reference [33]

engulfment is often arrested at specific angular orientations. As with the macrophages, increasing the contact area of the nanoparticle with the cell membrane also increases the energy required for endocytosis [39]. For instance, when the maximum contact area of a nanoparticle is increased by doubling is radius, the force necessary for nanoparticle translocation is increased threefold. In correspondence with this calculation, it has been found in endothelial cells that the internalization rate of targeted nanodiscs is lower than targeted nanospheres. Similarly, in epithelial cells, it has been found that the uptake of disk-shaped nanoparticles is 1.5–2 times higher than the uptake of rod-shaped nanoparticles. In agreement with the measured uptake rates, nearly double the energy was required to internalize the rod-shaped nanoparticles. Thus, careful experimentation must be conducted to identify the ideal shape that simultaneously provides extended blood circulation, maximized binding, and efficient and rapid internalization.

3.3 Effect of Nanoparticle Surface Chemistry on Biodistribution and Targeting

While size and shape are critical parameters that govern a nanoparticle's pharmacokinetics and biodistribution, the surface chemistry is a parameter that is equally important for consideration. To prolong the circulation half-life of a nanoparticle, hydrophilic polymers such as PEG are conjugated to the particle surface. Imparting hydrophilicity to the nanoparticle reduces recognition by the body's immune system, which allows it to circulate for a longer period of time. In addition to the type of polymer, the length and density of the polymer also play a role in dictating the nanoparticle's pharmacokinetics [40]. An excess of functional groups may augment immunogenicity, while sufficient polymer shielding must be present for aqueous stability.

At the same time, the characteristics of the polymer dictate the nanoparticle's binding avidity. As described previously, the binding efficiency can be expressed through the AFAC parameter, which is a function of nanoparticle aspect ratio, polymer length, and polymer flexibility. Increasing the polymer density, which simultaneously increases the density of the targeting ligand, also affects the nanoparticle's rate of cellular uptake. In addition, receptors, which are often presented in clusters, are more likely to interact with nanoparticles with a higher ligand surface density. Care must be taken, however, not to use an overwhelming number of targeting ligands. A very high number of targeting ligands could saturate the cell surface receptors. In response to an excess of ligand, cells have a tendency to decrease the recycling rate of receptors back to the cell surface. As a result, fewer receptors will be available to bind to extracellular nanoparticles. This saturation effect has been observed with HER2-targeted immunoliposomes, with which an increase of ligand surface density from 1 to 2 % doubled nanoparticle uptake in BT-474 cells [41]. A further increase of ligand surface density from 2 to 3 %, however, only led to a 10 % increase in BT-474 cells.

It is important to note that the ligand density which maximizes nanoparticle uptake depends on both the type of surface ligand and cell which overexpresses the receptor. In another study, an optimal ligand density of 14 mol% was identified for prostate-specific membrane antigen (PSMA) nanoparticles—both lower and higher ligand densities resulted in a decrease in uptake of the PSMA nanoparticles. Therefore, the ideal ligand density must be identified in a case-by-case basis.

3.4 Design Criteria of a Paramagnetic Nanoparticle

To recap the principal lessons from this section, several questions must be asked to appropriately design a paramagnetic nanoparticle contrast agent for its desired application. First, should the circulation of the nanoparticle be long or short? The answer to this question depends on whether the nanoparticle is a blood pool agent or a site-specific, targeted agent. Also, the window for therapeutic effectiveness must also be considered in optimization of the nanoparticle's pharmacokinetics. For a targeted agent, a nanoparticle, which is capable of marginating towards the blood vessel wall is necessary. To obtain the desired circulation half-life, the effect of size and shape should be carefully investigated for a particular nanoparticle in terms of its material and surface coating. With respect to surface coating, material, length, and density all critically affect nanoparticle pharmacokinetics. Second, what are the characteristics of the target site's microenvironment? The biobarriers at the target site must be taken into account for the nanoparticle's design. Given that nanoparticle transport is governed by both diffusion and convection, it is essential to investigate how influential blood flow and interstitial pressures are at the target site. Third, if the agent is targeted, which receptor is overexpressed by the target cells and what are the receptor's internalization dynamics? To maximize nanoparticle internalization at the target site, understanding of the receptor dynamics is paramount. Ligand density must be chosen to maximize nanoparticle uptake without compromising nanoparticle pharmacokinetics. Taking into consideration the specific pattern of receptor expression for the cell type, the appropriate nanoparticle size and shape should be chosen to maximize internalization. This can be evaluated through in vitro cell uptake studies for different nanoparticle classes followed by in vivo imaging (e.g., MRI, fluorescent reflectance imaging, fluorescence molecular tomography) and biodistribution studies to confirm targeted nanoparticle localization. It should be emphasized that there will not be one size, shape, and surface chemistry that will optimize the performance of all paramagnetic nanoparticles. Each of these three questions must be answered on a case-by-case basis to maximize the nanoparticle's diagnostic or therapeutic performance.

4 Biomedical Applications of Paramagnetic Nanoparticles

4.1 Targeted MR Imaging

In this section, the application of superparamagnetic lanthanide nanoparticles for T1-weighted targeted MR imaging and SPIO nanoparticles for T2-weighted targeted MR imaging will be discussed (Table 1). Although several lanthanides have been evaluated for their efficacy as T1 imaging agents, the majority of research focuses on targeted MR imaging agents formulated with gadolinium (Gd). As discussed, liposomes and dendrimers are the primary nano-structures used to ferry gadolinium to target sites. A primary use of Gd liposomes with targeted MR imaging is to evaluate tumor angiogenesis and inflammation [57, 63]. Receptors which are commonly targeted include intracellular adhesion molecule 1 (ICAM-1) [54], $\alpha_v\beta_3$ integrin [50, 58, 59], vascular cell adhesion molecule 1 (VCAM-1) [64], and CD105 [55]. The branched structure and narrow size distribution (~5–10 nm) of dendrimers enable the presentation of multiple contrast agents and/or targeting ligands. Design of Gd-based agents requires knowledge of several factors because signal intensity is not linearly related to the concentration of the imaging agent. When designing Gd-based agents, several factors need to be considered since

Table 1
Summary of nanoparticle platforms utilized for development of targeted paramagnetic nanoparticles

Nanoparticle platform	Ligand type	Target	Reference
Iron oxide nanoparticles	Peptide	Integrins	[42]
		uPA receptor	[43]
		EDB	[44]
	Antibody	Chemokine Receptor	[45]
		VEGF	[46]
	Protein	Transferrin Receptor	[47]
Iron oxide nanochains	Peptide	Integrins	[48]
Capsules (iron oxide)	Peptide	Integrins	[49]
Lipid-based (gadolinium)	Peptide	Integrin	[50, 51]
		Integrin/galectin-1	[52, 53]
	Antibody	ICAM-1	[54]
		CD105	[55]
	Small molecule	FA Receptor	[56]
Perfluorocarbon nanoparticles	Various	Various	[57]
	Peptide	Integrin	[58]
	Antibody	Integrin	[59]
LipoCEST	Peptide	Integrin	[60]
Dendrimers (Gd)	Small molecule	FA Receptor	[61, 62]

signal intensity at the target site is not linearly related to the concentration of the imaging moiety. For instance, the presentation of Gd atoms in a nanoparticle structure impacts the efficiency of nanoparticle MR probes [10, 65, 66]. "Activatable" Gd contrast agents also have been developed. In this application, an iron oxide core surrounded by a polymer coating containing Gd-DTPA quenches T1 contrast under normal physiological conditions. Inside an acidic environment, however, such as within the tumor microenvironment or inside a lysosome, Gd-DTPA, which generates T1 enhancement, is unquenched [67].

The notable advantages of SPIO nanoparticles include high micromolar detection thresholds, high T2* sensitivity, and the versatility to present a wide variety of ligands for cellular and molecular imaging [68]. The efficacy of iron oxide particles is governed by their magnetic properties that in turn are determined by their composition, size and morphology. To determine the optimal design parameters for SPIO nanoparticles, studies have been conducted to understand the effect of particle shape and size on the particle's magnetism and relaxivity [69, 70]. Deep tissue targeting with SPIOs has been used to image primary tumors by targeting urokinase plasminogen activator (uPA) [43, 44], transferrin receptors [47], HER2 receptors [71], chemokine receptor 4 [45]. In addition, vascular targeting of SPIO agents to integrins [42] or VEGFR [46] has been exploited for imaging of tumor-associated vasculature. A new nanoparticle class which is particularly effective for vascular targeting is a chain-like nanoparticle, which consists of several iron oxide nanospheres linked together in series [48]. The oblong shape of the iron oxide nanochain provides several advantages. First, margination, the ability of the nanoparticle to escape the blood flow and travel towards the blood vessel wall, is easier for oblong shaped nanoparticles. In fact, nanochains with an aspect ratio of about 3 were observed to marginate five times more than the parent constituent spheres (diameter = 20 nm) [48]. Second, the nanochain's oblong shape and high flexibility also imparts high binding avidity. In fact, a nanochain functionalized with RGD ligands was extremely effective in localizing at the site of micrometastatic lesions [48]. Third, the nanochain's magnetic relaxivity is higher than that of its spherical counterpart [20]. Indeed, this design has proven to be very accurate in finding and highlighting metastatic lesions via targeting of the $\alpha_v\beta_3$ integrin, which is overexpressed in the tumor vascular endothelium (Fig. 5) [72–78]. In a mouse model of breast cancer metastasis, 6 % of the nanochains injected in a mouse model congregated within a micrometastatic site of less than 1 mm in size [79]. On the contrary, less than 1 % of RGD-targeted iron oxide spheres was able to accumulate at the site of micrometastasis. This study emphasizes the need to rationally design the geometry of nanoparticles for tumor targeting to be successful.

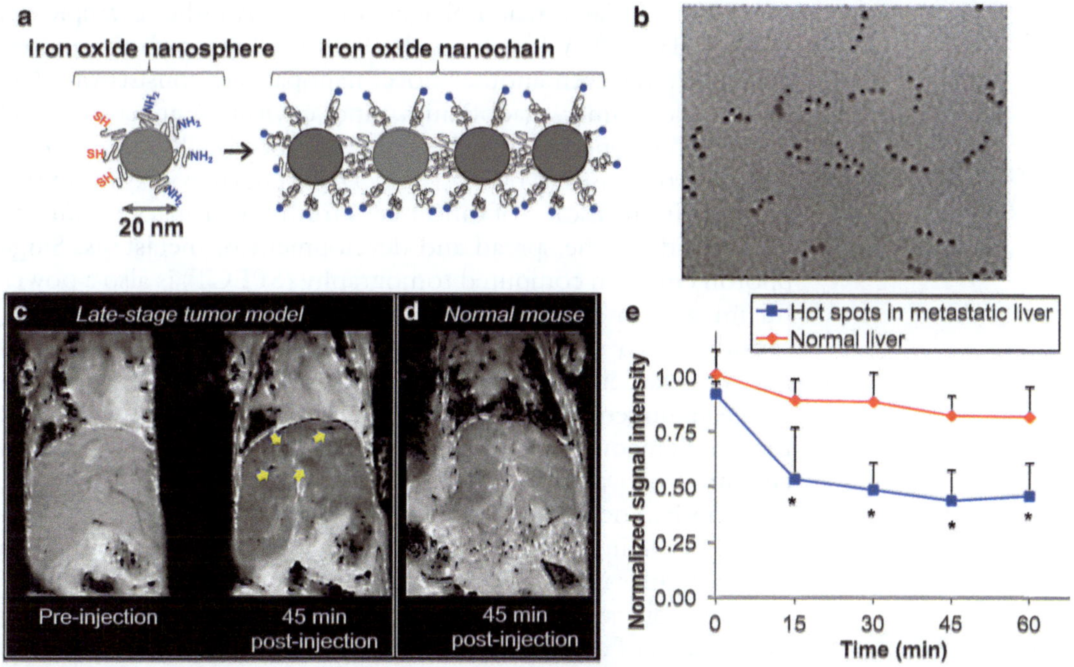

Fig. 5 Detection of breast cancer metastasis in liver using MRI and an iron oxide nanochain. (**a**) Illustration of the RGD-targeted nanochain particle and its constituent iron oxide nanospheres. (**b**) TEM image of the nanochain particles predominantly composed of four IO spheres. (**c**) Representative in vivo MR images of the liver in normal and metastasis-bearing mice were obtained using a 9.4 T MRI. Coronal *T*2-weighted images of the liver of a metastatic mouse before and 45 min after injection of the RGD-targeted nanochains. In the 45 min post-injection image, the *yellow arrows* show micrometastases of about 0.5 mm in size with increased contrast enhancement. (**d**) Coronal *T*2-weighted images of the liver of a normal mouse 45 min after injection of the nanochains. (**e**) Time course of the MR signal intensity in the liver hot spots was quantitatively evaluated. The absolute MR signal intensity in the metastatic lesions and the healthy liver was measured in manually drawn ROIs. The signal intensity in the hot spots or the entire healthy liver was normalized to the signal of an adjacent muscle (scale: 0–1). Since lower values indicate greater contrast in *T*2 images, normalized intensity values of 0 and 1 correspond to maximum and minimum contrast, respectively, compared to the pre-contrast intensity values (data presented as mean ± standard deviation; $n = 3$; each metastatic animal exhibited 2–4 hot spots; $^*P < 0.05$). Reproduced with permission from reference [48]

4.2 Multimodal Imaging with Enhanced Paramagnetic Nanoparticle Contrast Agents

The addition of radioactive tracers or optical probes to a paramagnetic nanoparticle further enhances its utility in medical diagnosis and imaging. With multimodal imaging using both positron emission tomography (PET) and MR imaging, treatment planning can be done with whole body imaging. Recent optical techniques enable the implementation of triggered therapeutic interventions, where the paramagnetic component of the nanoparticle enables tracking in vivo. For example, a dextran-coated SPIO nanoparticle co-labeled with ^{64}Cu and a near-infrared (NIR) fluorophore (Vivotag-680) was used to show the utility of combined Fluorescence Molecular Tomography (FMT) and PET for imaging of tumor associated macrophages [80, 81]. Another example of a multimodal PET-MR agent is the ^{111}In-perfluorocarbon nanoparticle [82]. Yet even another novel nanoparticle consists of a Cy5 labeled dendrimer, gadolinium, and environment-sensitive cell penetrating peptides, which is able to specifically target matrix metalloproteinases (MMPs) [83]. These enzymes play an important role in the escape of cancer cells from the primary tumor site, which leads to the spread and development of metastasis. Single photon emission computed tomography (SPECT) is also a powerful imaging modality of interest with extremely high contrast sensitivity. To enable use of this modality in conjunction with MR, $\alpha_v\beta_3$-targeted ^{99m}Tc-Gd nanoparticles have been developed to image angiogenesis. This powerful multimodal technique enabled the simultaneous visualization of the tumor mass and the neovasculature that was rapidly developing within the lesion [84].

Another new modality related to optical imaging is photoacoustic imaging (PAI), which has applications for both functional and molecular imaging [85]. PAI can generate images with endogeneous contrast that is obtained from differences in the absorption spectra of different tissue types. Molecular imaging, however, requires the use of exogenous contrast agents. A strong PAI agent will have strong light absorption. Examples of such agents are in the family of plasmonic nanoparticles, which include gold nanoshells, nanorods, and nanocages. PAI has been used in concert with MR imaging and Raman spectroscopy to acquire images of ovarian cancer (Fig. 6) [86]. In this study, NIRF-labeled SPIO nanoparticles targeted to Her-2/neu receptor generated significant contrast both with PAI and FMT.

4.3 Therapeutic Applications of Paramagnetic Nanoparticles

To comprehend the therapeutic potential, it is necessary to understand the response of a paramagnetic nanoparticle to an induced magnetic field. When magnetic nanoparticles are subjected to an external, oscillating magnetic field, there are two relaxation mechanisms (Brownian and Néel relaxation) that govern their magnetization response to align with the applied field. Brownian relaxation, the physical rotation of the entire nanoparticle, is typically the dominant relaxation mechanism for nanoparticles larger than about 25 nm. On the other hand, Néel relaxation (reorientation of the particle's magnetic moment with the applied field) is dominant for nanoparticles smaller than 15 nm. In addition, the dynamics of smaller nanoparticles are also dictated by superparamagnetism, which is the random flipping of magnetization in the absence of an external magnetic field [87]. This phenomenon is caused by the dominance of thermal fluctuations over dipole-dipole interactions on the particle's magnetization state. The critical size at which superparamagnetism plays a role is dependent on the material composition of the nanoparticle.

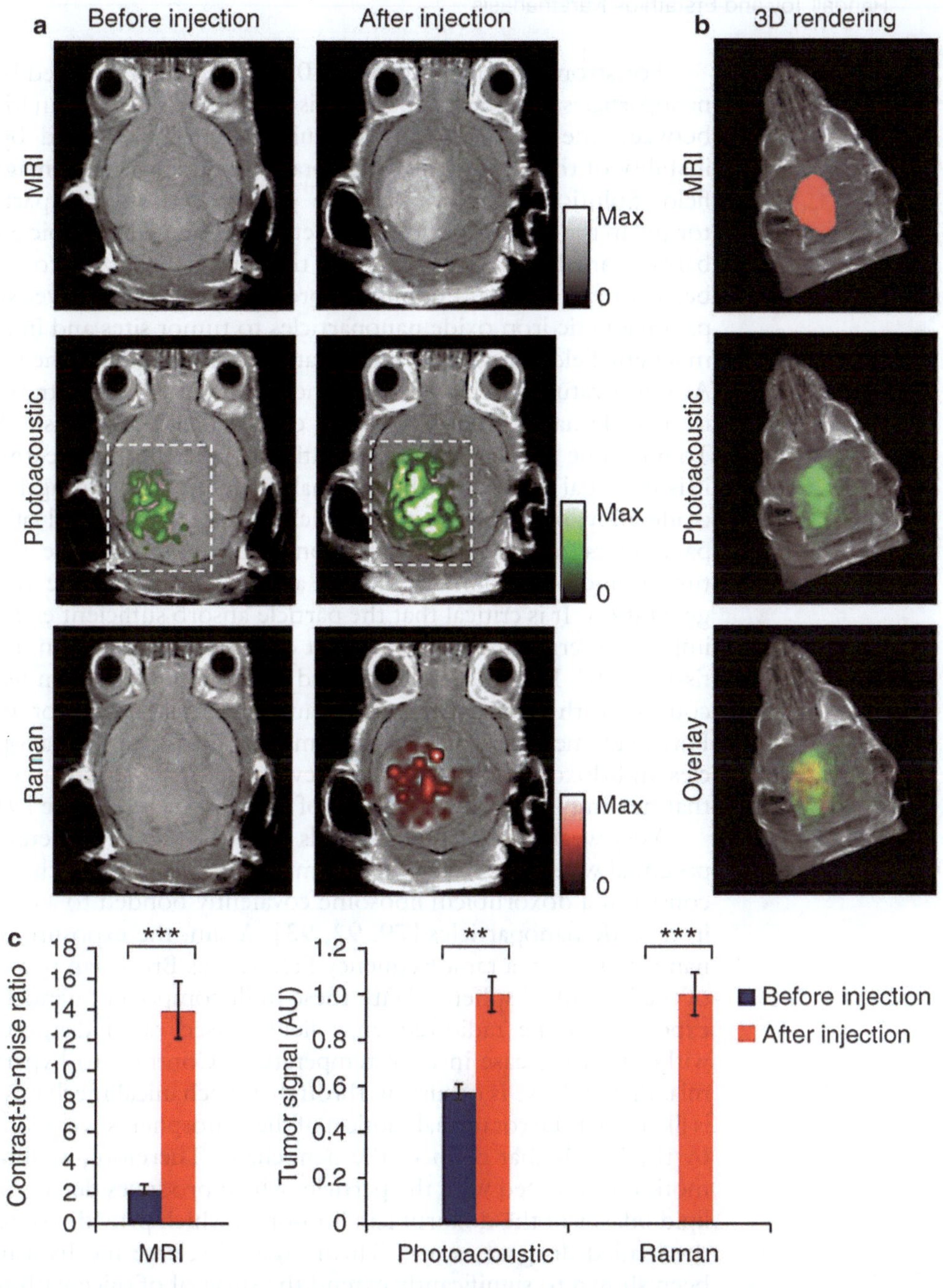

Fig. 6 A magnetic resonance imaging–photoacoustic imaging–Raman imaging (MPR) nanoparticle to delineate brain tumor margins in live mice. (**a**) Two-dimensional axial MIR, photoacoustic, and Raman images. The post-injection images for all modalities showed clear tumor visualization, where the imaging FOV is delineated by *dashed boxes*. (**b**) Three-dimensional rendering of MRI images with the tumor segmented (*red*, *top*), an overlay of 3D photoacoustic images (*green*) over the MRI (*middle*) and an overlay of MRI, the segmented tumor, and the photoacoustic images (*bottom*) demonstrate good co-localization of photoacoustic signal with the tumor. (**c**) Signal quantification reflects a significant increase from pre-injection to post-injection images in all three modalities ($n=4$ mice, data represent mean ± SEM, ***$P<0.001$, **$P<0.01$, 1-sided Student's *t*-test). Reproduced with permission from reference [86]

For strong magnetic fields (>10 mT), heat is generated by the nanoparticles. This heat generation is generated by Brownian friction between the particles and the fluid. Friction is caused by the inability of the nanoparticles to rotate in phase with the magnetic field. Solution viscosity, which is proportional to the particle's torque in the presence of the magnetic field, and anisotropic energy barriers are both responsible for this unsynchronized rotational behavior [88]. Thus, a popular approach has been to deliver superparamagnetic iron oxide nanoparticles to tumor sites and induce a magnetic field, which generates heat to thermally ablate the tumor. At temperatures of between 47 and 55 °C, the administration of iron oxide nanoparticles has been observed to ablate tissue [89]. To fine-tune the therapeutic potential of hyperthermia treatments, it is essential to choose the optimal magnetic field strength, iron oxide alloy, particle size, and particle surface coating. All of these parameters influence the interactions between the particle and the tumor microenvironment, which affects the magnitude of heat generation. It is critical that the particle absorb sufficient energy to impart a therapeutic effect without causing cytotoxicity in healthy tissues [90]. Hyperthermia-induced ablation has also been used in concert with chemotherapy to cause a larger antitumor effect. Polymersomes encapsulating paramagnetic iron oxide nanoparticles and doxorubicin have been developed; it has been suggested that heating improves the release of drug at the target site [91].

Very weak radiofrequency fields (<3 mT) also have therapeutic potential when used to energize a multicomponent nanochain that consist of a doxorubicin liposome covalently bonded to a chain of iron oxide nanoparticles [79, 92, 93]. Again, the exposure of the nanoparticles to a radiofrequency field causes Brownian relaxation of the individual spheres. With these multicomponent nanochains, exposure to the radiofrequency field caused rapid drug release without an increase in local temperature. Contrary to hyperthermia, drug release is occurring through a mechanical mechanism. It is likely that the rotational motion of the nanospheres is constrained by the bonds that connect the nanochain. Therefore, a vibratory motion is initiated with the particle, which produces defects in the lipid bilayer of the doxorubicin liposome, which provide routes for the loaded drug to escape. This triggered release mechanism has been shown to significantly extend the survival of mice with metastatic breast cancer [79].

Furthermore, magnetic targeting of iron oxide nanoparticles can significantly enhance selective deposition at a region of interest. Even though the concept of magnetic targeting exists for quite some time [94], it is not as simple as it appears. Major challenges include the attenuation of the magnetic field away from the magnet, which limits magnetic targeting to superficial tissues. Furthermore, these weak magnetic forces are appropriate only for relatively large magnetic particles with sizes in the range of microns.

However, a recent strategy utilized a combination of an external magnet and an embedded magnetizable micromesh to produce strong magnetic field gradients [95]. This system was successful in attracting individual 8-nm iron oxide nanoparticles in a human glioblastoma mouse model. Most notably, this magnetic targeting strategy synergistically amplified biochemical targeting of the nanoparticle to an overexpressed receptor. Magnetic targeting coupled to RGD-targeted magnetic nanoparticles resulted in significantly enhanced binding to $\alpha_v\beta_3$ integrins on angiogenic vessels in a glioma tumor model, which caused apoptosis of tumor blood vessels and promoted tumor regression (Fig. 7).

5 Future Prospects

The field of paramagnetic nanoparticles has an array of impactful applications, which include both highly sensitive diagnostic imaging and highly potent therapeutic strategies. There exist a large variety of paramagnetic materials, which allow for the fabrication of paramagnetic nanoparticles of different sizes and shapes.

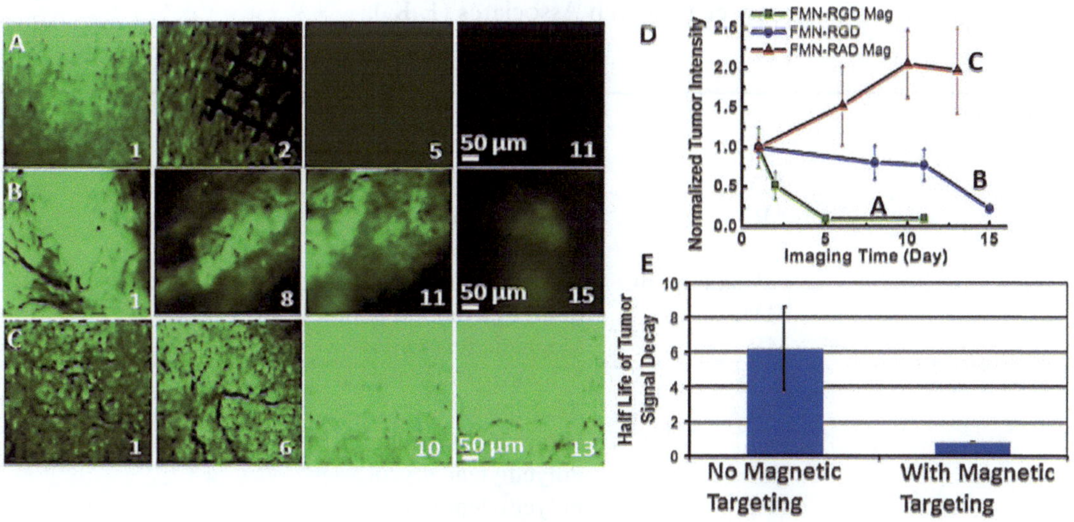

Fig. 7 RGD-targeted fluorescent magnetic nanoparticles (FMN-RGD) in combination with external magnetic targeting expedites tumor regression in a U87MG human glioblastoma xenograft mouse model. (**a–c**) EGFP-transfected tumor image channels show tumor intensity change within days of imaging for FMN-RGD together with magnetic targeting (**a**), FMN-RGD without magnetic targeting (**b**), and FMN-RAD under magnetic targeting (**c**). Day 1 is the day of FMN injection and magnetic targeting. The permanent magnet was placed for 2 h, and the Ni micromesh was removed the following day to better observe the imaging area. (**d**) The normalized tumor intensity vs. imaging time curves demonstrate that FMN-RGD together with magnetic targeting can expedite tumor regression ($n=3$, $P<0.05$). The fluorescence image intensity scales were set so that the brightest image within each series (**a–c**) was near saturation. (**e**) The half-lives of tumor signal decay demonstrate significantly faster tumor regression for FMN-RGD injection with magnetic targeting ($n=3$, 0.853 days) compared to without magnetic targeting ($n=3$, 6.197 days). Reproduced with permission from reference [95]

For progress to be made in this field, it is essential to consider not only the magnetic properties of the nanoparticle, but also how the nanoparticle's design affects its residence time and ability to interact with a target site. To enhance these properties, it is important to consider the surface chemistry, size, and the shape. For the utmost effectiveness, design parameters must be selected to take into account all of these considerations in relation to the microenvironment of the target site. To fully realize the potential of different classes of paramagnetic nanoparticles, it is essential that the particles be fully evaluated for pharmacokinetics, intravascular transport, cellular binding and uptake, and contrast sensitivity or therapeutic strength.

Acknowledgements

This work was supported by the National Cancer Institute of the National Institutes of Health (R01CA177716), the Clinical and Translational Science Collaborative of Cleveland (UL1TR000439) from the National Center for Advancing Translational Sciences component of the National Institutes of Health, and the Ohio Cancer Research Associates (E.K.).

Glossary

AFAC	Active fractional area of the nanoparticle
AR	Aspect ratio
FMT	Fluorescence molecular tomography
Gd gadolinium	iCAM-1 intracellular adhesion molecule 1
MMP	Matrix metalloproteinase
MR	Magnetic resonance
NHS	*N*-hydroxysuccinimide
NIR	Near-infrared
PAI	Photoacoustic imaging
PEG	Polyethylene glycol
PEI	Polyethylenimine
PET	Positron emission tomography
PSMA	Prostate-specific membrane antigen
RES	Reticuloendothelial system
SPECT	Single photon emission computed tomography
SPIO	Superparamagnetic iron oxide
uPA	Urokinase plasma activator
vCAM	Vascular cell adhesion molecule 1

References

1. Castelli DD et al (2014) Design and testing of paramagnetic liposome-based CEST agents for MRI visualization of payload release on pH-induced and ultrasound stimulation. J Biol Inorg Chem 19(2):207–214
2. Longmire MR et al (2014) Dendrimers as high relaxivity MR contrast agents. Wiley Interdiscip Rev Nanomed Nanobiotechnol 6(2):155–162
3. Kobayashi H, Brechbiel MW (2005) Nano-sized MRI contrast agents with dendrimer cores. Adv Drug Deliv Rev 57(15):2271–2286
4. Cheng Z, Thorek DL, Tsourkas A (2010) Gadolinium-conjugated dendrimer nanoclusters as a tumor-targeted T1 magnetic resonance imaging contrast agent. Angew Chem Int Ed Engl 49(2):346–350
5. Huang CH et al (2012) Biodegradable polydisulfide dendrimer nanoclusters as MRI contrast agents. ACS Nano 6(11):9416–9424
6. Mulder WJ et al (2004) A liposomal system for contrast-enhanced magnetic resonance imaging of molecular targets. Bioconjug Chem 15(4): 799–806
7. Tilcock C et al (1989) Liposomal Gd-DTPA: preparation and characterization of relaxivity. Radiology 171(1):77–80
8. Ghaghada K et al (2008) T1 relaxivity of core-encapsulated gadolinium liposomal contrast agents--effect of liposome size and internal gadolinium concentration. Acad Radiol 15(10):1259–1263
9. Storrs RW et al (1995) Paramagnetic polymerized liposomes as new recirculating MR contrast agents. J Magn Reson Imaging 5(6): 719–724
10. Ghaghada KB et al (2009) New dual mode gadolinium nanoparticle contrast agent for magnetic resonance imaging. PLoS One 4(10): e7628
11. Lee SH et al (2014) Paramagnetic inorganic nanoparticles as T1 MRI contrast agents. Wiley Interdiscip Rev Nanomed Nanobiotechnol 6(2):196–209
12. Ponce AM et al (2007) Magnetic resonance imaging of temperature-sensitive liposome release: drug dose painting and antitumor effects. J Natl Cancer Inst 99(1):53–63
13. Chen JS et al (2010) Top-down fabrication of alpha-Fe2O3 single-crystal nanodiscs and microparticles with tunable porosity for largely improved lithium storage properties. J Am Chem Soc 132(38):13162–13164
14. Yathindranath V et al (2013) One-pot synthesis of iron oxide nanoparticles with functional silane shells: a versatile general precursor for conjugations and biomedical applications. Langmuir 29(34):10850–10858
15. McCarthy SA, Davies GL, Gun'ko YK (2012) Preparation of multifunctional nanoparticles and their assemblies. Nat Protoc 7(9): 1677–1693
16. Park JH et al (2008) Magnetic iron oxide nanoworms for tumor targeting and imaging. Adv Mater 20(9):1630–1635
17. Gossuin Y et al (2010) NMR relaxation and magnetic properties of superparamagnetic nanoworms. Contrast Media Mol Imaging 6:318. doi:10.1002/cmmi.387
18. Lu J et al (2009) Manganese ferrite nanoparticle micellar nanocomposites as MRI contrast agent for liver imaging. Biomaterials 30(15): 2919–2928
19. Ai H et al (2005) Magnetite-loaded polymeric micelles as ultrasensitive magnetic-resonance probes. Adv Mater 17(16):1949–1952
20. Peiris PM et al (2011) Assembly of linear nano-chains from iron oxide nanospheres with asymmetric surface chemistry. PLoS One 6(1): e15927
21. Owens DE 3rd, Peppas NA (2006) Opsonization, biodistribution, and pharmacokinetics of polymeric nanoparticles. Int J Pharm 307(1):93–102
22. Moghimi SM, Szebeni J (2003) Stealth liposomes and long circulating nanoparticles: critical issues in pharmacokinetics, opsonization and protein-binding properties. Prog Lipid Res 42(6):463–478
23. Litzinger DC et al (1994) Effect of liposome size on the circulation time and intraorgan distribution of amphipathic poly(ethylene glycol)-containing liposomes. Biochim Biophys Acta 1190(1):99–107
24. Mayer LD et al (1989) Influence of vesicle size, lipid composition, and drug-to-lipid ratio on the biological activity of liposomal doxorubicin in mice. Cancer Res 49(21):5922–5930
25. Nagayasu A, Uchiyama K, Kiwada H (1999) The size of liposomes: a factor which affects their targeting efficiency to tumors and therapeutic activity of liposomal antitumor drugs. Adv Drug Deliv Rev 40(1-2):75–87
26. Toy R et al (2011) The effects of particle size, density and shape on margination of nanoparticles in microcirculation. Nanotechnology 22(11):115101
27. Toy R et al (2013) Multimodal in vivo imaging exposes the voyage of nanoparticles in tumor microcirculation. ACS Nano 7(4): 3118–3129

28. Kibria G et al (2013) The effect of liposomal size on the targeted delivery of doxorubicin to Integrin alphavbeta3-expressing tumor endothelial cells. Biomaterials 34(22):5617–5627
29. Champion JA, Mitragotri S (2006) Role of target geometry in phagocytosis. Proc Natl Acad Sci U S A 103(13):4930–4934
30. Arnida et al (2011) Geometry and surface characteristics of gold nanoparticles influence their biodistribution and uptake by macrophages. Eur J Pharm Biopharm 77(3):417–423
31. Huang X et al (2011) The shape effect of mesoporous silica nanoparticles on biodistribution, clearance, and biocompatibility in vivo. ACS Nano 5(7):5390–5399
32. Lee SY, Ferrari M, Decuzzi P (2009) Shaping nano-/micro-particles for enhanced vascular interaction in laminar flows. Nanotechnology 20:495101 (11pp)
33. Toy R et al (2014) Shaping cancer nanomedicine: the effect of particle shape on the in vivo journey of nanoparticles. Nanomedicine (Lond) 9(1):121–134
34. Gave E, Shapiro M (1997) Particles in a shear flow near a solid wall: effect of nonsphericity on forces and velocities. Int J Multiphas Flow 23:155
35. Adriani G et al (2012) The preferential targeting of the diseased microvasculature by disk-like particles. Biomaterials 33(22):5504–5513
36. Doshi N et al (2010) Flow and adhesion of drug carriers in blood vessels depend on their shape: a study using model synthetic microvascular networks. J Control Release 146(2): 196–200
37. Ghaghada KB et al (2005) Folate targeting of drug carriers: a mathematical model. J Control Release 104(1):113–128
38. Kolhar P et al (2013) Using shape effects to target antibody-coated nanoparticles to lung and brain endothelium. Proc Natl Acad Sci U S A 110:10753
39. Dasgupta S, Auth T, Gompper G (2014) Shape and orientation matter for the cellular uptake of nonspherical particles. Nano Lett 14(2): 687–693
40. Valencia PM et al (2013) Microfluidic platform for combinatorial synthesis and optimization of targeted nanoparticles for cancer therapy. ACS Nano 7(12):10671–10680
41. Stefanick JF et al (2013) A systematic analysis of peptide linker length and liposomal polyethylene glycol coating on cellular uptake of peptide-targeted liposomes. ACS Nano 7(4): 2935–2947
42. Zhang C et al (2007) Specific targeting of tumor angiogenesis by RGD-conjugated ultrasmall superparamagnetic iron oxide particles using a clinical 1.5-T magnetic resonance scanner. Cancer Res 67(4):1555–1562
43. Lee GY et al (2013) Theranostic nanoparticles with controlled release of gemcitabine for targeted therapy and MRI of pancreatic cancer. ACS Nano 7(3):2078–2089
44. Park J et al (2012) Fibronectin extra domain B-specific aptide conjugated nanoparticles for targeted cancer imaging. J Control Release 163(2):111–118
45. He Y et al (2012) Anti-CXCR4 monoclonal antibody conjugated to ultrasmall superparamagnetic iron oxide nanoparticles in an application of MR molecular imaging of pancreatic cancer cell lines. Acta Radiol 53(9):1049–1058
46. Hsieh WJ et al (2012) In vivo tumor targeting and imaging with anti-vascular endothelial growth factor antibody-conjugated dextran-coated iron oxide nanoparticles. Int J Nanomedicine 7:2833–2842
47. Kresse M et al (1998) Targeting of ultrasmall superparamagnetic iron oxide (USPIO) particles to tumor cells in vivo by using transferrin receptor pathways. Magn Reson Med 40: 236–242
48. Peiris PM et al (2012) Imaging metastasis using an integrin-targeting chain-shaped nanoparticle. ACS Nano 6(10):8783–8795
49. John R et al (2012) Targeted multifunctional multimodal protein-shell microspheres as cancer imaging contrast agents. Mol Imaging Biol 14(1):17–24
50. Mulder WJ et al (2005) MR molecular imaging and fluorescence microscopy for identification of activated tumor endothelium using a bimodal lipidic nanoparticle. FASEB J 19(14): 2008–2010
51. Mulder WJ et al (2007) Early in vivo assessment of angiostatic therapy efficacy by molecular MRI. FASEB J 21(2):378–383
52. Kluza E et al (2012) Dual-targeting of alphavbeta3 and galectin-1 improves the specificity of paramagnetic/fluorescent liposomes to tumor endothelium in vivo. J Control Release 158(2): 207–214
53. Kluza E et al (2010) Synergistic targeting of alphavbeta3 integrin and galectin-1 with heteromultivalent paramagnetic liposomes for combined MR imaging and treatment of angiogenesis. Nano Lett 10(1):52–58
54. Paulis LEM et al (2012) Targeting of ICAM-1 on vascular endothelium under static and shear stress conditions using a liposomal Gd-based MRI contrast agent. J Nanobiotechnol 10:25
55. Zhang D et al (2009) MR imaging of tumor angiogenesis using sterically stabilized

Gd-DTPA liposomes targeted to CD105. Eur J Radiol 70(1):180–189

56. Kamaly N et al (2009) Folate receptor targeted bimodal liposomes for tumor magnetic resonance imaging. Bioconjug Chem 20:648–655
57. Kaneda MM et al (2009) Perfluorocarbon nanoemulsions for quantitative molecular imaging and targeted therapeutics. Ann Biomed Eng 37(10):1922–1933
58. Schmieder AH et al (2008) Three-dimensional MR mapping of angiogenesis with alpha5beta1(alpha nu beta3)-targeted theranostic nanoparticles in the MDA-MB-435 xenograft mouse model. FASEB J 22(12): 4179–4189
59. Boles KS et al (2010) MR angiogenesis imaging with Robo4- vs. alphaVbeta3-targeted nanoparticles in a B16/F10 mouse melanoma model. FASEB J 24(11):4262–4270
60. Flament J et al (2013) In vivo CEST MR imaging of U87 mice brain tumor angiogenesis using targeted LipoCEST contrast agent at 7 T. Magn Reson Med 69(1):179–187
61. Konda SD et al (2001) Specific targeting of folate-dendrimer MRI contrast agents to the high affinity folate receptor expressed in ovarian tumor xenografts. MAGMA 12:104–113
62. Swanson SD et al (2008) Targeted gadolinium-loaded dendrimer nanoparticles for tumor-specific magnetic resonance contrast enhancement. Int J Nanomedicine 3(2): 201–210
63. Langereis S et al (2013) Paramagnetic liposomes for molecular MRI and MRI-guided drug delivery. NMR Biomed 26(7):728–744
64. Kelly KA et al (2005) Detection of vascular adhesion molecule-1 expression using a novel multimodal nanoparticle. Circ Res 96(3): 327–336
65. Laurent S et al (2008) Paramagnetic liposomes: inner versus outer membrane relaxivity of DPPC liposomes incorporating lipophilic gadolinium complexes. Langmuir 24:4347–4351
66. Laurent S et al (2008) Relaxivities of paramagnetic liposomes: on the importance of the chain type and the length of the amphiphilic complex. Eur Biophys J 37(6):1007–1014
67. Santra S et al (2012) Gadolinium-encapsulating iron oxide nanoprobe as activatable NMR/MRI contrast agent. ACS Nano 6(8):7281–7294
68. Bulte JW, Kraitchman DL (2004) Iron oxide MR contrast agents for molecular and cellular imaging. NMR Biomed 17(7):484–499
69. Jun Y-W, Seo J-W, Cheon J (2008) Nanoscaling laws of magnetic nanoparticles and their applicabilities in biomedical sciences. Acc Chem Res 41(2):179–189
70. Smolensky ED et al (2013) Scaling laws at the nano size: the effect of particle size and shape on the magnetism and relaxivity of iron oxide nanoparticle contrast agents. J Mater Chem B Mater Biol Med 1(22):2818–2828
71. Artemov D et al (2003) MR molecular imaging of the Her-2/neu receptor in breast cancer cells using targeted iron oxide nanoparticles. Magn Reson Med 49(3):403–408
72. Gay LJ, Felding-Habermann B (2011) Contribution of platelets to tumour metastasis. Nat Rev Cancer 11(2):123–134
73. Felding-Habermann B et al (1996) Role of beta3 integrins in melanoma cell adhesion to activated platelets under flow. J Biol Chem 271(10):5892–5900
74. McCarty OJ et al (2000) Immobilized platelets support human colon carcinoma cell tethering, rolling, and firm adhesion under dynamic flow conditions. Blood 96(5):1789–1797
75. Arnaout MA, Mahalingam B, Xiong JP (2005) Integrin structure, allostery, and bidirectional signaling. Annu Rev Cell Dev Biol 21: 381–410
76. Felding-Habermann B et al (2001) Integrin activation controls metastasis in human breast cancer. Proc Natl Acad Sci U S A 98(4): 1853–1858
77. Lorger M et al (2009) Activation of tumor cell integrin alphavbeta3 controls angiogenesis and metastatic growth in the brain. Proc Natl Acad Sci U S A 106(26):10666–10671
78. Desgrosellier JS, Cheresh DA (2010) Integrins in cancer: biological implications and therapeutic opportunities. Nat Rev Cancer 10(1):9–22
79. Peiris PM et al (2014) Treatment of cancer micrometastasis using a multicomponent chain-like nanoparticle. J Control Release 173:51–58
80. Nahrendorf M et al (2008) Nanoparticle PET-CT imaging of macrophages in inflammatory atherosclerosis. Circulation 117(3): 379–387
81. Nahrendorf M et al (2010) Hybrid PET-optical imaging using targeted probes. Proc Natl Acad Sci U S A 107(17):7910–7915
82. Hu G et al (2007) Imaging of Vx-2 rabbit tumors with alpha(nu)beta3-integrin-targeted 111In nanoparticles. Int J Cancer 120(9): 1951–1957
83. Olson ES et al (2010) Activatable cell penetrating peptides linked to nanoparticles as dual probes for in vivo fluorescence and MR imaging

of proteases. Proc Natl Acad Sci U S A 107(9):4311–4316
84. Lijowski M et al (2009) High sensitivity: high-resolution SPECT-CT/MR molecular imaging of angiogenesis in the Vx2 model. Invest Radiol 44(1):15–22
85. Kim G et al (2007) Indocyanine-green-embedded PEBBLEs as a contrast agent for photoacoustic imaging. J Biomed Opt 12(4): 044020
86. Kircher MF et al (2012) A brain tumor molecular imaging strategy using a new triple-modality MRI-photoacoustic-Raman nanoparticle. Nat Med 18(5):829–834
87. Rumenapp C, Gleich B, Haase A (2012) Magnetic nanoparticles in magnetic resonance imaging and diagnostics. Pharm Res 29(5): 1165–1179
88. Reeves DB, Weaver JB (2012) Simulations of magnetic nanoparticle Brownian motion. J Appl Phys 112(12):124311
89. Hilger I et al (2002) Thermal ablation of tumors using magnetic nanoparticles: an in vivo feasibility study. Invest Radiol 37(10):580–586
90. Giustini AJ et al (2010) Magnetic nanoparticle hyperthermia in cancer treatment. Nano Life 1(01n02):17
91. Oliveira H et al (2013) Magnetic field triggered drug release from polymersomes for cancer therapeutics. J Control Release 169(3): 165–170
92. Peiris PM et al (2012) Enhanced delivery of chemotherapy to tumors using a multicomponent nanochain with radio-frequency-tunable drug release. ACS Nano 6(5):4157–4168
93. Peiris PM et al (2014) On-command drug release from nanochains inhibits growth of breast tumors. Pharm Res 31:1460
94. Meyers PH, Cronic F, Nice CM Jr (1963) Experimental approach in the use and magnetic control of metallic iron particles in the lymphatic and vascular system of dogs as a contrast and isotopic agent. Am J Roentgenol Radium Ther Nucl Med 90:1068–1077
95. Fu A et al (2012) Fluorescent magnetic nanoparticles for magnetically enhanced cancer imaging and targeting in living subjects. ACS Nano 6(8):6862–6869

Chapter 7

Silica Nanomaterials

Katsuhiko Ariga and Qingmin Ji

Abstract

Ultrafine mechanisms are efficiently working in biological systems. Fabrication of desired nanostructured materials has been paid much attention in biology, biochemistry, and pharmaceutical sciences. For these demands, nanostructured inorganic materials have to be more utilized in biological pharmaceutical fields. Among numerous candidates of inorganic materials, silica is the strongest candidate for use because silica is very abundant in nature and has low toxicity with huge knowledge on nanostructure fabrication. In this chapter, mesoporous silica and layer-by-layer assembly are first introduced, followed by description of emerging materials such as silica flake-shell capsule and silica nanostructure plate with examples for their usages in drug delivery and gene transfections.

Key words Mesoporous silica, Layer-by-layer assembly, Nanostructure, Drug delivery, Gene transfection

1 Introduction

Ultrafine mechanisms are efficiently working in biological systems. With understanding these activities more deeply, the importance of micro and nanostructures in life activities has been realized. Therefore, fabrication of desired nanostructured materials has been paid much attention in biology, biochemistry, and pharmaceutical sciences [1–6].

Not limited to such biological fields, considerable amounts of efforts have been made for fabrication of nanometer-scale structures for ultrafine devices. Accumulated technologies have been well combined with demands from biological sciences. Several excellent top-down-type approaches including photolithography and electron-beam lithography have been so far used to provide fine micro-structures. In addition, bottom-up approaches, which rely on molecular-self assemblies in supramolecular process, have been also actively investigated [7–19].

Especially, organic materials have huge varieties in their properties that are related with many interesting chemical, physical, and biological functions. However, they do not always have mechanical

Zheng-Rong Lu and Shinji Sakuma (eds.), *Nanomaterials in Pharmacology*, Methods in Pharmacology and Toxicology,
DOI 10.1007/978-1-4939-3121-7_7, © Springer Science+Business Media New York 2016

stability necessary for application under harsh conditions and hardness required for precise fabrication. In contrast, most of inorganic substances have high mechanical strength. Nanostructured inorganic materials have to be more aggressively utilized in biological pharmaceutical fields.

Among numerous candidates of inorganic materials for biorelated application, silica is the strongest candidate for use. Silica is very abundant in nature and has low toxicity. Fabrication of nanostructured silica has been widely researched. From these advantageous features, we focus on nanostructured silica in this chapter. We first introduce general silica nanostructures: mesoporous silica, and then the novel nanostructures from layer-by-layer assembly. Finally we emphasize on new developed emerging materials such as silica flake-shell capsule and silica nanostructure plate. Their several functions including drug delivery and gene transfections are described.

2 Mesoporous Silica

Mesoporous materials such as mesoporous silica have been widely used as drug carriers. To guarantee the therapeutic efficacy, control release of drugs from pores to outside is preferred through tailoring silica channels.

2.1 Fundamentals of Mesoporous Silica

Not limited to pharmacological science and technology, mesoporous materials with well-defined geometry have been recently paid more attention due to their large potential in practical applications such as catalysis, adsorption, separation, and so on [20–26]. According to the IUPAC classification, these materials are defined as a porous material having a diameter in the size range of from 2 to 50 nm (Fig. 1). In 1990, Kuroda and coworkers reported preparation of the mesoporous silica from folded sheet material (FSM-16) [27]. Great progress of the mesoporous material was brought by Mobil group who invented the M41S family of materials such as hexagonal MCM-41 and cubic MCM-48 [28]. These materials have high specific surface area and pore volume. These findings have been followed by research efforts on various types of mesoporous materials.

Recent studies have revealed that new categories of mesoporous materials can be synthesized by wise selection of structure-directing molecules and/or silica-source materials. One typical example is periodic mesoporous organosilicate (PMO) [29]. Synthesis of this category of materials uses organic molecules that have a multiple alkoxysilane groups as a silicate source with variety of organic functional moieties. According to this approach, mesoporous structures with organic functional group can be obtained.

Preparation of non-silica material with a mesoporous structure also played an important role particularly in advancements of

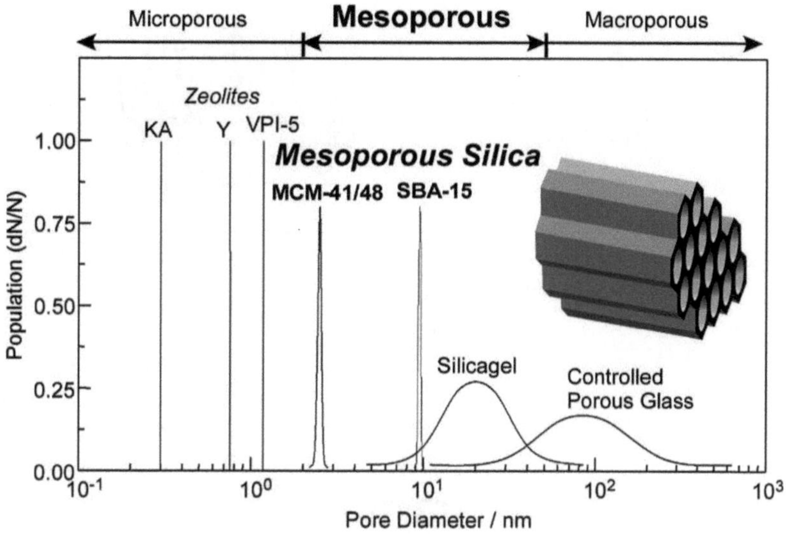

Fig. 1 Classification of porous materials: MCM-41, MCM-48, and SBA15 representative mesoporous silica materials

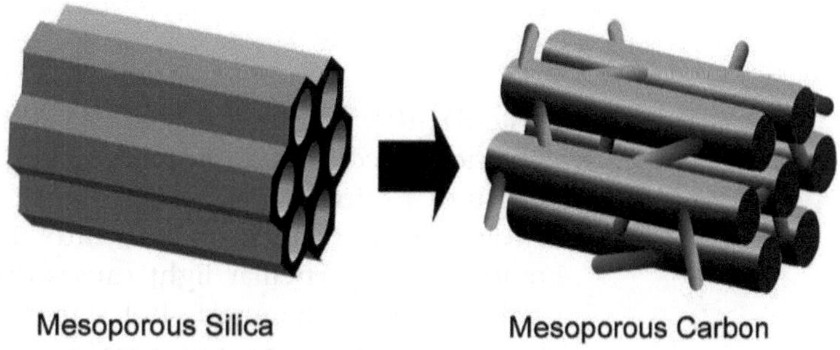

Fig. 2 Conversion from mesoporous silica to mesoporous carbon

mesoporous materials. For example, mesoporous carbon materials prepared as replica of mesoporous silica have been widely used (Fig. 2) [30–33]. Not limited to mesoporous carbon, preparation of mesoporous material of non-oxide material containing carbon nitride [34], boron nitride [35], and metals [36, 37] have been reported. In addition, a mesoporous hybrid material with bio-related components has been also researched as materials related with pharmacological science and technology.

2.2 Gate-Controlled Materials Release

Well-defined pore structures with larger specific volumes of pore spaces in mesoporous materials are apparently suitable for carriers for drug delivery. Addition of gate opening/closure functions at the pore entrance on the material would lead to development of controlled drug delivery systems [38, 39].

As a pioneering work, Fujiwara and coworkers achieved photo-control of release of drug molecules stored in mesoporous silica

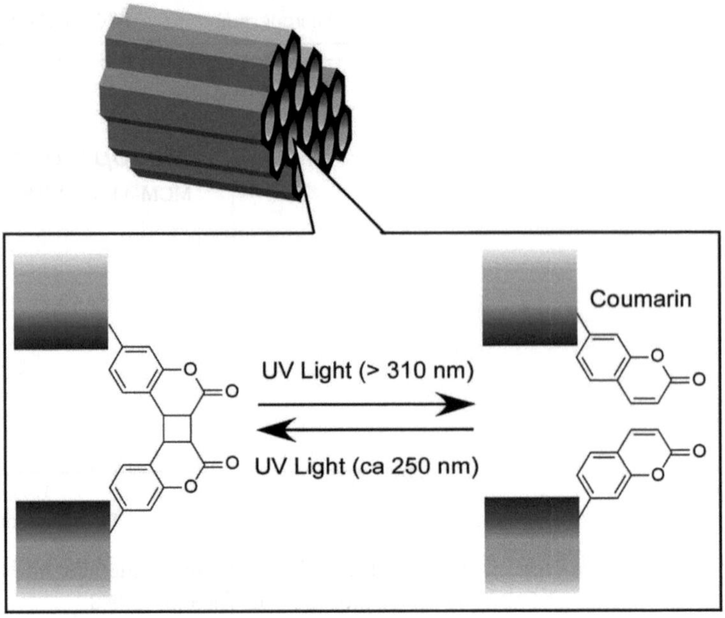

Fig. 3 Gate control at mesoporous media through photoactive coumarin dimerization

(Fig. 3) [40]. They prepared MCM-41 mesoporous silica, which was functionalized with a photoactive coumarin as a gate component through grafting only in mesopore exit. Guest drugs such as cholestane were incorporated into the mesopores of silica. The radiation by particular light causes dimerization of coumarin for stably trapping the guest cholestane. Release of cholestane can be induced through de-dimerization of the coumarin moieties by radiation due to light with different wavelength.

Lin and coworkers applied colloid-gate systems for controlled release of drugs such as a neurotransmitter vancomycin from functionalized mesoporous silica (Fig. 4) [41]. The mesoporous silica functionalized with thiol-related groups can trap drugs such as neurotransmitter molecules through formation of covalent disulfide linkage with thiol-functionalized CdS nanoparticles. Cleavage of the disulfide linkage with appropriate reducing reagents such as mercaptoethanol and dithiothreitol removes CdS capping to release drugs to outside. Biocompatibility of the proposed systems was also confirmed.

Martínez-Máñez and coworkers developed mesoporous silica MCM-41 functionalized with polyamine segments as a plunge of release of model drugs such as $[Ru(bipy)_3]^{2+}$ [42]. The polyamine moieties are fully protonated at low pH conditions where release of cationic guest molecules was completely blocked. In contrast, partial protonation of the polyamines are induced at neutral and slightly basic pH conditions, much suppressing pore blockage

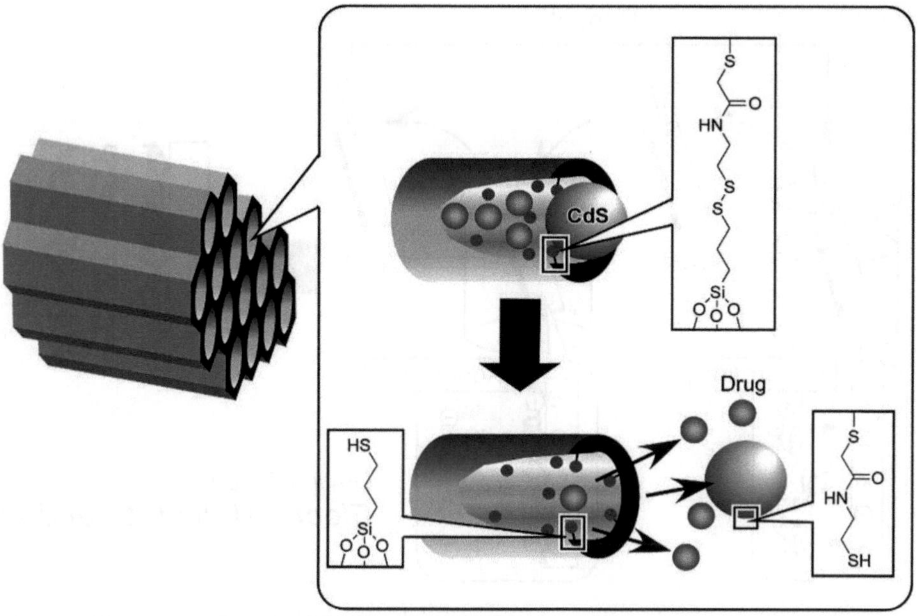

Fig. 4 Gate-control at mesoporous media by colloid-capping

effects and inducing a massive delivery of the $[Ru(bipy)_3]^{2+}$ guest from the pores to the solution.

Not limited to these pioneering examples, functional mesoporous silica materials are attractive materials to realize gate-controlled drug delivery. Especially, functionalization of silica surface is well established, and thus, huge variety in designing these functional materials is ensured.

3 Layer-by-Layer Assembly

When we design sophisticated drug release systems, organization of functional materials into hierarchic structures is often required. Layer-by-layer (LbL) assembly technique is one of the most frequently used methods in organization of functional materials [43–52].

3.1 Fundamentals of Layer-by-Layer Assembly

The principle of LbL assembly is based on alternate adsorption of functional components between which certain kinds of interactions such as electrostatic interaction, hydrogen bonding and metal coordination play key roles in selective adsorption (Fig. 5). Although basic principles and related mechanism of this method was previously suggested by several researchers [53, 54], Decher and Hong first reported LbL films composed of positively and negatively charged bola-amphiphiles [55], that was soon applied to LbL assembly of positively and negatively charged polyelectrolytes [56]. Since its assembly mechanism is very simple, the method

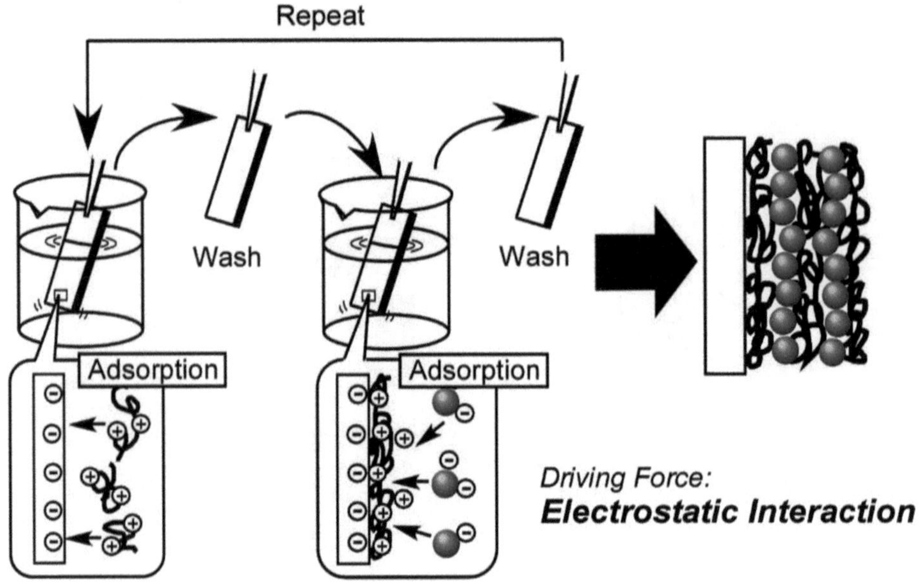

Fig. 5 Layer-by-layer (LbL) assembly where electrostatic interaction plays a role of adsorption driving force

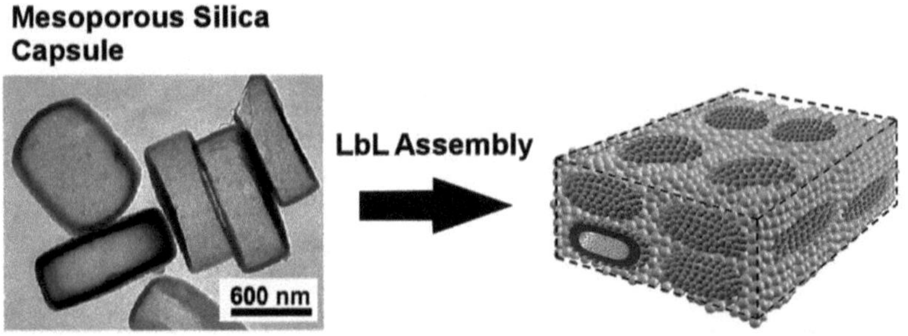

Fig. 6 Layer-by-layer assembly of mesoporous silica capsule with silica nanoparticle and polyelectrolyte

requires only minimum required apparatus such as tweezers and beaker. This simplicity in assembling principle is also advantageous to expand choice of applicable materials, including conventional and functional polymers, biomolecules (proteins, DNA, polysaccharides, etc.), inorganic substances (nanoparticle, nanotube, nanosheet, graphene, quantum dots, etc.) and molecular assemblies (lipid bilayer, Langmuir–Blodgett (LB) films, dye assemblies, etc.). Even virus and cells can be assembled into thin films and/or capsules with the LbL method.

3.2 Automodulated Materials Release

The following examples demonstrate unusual automodulated material release by LbL assembly of mesoporous silica capsules (Fig. 6). The use capsules have interior space (1000 × 700 × 300 nm) at the capsule inside and mesoporous nanospace (average pore diameter of 2.2 nm) at the silica shell [57, 58]. The mesoporous

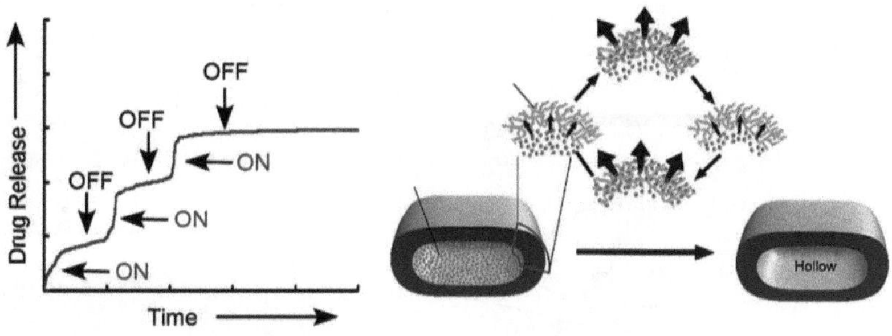

Fig. 7 Stepwise material release (*left*) and plausible mechanism (*right*)

silica capsules were mixed with silica nanoparticles and the formed mixtures were then assembled with cationic polyelectrolytes through LbL assembling method on appropriate solid supports such as quartz crystal microbalance (QCM).

As an initial investigation of material release from the LbL assembly of mesoporous silica capsules, a quantitative analysis of water release from the LbL film compartment under various conditions were investigated using QCM apparatus. After introducing water into the LbL films of mesoporous silica capsules on a QCM plate through immersing the system in water phase, release of water from the silica capsule films were evaluated in air upon frequency shifts of the QCM system. Surprisingly, frequency shifts upon water release from the capsule film exhibited stepwise behavior (release and stop) even without applying any external stimuli (automodulated material release) (Fig. 7).

Plausible mechanism of the observed automodulated water release can be briefly explained as follows. Water molecules entrapped in mesoporous channels at the outer shell were first evaporated, corresponding to the first release step. Only when most of the water was released from the mesopore channel, water can enter into the mesopore nanospace from interior space through introduction of air from external environment to capsule interior. Therefore, water release becomes slow down (the first stop step). However, enough sully of water from the capsule interior to mesopore channels can restart water release process, resulting in periodic repetition of release and stop without supplying external stimuli.

The similar release profiles were demonstrated in case of material release of various fluid medicines such as liquid volatile drug molecules. The reported release system is different from most of the current drug delivery systems with necessity of stimuli-application. It may lead to development of patient friendly drug release systems that does not require any external stimuli application. In addition, strategy of LbL assemblies of mesoporous capsules can be applied to the other functions with non-silica materials. It was actually demonstrated that LbL films of mesoporous carbon capsules can be applied to sensing applications of bioactive substances and toxic materials (Fig. 8) [59–61].

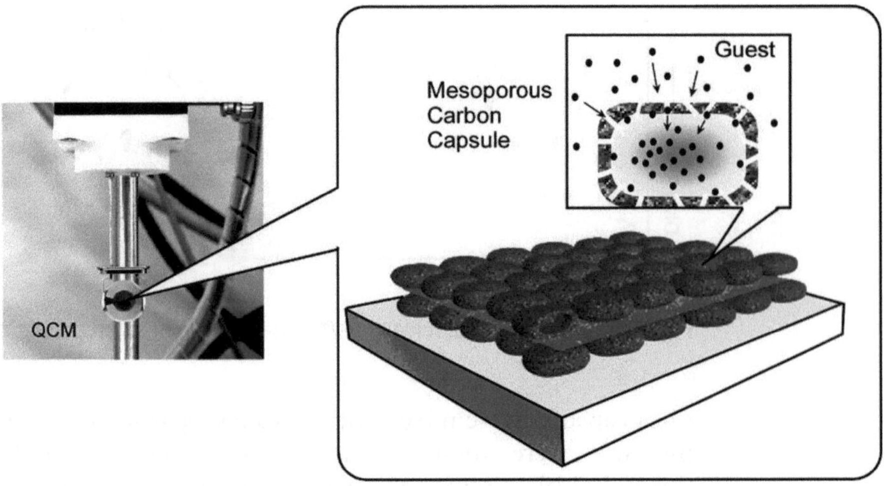

Fig. 8 Layer-by-layer assembly of mesoporous carbon capsule for sensor application

4 Emerging Materials

Not limited to typical nanomaterials nanostructures such as mesoporous materials and LbL assemblies, various kinds of silica nanostructures have been investigated in drug delivery and gene transfection. In the following sections, a few examples of emerging materials are introduced.

4.1 Drug Delivery from Flake-Shell Capsule

Various capsule materials have been investigated as drug carriers in controlled drug release. Basically capsules composed of organic materials such as LbL capsules have flexible and soft natures but may be inferior in mechanical strength. On the other hand, inorganic capsules and spheres including mesoporous silica spheres ensure their excellent robustness that could be disadvantageous in flexibility for certain kinds of controlled drug release. Therefore, the development of a drug-carrier capsule structure with the advantages of both types had been desired.

Recently, a soft capsule was developed by creating a fluffy assembly of nanosheets of silica [62–64]. While this capsule consists of a mechanically stable inorganic material, free control of its structure is also possible. This capsule was named as flake-shell capsules. They can expand and contract when heated and cooled, and the size of the pores in the outer wall, which are formed by the spaces between the nanosheets and serve as passages for drug release, can be controlled over a wide range by adjusting pH to various levels. As a result, the sustained release time of the anticancer drug DOX was successfully extended by several times in comparison with conventional porous capsules having a simple structure. It was also possible to control the drug release duration and drug

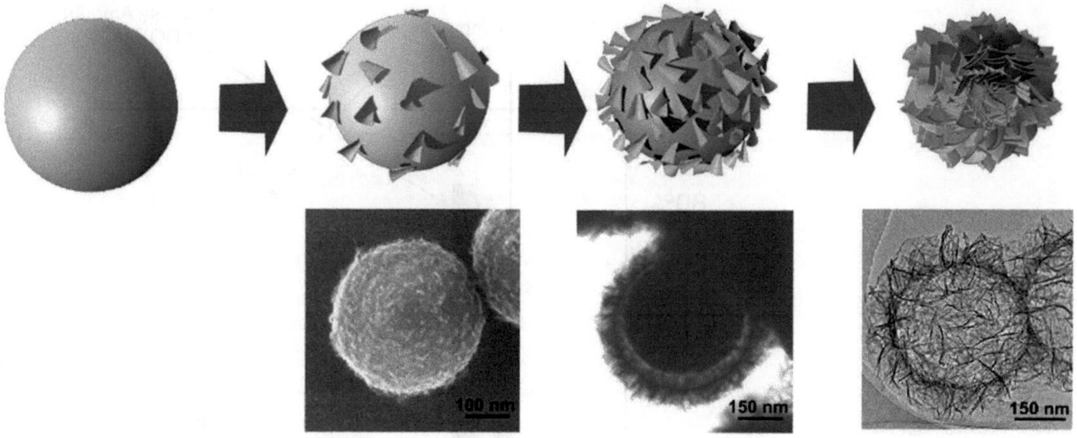

Fig. 9 Formation of flake-shell capsule

storage amount by changing the pore structure of the capsule, thereby changing the drug release routes, by advance treatment of the capsule under appropriate pH conditions.

The flake-shell capsules can be fabricated spontaneously by self-templating approach through exposing silica nanoparticles in hydrothermal conditions. Gradual dissolution of silica from the nanoparticle surface and precipitation as nanosheets at vicinity of the original nanoparticles result in formation of flexible hollow capsules with assembly of numerous silica nanosheets (Fig. 9). The structural flexibility of the flake-shell capsule was confirmed in scanning electron microscopic (SEM) observation. The diameter of flake shell capsule decreased from 560 to 440 nm (shrinkage of the capsule) was induced by the emission of the electron beam for 5 min. Similar structural modification can be done with modulation of Si-O-Si connections under various pH conditions.

The flake-shell capsules can entrap various drugs in their interior space and release them from the capsule interior upon diffusion through integrated assemblies of silica nanosheets. Therefore, pH modulation of assembled structures of silica nanosheet would result in control of drug storage and release. The comparison between structure-fixed mesoporous silica sphere and structure-flexible flake-shell capsules was made using anticancer drug, DOX (Fig. 10). While only 20 % (per weight) of drug can be stored into structurally inflexible mesoporous silica sphere, storage efficiency exceeds 80 % for the flake-shell capsules under the same condition. This high loading efficiency was achieved through pH modification of nanosheet assembly. To keep opening of pores between nanosheet assemblies leads to high loading of drugs into capsule inside. After loading of DOX molecules, capsule shell structures can be tuned again by the next pH treatment. By closing pores between silica nanosheet assemblies, release rate of DOX from the capsule to external environment can be drastically decreased.

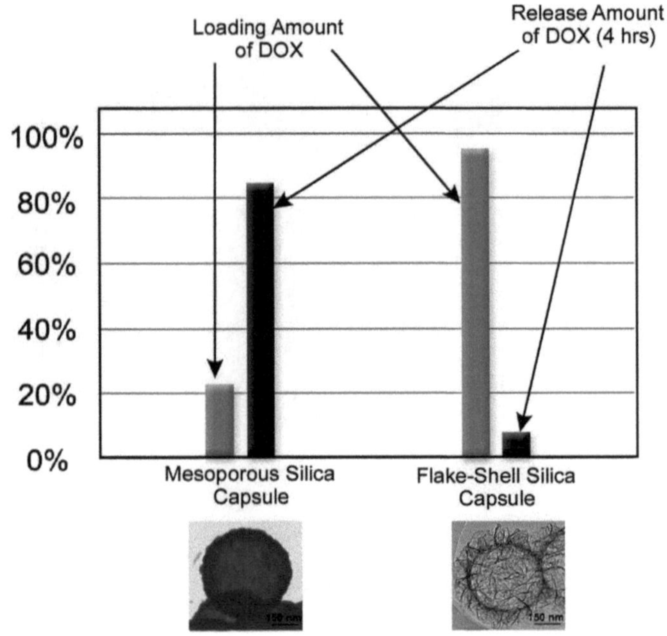

Fig. 10 Comparison between mesoporous silica capsule and flake-shell capsule in sustained release of DOX

At fixed condition, more than 90 % of the stored DOX was released within 4 h from nonflexible silica capsules. In contrast, only 10 % of the loaded drug was released from flake-shell capsules under the same conditions. As the results, drug release continued in day-scales when the flake-shell capsules were used.

With the flexible and adjustable structure of the flake-shell capsules, both high drug loading and slow drug release can be attained. This nature is advantageous for sustainable drug release with adjusting release rate of drugs. Optimum drug release rate depends much on diseases and conditions. Therefore, such high adjustable nature of drug release rate in flake-shell capsules would have high applicability to various kinds of medical needs.

4.2 DNA Transfection from Silica Nanostructure

Introduction of desirable genes into cells would contribute to various therapies. However, the existing technology needs complicated operation as well as insufficient introductory efficiency of a gene and safety. Therefore, certain breakthrough of the related technologies has been awaited. Methods for gene deriver can be classified into two categories, strategies with virus vectors and non-virus technique. The former one always includes safety problems of virus origins. Some of the latter methods may have low efficiency in delivery of genes into cells. As alternate methodology, reverse transfection has been proposed [65–67]. In this strategy, genes are immobilized on surface of designed materials and contact of cells at the surface induces gene transfer to cells. It has several advantages

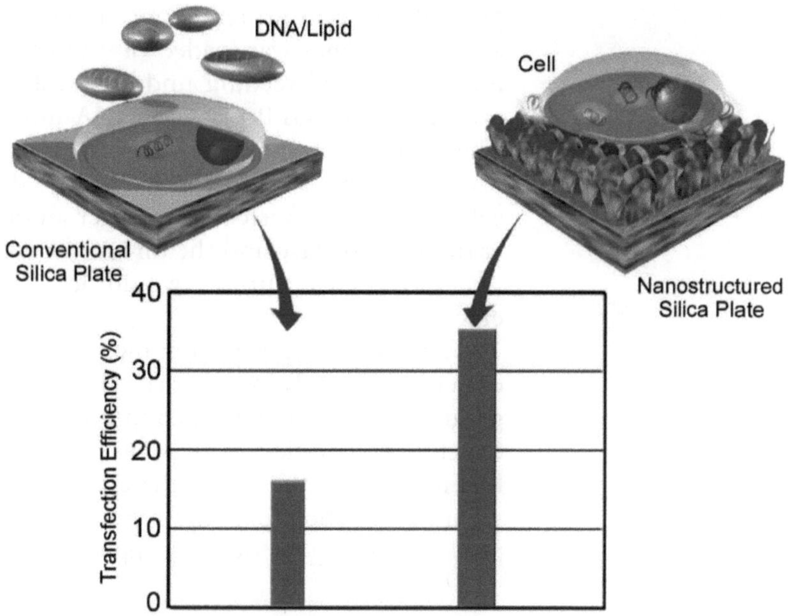

Fig. 11 Comparison of transfection efficiency between conventional silica plate and nanostructured silica plate

including lower necessary amounts of genes and lower toxicity. In addition, delivery of multiple gene species into small amount cells becomes possible upon combining this reverse transfection strategy with microarray fabrication. However, most current delivery platforms of the reverse transfection are still limited to cell types, with suppressed transfection efficiency, and still have risk in safety or unexpected adverse effects.

In contrast to the preexisting methods, we have developed a novel reverse transfection methods using silica surface (Fig. 11) [68]. Nanostructures advantageous for efficient reverse transfection can be fabricated as vertical fin silica sheets that can be spontaneously grown from silica surface under controlled hydrothermal conditions. The formed vertical silica fin walls have thickness of only 5 nm and their density on the silica surface can be tuned by selecting appropriate reaction conditions.

Immobilization of plasmid DNA was also demonstrated. Loading efficiency of the plasmid DNA can be adjusted through density control of the vertical fin walls. At optimized condition, gene loading efficiency in silica surface with vertical nanostructures becomes ca. 5.5 times larger than flat silica surface, indicating that formation of vertical fin structures effectively promote gene loading to the silica surface.

Contact of cell to the nanostructured silica surface is also possible, and thus gene delivery from the silica surface to cells was realized. The in vitro transfection experiments were carried out with the human embryonic kidney mammalian cell line with the green fluorescent protein reporter genes. Complex of cationic lipid and target genes was loaded on the nanostructured silica surface, followed by cell seeding under typical cell cultivation. Successful transfection of GFP plasmid DNA into the cells was confirmed. The transfection efficacy in the case of this silica reverse transfection becomes 35 %, approximately double that obtained by solution-based transfection. Larger amount of immobilized DNA at the silica surface and the direct contact of the cells to the nanostructured silica surface would lead to enhanced transfection efficacy.

This reverse transfection method can introduce multiple kinds of genes efficiently into animal cells. This nature would be advantageous for cell profiling. In addition, this method can be utilized for effective preparation of iPS cells. It is sure that silica materials are less toxic than the other materials used for reverse transfection techniques. Therefore, the reported method would have various possibilities in gene delivery applications.

5 Conclusion

In this chapter, usages of nanostructured silica in biological and pharmaceutical fields are explained. As seen in several examples of mesoporous silica and layer-by-layer assemblies as well as newly developed silica nanostructures, silica materials have high potential to have variously structured materials with nanometer-scale precision. In addition, many applications including drug delivery and gene transfection have been realized because of high biocompatibility of these silica materials. Therefore, nanostructured silica materials will play essential roles in application of inorganic stuffs in biological and pharmaceutical fields.

Acknowledgement

This work was partly supported by World Premier International Research Center Initiative (WPI Initiative), MEXT, Japan and Core Research for Evolutional Science and Technology (CREST) program of Japan Science and Technology Agency (JST), Japan.

References

1. Ariga K, Ji Q, Hill JP, Kawazoe N, Chen G (2009) Supramolecular approaches to biological therapy. Expert Opin Biol Ther 9:307
2. Ruiz-Hitzky E, Darder M, Aranda P, Ariga K (2010) Advances in biomimetic and nanostructured biohybrid materials. Adv Mater 22:323
3. Ariga K, Hill JP (2011) Monolayers at air-water interfaces: from origins-of-life to nanotechnology. Chem Rec 11:199
4. Ariga K, Ji Q, McShane MJ, Lvov YM, Vinu A, Hill JP (2012) Inorganic nanoarchitectonics for biological applications. Chem Mater 24:728

5. Ariga K, Ishihara S, Abe H, Li M, Hill JP (2012) Materials nanoarchitectonics for environmental remediation and sensing. J Mater Chem 22:2369
6. Ariga K, Ji Q, Mori T, Naito M, Yamauchi Y, Abe H, Hill JP (2013) Enzyme nanoarchitectonics: organization and device application. Chem Soc Rev 42:6322
7. Ariga K, Hill JP, Lee MV, Vinu A, Charvet R, Acharya S (2008) Challenges and breakthroughs in recent research on self-assembly. Sci Technol Adv Mater 9:014109
8. Ariga K, Hu X, Mandal S, Hill JP (2010) By what means should nanoscaled materials be constructed: molecule, medium, or human? Nanoscale 2:198
9. Ariga K, Lee MV, Mori T, Yu X-Y, Hill JP (2010) Two-dimensional nanoarchitectonics based on self-assembly. Adv Colloid Interface Sci 154:20
10. Ariga K, Ji Q, Hill JP, Vinu A (2010) Supramolecular materials from inorganic building blocks. J Inorg Organomet Polym 20:1
11. Ariga K, Li M, Richards GJ, Hill JP (2011) Nanoarchitectonics: a conceptual paradigm for design and synthesis of dimension-controlled functional nanomatcrials. J Nanosci Nanotechnol 11:1
12. Ariga K, Mori T, Hill JP (2012) Mechanical control of nanomaterials and nanosystems. Adv Mater 24:158
13. Ramanathan M, Kilbey Michael S II, Ji Q, Hill JP, Ariga K (2012) Materials self-assembly and fabrication in confined spaces. J Mater Chem 22:10389
14. Li M, Ishihara S, Ji Q, Akada M, Hill JP, Ariga K (2012) Paradigm shift from self-assembly to commanded assembly of functional materials: recent examples in porphyrin/fullerene supramolecular systems. Sci Technol Adv Mater 13:053001
15. Ramanathan M, Shrestha LK, Mori T, Ji Q, Hill JP, Ariga K (2013) Amphiphile nanoarchitectonics: from basic physical chemistry to advanced applications. Phys Chem Chem Phys 15:10580
16. Ariga K, Mori T, Hill JP (2013) Interfacial nanoarchitectonics: lateral and vertical, static and dynamic. Langmuir 29:8459
17. Shrestha LK, Ji Q, Mori T, Miyazawa K, Yamauchi Y, Hill JP, Ariga K (2013) Fullerene nanoarchitectonics: from zero to higher dimensions. Chem Asian J 8:1662
18. Ariga K, Mori T, Akamatsu M, Hill JP (2014) Two-dimensional nanofabrication and supramolecular functionality controlled by mechanical stimuli. Thin Solid Films 554:32
19. Hill JP, Shrestha LK, Ishihara S, Ji Q, Ariga K (2014) Self-assembly: from amphiphiles to chromophores and beyond. Molecules 19:8589
20. Vinu A, Mori T, Ariga K (2006) New families of mesoporous materials. Sci Technol Adv Mater 7:753
21. Ariga K, Ji Q, Hill JP, Vinu A (2009) Coupling of soft technology (layer-by-layer assembly) with hard materials (mesoporous solids) to give hierarchic functional structures. Soft Matter 5:3562
22. Alam S, Anand C, Ariga K, Mori T, Vinu A (2009) Unusual magnetic properties of size-controlled iron oxide nanoparticles grown in a nanoporous matrix with tunable pores. Angew Chem Int Ed 48:7358
23. Ariga K, Vinu A, Yamauchi Y, Ji Q, Hill JP (2012) Nanoarchitectonics for mesoporous materials. Bull Chem Soc Jpn 85:1
24. Shrestha LK, Yamauchi Y, Hill JP, Miyazawa K, Ariga K (2013) Fullerene crystals with bimodal pore architectures consisting of macropores and mesopores. J Am Chem Soc 135:586
25. Ariga K, Yamauchi Y, Ji Q, Yonamine Y, Hill JP (2014) Mesoporous sensor nanoarchitectonics. APL Mat 2:030701
26. Chaikittisilp W, Muraoka K, Ji Q, Ariga K, Yamauchi Y (2014) Mesoporous architectures with highly crystallized frameworks. J Mater Chem A 2:12096
27. Yanagisawa T, Shimizu T, Kuroda K, Kato C (1990) The preparation of alkyltrimethulammonium kanemite complexes and their conversion to microporous materials. Bull Chem Soc Jpn 63:988
28. Kresge CT, Leonowicz ME, Roth WJ, Vartuli JC, Beck JS (1992) Ordered mesoporous molecular-sieves synthesized by a liquid-crystal template mechanism. Nature 359:710
29. Kapoor MP, Inagaki S (2006) Highly ordered mesoporous organosilica hybrid materials. Bull Chem Soc Jpn 79:1463
30. Ariga K, Vinu A, Miyahara M, Hill JP, Mori T (2007) One-pot separation of tea components through selective adsorption on pore-engineered nanocarbon, carbon nanocage. J Am Chem Soc 129:11022
31. Datta KKR, Subba Reddy BV, Ariga K, Vinu A (2010) Gold nanoparticles embedded in a mesoporous carbon nitride stabilizer for highly efficient three-component coupling reaction. Angew Chem Int Ed 49:5961
32. Hu M, Reboul J, Furukawa S, Torad NL, Ji Q, Srinivasu P, Ariga K, Kitagawa S, Yamauchi Y (2012) Direct carbonization of Al-based porous coordination polymer for synthesis of nanoporous carbon. J Am Chem Soc 134:2864

33. Chaikittisilp W, Ariga K, Yamauchi Y (2013) A new family of carbon materials: synthesis of MOF-derived nanoporous carbons and their promising applications. J Mater Chem A 1:14
34. Vinu A, Ariga K, Mori T, Nakanishi T, Hishita S, Golberg D, Bando Y (2005) Preparation and characterization of well ordered hexagonal mesoporous carbon nitride. Adv Mater 17:1648
35. Vinu A, Terrones M, Golberg D, Hishita S, Ariga K, Mori T (2005) Synthesis of mesoporous BN and BCN exhibiting large surface areas via templating methods. Chem Mater 17:5887
36. Yamauchi Y, Kuroda K (2008) Rational design of mesoporous metals and related nanomaterials by a soft-template approach. Chem Asian J 3:664
37. Wang H, Ishihara S, Ariga K, Yamauchi Y (2012) All metal layer-by-layer films: bimetallic alternate layers with accessible mesopores for enhanced electrocatalysis. J Am Chem Soc 134:10819
38. Ariga K, Vinu A, Hill JP, Mori T (2007) Coordination chemistry and supramolecular chemistry in mesoporous nanospace. Coord Chem Rev 251:2562
39. Tarn D, Ashley CE, Xue M, Carnes EC, Zink JI, Brinker CJ (2013) Mesoporous silica nanoparticle nanocarriers: biofunctionality and biocompatibility. Acc Chem Res 46:792
40. Mal MK, Fujiwara M, Tanaka Y (2003) Photocontrolled reversible release of guest molecules from coumarin-modified mesoporous silica. Nature 421:350
41. Lai C-Y, Trewyn BG, Jeftinija DM, Jeftinija K, Xu S, Jeftinija S, Lin VS-Y (2003) A Mesoporous silica nanosphere-based carrier system with chemically removable CdS nanoparticle caps for stimuli-responsive controlled release of neurotransmitters and drug molecules. J Am Chem Soc 125:4451
42. Casasffls R, Aznar E, Marcos MD, Martínez-Máñez R, Sancenón F, Soto J, Amorós P (2006) New methods for anion recognition and signaling using nanoscopic gatelike scaffoldings. Angew Chem Int Ed 45:6661
43. Ariga K, Hill JP, Ji Q (2007) Layer-by-layer assembly as a versatile bottom-up nanofabrication technique for exploratory research and realistic application. Phys Chem Chem Phys 9:2319
44. Ariga K, Hill JP, Ji Q (2008) Biomaterials and biofunctionality in layered macromolecular assemblies. Macromol Biosci 8:981
45. Ariga K, Ji Q, Hill JP (2010) Enzyme-encapsulated layer-by-layer assemblies: current status and challenges toward ultimate nanodevices. Adv Polym Sci 229:51
46. Ji Q, Honma I, Paek S-M, Akada M, Hill JP, Vinu A, Ariga K (2010) Layer-by-layer films of graphene and ionic liquid for highly selective gas sensing. Angew Chem Int Ed 49:9737
47. Ariga K, McShane M, Lvov YM, Ji Q, Hill JP (2011) Layer-by-layer assembly for drug delivery and related applications. Expert Opin Drug Deliv 8:633
48. Li M, Ishihara S, Akada M, Liao M, Sang L, Hill JP, Krishnan V, Ma Y, Ariga K (2011) Electrochemical coupling layer-by-layer (ECC-LbL) assembly. J Am Chem Soc 133:7348
49. Ariga K, Lvov YM, Kawakami K, Ji Q, Hill JP (2011) Layer-by-layer self-assembled shells for drug delivery. Adv Drug Deliv Rev 63:762
50. Ariga K, Ji Q, Hill JP, Bando Y, Aono M (2012) Forming nanomaterials as layered functional structures towards materials nanoarchitectonics. NPG Asia Mater 4:e17
51. Ariga K, Yamauchi Y, Rydzek G, Ji Q, Yonamine Y, Wu KC-W, Hill JP (2014) Layer-by-layer nanoarchitectonics: invention, innovation, and evolution. Chem Lett 43:36
52. Rydzek G, Terentyeva TG, Pakdel A, Golberg D, Hill JP, Ariga K (2014) Simultaneous electropolymerization and electro-click functionalization for highly versatile surface platforms. ACS Nano 8:5240
53. Iler RK (1966) Multilayers of colloidal particles. J Colloid Interface Sci 21:569
54. Kirkland JJ (1965) Porous thin-layer modified glass bead supports for gas liquid chromatography. Anal Chem 37:1458
55. Decher G, Hong J-D (1991) Buildup of ultrathin multilayer films by a self-assembly process, 1 consecutive adsorption of anionic and cationic bipolar amphiphiles on charged surfaces. Makromol Chem Macromol Symp 46:321
56. Decher G, Hong JD (1991) Buildup of ultrathin multilayer films by a self-assembly process: II consecutive adsorption of anionic and cationic bipolar amphiphiles and polyelectrolytes on charged surfaces. Ber Bunsen-Ges Phys Chem 95:1430
57. Ji Q, Miyahara M, Hill JP, Acharya S, Vinu A, Yoon SB, Yu J-S, Sakamoto K, Ariga K (2008) Stimuli-free auto-modulated material release from mesoporous nanocompartment films. J Am Chem Soc 130:2376
58. Ji Q, Acharya S, Hill JP, Vinu A, Yoon SB, Yu J-S, Sakamoto K, Ariga K (2009) Hierarchic nanostructure for auto-modulation of material release: mesoporous nanocompartment films. Adv Funct Mater 19:1792
59. Ariga K, Vinu A, Ji Q, Ohmori O, Hill JP, Acharya S, Koike J, Shiratori S (2008) A layered mesoporous carbon sensor based on

nanopore-filling cooperative adsorption in the liquid phase. Angew Chem Int Ed 47:7254

60. Ji Q, Yoon SB, Hill JP, Vinu A, Yu J-S, Ariga K (2009) Layer-by-layer films of dual-pore carbon capsules with designable selectivity of gas adsorption. J Am Chem Soc 131:4220
61. Ji Q, Guo C, Yu X, Ochs CJ, Hill JP, Caruso F, Nakazawa H, Ariga K (2012) Flake-shell capsules: adjustable inorganic structures. Small 8:2345
62. Manoharan Y, Ji Q, Yamazaki T, Chinnathambi S, Chen S, Singaravelu G, Hill JP, Ariga K, Hanagata N (2012) Effect of molecular weight of polyethyleneimine on loading of CpG oligodeoxynucleotides onto flake-shell silica nanoparticles for enhanced TLR9-mediated induction of interferon-α. Int J Nanomedicine 7:3625
63. Terentyeva TG, Matras A, Van Rossom W, Hill JP, Ji Q, Ariga K (2013) Bioactive flake-shell capsules: soft silica nanoparticles for efficient enzyme immobilization. J Mater Chem B 1:3248
64. Ji Q, Hill JP, Ariga K (2013) Shell-adjustable hollow 'soft' silica spheres as a support for gold nanoparticles. J Mater Chem A 1:3600
65. Erfle H, Neumann B, Liebel U, Rogers P, Held M, Walter T, Ellenberg J, Pepperkok R (2007) Reverse transfection on cell arrays for high content screening microscopy. Nat Protoc 2:392
66. Fujita S, Ota E, Sasaki C, Takano K, Miyake M, Miyake J (2007) Highly efficient reverse transfection with siRNA in multiple wells of microtiter plates. J Biosci Bioeng 104:329
67. Villa-Diaz LG, Garcia-Perez JL, Krebsbach PH (2010) Enhanced transfection efficiency of human embryonic stem cells by the incorporation of DNA liposomes in extracellular matrix. Stem Cells Dev 19:1949
68. Ji Q, Yamazaki T, Hanagata N, Lee MV, Hill JP, Ariga K (2012) Silica-based gene reverse transfection: upright nanosheet network for promoted DNA delivery to cell. Chem Commun 48:8496

Chapter 8

Silicon Nanoparticles and Microparticles

Chaofeng Mu and Haifa Shen

Abstract

Porous silicon nanoparticles and microparticles have great potential as drug delivery carriers of a variety of therapeutic agents in chemotherapeutics, gene delivery, molecular diagnostics, and immunotherapy due to their biodegradability, biocompatibility, and unique structural properties. The in vivo toxicological properties and biosafety of porous silicon (pSi) particles highly depend on the particles' surface properties (size and geometries), preparation processes, administration routes and dosage. Versatile composite pSi particles can be fabricated via functionalizing them with organic and/or inorganic components to satisfy the effectiveness of different in vivo therapeutic purposes such as stimuli-responsive drug release, active drug targeting, and diagnostic imaging. This chapter focuses on the fabrication and surface functionalization of pSi nanoparticles and microparticles as drug delivery vehicles, in vivo toxicological properties and biosafety, and the therapeutic and diagnostic imaging applications.

Key words Porous silicon, Nanoparticles, Biocompatibility, Drug delivery, Cancer therapy

1 Introduction

In nanotechnology, nanoparticles are often defined as microscopic particles with at least one dimension between 1 and 100 nm, which were fabricated from organic, inorganic, and inorganic–organic hybrid materials. However, the nanoscale is accepted to rise up to 200–300 nm in biomedical and pharmaceutical application. In particulate drug delivery, microparticles refer to the micrometer dimensions of the particles. In the biomedical and pharmaceutical areas, nanoparticles and microparticles were explored for drug delivery application as a means of effectively treating and precisely diagnosing disease. As therapeutic delivery systems, particles allow for the controlled release of entrapped drugs and targeted delivery. The advantages of particulate drug delivery include several aspects: improving the solubility of poorly water-soluble drugs; reducing the systemic toxicity or side effects of the incorporated drugs; increasing circulation time by controlled drug release; protecting siRNA/proteins from degradation; compatibility with multiple administration routes (oral, inhalation, etc.) [1–4]. All of these

Zheng-Rong Lu and Shinji Sakuma (eds.), *Nanomaterials in Pharmacology*, Methods in Pharmacology and Toxicology, DOI 10.1007/978-1-4939-3121-7_8, © Springer Science+Business Media New York 2016

advantages could result in improvements in drug bioavailability and resolve noncompliance with prescribed therapies.

With the great progress of nanomaterials, particles fabricated with inorganic or organic–inorganic hybrid biomaterials were developed for drug delivery, molecular diagnostics and immunotherapy. However, the toxicological properties and biosafety of inorganic or hybrid particles, especially the biodegradability and accumulation toxicity in the animal or human body, are one of the crucial issues now under consideration and debate, which greatly limits the bench-to-bedside translation possibilities [5–8].

Silicon, one of the most abundant chemical elements, is essential in living organisms and naturally present in human tissues such as bone, blood vessels and cartilages [9]. Porous silicon (pSi) was discovered over 60 years ago and its optical and biomedical applications were increased during the 1990s. Si based materials are widely utilized for biomedical products such as bandages, dental fillers, implants, and contact lenses [10–12]. In the past several decades, Si-based nano- and micro-materials were broadly investigated as drug delivery vehicles for improving the delivery efficiency of therapeutic agents and diagnostic imaging in the pharmaceutical field [13, 14]. Silicon particles as one type of inorganic particles have attracted increasing attention due to their unprecedented advantages.

For in vivo therapeutic application purposes, the high surface-to-volume ratio of nanostructured silicon materials is the essential characteristic of silicon nano- or micro-materials. The tunable pore size (2–50 nm) and high pore volume are available for loading many types of therapeutic and diagnostic molecules with high capacity. pSi nanocarriers are developed for controlled-release to enhance drug therapy by protecting the drug from degradation and elimination in blood circulation before reaching the specific action site, thus finally achieving desired effective concentrations at targeted sites in the body. The silicon particles also provide large surfaces for functionalization by different reaction groups such as amine, carboxyl and end groups attached to polyethylene glycol, allowing for manifold biomedical applications.

This chapter highlights the preparation and functionalization methods, and in vivo biodistribution and biosafety of silicon particles and their potential applications in the biomedical and pharmaceutical fields for disease therapeutics and diagnostics.

2 Fabrication and Surface Functionalization of Porous Silicon Particles

2.1 Fabrication Methods

Porous silicon can be fabricated by a range of methods, including chemical vapor etching [15], microwave plasma decomposition [16], laser-stimulated etching [17], and spark erosion etching [18]. Currently, porous silicon has been mainly fabricated by the

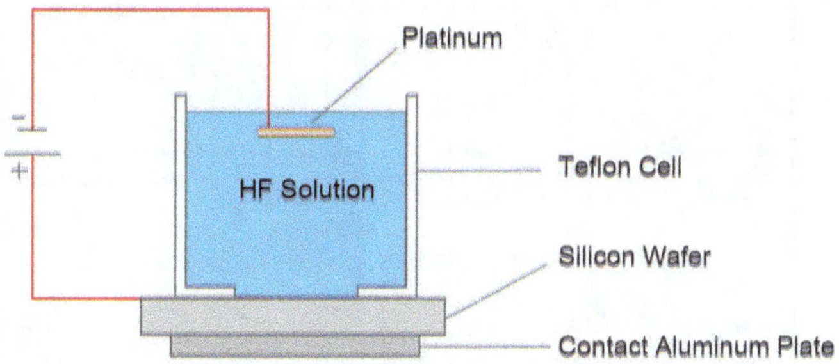

Fig. 1 Schematic electrochemical anodization for porous silicon fabrication

electrochemical anodization method for biomedical applications purposes. Electrochemical anodization is a popular "top-down" approach for porous pSi materials fabrication from single bulk crystalline Si wafers in a hydrofluoric acid electrolyte solution [19, 20]. Anodization to produce porous silicon was conducted between the silicon wafer (anode) and the platinum wire (cathode) via immersion in electrochemical aqueous or ethanoic hydrofluoric acid/ ethanol. A schematic of the anodization process for porous silicon formation is shown in Fig. 1. The typical anodization parameters, such as hydrofluoric acid concentration, current density, etching time, temperature, and wafer resistivity, are able to affect the final silicon porous structures during etching process.

In the next step, pSi materials were converted into nanoparticles or microparticles using ultrasonic fracture or ball-milling [21, 22]. However, these pulverization techniques were employed for obtaining pSi particles of broad size distribution and irregular shape, which could greatly influence the particles' biological performance.

Recently, photolithography and electrochemical etching of patterned silicon trenches were developed to fabricate highly reproducible, monodisperse porous pSi particles of submicron and micron size (Fig. 2) [23–25]. The trench was constructed into the 100 mm p++ silicon wafer by a second dry- or wet-etch step. Finally, pSi particles were released from the wafer by sonication in isopropanol. Pore size (5–50 nm), porosity (47 % to over 80 %), and shape (discoidal, hemispherical to tubular) of the pSi particles were controlled by varying the related parameters during etching.

The freshly etched pSi surface was anodized and subsequently oxidized slowly with ambient air. The hydrogen-terminated groups (Si-H*n*) on the surface were unstable, and subsequent surface treatment was always needed to apply diverse optical and biomedical application. The most common surface treatments contain thermal oxidation (OSiH, OSiOH, and O-Si-O bonds), carbonization (Si-C, C-H bonds), and hydrosilylation (Si-C-C, Si-C-O bonds), which tailor surface properties of pSi (hydrophilic or hydrophobic) [26].

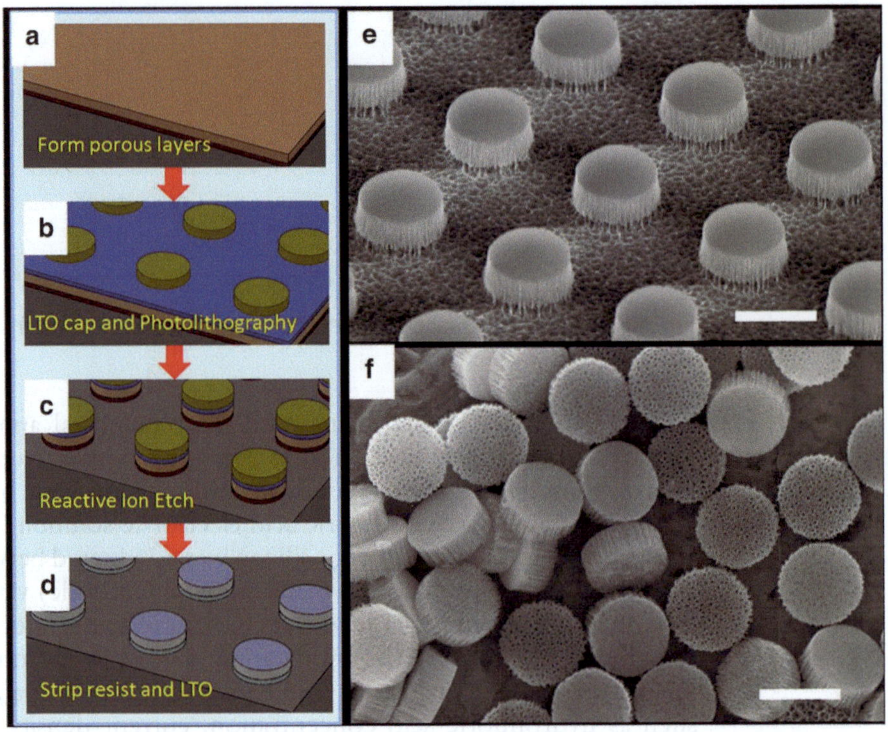

Fig. 2 Description of pSi particles by photolithography and electrochemical etching. (**a–d**) Schematic process flowchart (LTO: low temperature oxide). (**e**) Scanning transmission microscopy image of discoidal pSi particle (1000 nm × 400 nm) array retained on wafer. (**f**) Released monodispersed discoidal pSi particles (Scale bar is 1 μm). Reprinted from Godin et al. [25], with permission from Wiley

2.2 Surface Functionalization

Surfaces functionalization can be done by post-etching chemical modification. The siloxane and silanol groups inside the nanopores or on the surface of the pSi particles are available to react with various linkers to form carboxyl, amine, and thiol groups. The versatility of SiO chemistry allows for an unlimited possibility of surface modifications using different biomolecules. In the grafting method, major functionalization reactions take place between native Si-H and organic linkers at the exterior surface and interior pore-walls of the pSi particles. Grafted pSi materials still retained their porous structures and rigid stability. The attachment of functional groups was preferentially conjugated to the external surface. Locations of functional groups cannot be regulated accurately. Surface functionalization aims to diversify the surface characteristics to satisfy manifold biomedical demands. The proper surface functionalization of pSi particles could modify their degradation rate, improve their biocompatibility, and allow for their bioconjugation to targeting moieties and covalent coupling to drugs.

Short-chain poly(ethylene glycol) (PEG) was attached to the pSi particles' surface by using undecylenic acid as a spacer, creating a hydrophilic surface used to prevent nonspecific binding in biological applications [27]. The surface of multistage vehicles (MSVs) prepared with pSi particles was negatively charged, and conjugation with amino silanes (e.g., 3-Aminopropyltriethoxysilane (APTES)) can invert its zeta potential to positive. Negatively charged siRNA-liposomes were able to load into this positively charged MSV with high capacity [28]. Chitosan oligomers-functionalized porous silicon films were utilized to detect carboxylic acid-containing drugs in water [29]. E-selectin thioaptamer was conjugated with APTES-modified MSV for the specific targeting of bone marrow vascular endothelium in the treatment of breast cancer bone metastasis [30]. Arginine-polyethyleneimine (Arg-PEI) was conjugated to APTES-modified nanoporous silicon particles. siRNA oligos were loaded into nanopores of positively charged pSi particles with high capacity [31].

2.3 Pore Structure

Structured porous materials are classified by International Union of Pure and Applied Chemistry (IUPAC) into three categories based on their pore diameter: nanoporous (microporous, less than 2 nm), mesoporous (2–50 nm), and macroporous (above 50 nm) [32]. The organized porosity, pore size and volume, and pore morphology determine its chemical and mechanical stability, and optical and biochemical properties [33]. Mesoporous pSi particles exhibit high pore volume, tunable pore size, and structural stability, which make them suitable drug vehicles for controlled drug release. Porosity means the volumetric fraction of air within nanomaterials. For pSi particles, it can reach over 80 %. The pSi internal surface of per unit volume can be very large and on the order of 500 m^2/cm^3.

Among them, pore morphology is a critical parameter for drug loading. It influences the docking location and absorption capability of non-crystallized drugs or secondary drug-vehicles in the pores. Pore morphology mainly refers to the shape and orientation (branched, facetted, etc.) of interconnected pores. For nanoporous and mesoporous pSi, it typically exhibits a sponge-like structure with randomly branched pores and does not show a clear orientation (Fig. 3).

3 Drug Loading, Release, and Intracellular Trafficking of Porous Silicon Particles

3.1 Drug Loading

The nanostructures of porous silicon particles are highly ordered and have empty irregular channels. One attractive characteristic of porous nanomaterials is the desired drug loading capacity. The high surface areas and pore volumes allow for a large payload of drug molecules. The interior pore physicochemical environment can be tailored by modification with multiple functional groups according to different properties of drug molecules in order to enhance drug loading and retention capability, as well as reduce carrier amounts for drug

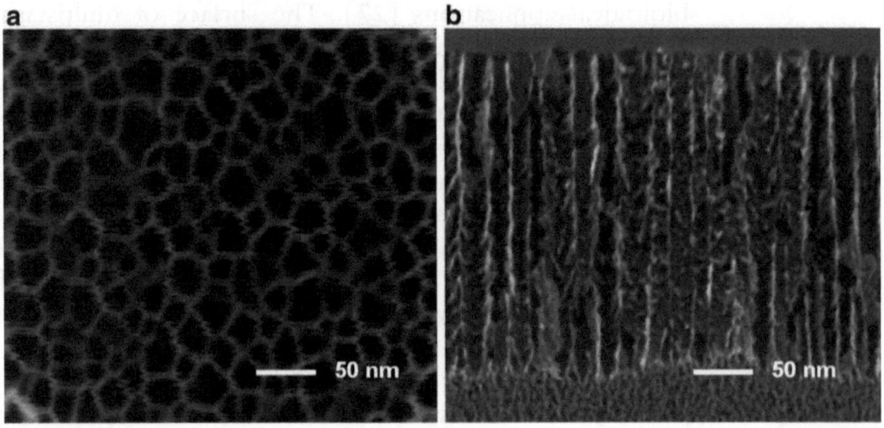

Fig. 3 SEM images of pore structure on surface (**a**) and interior pore morphology by cross-cutting (**b**) of pSi particles

delivery. The drug loading into the pSi nanostructure can be achieved by different encapsulation methods. The loading mechanisms mainly include physical adsorption and covalent attachment.

3.1.1 Physical Adsorption

The physical adsorption of drugs into the porous structure was performed mainly through capillary force within numerous irregular nano-channels and other forces such as electrostatic interaction and sonication driving. This process can be achieved by immersing dry pSi nanoparticles into a high concentration drug solution and then sonicating for enough time at room temperature. The unbound drugs are removed by washing. The randomly branched pores with sponge-like structures are available for drug docking.

5.6 % (w/w) of indomethacin was loaded into the nanopores of thermally oxidized mesoporous silicon microparticles (13.6 μm) via immersion in a concentrated drug chloroform solution and subsequent solvent evaporation [34]. The indomethacin confined in the nanopores in a noncrystalline state due to the sponge-like pore structure was characterized by various physicochemical methods including Fourier-transform infrared spectroscopy (FTIR), powder X-ray diffraction (XRD), differential scanning calorimetry (DSC), and thermal GraVimetric analysis (TGA). The drug in noncrystalline state was able to be stored for several months in accelerated stability environments.

The undecylenic acid modified pSi microparticles (4 μm) were synthesized for loading anticancer drugs cis-dichlorodiamine (cisplatin), transplatin, and Pt (IV) pro-drug by physical adsorption methods [35]. The surface properties of the pSi particles and the drug's chemical state greatly influenced the loading efficiency. Pt was deposited on the particles' surfaces for capping the nanostructures and trapping the unreduced cisplatin.

A large amount of insulin (about 22 %, w/w) was loaded into annealed thermally hydrocarbonized and undecylenic acid-modified pSi microparticles for oral insulin delivery [36]. 14.3 % (w/w) of splice-correcting oligonucleotides (SCOs, negatively charged) were rapidly loaded into positively charged aminosilanes-grafted thermal oxidation pSi nanoparticles with electrostatic interactions [37]. Both indomethacin (hydrophobic) and peptide YY3-36 (PYY3-36, hydrophilic) were co-loaded into the surface-treated pSi nanoparticles by an immersion method with high loading capability for simultaneous multidrug delivery within a single delivery system [38].

3.1.2 Covalent Attachment

For covalent attachment, a spacer arm such as an aliphatic chain containing carboxyl or amino group is usually needed for grafting by gentle chemistry. Spacer attachments are usually made through an amide linkage but other functionalities are possible. These gentle reactions take place between native Si-H and organic linkers on the exterior surfaces and interior pore-walls of pSi particles. The design and optimization of linkers depends on the properties (molecular weight and chemical stability) of the covalent drugs and the expected release mechanisms and kinetics profiles. The locations of spacers in pSi particles cannot be regulated accurately by chemical reaction. Daunorubicin was covalently attached to hydrosilylated porous silicon photonic crystal particles of dimensions 12 μm thick and 35 μm across via undecylenic acid as a linker. This system was developed for intravitreally local administration [39]. The anticancer drug doxorubicin (4.5 % (w/w)) was conjugated to the surfaces and inner pores of the porous Si particles (30–50 μm) by covalent attachment using an undecenoic acid linker [40].

3.2 Drug Release

Generally, pSi nanocarriers are developed for controlled-release to enhance drug therapies by assisting drugs in traversing physiological barriers, shielding drug from premature degradation and elimination, minimizing drug exposure to untargeted sites, and finally achieving the desired effective concentration on targeted sites in the body. Drugs are released from pSi particles in a controlled manner through several combinations of mechanisms including desorption, diffusion and degradation at different stages. This process is highly correlated to the drug loading methods, pore size and porosity, surface amphiphilicity of the pSi particles, and release environment. A sustained release profile can be achieved by either physical absorption or covalent attachment. However, a premature burse release always happens when using physical absorption loading. The amphiphilicity of pSi particles can control the degradation rate of pSi nanostructures in saline buffer. Daunorubicin was covalently conjugated to the inner surface of porous silicon photonic crystal particles of size 12 μm thick and 35 μm across. The conjugated drug release can be controlled in a zero-order model for 30 days via porous Si matrix degradation, which is significantly longer than that of free drug injection [41]. Noncrystalline indomethacin (poorly soluble BCS type II drug) loaded into porous

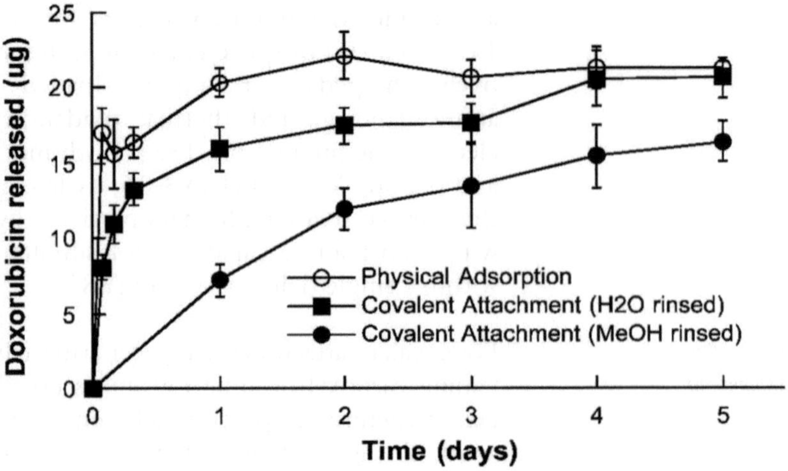

Fig. 4 Doxorubicin release from pSi microparticles in phosphate-buffered saline (PBS buffer) by different loading methods. Approximately 80 % of the drug was released at 8 h and complete drug release occurred within 1 day for doxorubicin loaded by physical absorption. However, the covalently attached drug was sustainedly released in 5 days. Reprinted from Wu et al. [40], with permission from American ACS

silicon microparticles could greatly improve its release profile in comparison with that of a crystalline-state drug by enhancing the indomethacin dissolution in the gastrointestinal tract. Doxorubicin released from pSi microparticles by covalent attachment is triggered by the oxidation of particles. The drug release rate can be accelerated by the introduction of peroxynitrite (oxidizing species) into the release medium. The explanation is that doxorubicin mainly existed on the porous surface. The controlled release profiles showed that the release of doxorubicin was delayed by covalent attachment compared to that loaded by physical adsorption (Fig. 4). The oxidation-triggered release was also demonstrated in Hela cells [40].

The prominent advantage of pSi nanoparticles as drug delivery carriers is the near zero premature controlled release by entrapping drugs inside their pores. This is the prerequisite for achieving long blood circulation time and targeting cells or tissues for stimuli-responsive drug release via intravenous administration. Hence, the drug release takes place only when pSi nanocarriers are triggered by external or internal stimuli that are manipulated at a desired location and time. Furthermore, pSi particles have been widely used for controlling the intracellular delivery of anticancer drugs and DNA and RNA oligonucleotides due to their unique properties. The intracellular delivery highly depends on the precisely manipulated release behaviors controlled by the external surroundings of cells and the fine microenvironments in different cellular organelles, such as pH, oxidation–reduction, and enzymatic degradation.

Rod-shaped porous silicon nanoparticles (200–400 nm high and 100–200 nm in diameter) were synthesized and derivatized with a cyclodextrin-based nanovalve as a gatekeeper agent [42]. This cyclodextrin-based nanovalve was closed at the physiological pH of 7.4, and the cap was opened by protonation at pH less than 6.0. Hoechst 33342 released from pSi nanoparticles showed obvious pH-dependent characteristics, which was premature zero release at pH 7.4 and controlled release in acidified release medium (pH 5). This will benefit the intracellular release of cargo-loaded pSi nanoparticles under lysosomal acidity conditions.

3.3 Intracellular Uptake and Cell Trafficking

In order to understand the response of biological cells to particles, it is crucial to figure out the mechanisms of cellular uptake and intracellular trafficking. The internalization mainly includes physical proximity and specific interactions between ligands-particles and receptors on the cell membrane. This process always takes place via internalization of early endosomes (intracellular vesicles). Generally, the intracellular process will be decisive for nanoparticles and the encapsulated drugs, leading to their degradation, translocation into other cytoplasmic compartments, or pumping out to the extracellular environment [43]. The size and surface characteristics of pSi particles determine the cellular uptake mechanisms and any further form of intracellular transport, thereby significantly affecting the release and efficacy of encapsulated drugs. Nanoparticles smaller than 200 nm are mainly internalized by endocytosis, whereas bigger particles (above 200 nm) undergo uptake by either endocytosis or phagocytosis, which are also influenced by cell types (Fig. 5). The pSi microparticles were demonstrated to be internalized by phagocytosis and/or macropinocytosis [44]. The surface properties

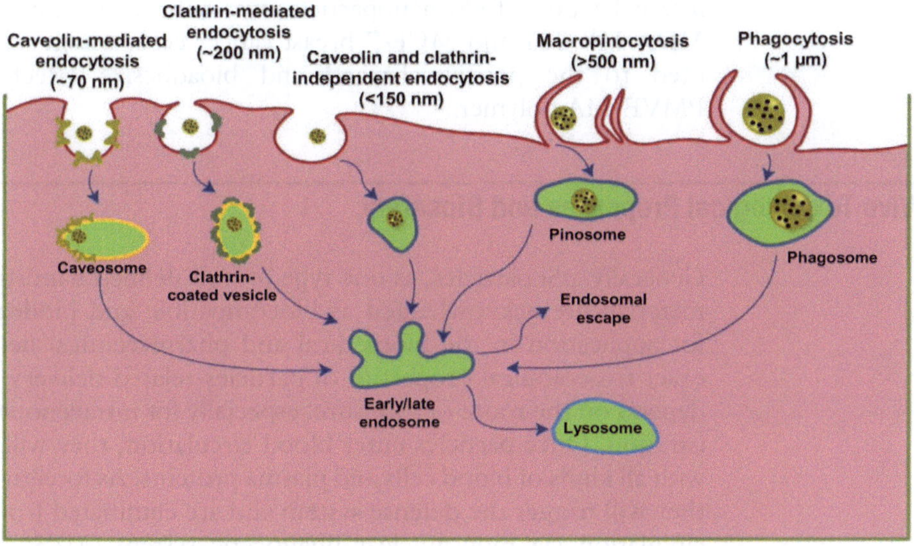

Fig. 5 Mechanisms of intracellular internalization of silicon particles in a typical cell

of pSi particles refer to their shape, charge, hydrophobicity and biological compatibility. The binding and uptake of positively charged nanoparticles to the cell surface is the result of a nonspecific ionic interaction between the positive charge of the nanoparticles and the negative charge of the cell surface. Negatively charged cell surface constituents, such as heparan sulfate proteoglycans and integrins, play a role in the cellular binding of positively charged nanoparticles [45]. The cellular uptake improves with the hydrophobicity increase of the particle's surface. For nanoparticles as siRNA delivery vehicles, the endosomes often mature into increasingly acidic vesicles, which may or may not fuse with lysosomes, where hydrolytic and enzymatic reactions may lead to the complete destruction of the endocyted siRNA. However, responsive surface modification of pSi nanoparticles may interfere with this mechanism and exploit acidification to cause cytoplasmic release by means of a pH-dependent endosomal disruption. The amino groups on the surface of nanoparticles have the ability to create a proton sponge effect by proton osmotic influx inside the endosome, allowing the escape of the particles.

Cell penetrating peptides, also known as protein transduction domains, consist of less than 40 amino acids and have the ability to translocate through almost any cellular plasma membrane. A cell penetrating peptide (NF51) was functionalized on the surface of splice-correcting oligonucleotides loaded aminosilanes-grafted pSi nanoparticles [37]. This delivery system could promote the release of oligonucleotides into the cytosol and protect them from endosome-mediated degradation.

The positively charged pSi nanoparticles (+33 mV) were fabricated by covalently attaching of poly(methyl vinyl ether- *co* -maleic acid) (PMVE-MA) copolymer to the surface of (3-aminopropyl) triethoxysilane-modified porous silicon nanoparticles [46]. The internalization of pSi nanoparticles was enhanced greatly in both MDA-MB-231 and MCF-7 breast cancer cells, which was attributed to the positive-charged and bioadhesive effect of the PMVE-MA polymer.

4 In Vivo Toxicological Properties and Biosafety

Generally, pSi particles, as one type of well-defined nanostructures materials are acknowledged as biocompatible and biodegradable for application in the biomedical and pharmaceutical fields. The exact toxicological properties of particles-related delivery vehicles depend on the route of exposure, especially for intravenous administration. Once particles enter blood circulation, they will contact with all kinds of blood cells and plasma proteins. As foreign objects, they will trigger the defense system and are eliminated from blood circulation via mononuclear phagocytic system (MPS). On the other hand, nanoparticles also bind to and are coated with serum proteins in blood fluids, which could modulate the particles' uptake and lead to complement system activation. Therefore, the toxicological properties and biosafety are highly correlated with to the exposure route and particles' characteristics, such as size, surface morphology, composition, and dose metrics, etc. All these parameters need be taken into account when designing and fabricating pSi particles especially for intravenous injection so as to minimize the systemic toxicity and improve in vivo performance.

4.1 In Vivo Biodistribution

As ideal particles for systemic drug delivery, pSi particles are assumed to be able to arrive and release entrapped drug at targeted sites (such as specific organs, tissues or cells) by easily traversing tissues, cells and organelles through body circulation. However, in the journey of particles to targeted sites, multiple biological barriers exist that would filtrate and opsonize particles and influence their biodistribution and therapeutic effect [47]. The pSi particles are similar to the others organic polymeric particles, and their time-dependence biodistribution strongly depends on their size, surface charge, shape, and composition. The accumulation of pSi particles in healthy tissues should be minimalized to guarantee the maximum targeted accumulation of entrapped drugs so as to achieve the desired pharmacological effect and mitigate the potential systemic toxicity.

4.1.1 Size and Geometry Effect

In the blood circulation, particle size mainly impacts the efficacy of lung and hepatic filtration, kidney excretion, tissue extravasation and diffusion. In some ways, the biodistribution of pSi particles is the combination filtration outcome of these physiological barriers. Along with size, the geometry of pSi nanostructures can determine their behaviors in the body. Unlike spherical particles, nonspherical particles (size, shape, and orientation) exhibit more complex motions with tumbling and rolling in flowing blood. The probability of cellular adhesion is also decreased as a result of the increased particle size and shear stress at the vessel walls [48].

For intravenous administration, approximately above 80 % dose of luminescent porous silicon nanoparticles (LPSiNPs, 20 mg/kg) with 126 nm was accumulated in the liver and spleen 24 h after I.V. injection. The distribution silicon content in the spleen was almost threefold compared to that in the liver in Park's study [49]. This distribution ratio of liver to spleen is quite different for pSi microparticles, which mainly accumulated in the liver other than in the spleen [50]. The accumulation of pSi particles in the lungs increased as the particle size increased.

Different shapes of porous pSi particles (discoidal, spherical, hemispherical and cylindrical) were intravenously injected into MDA-MB-231 breast tumor bearing mice [50]. Si content in major organs was detected by inductively coupled plasma atomic emission spectrometer (ICP-AES). The biodistribution results at 6 h

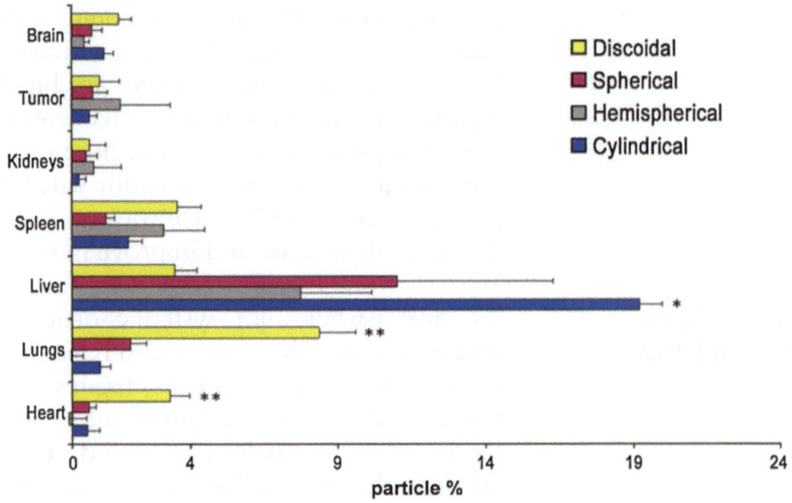

Fig. 6 In vivo biodistribution of pSi particles with different geometries. The percentage of silicon is proportional to the number of particles accumulating in each organ 6 h after intravenous administration into breast tumor burdened mice. Reprinted from Decuzzi et al. [50], with permission from Elsevier

showed shape-dependent accumulation of pSi in major organs and around 2 % of particles existed in tumor tissue (Fig. 6). In the heart and lungs, discoidal particles indicated relatively high accumulation compared to the other shape particles. Hemispherical particles showed more than twofold accumulation in the liver, with small amount of distribution in the heart and lungs.

For oral delivery, pSi particles was designed and fabricated to prevent the encapsulated active ingredients from enzymatic degradation and enhance their oral dissolution properties. The loaded drugs should always release in gastrointestinal (GI) tract. The pSi drug vehicle's distribution behaviors in the GI tract are much more important than that in the organs reached by I.V. injection. 18F-labeled hydrocarbonized pSi nanoparticles (188 nm) could partially pass through the gastrointestinal tract after oral administration and were not absorbed from a subcutaneous deposit. They mainly accumulated in the liver and spleen 4 h after intravenous injection [51].

4.1.2 Surface Composition

The hydrophilicity of the pSi particles surface has great impacts on opsonized phagocytosis and complement activation. The mechanism involved in nanoparticle opsonization is receptor-mediated by interactions of specific proteins absorbed onto the surface of the nanoparticles with phagocytes [52]. In Sarparanta's study, they coated hydrophobic thermally hydrocarbonized porous silicon (THCPsi) nanoparticles with *Trichoderma reesei* HFBII protein [53]. The size of THCPsi NPs increased slightly (215–324 nm) by protein coating. This surface composition transfer significantly reduced THCPsi nanoparticles accumulation in the spleen (about 2.5-fold at 60 min), even though blood circulation time of protein modified pSi nanoparticles showed no significant improvement. This was attributed to the difference of protein types absorbed onto THCPsi NPs and HFBII-THCPsi NPs after incubation in plasma.

All the evidence demonstrated that the biodistribution of pSi particles can be optimized by proper particle size, geometry and surface composition design.

4.2 In Vivo Degradation and Clearance

The pSi particles are readily degraded into monomeric silicic acid through hydrolysis of Si-O bonds in a physiological environment, which is naturally found in human body such as bone and other human tissues. The pSi degradation rate is directly correlated with the particles' porosity, surface area and surface modifications. The surface properties of pSi are the determinant of degradation kinetics among these factors. The surface of untreated pSi particles is hydrogen-terminated. In physiological fluid, they are able to degrade in hours, which is unfavorable for controlled drug release and long circulation time in blood required for drug delivery vehicles. Thus, the surface stabilization of pSi particles should be conducted. The stabilization strategies mainly include functional groups replacement, long chain polymer grafting and surface-protein coating.

Two thermal oxidation processes were developed by Hon et al., which were able to increase the degradation half-life of 100 nm pSi nanoparticles from 10 min to 3 h [54]. It can be extended up to 8 h by using silica coating. The formation of an inert silica layer in the oxidation processes resulted in preventing the Si core from degradation. Modification of porous silicon particles with APTES also could limit surface attack by water molecules and thus prevented the particle from rapid degradation [31]. Godin et al. modified the surface of hemispherical pSi microparticles by covalent conjugation using different molecular weights of PEGs. This PEGylation precisely tuned the degradation kinetics of pSi particles, which can prolong the degradation over 3 days [55]. The degradation rate was prolonged as the PEG length increased.

The degradation kinetics was independent of the particle diameters, while the total specific surface area and porosity dominated the degradation process. The pSi particles with high porosity (above 50 %) are gradually degraded in the majority of the simulated physiological fluids, including phosphate-buffered saline (PBS) and proteins-contained solutions and excluding simulated acidic gastric fluid (pH less than 5.0). The degradation proceeded from the outer surfaces of particles and simultaneously from the inner cores, and the degradation process was heterogeneous. The biodegradation properties of the pSi nanoparticles provide safe clearance from the body.

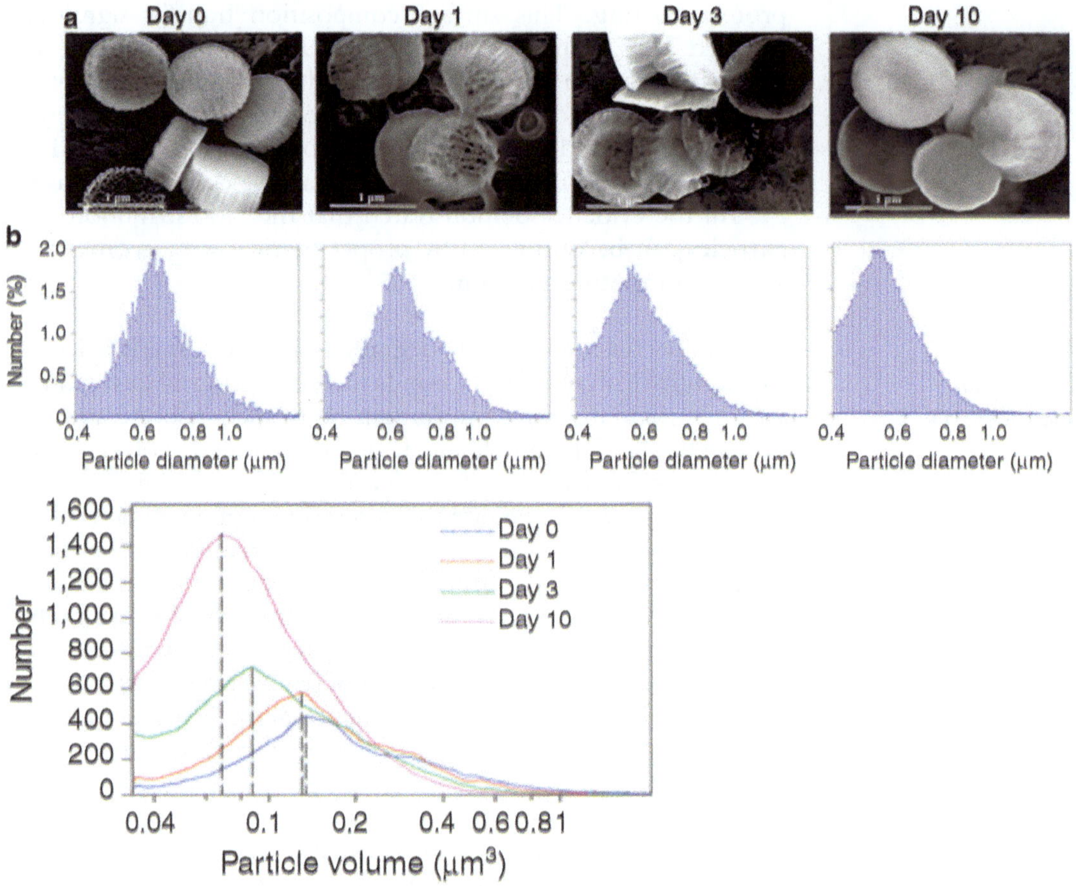

Fig. 7 The degradation of pSi particles in serum. (**a**) Discoidal pSi microparticles (1000 × 400 nm) were incubated in fetal bovine serum (FBS), pH 5.7. The structures of particles were visualized by SEM after 1, 3, and 10 days incubation. (**b**) The particle size was measured with a Multisizer instrument and displayed on the basis of diameter and volume. Reprinted from Shen et al. [56], with permission from American Association for Cancer Research

The degradation of APTES-modified porous silicon microparticles was conducted in PBS containing 10 % fetal bovine serum (FBS) and characterized by scanning electronic microscope (SEM) images and size measurements (Fig. 7). The pSi particles gradually lost their porous layer and were only left with the high-density layer after incubation for 3 days. 46 % of the median sizes of the particles were observed to drop after 10 days of incubation [56].

It is noted that the in vitro degradation performed in simulated buffers cannot fully simulate the in vivo biodegradation behavior because of the complexity of the biological environment. However, there is not a well-rounded in vivo degradation assay available for determining the biodegradation behaviors of pSi particles in vivo. To date, no systematic in vivo results about the degradation processes of pSi particles have been reported. It is unpractical to discriminate the degraded products from the total administrated Si content.

The soluble degradation product-silicic acid can be absorbed by the human body or removed from body through renal clearance. The clearance rate of pSi particles in vivo mainly depends on the degradation rate. Park et al. demonstrated that the LPSiNPs of 126 nm size that accumulated in monocuclear phagocytic system-related organs (liver and spleen) could be cleared completely in a month [49]. Bovine serum albumin (BSA) coated alkyl-terminated pSi nanoparticles via hydrophobic interactions greatly prolonged the nanoparticles in vivo blood circulation time and delayed their clearance from body [57]. The half-life of BSA-pSi nanoparticles was 262.4 min, while that of bare pSi nanoparticles was only 28.6 min. The influence of the surface charge on the in vivo clearance of the pSi particles was still not clear. For the silica nanoparticles, their excretion in vivo is strongly dependent on their surface charge, which results from the charge-dependent proteins adsorption effects on hepatobiliary excretion [58].

4.3 In Vivo Tolerance and Toxicological Properties

When porous silicon particles are introduced into the body, their aqueous dispersibility and biodegradability determine their disposition and elimination routes, which highly influence their in vivo tolerance and toxicological properties. Due to the versatility of pSi synthesis and modification methods for meeting diverse demands, the availability of general systemic toxicological data is limited currently. The pSi particles' tunable size and high porosity largely govern the body's reaction to them. As particulate matters, the pSi particles are able to cause an acute or subacute inflammatory response by macrophage recognition and ingestion after entering human body due to their structural features. On the other hand, the magnitude and accuracy of toxicological evaluation of pSi particles depend on the in vitro validation methods, which should have high relevancy to their conditions of exposure in vivo.

The in vivo safety of negatively and positively charged nanoporous pSi particles was evaluated by acute single and subchronic multiple dose intravenous injection in FBV mice [28]. The renal (BUN and creatinine), hepatic (LDH), and 23 cytokines levels in plasma were not changed compared to those of control animals. The LDH (Lactate Dehydrogenase) levels in the liver and spleen were not altered and there was no leukocytes infiltration into the major organs. This indicated that porous pSi particles did not induce immunoreactivity in mice.

For the pSi particles, the biodegradation properties offer a nontoxic clearance from the body. An effective clearance can prevent toxicity induced by residual impurities and foreign materials in the body. Luminescent pSi nanoparticles could be removed by renal clearance within weeks with no toxic effect and could overcome the toxicity of residual particles of smaller nanocrystals (carbon nanotubes, quantum dots etc.) for in vivo imaging that do not escape phagocytic uptake [49]. Hydrocarbonized pSi particles with around 150 nm diameters did not induce cell toxicity, oxidative stress, or inflammatory response in human colon carcinoma Caco-2 and murine macrophage cells, which indicated that they could be applicable as oral drug delivery vehicles [51].

The major concern for using pSi particles was that mechanical obstruction in the vasculature was possible and could cause congestion in major organs after long-term accumulation in repeated administration [59]. Thus, the in vivo degradation and clearance kinetics should be closely monitored when determining the repeated dose time intervals.

For intravenous administration, the silanol groups in porous SiO_2 nanoparticles surfaces are able to interact with the surface of the phospholipids of the red blood cell membranes resulting in hemolysis [60]. Shahbazi et al. demonstrated that the morphological changes of red blood cells and the amount of particles adsorption into red blood cells were high correlated with the surface chemistry of pSi nanoparticles (hydrophilicity, surface charge, etc.) [61]. Godin's study demonstrated that pSi microparticles did not cause erythrocyte lysis by incubation them with the whole mouse blood [62].

4.4 Summary

In vivo biobehaviors of pSi particles, such as the biodistribution, biodegradation, and toxicological properties, are determined by the synthetic processes, particle sizes, morphologies, surface modifications and dose metrics. The biodistribution and clearance assessment of pSi nano/microparticles found that the particles mainly accumulate in the liver and spleen. There are few particles accumulated in the lungs and even fewer in the kidneys and heart. The degradation and clearance rate of pSi particles depends on their surface composite, which can be tuned by surface modification. More importantly, the long term in vivo biosafety issue and relevant data should be addressed in big mammals such as dogs or pigs for future clinical translation.

5 Therapeutic Applications of pSi Particles

Chemotherapeutic drugs (doxorubicin, paclitaxel, etc.) for cancer therapy currently in clinic have low solubility and are always associated with unexpected chemoresistance and nonselective dose-limiting toxicity, such as myelosuppression, gastrointestinal dysfunctions, neurologic toxicities and immune suppression [63]. Proteins/peptides and DNA/RNA oligonucleotides are two new generations of drugs in biotechnology. Their limitations to in vivo therapies include high molecular weight impeded transportation through tissues and intracellular barriers and enzymatic degradation-caused rapid clearance [64]. The imperative task is to improve their bioavailability and minimize undesirable side effects for systemic application. Nanocarriers such as liposomes, micelles and inorganic nanoparticles have been extensively investigated for improving the pharmacokinetics and pharmacodynamics properties of chemotherapeutic, protein and gene drugs, thus increasing their safety and maximizing the therapeutic effect.

The biocompatibility and biodegradability of pSi particles make them suitable and safe as emerging drug delivery carriers. In contrast to conventional organic nanomaterials-based drug delivery carriers, the prominent advantages of pSi particles mainly include their high porosity, controlled size distribution, tunable degradation kinetics, convenient surface chemistry, and good aqueous dispersion capability. Additionally, the versatility of silicon-based chemistry offers composite nanoparticles systems by inorganic or organic/inorganic hybridization, which are able to be employed for multiple biomedical applications such as immunotherapy, photothermal and photodynamic therapy, diagnostic imaging, and combined diagnostics and therapy.

5.1 In Vivo Chemical Drug Therapy

As previously described, pSi particles can be chemotherapeutic drug carriers with high payload capacities, near zero premature release, and excellent aqueous stability. Thus, they are able to protect the encapsulated chemotherapeutic agents within the nanopores before reaching targeted sites, minimize nonselective toxicity and maximize the therapeutic effect for systemic circulation. A tumor homing peptide (CooP) biofunctionalized thermally hydrocarbonized pSi (THCPSi) nanoparticles (180 nm) was utilized to targeting mammary-derived growth inhibitor (MDGI) expressing tumor in vivo [65]. The CooP-THCPSi nanoparticles showed around ninefold tumor accumulation efficiency compared to the unmodified THCPSi particles. Paclitaxel-containing poly(ethylene glycol)-block-poly(ε-caprolactone) micelles was loaded within the pores of pSi microparticles. The pSi particles greatly delayed the paclitaxel release in vitro and significantly improved the antitumor efficacy in mice bearing MDA-MB-468 breast tumors compared to that of commercial formulation [66].

The high payload capacities and sustained-release properties of pSi particles are critical characteristics for local delivery, such as in subcutaneous and intravitreal applications. Daunorubicin-attached porous silicon microparticles were developed for long-term intravitreally local administration [67, 68]. The covalently loaded daunorubicin was sustainedly released for 3 months without ocular toxicity after intravitreal injection.

For oral administration, the dissolution kinetics of poorly soluble drugs in the GI tract was hugely improved by the altered crystalline behaviors of drugs in the irregular sponge-like nanopores of pSi particles. Indomethacin-loaded mesoporous silicon microparticles could promote the immediate release of non-crystal drugs and greatly alter the in vivo pharmacokinetic behaviors of

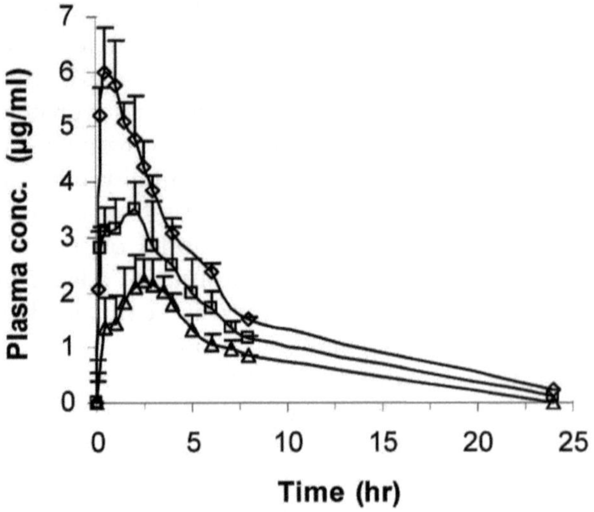

Fig. 8 Time-plasma concentration profiles of indomethacin-loaded pSi microparticles by oral administration in fasted Sprague–Dawley rats. Free indomethacin (*open triangle*), Indocid® (*open square*), and indomethacin in oxidized pSi particles (*open diamond*). Reprinted from Wang et al. [34], with permission from American ACS

the drugs via oral administration, as compared with crystalline indomethacin (Fig. 8). The critical pharmacokinetic parameters: Cmax was increased twofold, AUC was enhanced 77 %, and Tmax was shortened from 2 to 0.6 h [34].

5.2 In Vivo siRNA Delivery

Small interfering RNA (siRNA) and microRNA are gene silencing agents that have the clinical potential to modulate gene expression for the treatment of human diseases, including cancer. Because of the unfavorable physicochemical properties of siRNA, including its negative charge, high molecule weight and instability (plasma half-life: about 10 min), the barriers for systemic siRNA delivery are multiple. They mainly refers to difficulties in the distribution to organs, penetration to the interstitium, internalization by target cells, escape from endosomes, and release of siRNA into cytosol from carriers [69]. Therefore, as the effective siRNA delivery vehicles, pores and surface modification of pSi particles are always crucial for loading siRNA and controlling its release behaviors in vivo.

Shen et al. developed a high capacity polycation-functionalized nanoporous silicon particles (PCPS) platform, which was based on Arg-PEI modified nanoporous silicon microparticles (1 µm in diameter and 400 nm in height) as gene silencing agents (Fig. 9a) [31]. Negatively charged siRNA and microRNA were bound to positively charged Arg-PEI modified pSi particles with high payload. The size of released siRNA nanocomplex was around 100 nm (Fig. 9d, e) under in vitro release condition.

Over 80 % of protein knockdowns were accomplished using STAT3 or GRP78 siRNA-loaded PCPS in MDA-MB-231 human

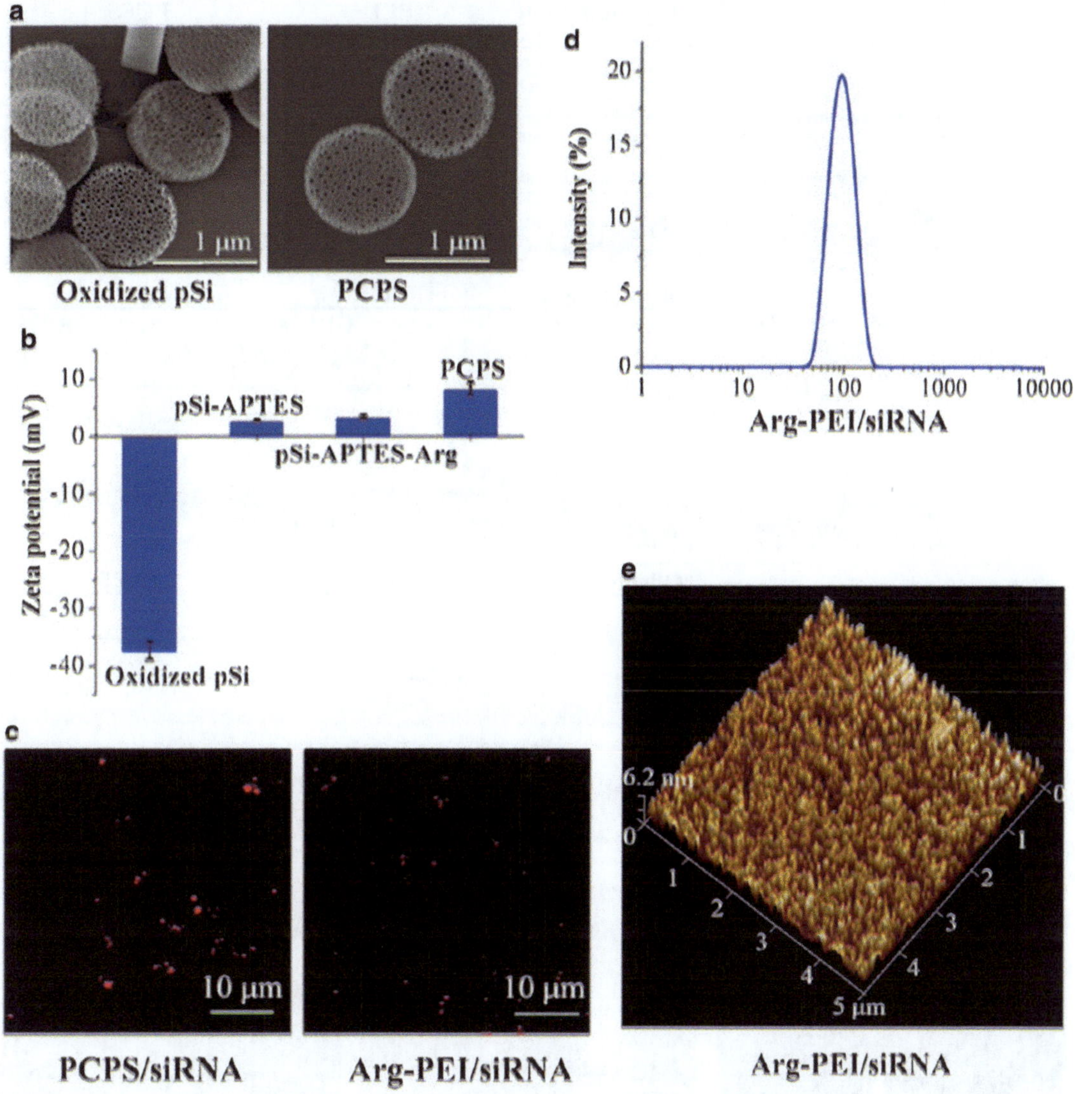

Fig. 9 Characterization of polycation-functionalized pSi particles (PCPS) as delivery carriers for gene silencing agents. (**a**) SEM images of pSi particles and PCPS. (**b**) Changes of zeta potential at each stage of PCPS fabrication. (**c**) Confocal microscopy images of PCPS/Alexa 555-siRNA (*left*) and the released Arg-PEI-siRNA nanocomplex (*right*). (**d**) Size distribution of released siRNA nanocomplex measured by dynamic light scattering (DLS). (**e**) Atomic force microscopy (AFM) image of siRNA nanocomplex. Reprinted from Shen et al. [31], with permission from American ACS

breast cancer cells in vitro. MicroRNA-18a in PCPS also knocked down 90 % of the microRNA-18a target gene ATM expression (Fig. 10). In vivo STAT3 gene expression knockdown caused great reduction of cancer stem cells in MDA-MB-231 tumor tissue by systemic delivery of PCPS/STAT3 siRNA.

The acute immune response and subacute toxicity results demonstrated the biosafety of the PCPS gene delivery system in

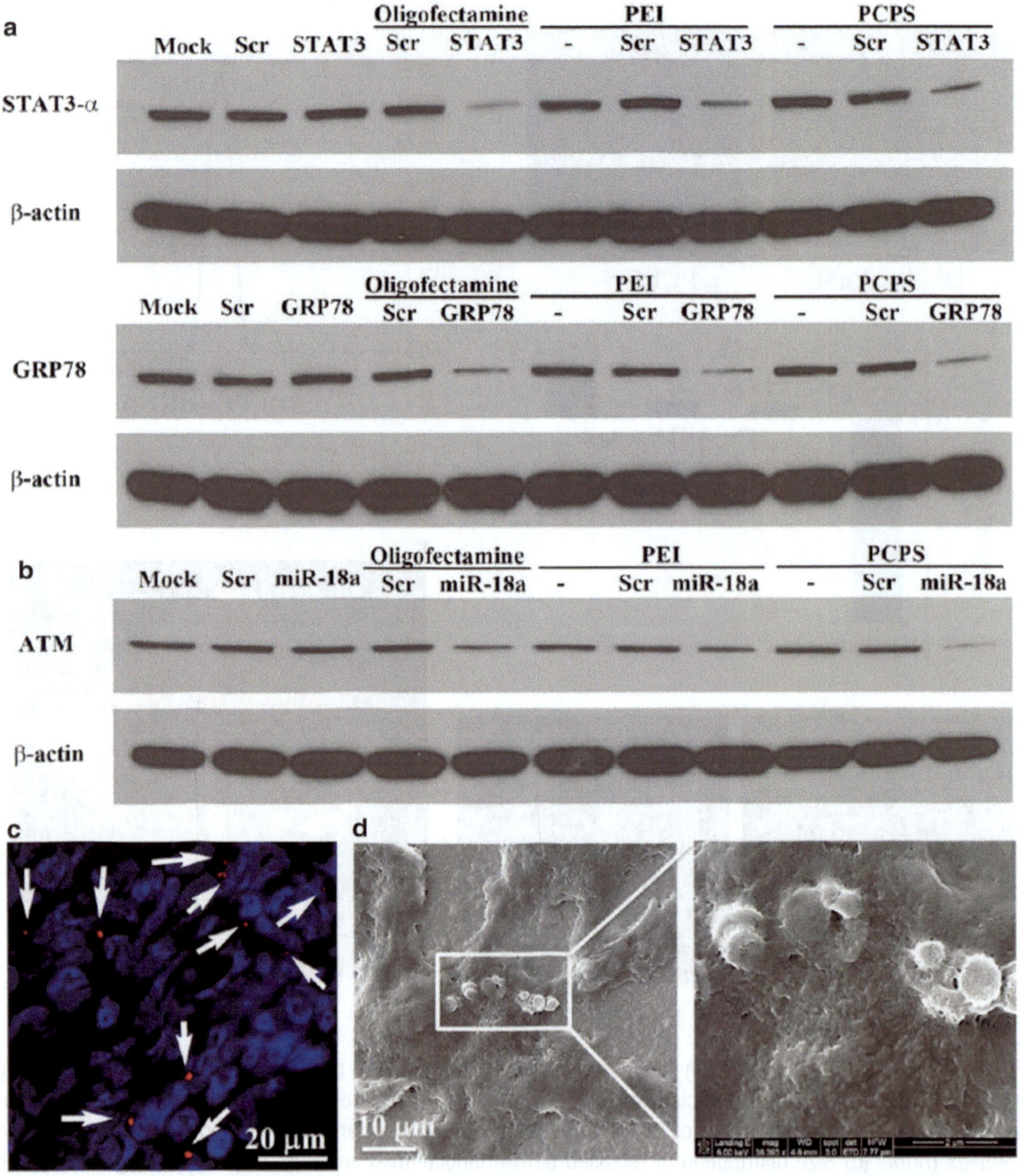

Fig. 10 Gene knockdown in two breast cancer cells via PCPS in vitro. (**a**) Western blot on knockdown of STAT3 and GRP78 expression in MDA-MB-231 cells following treatment with the corresponding siRNA for 72 h. (**b**) Knockdown of ATM expression in MCF-7 cells. (**c**) Accumulation of PCPS/siRNA in primary MDA-MB-231 tumor 6 h after intravenous administration of 150×10^6 Alexa 555 PCPS/siRNA. (**d**) SEM images of PCPS/siRNA in tumor tissue. Reprinted from Shen et al. [31], with permission from American ACS

FVB mice by detecting the related cytokines, colony-stimulating factors, hematology, blood chemistry, and major organ histology changes.

5.3 Proteins and Peptides Delivery

Proteins and peptides show high molecular weight, hydrophilicity and structural fragility. They are easily degraded, denaturated and inactivated during formulation, storage, and delivery. Their formulations always include structure stabilizers, salt buffers and preservatives for improving their in vitro and in vivo stabilities [70]. The intramuscular, intravenous and subcutaneous injections are common administration routes for protein and peptide deliveries.

For oral administration, the degradation by the proteolytic enzymes located in the gastrointestinal tract and the poor intestinal mucosa permeability strongly limit oral protein bioavailability. Chitosan (CS) modified undecylenic acid-attachment hydrocarbonized pSi microparticles were able to protect insulin from degradation by enzymes in the GI tract and greatly increased the interactions between microparticles with Caco-2/HT-29 cell monolayers, which was expected to enhance the permeation capability of insulin across intestinal mucosa [36].

One gut hormone peptide YY3-36, a potential candidate for obesity therapy was absorbed into three kinds of modified pSi nanoparticles (~160 nm): hydrophilic thermally oxidized (TOPSi), moderately hydrophilic undecylenic acid-treated thermally hydrocarbonized (UnTHCPSi), and hydrophobic thermally hydrocarbonized (THCPSi). PYY3-36 was sustainedly released for 4 days, and the different surface modification of pSi nanoparticles did not change its bioavailability via subcutaneous injection (Fig. 11) [71]. However, the free YY3-36 was rapidly cleared in mice and undetectable 12 h after subcutaneous administration. The surface hydrophilicity promoted the peptide release in blood circulation by intravenous injection. The bioavailability of peptide pSi formulations was increased around three times compared to that of solution formulation in both administration routes, which was attributed to the controlled release and peptide's protection from rapid elimination by encapsulation of drug in pSi nanocarriers.

5.4 In Vivo Imaging

Biocompatible and functionalized nanoparticles have been widely investigated for fluorescence, magnetic, and radioactive signals for enhancing the sensitivity and specificity of noninvasive imaging [72–74]. Visible photoluminescence of porous silicon used in biomedical applications was first reported by Canham in 1990s [75]. The unique features of pSi nanoparticles for imaging include their ample surface modification area, capability for multiple conjugations to tumor-targeting ligands and relatively in vivo long-circulation properties [76, 77]. The degradation of pSi particles and loaded drug release can be monitored in situ by digital imaging. The optical reflectance spectrum shift change has a good correlation with the released drug amount as measured by photonic resonance. Luminescent porous silicon nanoparticles (130–180 nm, LPSiNPs) were applied for monitoring in vivo degradation and accumulation by using their intrinsic near-infrared

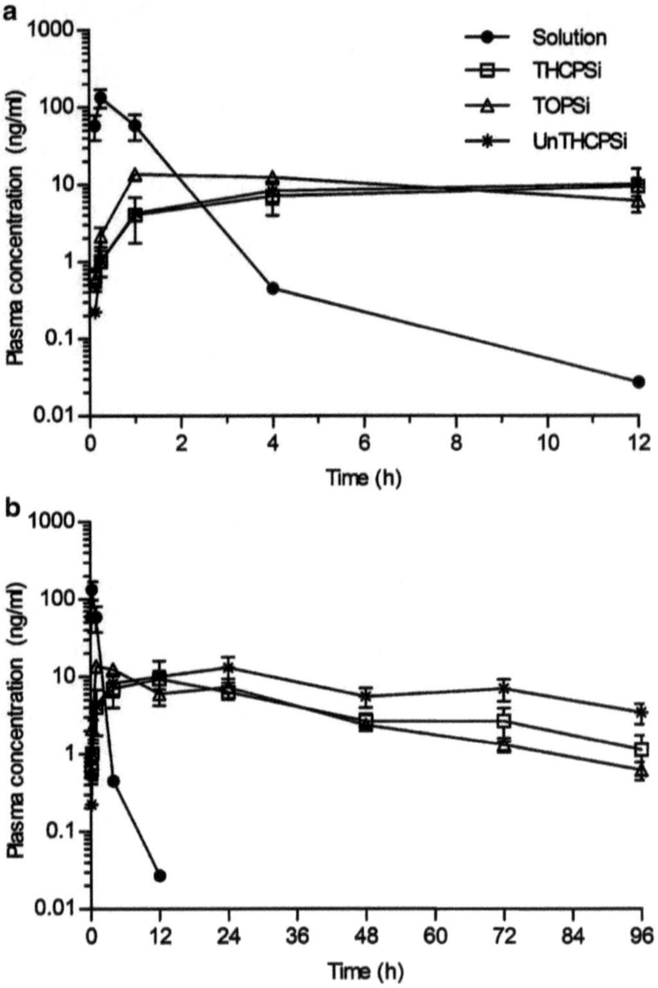

Fig. 11 Time-plasma concentration profiles of Peptide YY3-36 pSi nanoparticles or solution (20 μg) up to 12 h (**a**) and 4 days (**b**) after subcutaneous administration in mice. Reprinted from Kovalainen et al. [71], with permission from American ACS

photoluminescence. The quantum yield of LPSiNPs is sufficient for observation in internal organs using fluorescence imaging systems [49].

Luminescent PEG5000-porous silicon nanoparticles (PEG-LPSiNPs) with 150 nm diameters were prepared for in vivo tumor imaging by the enhanced permeability and retention (EPR) effect promoted nanoparticles accumulation in tumor of human ovarian cancer xenografted mice [78]. The rationale is that the long emission lifetime of photo-luminescent PEG-LPSiNPs (5–13 ms) can eliminate the shorter-lived emission signals from tissue auto-fluorescence (less than 10 ns). This type of time-gating imaging tools could greatly improve the signal-to-background contrast ratio by around 400-fold both in vitro and in vivo (Fig. 12).

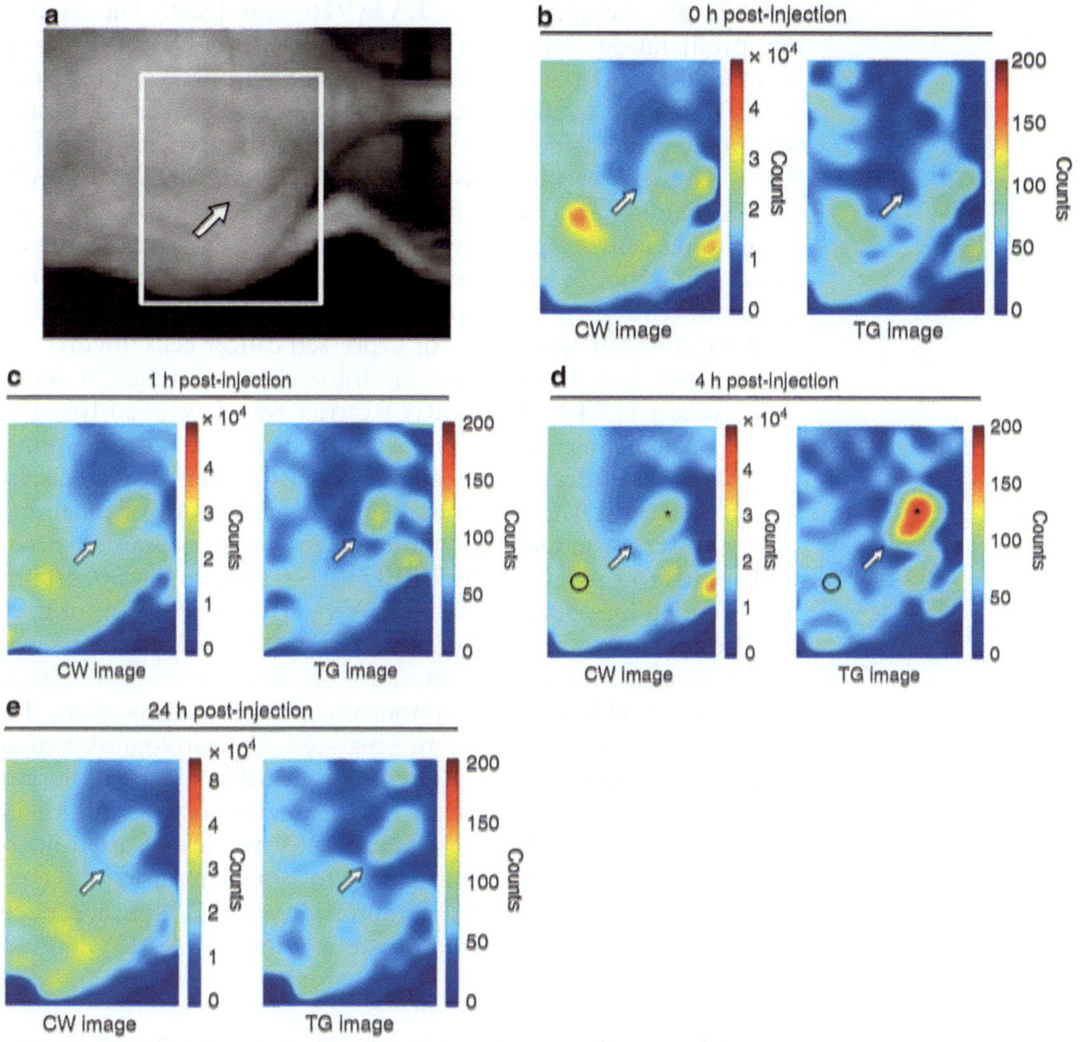

Fig. 12 Time-gated (TG) fluorescence images of mice bearing SKOV3 ovarian tumor after intravenous administration of PEG-LPSiNPs. (**a**) Bright-field image of nude mouse bearing tumor at the flank. The *arrow* indicated the tumor site. (**b–e**) continuous wave (CW) and TG fluorescence images of the region indicated with the *white box* in (**a**). immediately (**b**), 1 h (**c**), 4 h (**d**), or 24 h (**e**) after intravenous injection of PEG-LPSiNPs (10 mg/kg). Reprinted from Gu et al. [78], with permission from Macmillan Publishers Limited

5.5 Targeted Delivery

The surface of pSi particles provides one suitable vehicle for covalent conjugation and electrostatic attachment of a vast spectrum of targeting ligands. Currently, the targeting ligands under active investigation include small chemicals, peptides, aptamers, and antibodies, which have the most clinical potential [79].

Two arginylglycylaspartic acid derivatives (RGDS and iRGD) as targeting moieties were conjugated to APTES-modified thermally carbonized pSi (APS-TCPSi) nanoparticles, which size was increased around 20 nm. The cellular uptake efficiency of RGD-pSi nanoparticles was increased around 1.5 times compared to that of APS-pSi nanoparticles in EA.hy926 cells [80]. The in vitro antiproliferation activity of sorafenib was also enhanced by drug-containing RGD-pSi nanoparticles. Three periodate-oxidized antibodies targeted to different types of cancer cells were conjugated to the semicarbazide functionalized pSi nanoparticles (115 nm) [81]. These three monoclonal antibodies were MLR2, mAb528, and Rituximab, targeting glioblastoma, neuroblastoma, and B cell lymphoma cells, respectively. Camptothecin was loaded into the pores of antibody-pSi nanoparticles via a physical absorption method. The drug containing antibody-pSi nanoparticles exhibited selective killing of receptor expressed cancer cells in vitro.

In our group, an E-selectin thioaptamer-conjugated multistage vector (ESTA-MSV) siRNA carrier was developed based on porous silicon microparticles (1 μm in diameter and 400 nm in height) for the effective treatment of breast cancer bone metastasis [30]. E-selectin is overexpressed in the vasculature of inflammatory and tumor tissues. The targeting moiety thioaptamer specifically binds to E-selectin. PEG-PEI/siRNA polyplexes (30–40 nm) were loaded into porous ESTA-MSV by sonication absorption.

Bone marrow accumulation of ESTA-MSV was evaluated with Cy5-labeled ESTA-MSV by immunohistology in mice bearing bone metastatic MDA-MB-231 tumors via intravenous injection. The femur and spine of mice were separated for histological analysis after 4 h. Compared with untargeted Cy5-MSV, more red fluorescent particles co-localized with the E-selectin-positive endothelial cells (green) (Fig. 13b). Most ESTA-MSV particles existed in the perivascular region following binding to E-selectin inside the medullary cavity (Fig. 13c). STAT3 expression in 48.7 % of cancer cells in bone marrow showed knockdown by using ESTA-MSV targeted delivery system.

5.6 Multistage Drug Delivery

Recently, a multistage drug delivery system called multistage vector (MSV) was designed and employed for diverse applications in the biomedical field based on porous silicon microparticles [82]. The dominating parameters in the intravascular journey of nanoparticles in blood were intensively studied on the basis of three fundamental events: the margination dynamics, firm adhesion, and control of internalization. Along with size, the geometry of the pSi nanostructure can determine a NP's behavior in the body. Nonspherical porous silicon particles show more complex motions of tumbling and rolling in flowing blood compared with spherical particles, which influences the tissue penetration and vascular adhesion ability in body circulation [48]. Hemispherical and quasi-hemispherical porous silicon particles (pore size: 30–60 nm) were designed and fabricated as the stage one particles by combination of photolithographic techniques and electrochemical etch. The secondary nanoparticles of size smaller than 30 nm (liposomes, quantum dots, gold nanoshells, micelles, etc.) can be loaded within the pores by using dry silicon particles through simple capillary

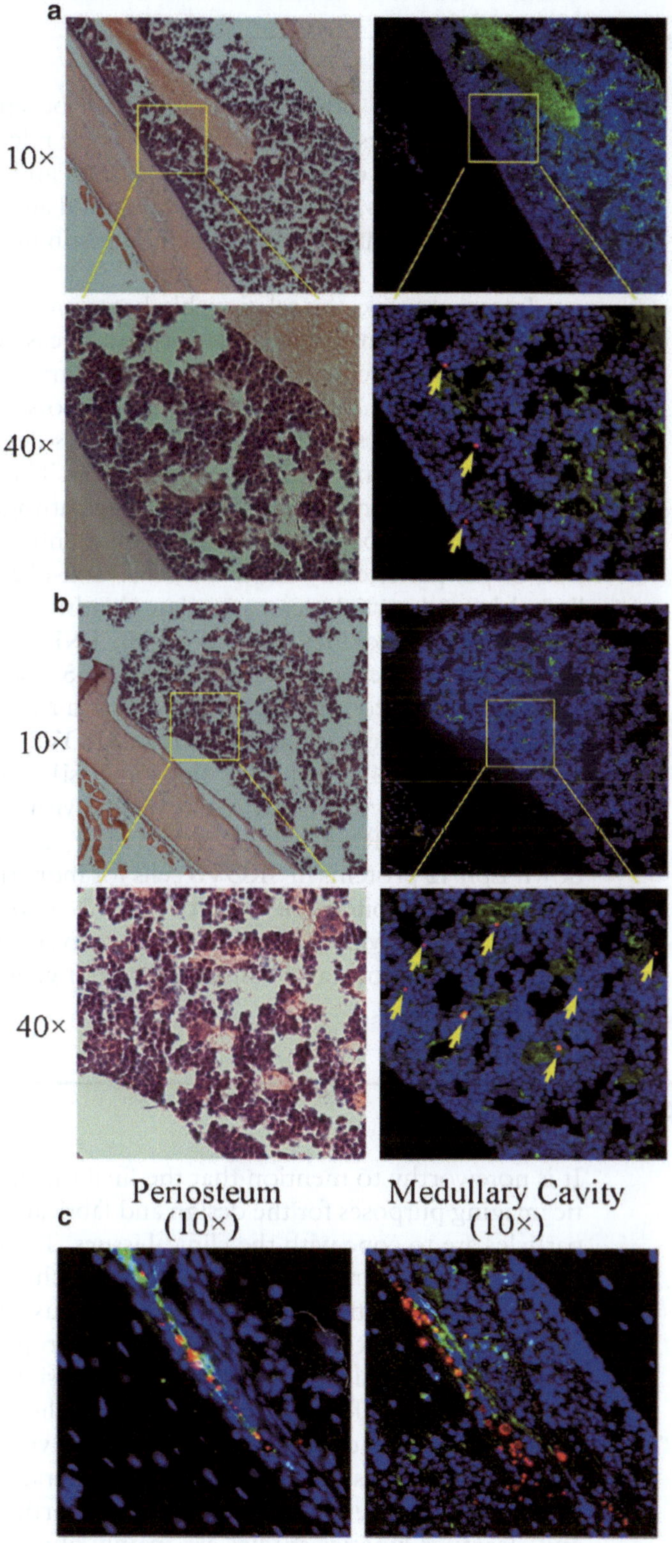

Fig. 13 Accumulation and distribution of multistage vector (pSi particles, MSV) in the bone marrow by histological analysis. (**a**) Free MSV particles. *Left panel*: H&E staining. *Right panel*: E-selectin Staining (in *green*) for E-selectin expression inside the bone marrow. Nuclei are stained in blue with 4′,6-diamidino-2-phenylindole (DAPI) and Cy5-labeled MSV particles in *red* (indicated by *arrows*). (**b**) ESTA-MSV particles. (**c**) Fluorescent microscopy images of ESTA-MSV particles inside and outside of bone marrow. Endothelial cells are stained in *green*, and nuclei in *blue*. The cy5-ESTA-MSV particles are stained in *red*. Reprinted from Mai et al. [30], with permission from Elsevier

force. Drugs and other therapeutics can be encapsulated in the secondary particles. Secondary nanoparticle release from stage one particles depends on the degradation rates and surface coating of stage one particles, and the physicochemical and biological properties of stage two nanoparticles including stimuli-sensitive response techniques.

In recent work, the relationship between variations in pore size and the impact on the degradation and release of multistage vectors (MSVs) was elucidated [83]. The degradation rate of MSVs was accelerated and the loaded quantum dots' release was slowed down as the pore size increased. The MSVs degradation occurred heterogeneously in a multistep progression. The pSi microparticles as MSVs were demonstrated to present pathogen-associated patterns and mimic pathogens, which could enhance the internalization of pSi particles by dendritic cells. Toll-like receptor (TLR)-4 ligand-bound particles can stimulate dendritic cells to secrete pro-inflammatory cytokines, such as IL-1β, TNF-α, and IL-6 [44].

As siRNA delivery vehicles, Alexa 555 siRNA-DOPC liposomes were loaded into the 1000×400 nm MSVs. A large number of MSVs underwent uptake in human SKOV3ip2 and HeyA8 cancer cells (Fig. 14) [56]. The liposomal siRNA were sustainedly released in the cytosol and could still be visualized on day 2 and day 7. EphA2 siRNA loaded MSV (MSV/EphA2) could knockdown EphA2 proteins in SKOV3 cells for more than 9 days. EphA2 knockdown inhibited cell viability by 40 % on day 9. Combination treatment with MSV/EphA2 and docetaxel effectively inhibited HeyA8-MDR (docetaxel-resistance) tumor growth in mice models of ovarian cancer.

6 Future Prospects

It is noteworthy to mention that the final therapeutic and diagnostic imaging purposes for the design and fabrication of porous silicon particles are to cope with the clinical issues. The compositional and structural characteristics of pSi particles (such as particle size, pore structure, aggregation state and surface status) should be designed and tuned to meet the biopharmaceutical properties of the encapsulated drug, administration route and physiological environment in the body. Therefore, the correlation establishment of in vitro pSi particles' physiochemical properties and in vivo pharmacokinetic-pharmacodynamics behaviors becomes imperative.

Nowadays, the results for in vivo pSi particles' biodistribution and clearance kinetics studies are mainly obtained by fluorescence intensity or the ICP detection of silicon amounts. However, the fluorescence may suffer from quenching after administration in vivo. The unstable in vivo silicon background could interfere with the accuracy of silicon quantitative analysis by ICP. Therefore, there is an urgent need for the development of reliable and robust

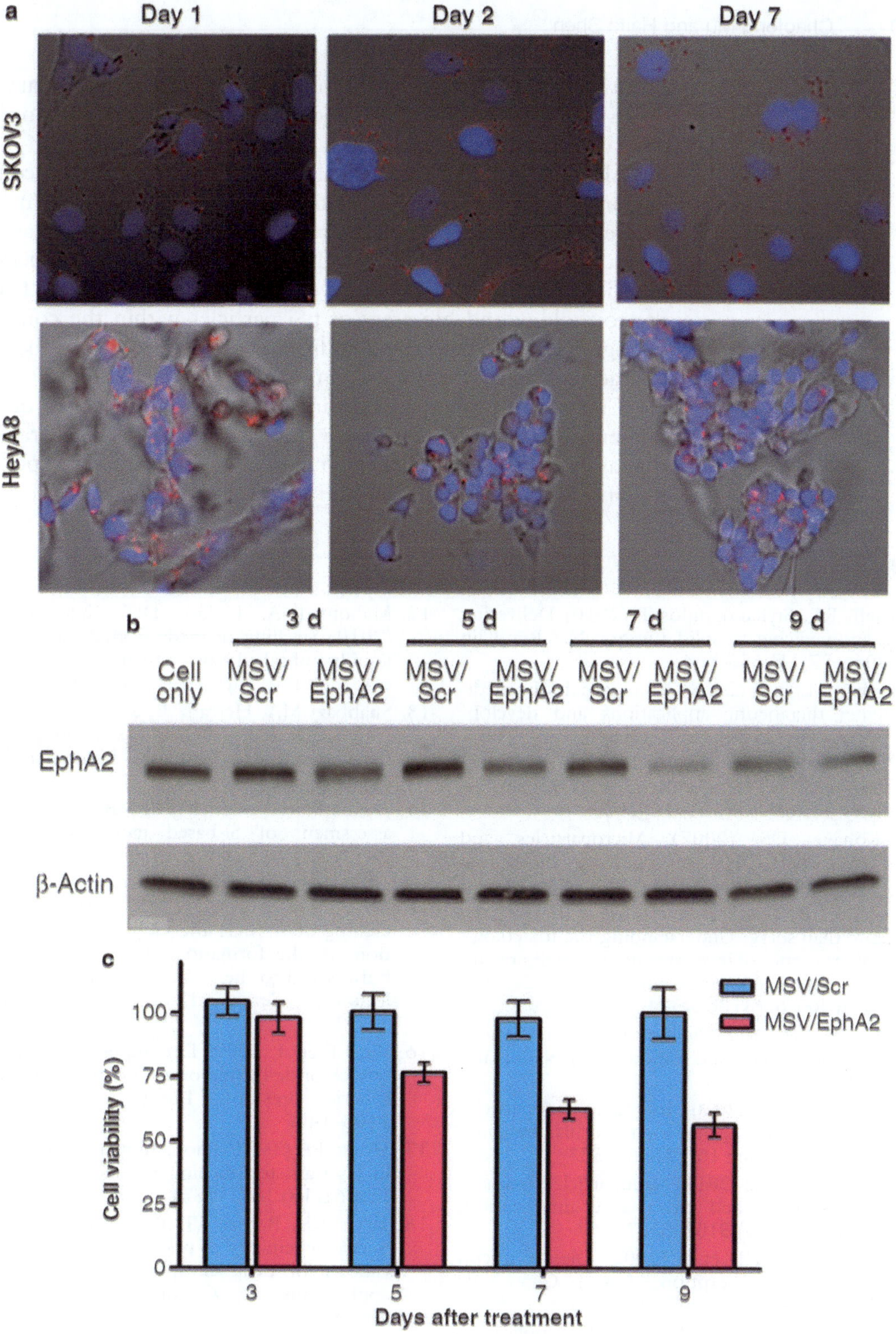

Fig. 14 Sustained release of liposomal siRNA from MSV in tumor cells. (**a**) Alexa 555-labeled siRNAs were encapsulated in DOPC liposomes and loaded into MSV (MSV/Alexa 555 siRNA). Human ovarian tumor cells SKOV3ip2 and HeyA8 were incubated with MSV/Alexa 555 siRNA and the release of Alexa 555 siRNA from MSV was monitored by confocal microscopy over the next 7 days. Nuclei were stained in *blue* with DAPI, and Alexa 555 siRNA was in *red*. (**b**) Western blot analysis of EphA2 expression in SKOV3 cells incubated with MSV/EphA2 siRNA. (**c**) Cell viability measurement after treatment with MSV/EphA2. Reprinted from Shen et al. [56], with permission from American Association for Cancer Research

quantitative analytical methods in order to collect accurate data for the in vivo biodistribution, degradation processes, and clearance of pSi particles in biological tissues.

Although many in vivo animal model results have confirmed the biocompatibility of pSi particles, the conducted studies have mainly focused on limited acute and subacute toxicities. It is necessary to extend the biocompatibility studies to include chronic toxicities, specific neurotoxicity, reproductive toxicity, etc. On the other hand, the toxicology and biosafety of pSi particles within the complex biological environment is still far from being defined due to the lack of practical clinical trials in human bodies.

Current findings are promising and meaningful for the development of effective and safe pSi particles and the clinical translation as they move from bench to beside, which is greatly expected to contribute to human health in the near future.

References

1. Jain RK, Stylianopoulos T (2010) Delivering nanomedicine to solid tumors. Nat Rev Clin Oncol 7(11):653–664
2. Zhang L et al (2008) Nanoparticles in medicine: therapeutic applications and developments. Clin Pharmacol Ther 83(5):761–769
3. Solaro R, Chiellini F, Battisti A (2010) Targeted delivery of protein drugs by nanocarriers. Materials 3(3):1928–1980
4. Kohane DS (2007) Microparticles and nanoparticles for drug delivery. Biotechnol Bioeng 96(2):203–209
5. Fadeel B, Garcia-Bennett AE (2010) Better safe than sorry: Understanding the toxicological properties of inorganic nanoparticles manufactured for biomedical applications. Adv Drug Deliv Rev 62(3):362–374
6. Li XM et al (2012) Biocompatibility and toxicity of nanoparticles and nanotubes. J Nanomater 2012, 548389
7. Cho EC et al (2010) Inorganic nanoparticle-based contrast agents for molecular imaging. Trends Mol Med 16(12):561–573
8. Bogart LK et al (2014) Nanoparticles for imaging, sensing, and therapeutic intervention. ACS Nano 8(4):3107–3122
9. Jugdaohsingh R et al (2002) Dietary silicon intake and absorption. Am J Clin Nutr 75(5):887–893
10. Luhrs AK, Geurtsen W (2009) The application of silicon and silicates in dentistry: a review. Prog Mol Subcell Biol 47:359–380
11. Leslie LJ et al (2008) The effect of the environment on the mechanical properties of medical grade silicones. J Biomed Mater Res B Appl Biomater 86(2):460–465
12. Mahomed A, Hukins DW, Kukureka SN (2010) Swelling of medical grade silicones in liquids and calculation of their cross-link densities. Med Eng Phys 32(4):298–303
13. Shahbazi MA, Herranz B, Santos HA (2012) Nanostructured porous Si-based nanoparticles for targeted drug delivery. Biomatter 2(4): 296–312
14. Jaganathan H, Godin B (2012) Biocompatibility assessment of Si-based nano- and microparticles. Adv Drug Deliv Rev 64(15): 1800–1819
15. Bogumilowicz Y et al (2005) Chemical vapour etching of Si, SiGe and Ge with HCl; applications to the formation of thin relaxed SiGe buffers and to the revelation of threading dislocations. Semicond Sci Technol 20(2): 127–134
16. Wu LF et al (2009) Decomposition of silicon tetrachloride by microwave plasma jet at atmospheric pressure. Inorg Mater 45(12): 1403–1407
17. Houle FA (1988) Photostimulated desorption in laser-assisted etching of silicon. Phys Rev Lett 61(16):1871–1874
18. Jarvis KL, Barnes TJ, Prestidge CA (2012) Surface chemistry of porous silicon and implications for drug encapsulation and delivery applications. Adv Colloid Interface Sci 175: 25–38
19. Eckhoff DA et al (2005) Optical characterization of ultrasmall Si nanoparticles prepared through electrochemical dispersion of bulk Si. J Phys Chem B 109(42):19786–19797
20. Bisi O, Ossicini S, Pavesi L (2000) Porous silicon: a quantum sponge structure for silicon

based optoelectronics. Surf Sci Rep 38(1-3): 1–126

21. Pace S, Sciacca B, Geobaldo F (2013) Surface modification of porous silicon microparticles by sonochemistry. RSC Adv 3(41): 18799–18802
22. Russo L et al (2011) A mechanochemical approach to porous silicon nanoparticles fabrication. Materials 4(6):1023–1033
23. Chiappini C et al (2010) Tailored porous silicon microparticles: fabrication and properties. ChemPhysChem 11(5):1029–1035
24. Godin B et al (2011) Multistage nanovectors: from concept to novel imaging contrast agents and therapeutics. Acc Chem Res 44(10): 979–989
25. Godin B et al (2012) Discoidal porous silicon particles: fabrication and biodistribution in breast cancer bearing mice. Adv Funct Mater 22(20):4225–4235
26. Santos HA et al (2014) Porous silicon nanoparticles for nanomedicine: preparation and biomedical applications. Nanomedicine 9(4):535–554
27. Schwartz MP et al (2005) Chemical modification of silicon surfaces for biological applications. Phys Status Solidi A 202(8):1380–1384
28. Tanaka T et al (2010) In vivo evaluation of safety of nanoporous silicon carriers following single and multiple dose intravenous administrations in mice. Int J Pharm 402(1-2): 190–197
29. Sciacca B et al (2011) Chitosan-functionalized porous silicon optical transducer for the detection of carboxylic acid-containing drugs in water. J Mater Chem 21(7):2294–2302
30. Mai J et al (2014) Bone marrow endothelium-targeted therapeutics for metastatic breast cancer. J Control Release 187C:22–29
31. Shen J et al (2013) High capacity nanoporous silicon carrier for systemic delivery of gene silencing therapeutics. ACS Nano 7(11): 9867–9880
32. Vernimmen J, Meynen V, Cool P (2011) Synthesis and catalytic applications of combined zeolitic/mesoporous materials. Beilstein J Nanotechnol 2:785–801
33. Fine D et al (2013) Silicon micro- and nanofabrication for medicine. Adv Healthc Materials 2(5):632–666
34. Wang F et al (2010) Oxidized mesoporous silicon microparticles for improved oral delivery of poorly soluble drugs. Mol Pharm 7(1): 227–236
35. Park JS et al (2011) Cisplatin-loaded porous Si microparticles capped by electroless deposition of platinum. Small 7(14):2061–2069
36. Shrestha N et al (2014) Chitosan-modified porous silicon microparticles for enhanced permeability of insulin across intestinal cell monolayers. Biomaterials 35(25):7172–7179
37. Rytkonen J et al (2014) Porous silicon-cell penetrating peptide hybrid nanocarrier for intracellular delivery of oligonucleotides. Mol Pharm 11(2):382–390
38. Liu D et al (2013) Co-delivery of a hydrophobic small molecule and a hydrophilic peptide by porous silicon nanoparticles. J Control Release 170(2):268–278
39. Chhablani J et al (2013) Oxidized porous silicon particles covalently grafted with daunorubicin as a sustained intraocular drug delivery system. Invest Ophthalmol Vis Sci 54(2):1268–1279
40. Wu EC et al (2008) Oxidation-triggered release of fluorescent molecules or drugs from mesoporous Si microparticles. ACS Nano 2(11):2401–2409
41. Wu EC et al (2011) Real-time monitoring of sustained drug release using the optical properties of porous silicon photonic crystal particles. Biomaterials 32(7):1957–1966
42. Xue M et al (2011) pH-Operated mechanized porous silicon nanoparticles. J Am Chem Soc 133(23):8798–8801
43. Khalil IA et al (2006) Uptake pathways and subsequent intracellular trafficking in nonviral gene delivery. Pharmacol Rev 58(1):32–45
44. Meraz IM et al (2012) Activation of the inflammasome and enhanced migration of microparticle-stimulated dendritic cells to the draining lymph node. Mol Pharm 9(7): 2049–2062
45. Zaki NM, Tirelli N (2010) Gateways for the intracellular access of nanocarriers: a review of receptor-mediated endocytosis mechanisms and of strategies in receptor targeting. Expert Opin Drug Deliv 7(8):895–913
46. Shahbazi MA et al (2014) Poly(methyl vinyl ether-alt-maleic acid)-functionalized porous silicon nanoparticles for enhanced stability and cellular internalization. Macromol Rapid Commun 35(6):624–629
47. Alexis F et al (2008) Factors affecting the clearance and biodistribution of polymeric nanoparticles. Mol Pharm 5(4):505–515
48. Serda RE et al (2011) Multi-stage delivery nano-particle systems for therapeutic applications. Biochim Biophys Acta 1810(3):317–329
49. Park JH et al (2009) Biodegradable luminescent porous silicon nanoparticles for in vivo applications. Nat Mater 8(4):331–336
50. Decuzzi P et al (2010) Size and shape effects in the biodistribution of intravascularly injected particles. J Control Release 141(3):320–327

51. Bimbo LM et al (2010) Biocompatibility of thermally hydrocarbonized porous silicon nanoparticles and their biodistribution in rats. ACS Nano 4(6):3023–3032
52. Moghimi SM, Hunter AC, Murray JC (2001) Long-circulating and target-specific nanoparticles: theory to practice. Pharmacol Rev 53(2):283–318
53. Sarparanta M et al (2012) Intravenous delivery of hydrophobin-functionalized porous silicon nanoparticles: stability, plasma protein adsorption and biodistribution. Mol Pharm 9(3):654–663
54. Hon NK et al (2012) Tailoring the biodegradability of porous silicon nanoparticles. J Biomed Mater Res A 100A(12):3416–3421
55. Godin B et al (2010) Tailoring the degradation kinetics of mesoporous silicon structures through PEGylation. J Biomed Mater Res A 94(4):1236–1243
56. Shen H et al (2013) Enhancing chemotherapy response with sustained EphA2 silencing using multistage vector delivery. Clin Cancer Res 19(7):1806–1815
57. Xia B et al (2013) Engineered stealth porous silicon nanoparticles via surface encapsulation of bovine serum albumin for prolonging blood circulation in vivo. ACS Appl Mater Interfaces 5(22):11718–11724
58. Souris JS et al (2010) Surface charge-mediated rapid hepatobiliary excretion of mesoporous silica nanoparticles. Biomaterials 31(21): 5564–5574
59. Yu T et al (2012) Influence of geometry, porosity, and surface characteristics of silica nanoparticles on acute toxicity: their vasculature effect and tolerance threshold. ACS Nano 6(3):2289–2301
60. Rosenholm JM et al (2012) Nanoparticles in targeted cancer therapy: mesoporous silica nanoparticles entering preclinical development stage. Nanomedicine 7(1):111–120
61. Shahbazi MA et al (2013) The mechanisms of surface chemistry effects of mesoporous silicon nanoparticles on immunotoxicity and biocompatibility. Biomaterials 34(31):7776–7789
62. Godin B et al (2008) Multistage mesoporous silicon-based nanocarriers: biocompatibility with immune cells and controlled degradation in physiological fluids. Control Release Newsl 25(4):9–11
63. Beija M et al (2012) Colloidal systems for drug delivery: from design to therapy. Trends Biotechnol 30(9):485–496
64. Zhang Y, Satterlee A, Huang L (2012) In vivo gene delivery by nonviral vectors: overcoming hurdles? Mol Ther 20(7):1298–1304
65. Kinnari PJ et al (2013) Tumour homing peptide-functionalized porous silicon nanovectors for cancer therapy. Biomaterials 34(36): 9134–9141
66. Blanco E et al (2013) Multistage delivery of chemotherapeutic nanoparticles for breast cancer treatment. Cancer Lett 334(2):245–252
67. Hou H et al (2014) Tunable sustained intravitreal drug delivery system for daunorubicin using oxidized porous silicon. J Control Release 178:46–54
68. Hartmann KI et al (2013) Hydrosilylated porous silicon particles function as an intravitreal drug delivery system for daunorubicin. J Ocul Pharmacol Ther 29(5):493–500
69. Wang J et al (2010) Delivery of siRNA therapeutics: barriers and carriers. AAPS J 12(4): 492–503
70. Almeida AJ, Souto E (2007) Solid lipid nanoparticles as a drug delivery system for peptides and proteins. Adv Drug Deliv Rev 59(6):478–490
71. Kovalainen M et al (2013) Development of porous silicon nanocarriers for parenteral peptide delivery. Mol Pharm 10(1):353–359
72. Kelly K et al (2004) Detection of invasive colon cancer using a novel, targeted, library-derived fluorescent peptide. Cancer Res 64(17): 6247–6251
73. Wu PC et al (2008) Modularly assembled magnetite nanoparticles enhance in vivo targeting for magnetic resonance cancer imaging. Bioconjug Chem 19(10):1972–1979
74. Woodward JD et al. (2008) INOR 302-In vivo SPECT/CT imaging and biodistribution using radioactive CdTe-125mTe/ZnS nanoparticles. Abstracts of Papers of the American Chemical Society, 236
75. Canham LT (1990) Silicon quantum wire array fabrication by electrochemical and chemical dissolution of wafers. Appl Phys Lett 57(10): 1046–1048
76. von Behren J et al (1998) Quantum confinement in nanoscale silicon: the correlation of size with bandgap and luminescence. Solid State Commun 105(5):317–322
77. Cullis AG, Canham LT, Calcott PDJ (1997) The structural and luminescence properties of porous silicon. J Appl Phys 82(3): 909–965
78. Gu L et al (2013) In vivo time-gated fluorescence imaging with biodegradable luminescent porous silicon nanoparticles. Nat Commun 4:2326
79. Friedman AD, Claypool SE, Liu R (2013) The smart targeting of nanoparticles. Curr Pharm Des 19(35):6315–6329

80. Wang CF et al (2014) Copper-free azide-alkyne cycloaddition of targeting peptides to porous silicon nanoparticles for intracellular drug uptake. Biomaterials 35(4):1257–1266
81. Secret E et al (2013) Antibody-functionalized porous silicon nanoparticles for vectorization of hydrophobic drugs. Adv Healthc Mater 2(5):718–727
82. Savage DJ et al (2013) Porous silicon advances in drug delivery and immunotherapy. Curr Opin Pharmacol 13(5):834–841
83. Martinez JO et al (2013) Engineering multi-stage nanovectors for controlled degradation and tunable release kinetics. Biomaterials 34(33):8469–8477

Chapter 9

Biocompatibility of Nanomaterials

Yasuo Yoshioka, Kazuma Higashisaka, and Yasuo Tsutsumi

Abstract

Remarkable progress has been made in the field of nanotechnology in the past decade. Many new nanoparticles, which are defined as particles with at least one dimension between 1 and 100 nm, have been created, and new medical applications for these nanoparticles are now expected. To be able to create effective and safe nanomedicines, more information is needed about the effects and safety of nanoparticles in vivo because physical properties such as material composition, particle size, surface area, surface chemistry, surface charge, and agglomeration state all influence nanoparticle biocompatibility, particularly with regard to activation of the complement, coagulation, and immune systems. In this chapter, we introduce the most recent developments in our understanding of the biocompatibility of nanoparticles and discuss how our current understanding translates to the field of nanomedicine.

Key words Coagulation, Complement, Immune response, Nanomedicine, Protein corona, Safety, Surface property, Toxicity

1 Introduction

Recent progress in the field of nanotechnology means that it is now possible to produce a wide variety of nanoparticles, which are particles that have at least one dimension between 1 and 100 nm. Compared with larger particles of the same material, nanoparticles have a larger surface area per unit weight, which produces desirable properties such as enhanced electrical conductivity, tensile strength, and chemical reactivity. Nanoparticles are already being used in the electronics, food, cosmetics, and medical industries. In the medical industry, the application of nanotechnology (nanomedicine) is expected to provide novel diagnostic and imaging technologies, photothermal therapies, and vaccine and drug delivery systems for poorly soluble or unstable drugs. Unlike larger, micrometer-sized particles, nanoparticles are small enough to be absorbed through biological barriers and therefore can enter almost all of the body's compartments, including cells and intracellular organelles. Furthermore, the targeting of nanoparticles to specific pathological sites may reduce the incidence of side effects by increasing drug

Zheng-Rong Lu and Shinji Sakuma (eds.), *Nanomaterials in Pharmacology*, Methods in Pharmacology and Toxicology,
DOI 10.1007/978-1-4939-3121-7_9, © Springer Science+Business Media New York 2016

exposure at target sites while decreasing systemic exposure. Biodegradable lipid nanoparticles and biopolymer-based nanoparticles are already being used as drug delivery systems; however, applications using non-biodegradable nanoparticles are still in development and are yet to be authorized for the use in humans.

Our current knowledge of the factors that affect the safety of nanoparticles is insufficient for the development of safe and efficacious nanomedicines. Since nanoparticles can penetrate cells and tissues that are remote from the portal of entry to the body, we must further examine the potential risks to human health posed by nanoparticles. If nanoparticles are to be used successfully as next-generation medicines, it will also be essential to address the concerns expressed in the literature regarding nanoparticle toxicity by collecting as much information as possible on the pharmacological and toxicological profiles of nanoparticles. The toxicity of nanoparticles is related not only to the effects of the nanomaterial itself but also to the concentration and length of time the nanoparticle spends in the body's tissues. Therefore, in addition to analyses of toxicity, systematic and thorough analyses of the absorption, distribution, metabolism, and excretion profiles of nanoparticles are needed to determine which nanoparticles pose a risk to human health.

Biocompatibility is the ability of a material to produce an appropriate host response in a specific situation. The body responds to nanoparticles, as it does to any foreign substance that enters it, by initiating biological responses that result in clearance of the nanoparticles. If these biological responses are unwanted, they can result in toxicity and bio-incompatibility. A high degree of biocompatibility is achieved when a material interacts with the body without inducing unacceptable toxic, immunogenic, thrombogenic, or carcinogenic responses. The levels of these responses are determined in part by how the nanoparticle interacts with various biological substances such as immune cells, proteins, and lipids (Fig. 1). Parameters such as structure, size distribution, surface area, surface chemistry, surface charge, and agglomeration state, as well as sample purity, also contribute to the biocompatibility of

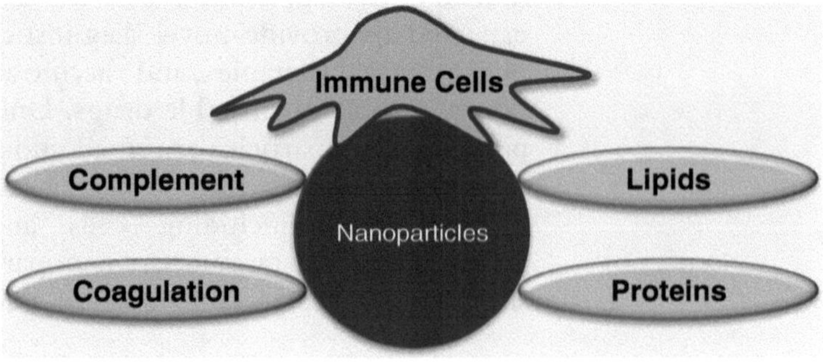

Fig. 1 Nanoparticles interact with various biological substances

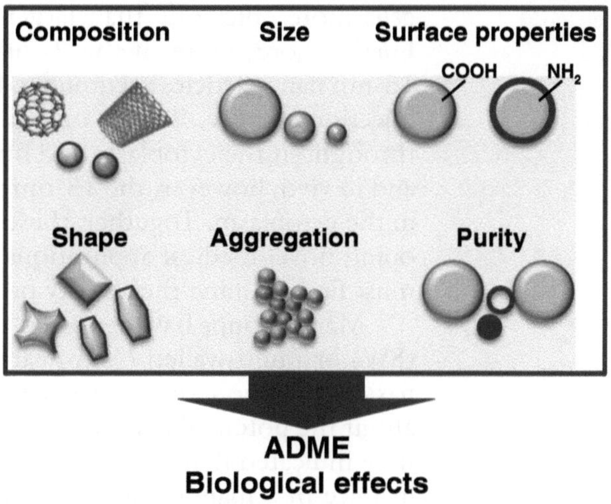

Fig. 2 Several parameters contribute to the biocompatibility of nanoparticles

nanoparticles (Fig. 2). Therefore, to understand the biocompatibility of a particular nanoparticle, we must first comprehensively understand the interrelationships among the physical properties of the nanoparticle and its interactions with biological substances.

2 Particle Size and Surface Charge

The biocompatibility of a nanoparticle is greatly influenced by its physicochemical properties [1, 2]. Therefore, to better understand the effects of nanoparticles in vivo, each type of nanoparticle must be evaluated individually. Particle size and surface charge are key parameters that affect the cellular uptake and biological interactions of nanoparticles. For example, Qiu et al. have shown that among gold nanorods with similar surface charges, shorter nanorods are internalized to a greater degree than longer nanorods, suggesting that the length of gold nanorods influences their cellular uptake [3]. In addition, we detected 70-nm silica nanoparticles (nSP70) in the maternal liver, placenta, and brain of pregnant mice and in the fetal liver, after intravenous injection, whereas we did not detect larger, micro-sized silica particles [2]. Furthermore, nSP70 induced miscarriage and fetal growth restriction in pregnant mice, whereas micro-sized silica particles did not. These results demonstrate the importance of evaluating the relationship between a nanoparticle's size and its reproductive toxicity.

Recently, ultra-small nanoparticles (diameter, <10 nm) have been investigated for their potential use as nanomedicines. Huang et al. compared the localization and penetration of gold nanoparticles (diameter, 2, 6, or 15 nm) in vitro and in vivo and showed that smaller gold nanoparticles internalized into cancer cells more efficiently than larger gold nanoparticles in vitro [4]. Furthermore, more of the 2- or 6-nm nanoparticles than of the 15-nm nanoparticles accumulated in tumor tissue after intravenous injection in mice. The 2- or 6-nm nanoparticles were distributed throughout the cytoplasm and nucleus of cancer cells both in vitro and in vivo; however, the 15-nm nanoparticles were observed only in the cytoplasm. Together, these results suggest that before developing novel medical applications for ultra-small nanoparticles, we must first examine their safety profiles in vitro and in vivo.

Many groups have reported that certain types of single-walled (SW) or multi-walled (MW) carbon nanotubes (CNTs) are cytotoxic and genotoxic in vitro, prompting concern in the literature about the potential risks of CNTs to human health. Recent reports have indicated that certain CNTs induce mesothelioma-like lesions in mice in a manner similar to that observed in asbestos-induced mesothelioma. For example, Takagi et al. showed that intraperitoneally administered pristine MW-CNTs induced mesothelioma in a p53 (+/−) mouse carcinogenesis model, which was attributed to both biopersistence and geometric resemblance to asbestos of the MW-CNTs [5]. Poland et al. have also reported the asbestos-like pathogenic behavior of long, pristine MW-CNTs, which was associated with the needlelike fiber shape of the MW-CNTs, and established a structure–activity relationship based on the length of the MW-CNTs [6]. Furthermore, long, fibrous MW-CNTs were shown to produce inflammation and fibrosis in the peritoneal cavity at a level that is similar to, or greater than, that produced by long asbestos fibers; however, neither short asbestos fibers nor short, tangled MW-CNTs caused any significant inflammation [7], suggesting that length, diameter, and physicochemical properties are related only to the safety profile of pristine MW-CNTs.

Size-independent effects of nanoparticles have also been reported. Jiang et al. examined the effects of gold and silver nanoparticles coated with antibodies that bind to the ErbB family of protein kinases during signaling processes such as cell death [8]. Nanoparticles with diameters in the 2- to 100-nm range were all shown to affect basic cellular signaling processes, with those with diameters of 40 or 50 nm having the greatest effect, suggesting that when designing nanomedicines we must optimize the particle size depending on how the nanomedicine will be used.

Aggregation is a phenomenon associated with most nanoparticles; however, few studies have examined the influence of aggregation on cellular uptake and toxicity. One study by Albanese et al. has shown that aggregation influences the uptake patterns of different gold nanoparticles [9].

Being able to manipulate the surface chemistry of nanoparticles, such as by adding functional groups to reduce surface reactivity or enhance stability, will be indispensable in the future for the development of nanoparticles for the use as nanomedicines.

Positively charged particles are more efficiently internalized into cells than neutral- or negatively charged nanoparticles because they bind more effectively to negatively charged groups on the cell surface. Jiang et al. examined the cellular internalization of plain polystyrene nanoparticles and amino-functionalized polystyrene nanoparticles in mesenchymal stem cells and found that amino-functionalized polystyrene was internalized more rapidly than pristine polystyrene [10]. In addition, they found that amino-functionalized polystyrene was internalized via clathrin-mediated endocytosis, whereas plain polystyrene was internalized mainly via a clathrin-independent endocytotic pathway. Therefore, the surface coating or surface charge of nanoparticles influences not only the degree of internalization but also the mechanism through which the nanoparticles are internalized.

Li et al. compared the inflammatory and fibrogenic effects of MW-CNTs functionalized to create different surface charges [11]. Whereas the pulmonary fibrogenic potential of anionic-functionalized MW-CNTs was lower than that of pristine MW-CNTs, strong cationic-functionalized MW-CNTs induced greater pulmonary fibrosis than that of pristine MW-CNTs via activation of the NLRP3 inflammasome. Furthermore, Qiu et al. compared the cytotoxicity of three gold nanoparticles each coated with a different polymer (i.e., cetyltrimethylammonium bromide, polystyrene sulfonate, or poly(diallyldimethylammonium chloride) [3]. Poly(diallyldimethylammonium chloride)-coated gold nanoparticles exhibited a much greater degree of cellular internalization but were not cytotoxic.

Together, these results show that surface charge and functional groups play an important role in the toxicity of nanoparticles. Since a wide variety of nanoparticles with different functional groups have now been developed, we will be able to further investigate the effects of size and surface charge on the systemic biological effects of nanoparticles.

3 Shape

Although the influences of particle size, surface charge, and material composition on the biological effects and cellular uptake of nanoparticles have been extensively studied, the effects of particle geometry are much less understood. Chan's group have shown that fewer rod-shaped gold nanoparticles enter cells compared with spherical gold nanoparticles because of the longer membrane wrapping time required for the rod-shaped nanoparticles [12, 13]. Agarwal et al. have shown that large or intermediate-sized nanodisks are internalized more efficiently compared with nanorods or small nanodisks and also that the mechanisms of uptake were shape and cell type specific [14]. These results suggest that cells can trigger unique uptake pathways in response to nanoscale geometry (both shape and size) and, therefore, that cells have different shape-dependent internalization efficiencies.

The results presented here and in the previous section show that synergism between size, surface chemistry, and shape must be taken into consideration when developing nanoparticles for biomedical applications.

4 Regulation of the Surface Properties of Nanoparticles for the Development of Nanomedicines

Foreign particles are removed from the body by phagocytes such as macrophages. For the medical application of nanoparticles, especially as part of passive targeted drug delivery systems, it will be important to improve the retention of nanoparticles in the blood. That is, systemically administered nanoparticles should not be cleared rapidly from the body and should instead remain in the circulation to allow the drug sufficient time to accumulate at the target site at a sufficiently high concentration. One way to prevent the clearance of nanoparticles from the circulation is to conjugate them with polyethylene glycol (PEG) or another water-soluble polymeric modifier. Covalent conjugation of PEG to the nanoparticle surface (through a process called pegylation) results in a longer plasma half-life and alters the tissue distribution of the conjugates compared with the native form because they avoid uptake by macrophages and renal clearance [15–18]. Furthermore, the prolonged circulation lifetime of the conjugates induces the enhanced permeability and retention effect, which results in increased delivery of conjugates to tumor tissue.

However, since the pegylation of nanoparticles may also prevent the delivery of drugs to targeted cells or the uptake of the nanoparticle into targeted cells, Rodriquez et al. have suggested an alternative approach to prolong the circulation lifetime of nanoparticles that uses CD47, which is a membrane protein and marker of self that is expressed on all cell membranes and prevents macrophage phagocytosis. Rodriquez et al. reported that nanoparticles conjugated to peptides designed from CD47 are not cleared by macrophages and are therefore retained longer in the circulation, resulting in enhanced dye and drug delivery to tumors [19]. In the future, other such homeostatic self-factors might similarly be used to prevent the clearance of nanoparticles by phagocytes, improve the targeting of specific tissues, or enhance the delivery of therapeutics and imaging agents.

Many groups have examined the use of carbon nanoparticle-based active targeted drug delivery systems for the treatment of cancer. Antibody-, folate-, arginine–glycine–aspartic acid peptide-, or epidermal growth factor-modified SW-CNTs have all been successfully used to actively target cancer cells [20–22]. The challenge in this approach is the identification of cancer cell-specific targets because conventional protein targets are often expressed by both normal and cancer cells. Therefore, the use of an integrated "omics" approach that utilizes proteomics, genomics, and metabolomics will be necessary to further identify potential cancer cell-specific targets.

5 Protein Corona

The adsorption of proteins on the surface of nanoparticles is an important factor that influences the biological effects of nanoparticles. When nanoparticles enter a biological fluid such as blood, they are rapidly coated with proteins and other biomolecules. For example, when nanoparticles are mixed with plasma, a protein corona is formed within 30 s [23]. The overall protein composition of the corona does not markedly change over time, although the concentration of a specific protein in the corona may change [23]. Which proteins bind to which nanoparticles depends on the physical properties of the nanoparticle; therefore, the size and surface properties of nanoparticles are important factors in determining the composition of the protein corona [24].

The binding of proteins to the surface of a nanoparticle changes the surface charge and alters the biological effects and rate of cellular uptake of the nanoparticle. Lesniak et al. showed that silica nanoparticles are more efficiently internalized into cells via a stronger adhesion to the cell membrane in the absence of serum compared with in the presence of serum when a protein corona is present on the nanoparticle surface [25]. Furthermore, Ge et al. have suggested that the binding of blood proteins to CNTs reduces CNT cytotoxicity [26].

The protein corona is also a major step in facilitating the phagocytosis of nanoparticles by macrophages. Deng et al. showed that negatively charged gold nanoparticles bind to fibrinogen causing it to unfold, which promotes the interaction of fibrinogen with Mac-1, an integrin receptor that is expressed on macrophages, in vitro [27]. The binding and activation of Mac-1 then induce the macrophage inflammatory response. In addition to proteins, nanoparticles can also be coated with lipids. The binding of lipids to MW-CNTs has been shown to influence the cellular uptake and toxicity of MW-CNTs [28–31].

Peng et al. have reported the successful use of the protein corona to regulate the biodistribution of nanoparticles [32]. By preforming a stable albumin corona around nanoparticles, they were able to inhibit plasma protein adsorption, prolong circulation lifetime, and reduce toxicity. This method is a simple yet potentially useful approach for optimizing nanoparticle drug delivery.

Many reports have described interactions between nanoparticles and extracellular proteins; however, nanoparticles also bind to intracellular proteins after being internalized into cells. Wang et al. showed that gold nanoparticles directly bind RNA polymerase, thereby suppressing RNA transcription in erythroid cells [33]. Furthermore, Falaschetti et al. have shown that several types of metal oxide nanoparticles bind to 20S proteasome subunits and increase 20S proteasome activity [34]. Proteasomes regulate intracellular protein degradation, and dysregulation of proteasome activity induces disorders such as cancer and neurodegenerative disease, suggesting that nanoparticles may provide a novel nanomedicine strategy against cancer and neurodegenerative disease. It will therefore be necessary to examine in more detail the effects of the nanoparticle protein corona on the cytosol.

6 Activation of Complement

It has been reported that the nanoparticle protein corona induces undesirable effects in vivo such as complement activation and blood clotting. Complement binds to foreign substances such as microbes and artificial materials that have entered the body to facilitate their clearance by macrophages. However, after engulfment, the nanoparticle protein corona may trigger unwanted inflammatory responses. Therefore, complement activation must be avoided to minimize the clearance of nanoparticles and induction of inflammatory responses.

Many studies have examined the relationship between nanoparticle size and degree of complement activation. For example, pegylated lipid nanocapsules with a diameter of 20, 50, or 100 nm have been shown to activate complement in a size-dependent manner [35, 36].

In contrast, some groups have also examined strategies to utilize the activation of complement by nanoparticles as a potential target for immunotherapeutics [37, 38]. Since the complement system plays an essential role in both adaptive and innate immunity, Reddy et al. designed a nanoparticle that strongly activates complement and successfully produces humoral and cellular immunity in mice [37]. Pluronic-stabilized polypropylene sulfide nanoparticles with a diameter of 25 nm were more efficiently translocated to lymphatic capillaries and their draining lymph nodes and accumulated in lymph node-residing dendritic cells than were larger particles (100 nm). Furthermore, the nanoparticles activated the complement cascade, which generated a danger signal in situ and possibly activated dendritic cells, and induced antigen-specific antibody responses and cellular immunity. In the future, it may be possible to harness these effects to produce novel vaccines for infectious diseases or cancer.

7 Activation of Coagulation

Some reports have suggested that nanoparticles activate the coagulant cascade. The blood coagulation system can be initiated via two pathways: the extrinsic cascade pathway, which is triggered by the release of tissue factor from a site of injury, or the intrinsic cascade pathway, which is triggered either by the activation of coagulation factors that have been brought into contact with a negatively charged substance or by the accumulation of activated platelets in the collagen layer under the vascular endothelium. Generally, the activation of platelets is associated with clot formation. The results of in vitro testing suggest that SW-CNTs and rutile titanium dioxide nanorods activate platelets and accelerate thrombus formation [39–41]. Burke et al. have also reported that some MW-CNTs directly activate platelets in vitro and that intravenous injection of some MW-CNTs reduces platelet count [42].

Our previous study showed that an excessive concentration of silica nanoparticles induced severe hepatotoxicity, lethal toxicity, and abnormal activation of the coagulation system in mice [43]. In addition, pretreatment with the anticoagulant heparin prior to the administration of silica nanoparticles reduced the induction of lethal toxicity and hepatotoxicity, suggesting that silica nanoparticle-mediated abnormal activation of the coagulant system was the main contributing factor to the lethal toxicity of silica nanoparticles.

We also examined the effects of silica nanoparticles on the coagulation system after intranasal exposure [44]. Hematological examination and coagulation tests showed that platelet count was decreased and activated partial thromboplastin time was prolonged in mice treated with silica nanoparticles, indicating that silica nanoparticles activate the coagulation cascade after intranasal exposure. In addition, in vitro activation tests showed that silica nanoparticles activate coagulation factor XII in a size-dependent manner, unlike micro-sized silica particles, suggesting that silica nanoparticles induce abnormal activation of the intrinsic cascade via activation of factor XII or platelets in the blood. Since a major factor in blood coagulation is the activation of coagulation factor XII via contact with hydrophilic activating particles, the abnormal activation of the coagulation system may be prevented by modifying the surface of silica nanoparticles to alter how they interact with coagulation factor XII.

8 Activation of Immune Responses

When foreign substances enter the body, the immune system recognizes them as foreign and initiates immune responses. In particular, macrophages, which are professional phagocytic cells, recognize and engulf nanoparticles as part of the body's defense mechanism. There are many reports showing the inflammatory effects of nanoparticles. It is known that nanoparticles are mainly recognized and phagocytosed by macrophages once they enter the bloodstream. We previously demonstrated that silica nanoparticles induce a strong inflammatory effect compared with micro-sized silica particles [45]. We compared the inflammatory effects of silica particles of various diameters (30–1000 nm) both in vitro and in vivo. Silica nanoparticles with a diameter of 30–70 nm induced greater cytokine production in macrophages than did larger silica nanoparticles in vitro. Furthermore, intraperitoneal injection of smaller silica nanoparticles induced stronger inflammatory responses as well as greater cytokine production than did larger silica nanoparticles. We also found that nSP70-mediated tumor necrosis factor alpha production was dependent on reactive oxygen species production and the activation of mitogen-activated protein kinases and that addition of a functional -COOH group to the surface of the silica nanoparticles suppressed silica nanoparticle-induced inflammatory responses.

9 Nanoparticle-Induced Immunosuppression

Urban air pollution is a major environmental problem in industrialized and developing countries. Indeed, increased levels of air pollution are associated with a wide range of health effects such as altered inflammatory responses in the respiratory system and cardiopulmonary disease [46, 47]. Urban air pollution is also associated with increased susceptibility to lung infection [48]. Similarly, exposure to nanoparticles has been shown to impair bacterial clearance from the lungs in mice. Shvedova et al. have shown that pharyngeal aspiration of SW-CNTs leads to increased susceptibility to infection by *Listeria monocytogenes* in mice due to decreased alveolar macrophage phagocytosis of bacteria and decreased phagocyte nitric oxide production [49]. Furthermore, Kim et al. have shown that inhalation or instillation of copper nanoparticles leads to increased susceptibility to infection by *Klebsiella pneumoniae* [50].

Although the precise mechanism of the increase in the risk of pulmonary infection has not yet been clarified, Kodali et al. have suggested a "ligand hijacking" theory [51]. Certain nanoparticles are known to bind to class A macrophage scavenger receptor (SR-A), a transmembrane glycoprotein whose natural ligands include bacterial cell wall components [52]. Kodali et al. have suggested that the endocytic internalization of SR-A following nanoparticle binding reduces the amount of cell surface SR-A available to interact with bacterial cell wall components, leaving macrophages unable to engulf bacteria. More studies are needed to clarify the mechanisms of this phenomenon.

Tsai et al. have shown that gold nanoparticles inhibit the Toll-like receptor (TLR)-mediated innate immune function activated by macrophages [53]. They have shown that gold nanoparticles accumulate in lysosomes after engulfment by macrophages and that they bind to high-mobility group box-1 in the lysosomal compartment, which is the general DNA sensor involved in the regulation of TLR9 signaling. This binding then leads to attenuation of TLR9 function. In addition, Sumbayev et al. have shown that gold nanoparticles neutralize extracellular interleukin (IL)-1β, leading to suppression of IL-1β-meditated inflammation [54].

The immunosuppressive effects of nanoparticles on dendritic cells (DCs) have also been shown. Tkach et al. have demonstrated that DC functions are modulated by SW-CNTs after pulmonary exposure [55], although the precise mechanism of this modulation remains unclear. They also showed that negatively charged graphene oxide suppresses the capacity of DCs to present antigens to T cells by decreasing the intracellular levels of immunoproteasome subunit LMP7, which is required for antigen processing, although non-charged "spherical" C_{60} fullerenes and negatively charged "spherical" C_{60}-TRIS fullerenes do not have this effect [56].

Together, these results suggest that the safety of nanoparticles is related not only to the inflammatory and immune system-activating effects of the nanoparticles but also their immunosuppressive effects. These data indicate potential opportunities for the utilization of nanoparticles as immunosuppressive therapeutics for the treatment of autoimmune disorders where it is desirable to inhibit antigen-specific immune responses.

10 Biodegradation of Nanoparticles

To understand the toxicity of nanoparticles, we must first fully understand how nanoparticles are metabolized, biodegraded, and excluded after being internalized into cells. There are many reports regarding the exclusion of nanoparticles from cells, although the precise mechanisms remain unclear. For example, Yanes et al. have shown that mesoporous silica nanoparticles are excluded from cells mainly via lysosomal exocytosis and that the cell-killing effect of anti-cancer-drug-loaded silica nanoparticles is enhanced by decreasing the rate of exocytosis [57]. These results suggest that it is necessary to consider the rate of exclusion of nanoparticles from cells when designing a nanomedicine.

Until recently, nanoparticles were thought to undergo little decomposition in vivo. However, recent studies have shown that CNTs are decomposed by natural enzymatic catalysis. Kagan et al. have shown that myeloperoxidase (MPO), an enzyme abundant in neutrophils, plays an important role in the oxidative biodegradation of SW-CNTs and that SW-CNTs degraded by MPO in vitro do not induce inflammatory and oxidative stress responses after pharyngeal aspiration in mice [58]. Consistent with these results, clearance of SW-CNTs from the lungs is decreased in MPO-deficient mice after pharyngeal aspiration, and the inflammatory responses in MPO-deficient mice are much more robust compared with those in wild-type mice [59].

An alternative mechanism for the degradation of CNTs in vivo has been suggested because neutrophils live for only a short time in the body. Kagan et al. have shown that superoxide/nitric oxide → peroxynitrite-driven oxidative pathways of activated macrophages are involved in the "digestion" of SW-CNTs and clearance of nanoparticles from the lungs [60].

Collectively, these studies suggest new ways to control the biopersistence of CNTs through genetic or pharmacological manipulations.

11 Conclusion

A range of toxicological studies have been conducted using various functionalized nanoparticles, cell lines, incubation conditions, agglomerations and aggregations, doses, and observation endpoints. It is therefore difficult to obtain systematic information about the interrelationships among the physicochemical properties and biological effects of nanoparticles. More rational methodologies must be developed to allow interpretation of the overarching information contained in the experimental data. Furthermore, since there is usually a difference between in vitro and in vivo results, an in vitro experimental system that mimics conditions in vivo is needed. Information collected by using this system would be useful for gaining a better understanding of the potential health risks of nanoparticles to humans. A detailed understanding of the toxicological properties of nanoparticles and balanced evaluations of risk–benefit ratios will be required before we can begin to develop safe and efficacious nanomedicines for routine clinical use.

References

1. He C, Hu Y, Yin L, Tang C, Yin C (2010) Effects of particle size and surface charge on cellular uptake and biodistribution of polymeric nanoparticles. Biomaterials 31:3657–3666
2. Yamashita K, Yoshioka Y, Higashisaka K, Mimura K, Morishita Y, Nozaki M, Yoshida T, Ogura T, Nabeshi H, Nagano K, Abe Y, Kamada H, Monobe Y, Imazawa T, Aoshima H, Shishido K, Kawai Y, Mayumi T, Tsunoda S, Itoh N, Yoshikawa T, Yanagihara I, Saito S, Tsutsumi Y (2011) Silica and titanium dioxide nanoparticles cause pregnancy complications in mice. Nat Nanotechnol 6:321–328
3. Qiu Y, Liu Y, Wang L, Xu L, Bai R, Ji Y, Wu X, Zhao Y, Li Y, Chen C (2010) Surface chemistry and aspect ratio mediated cellular uptake of Au nanorods. Biomaterials 31:7606–7619
4. Huang K, Ma H, Liu J, Huo S, Kumar A, Wei T, Zhang X, Jin S, Gan Y, Wang PC, He S, Zhang X, Liang XJ (2012) Size-dependent localization and penetration of ultrasmall gold

nanoparticles in cancer cells, multicellular spheroids, and tumors in vivo. ACS Nano 6:4483–4493

5. Takagi A, Hirose A, Nishimura T, Fukumori N, Ogata A, Ohashi N, Kitajima S, Kanno J (2008) Induction of mesothelioma in p53+/− mouse by intraperitoneal application of multi-wall carbon nanotube. J Toxicol Sci 33: 105–116
6. Poland CA, Duffin R, Kinloch I, Maynard A, Wallace WA, Seaton A, Stone V, Brown S, Macnee W, Donaldson K (2008) Carbon nanotubes introduced into the abdominal cavity of mice show asbestos-like pathogenicity in a pilot study. Nat Nanotechnol 3:423–428
7. Nagai H, Okazaki Y, Chew SH, Misawa N, Yamashita Y, Akatsuka S, Ishihara T, Yamashita K, Yoshikawa Y, Yasui H, Jiang L, Ohara H, Takahashi T, Ichihara G, Kostarelos K, Miyata Y, Shinohara H, Toyokuni S (2011) Diameter and rigidity of multiwalled carbon nanotubes are critical factors in mesothelial injury and carcinogenesis. Proc Natl Acad Sci U S A 108:E1330–E1338
8. Jiang W, Kim BY, Rutka JT, Chan WC (2008) Nanoparticle-mediated cellular response is size-dependent. Nat Nanotechnol 3:145–150
9. Albanese A, Chan WC (2011) Effect of gold nanoparticle aggregation on cell uptake and toxicity. ACS Nano 5:5478–5489
10. Jiang X, Dausend J, Hafner M, Musyanovych A, Rocker C, Landfester K, Mailander V, Nienhaus GU (2010) Specific effects of surface amines on polystyrene nanoparticles in their interactions with mesenchymal stem cells. Biomacromolecules 11:748–753
11. Li R, Wang X, Ji Z, Sun B, Zhang H, Chang CH, Lin S, Meng H, Liao YP, Wang M, Li Z, Hwang AA, Song TB, Xu R, Yang Y, Zink JI, Nel AE, Xia T (2013) Surface charge and cellular processing of covalently functionalized multiwall carbon nanotubes determine pulmonary toxicity. ACS Nano 7:2352–2368
12. Chithrani BD, Ghazani AA, Chan WC (2006) Determining the size and shape dependence of gold nanoparticle uptake into mammalian cells. Nano Lett 6:662–668
13. Chithrani BD, Chan WC (2007) Elucidating the mechanism of cellular uptake and removal of protein-coated gold nanoparticles of different sizes and shapes. Nano Lett 7:1542–1550
14. Agarwal R, Singh V, Jurney P, Shi L, Sreenivasan SV, Roy K (2013) Mammalian cells preferentially internalize hydrogel nanodiscs over nanorods and use shape-specific uptake mechanisms. Proc Natl Acad Sci U S A 110: 17247–17252
15. Mukai Y, Yoshioka Y, Tsutsumi Y (2005) Phage display and PEGylation of therapeutic proteins. Comb Chem High Throughput Screen 8:145–152
16. von Maltzahn G, Park JH, Agrawal A, Bandaru NK, Das SK, Sailor MJ, Bhatia SN (2009) Computationally guided photothermal tumor therapy using long-circulating gold nanorod antennas. Cancer Res 69:3892–3900
17. Lipka J, Semmler-Behnke M, Sperling RA, Wenk A, Takenaka S, Schleh C, Kissel T, Parak WJ, Kreyling WG (2010) Biodistribution of PEG-modified gold nanoparticles following intratracheal instillation and intravenous injection. Biomaterials 31:6574–6581
18. Yoshioka Y, Tsunoda S, Tsutsumi Y (2011) Development of a novel DDS for site-specific PEGylated proteins. Chem Cent J 5:25
19. Rodriguez PL, Harada T, Christian DA, Pantano DA, Tsai RK, Discher DE (2013) Minimal "Self" peptides that inhibit phagocytic clearance and enhance delivery of nanoparticles. Science 339:971–975
20. Ou Z, Wu B, Xing D, Zhou F, Wang H, Tang Y (2009) Functional single-walled carbon nanotubes based on an integrin alpha v beta 3 monoclonal antibody for highly efficient cancer cell targeting. Nanotechnology 20:105102
21. Wang CH, Chiou SH, Chou CP, Chen YC, Huang YJ, Peng CA (2011) Photothermolysis of glioblastoma stem-like cells targeted by carbon nanotubes conjugated with CD133 monoclonal antibody. Nanomedicine 7:69–79
22. Ruggiero A, Villa CH, Bander E, Rey DA, Bergkvist M, Batt CA, Manova-Todorova K, Deen WM, Scheinberg DA, McDevitt MR (2010) Paradoxical glomerular filtration of carbon nanotubes. Proc Natl Acad Sci U S A 107:12369–12374
23. Tenzer S, Docter D, Kuharev J, Musyanovych A, Fetz V, Hecht R, Schlenk F, Fischer D, Kiouptsi K, Reinhardt C, Landfester K, Schild H, Maskos M, Knauer SK, Stauber RH (2013) Rapid formation of plasma protein corona critically affects nanoparticle pathophysiology. Nat Nanotechnol 8:772–781
24. Tenzer S, Docter D, Rosfa S, Wlodarski A, Kuharev J, Rekik A, Knauer SK, Bantz C, Nawroth T, Bier C, Sirirattanapan J, Mann W, Treuel L, Zellner R, Maskos M, Schild H, Stauber RH (2011) Nanoparticle size is a critical physicochemical determinant of the human blood plasma corona: a comprehensive quantitative proteomic analysis. ACS Nano 5: 7155–7167
25. Lesniak A, Fenaroli F, Monopoli MP, Aberg C, Dawson KA, Salvati A (2012) Effects of the

presence or absence of a protein corona on silica nanoparticle uptake and impact on cells. ACS Nano 6:5845–5857

26. Ge C, Du J, Zhao L, Wang L, Liu Y, Li D, Yang Y, Zhou R, Zhao Y, Chai Z, Chen C (2011) Binding of blood proteins to carbon nanotubes reduces cytotoxicity. Proc Natl Acad Sci U S A 108:16968–16973
27. Deng ZJ, Liang M, Monteiro M, Toth I, Minchin RF (2011) Nanoparticle-induced unfolding of fibrinogen promotes Mac-1 receptor activation and inflammation. Nat Nanotechnol 6:39–44
28. Schleh C, Rothen-Rutishauser B, Kreyling WG (2011) The influence of pulmonary surfactant on nanoparticulate drug delivery systems. Eur J Pharm Biopharm 77:350–352
29. Gasser M, Rothen-Rutishauser B, Krug HF, Gehr P, Nelle M, Yan B, Wick P (2010) The adsorption of biomolecules to multi-walled carbon nanotubes is influenced by both pulmonary surfactant lipids and surface chemistry. J Nanobiotechnol 8:31
30. Konduru NV, Tyurina YY, Feng W, Basova LV, Belikova NA, Bayir H, Clark K, Rubin M, Stolz D, Vallhov H, Scheynius A, Witasp E, Fadeel B, Kichambare PD, Star A, Kisin ER, Murray AR, Shvedova AA, Kagan VE (2009) Phosphatidylserine targets single-walled carbon nanotubes to professional phagocytes in vitro and in vivo. PLoS One 4:e4398
31. Kapralov AA, Feng WH, Amoscato AA, Yanamala N, Balasubramanian K, Winnica DE, Kisin ER, Kotchey GP, Gou P, Sparvero LJ, Ray P, Mallampalli RK, Klein-Seetharaman J, Fadeel B, Star A, Shvedova AA, Kagan VE (2012) Adsorption of surfactant lipids by single-walled carbon nanotubes in mouse lung upon pharyngeal aspiration. ACS Nano 6: 4147–4156
32. Peng Q, Zhang S, Yang Q, Zhang T, Wei XQ, Jiang L, Zhang CL, Chen QM, Zhang ZR, Lin YF (2013) Preformed albumin corona, a protective coating for nanoparticles based drug delivery system. Biomaterials 34:8521–8530
33. Wang Z, Liu S, Ma J, Qu G, Wang X, Yu S, He J, Liu J, Xia T, Jiang GB (2013) Silver nanoparticles induced RNA polymerase-silver binding and RNA transcription inhibition in erythroid progenitor cells. ACS Nano 7:4171–4186
34. Falaschetti CA, Paunesku T, Kurepa J, Nanavati D, Chou SS, De M, Song M, Jang JT, Wu A, Dravid VP, Cheon J, Smalle J, Woloschak GE (2013) Negatively charged metal oxide nanoparticles interact with the 20S proteasome and differentially modulate its biologic functional effects. ACS Nano 7:7759–7772
35. Vonarbourg A, Passirani C, Saulnier P, Simard P, Leroux JC, Benoit JP (2006) Evaluation of pegylated lipid nanocapsules versus complement system activation and macrophage uptake. J Biomed Mater Res A 78:620–628
36. Vonarbourg A, Passirani C, Saulnier P, Benoit JP (2006) Parameters influencing the stealthiness of colloidal drug delivery systems. Biomaterials 27:4356–4373
37. Reddy ST, van der Vlies AJ, Simeoni E, Angeli V, Randolph GJ, O'Neil CP, Lee LK, Swartz MA, Hubbell JA (2007) Exploiting lymphatic transport and complement activation in nanoparticle vaccines. Nat Biotechnol 25: 1159–1164
38. Thomas SN, van der Vlies AJ, O'Neil CP, Reddy ST, Yu SS, Giorgio TD, Swartz MA, Hubbell JA (2011) Engineering complement activation on polypropylene sulfide vaccine nanoparticles. Biomaterials 32:2194–2203
39. Bihari P, Holzer M, Praetner M, Fent J, Lerchenberger M, Reichel CA, Rehberg M, Lakatos S, Krombach F (2010) Single-walled carbon nanotubes activate platelets and accelerate thrombus formation in the microcirculation. Toxicology 269:148–154
40. Meng J, Cheng X, Liu J, Zhang W, Li X, Kong H, Xu H (2012) Effects of long and short carboxylated or aminated multiwalled carbon nanotubes on blood coagulation. PLoS One 7:e38995
41. Nemmar A, Melghit K, Ali BH (2008) The acute proinflammatory and prothrombotic effects of pulmonary exposure to rutile TiO2 nanorods in rats. Exp Biol Med (Maywood) 233:610–619
42. Burke AR, Singh RN, Carroll DL, Owen JD, Kock ND, D'Agostino R Jr, Torti FM, Torti SV (2011) Determinants of the thrombogenic potential of multiwalled carbon nanotubes. Biomaterials 32:5970–5978
43. Nabeshi H, Yoshikawa T, Matsuyama K, Nakazato Y, Arimori A, Isobe M, Tochigi S, Kondoh S, Hirai T, Akase T, Yamashita T, Yamashita K, Yoshida T, Nagano K, Abe Y, Yoshioka Y, Kamada H, Imazawa T, Itoh N, Kondoh M, Yagi K, Mayumi T, Tsunoda S, Tsutsumi Y (2012) Amorphous nanosilicas induce consumptive coagulopathy after systemic exposure. Nanotechnology 23:045101
44. Yoshida T, Yoshioka Y, Tochigi S, Hirai T, Uji M, Ichihashi K, Nagano K, Abe Y, Kamada H, Tsunoda S, Nabeshi H, Higashisaka K, Yoshikawa T, Tsutsumi Y (2013) Intranasal exposure to amorphous nanosilica particles could activate intrinsic coagulation cascade and platelets in mice. Part Fibre Toxicol 10:41

45. Morishige T, Yoshioka Y, Inakura H, Tanabe A, Narimatsu S, Yao X, Monobe Y, Imazawa T, Tsunoda S, Tsutsumi Y, Mukai Y, Okada N, Nakagawa S (2012) Suppression of nanosilica particle-induced inflammation by surface modification of the particles. Arch Toxicol 86:1297–1307
46. Schwartz J (1994) Air pollution and hospital admissions for the elderly in Detroit, Michigan. Am J Respir Crit Care Med 150:648–655
47. Pope CA 3rd, Burnett RT, Thun MJ, Calle EE, Krewski D, Ito K, Thurston GD (2002) Lung cancer, cardiopulmonary mortality, and long-term exposure to fine particulate air pollution. JAMA 287:1132–1141
48. Neupane B, Jerrett M, Burnett RT, Marrie T, Arain A, Loeb M (2010) Long-term exposure to ambient air pollution and risk of hospitalization with community-acquired pneumonia in older adults. Am J Respir Crit Care Med 181:47–53
49. Shvedova AA, Fabisiak JP, Kisin ER, Murray AR, Roberts JR, Tyurina YY, Antonini JM, Feng WH, Kommineni C, Reynolds J, Barchowsky A, Castranova V, Kagan VE (2008) Sequential exposure to carbon nanotubes and bacteria enhances pulmonary inflammation and infectivity. Am J Respir Cell Mol Biol 38: 579–590
50. Kim JS, Adamcakova-Dodd A, O'Shaughnessy PT, Grassian VH, Thorne PS (2011) Effects of copper nanoparticle exposure on host defense in a murine pulmonary infection model. Part Fibre Toxicol 8:29
51. Kodali V, Littke MH, Tilton SC, Teeguarden JG, Shi L, Frevert CW, Wang W, Pounds JG, Thrall BD (2013) Dysregulation of macrophage activation profiles by engineered nanoparticles. ACS Nano 7:6997–7010
52. Chao Y, Karmali PP, Mukthavaram R, Kesari S, Kouznetsova VL, Tsigelny IF, Simberg D (2013) Direct recognition of superparamagnetic nanocrystals by macrophage scavenger receptor SR-AI. ACS Nano 7:4289–4298
53. Tsai CY, Lu SL, Hu CW, Yeh CS, Lee GB, Lei HY (2012) Size-dependent attenuation of TLR9 signaling by gold nanoparticles in macrophages. J Immunol 188:68–76
54. Sumbayev VV, Yasinska IM, Garcia CP, Gilliland D, Lall GS, Gibbs BF, Bonsall DR, Varani L, Rossi F, Calzolai L (2013) Gold nanoparticles downregulate interleukin-1beta-induced pro-inflammatory responses. Small 9:472–477
55. Tkach AV, Shurin GV, Shurin MR, Kisin ER, Murray AR, Young SH, Star A, Fadeel B, Kagan VE, Shvedova AA (2011) Direct effects of carbon nanotubes on dendritic cells induce immune suppression upon pulmonary exposure. ACS Nano 5:5755–5762
56. Tkach AV, Yanamala N, Stanley S, Shurin MR, Shurin GV, Kisin ER, Murray AR, Pareso S, Khaliullin T, Kotchey GP, Castranova V, Mathur S, Fadeel B, Star A, Kagan VE, Shvedova AA (2013) Graphene oxide, but not fullerenes, targets immunoproteasomes and suppresses antigen presentation by dendritic cells. Small 9:1686–1690
57. Yanes RE, Tarn D, Hwang AA, Ferris DP, Sherman SP, Thomas CR, Lu J, Pyle AD, Zink JI, Tamanoi F (2013) Involvement of lysosomal exocytosis in the excretion of mesoporous silica nanoparticles and enhancement of the drug delivery effect by exocytosis inhibition. Small 9:697–704
58. Kagan VE, Konduru NV, Feng W, Allen BL, Conroy J, Volkov Y, Vlasova II, Belikova NA, Yanamala N, Kapralov A, Tyurina YY, Shi J, Kisin ER, Murray AR, Franks J, Stolz D, Gou P, Klein-Seetharaman J, Fadeel B, Star A, Shvedova AA (2010) Carbon nanotubes degraded by neutrophil myeloperoxidase induce less pulmonary inflammation. Nat Nanotechnol 5:354–359
59. Shvedova AA, Kapralov AA, Feng WH, Kisin ER, Murray AR, Mercer RR, St Croix CM, Lang MA, Watkins SC, Konduru NV, Allen BL, Conroy J, Kotchey GP, Mohamed BM, Meade AD, Volkov Y, Star A, Fadeel B, Kagan VE (2012) Impaired clearance and enhanced pulmonary inflammatory/fibrotic response to carbon nanotubes in myeloperoxidase-deficient mice. PLoS One 7:e30923
60. Kagan VE, Kapralov AA, St Croix CM, Watkins SC, Kisin ER, Kotchey GP, Balasubramanian K, Vlasova II, Yu J, Kim K, Seo W, Mallampalli RK, Star A, Shvedova AA (2014) Lung macrophages "digest" carbon nanotubes using a superoxide/peroxynitrite oxidative pathway. ACS Nano 8:5610–5621

Chapter 10

Nanoparticle–Tissue Interaction

Xiaohui Wu and Zheng-Rong Lu

Abstract

Nanoparticles, particles with size at submicron scale, have brought tremendous advantages compared with microparticles or macroparticles. The research regarding nanoparticles in biomedical field has been focused on the fabrication method of nanoparticles, in vitro, and in vivo studies. Most of current reviews mainly introduced fabrication method and in vitro studies. To advance nanotechnology for clinic applications, it is of outmost importance to investigate and better understand how nanoparticles interact with in vivo environment and tissues including both healthy and malignant tissues after administration. In this chapter, we will extensively discuss the nanoparticle behavior when exposed to in vivo environment and the interaction between nanoparticles and tissues.

Key words Nanoparticles, In vivo environment, Tissues, Interaction

Abbreviations

BBB	Blood–brain barrier
CAM	Chick chorioallantoic membrane
EPR	Enhanced permeability and retention
GSH	Reduced glutathione
GSSG	Oxidized glutathione
LHRH	Luteinizing hormone-releasing hormone
MDP	Multidrug resistance-associated protein
MDR	Multidrug resistance
MPS	Mononuclear phagocytic system
MRI	Magnetic resonance imaging
MRP	Multidrug resistance-associated protein
P(MDS-co-CES)	Poly{(*N*-methyldietheneamine sebacate)-co-[(cholesteryl oxocarbonylamido ethyl) methyl bis(ethylene) ammonium bromide] sebacate}
PDLA	Poly(D,L-lactic acid)
PDT	Photodynamic therapy
PEG	Polyethylene glycol
PEI	Polyethylenimine
PIBCA	Poly-isobutyl cyanoacrylate
PLA	Poly(lactic acid)

Zheng-Rong Lu and Shinji Sakuma (eds.), *Nanomaterials in Pharmacology*, Methods in Pharmacology and Toxicology,
DOI 10.1007/978-1-4939-3121-7_10, © Springer Science+Business Media New York 2016

PLGA	Poly(D,L-lactic and glycolic acids)
PMMA	Poly(methyl methacrylate)
PS	Polystyrene
RES	Reticuloendothelial system
SOD	Superoxide dismutase
SPION	Superparamagnetic iron oxide nanoparticles
TLR	Toll-like receptor
VEGF	Vascular endothelium growth factor

1 Introduction

Numerous investigations in the past several decades have demonstrated that submicromic colloidal systems, namely, nanoparticles, could significantly modulate both cell and tissue distribution profiles of medical drugs by targeting the delivery of drugs more precisely, improving the solubility, extending the circulation time, improving therapeutic index, and meanwhile lowering the immunogenicity [1–7]. Nanoparticles widely studied for biomedical application represent a broad range of materials including, but not limited to, polymeric micelles [8], liposomes [9], dendrimers [2], quantum dots [10, 11], magnetic nanoparticles, [12–15] colloidal gold [16, 17], and silica nanoparticles [18]. Despite tremendous promising advantages that nanoparticles might bring, nanoparticles encounter difficulties to be used on the market (Table 1). The major reason is that the in vivo nanoparticle–tissue interaction can be complicated even though in vitro studies indicate that nanoparticles possess some many benefits. To advance nanotechnology for clinic applications, it is of outmost importance to investigate and better understand how nanoparticles interact with in vivo environment and tissues including both healthy and malignant tissues after administration. In this chapter, we will extensively discuss the nanoparticle behavior when exposed to in vivo environment and the interaction between nanoparticles and tissues.

2 Nanoparticle Interaction with In Vivo Environment

Once nanoparticles loaded with cargo are administrated into in vivo environment with whichever method (such as, tail vein, intravenous injection, oral or interstitial route, and inhalation) [5], the proteins or other biomolecules immediately attach nanoparticles upon contact with in vivo environment to form nano–bio interface. The nano–bio interface consists of three dynamical layers. The first layer is the nanoparticle surface, the characteristics of which are determined by the physicochemical composition. The second layer is the nanoparticle–liquid interface, and the third layer is the nanoparticle–liquid interface's interacting zone with the

Table 1
Nanoparticle therapeutics available on market

Products (year approved)	Components	Indication	Company	Reference
Zoladex (1989)	Goserelin acetate	Prostate cancer	AstraZeneca Pharmaceuticals	[75]
Taxol (1992)	Cremophor + paclitaxel	Solid tumor cancers	Tocris Bioscience	[75]
Oncaspar (1994)	PEG-asparaginase	Acute lymphoblastic leukemia	Enzon Pharmaceuticals	[76, 77]
Doxil/Caelyx (1995)	PEGylated liposomal doxorubicin	Ovarian cancer Multiple myeloma	Ortho Biotech	[78]
DaunoXome (1996)	Liposomal daunorubicin	Kaposi's sarcoma	Gilead Sciences	[79]
Gliadel	Biodegradable polymer with BCNU	Brain cancer	Arbor Pharms LLC	[75]
Copaxone	Biologically active polymer	Multiple sclerosis	Teva Neuroscience, Inc	[75]
DepoCyt (1999)	Liposomal cytarabine	Lymphomatous meningitis	SkyePharma	[55]
Myocet (2002)	Liposomal doxorubicin	Metastatic breast cancer	Elan Pharmaceuticals	[80]
Abraxane (2005)	Paclitaxel albumin bound nanoparticles	Metastatic breast cancer	Abraxis Bioscience	[81]

biological substrate. During formation of nano–bio interface, nanoparticle characteristics, media properties, solid–liquid interface, and nano–bio interface together shape the entire nano–bio interface and dominate its properties (Table 2) [19–25]. The interaction between nanoparticles and cells involves van der Waals, electrostatic, salvation, solvophobic, and depletion forces [25]. However, at nanoscale, nanoparticle–cell interaction seems to be more complicated than regular colloid (see details in Ref. [25]). Hence, it is believed that it is the nano–bio interface rather than nanoparticles interact with living system.

The immune system plays a significant role in the function of nanoparticle therapeutics. Nanoparticles are usually picked up by the mononuclear phagocytic system (MPS) cells of the immune system (such as macrophages) and undesirable consequences, such as immunostimulation or immunosuppression, may occur and devastate inflammatory or autoimmune disorders or increase the host's susceptibility to infections and cancer [26]. The major function of immune system is to recognize and protect the host from foreign

Table 2
Biophysicochemical factors determining the entire nano–bio interface

Nanoparticle	Media	Solid–liquid interface	Nano–bio interface
Chemical composition Functionalization Particle shape Porosity Crystallinity Heterogeneity Topography Hydrophilicity	Water molecules Acids and bases Salts and multivalent ions Natural organic matter Surfactants Polymers Polyelectrolytes	Surface hydration and dehydration Surface reconstruction and release of free surface energy Ion adsorption and charge neutralization Electrical double-layer formation, zeta potential, isoelectric point Sorption of steric molecules and toxins Electrostatic, steric, and electrosteric interactions Aggregation, dispersion, and dissolution Hydrophilic and hydrophobic interactions	Membrane interactions: specific and nonspecific forces Receptor–ligand binding interactions Membrane wrapping: resistive and promotive forces Biomolecule interactions (lipids, proteins, DNA) Free energy transfer to biomolecules Conformational change in biomolecules Oxidant injury to biomolecules Mitochondrial and lysosomal damage, decrease in ATP

substances. However, unwanted recognition of nanoparticles as foreign by the immune system might result in immune responses, which in turn causes toxicity in the host and lowers the therapeutic efficacy. As a matter of fact, the efficacy of nanoparticle drug delivery system is usually compromised due to recognition and clearance by the reticuloendothelial system (RES) before arriving at target sites as well as by inability of penetrating biological barriers, such as the vascular endothelium or the blood–brain barrier (BBB) [27]. Size, surface properties, targeting ligands, and distinguishing features of nanoparticle therapeutics are the key factors which affect pharmacokinetics and biodistribution and dominate the fate of nanoparticles upon administration. In the following section, we will focus on discussing how these factors influence nanoparticle–tissue interaction, which is also the emphasis of this chapter.

3 Characteristics of Nanoparticles Affecting Nanoparticle–Tissue Interaction

Tumor tissues comprised of three subcompartments, vascular, interstitial, and cellular, have some aspects similar to normal tissues, and, however, also possess special behavior compared with normal tissues [28]. Tumor cells collect nutrients via passive diffusion for growing up to 2 mm^3, and then angiogenesis is gradually developed to supply nutrients for tumor expansion [29]. However, the vascularized areas are not uniformly developed in the entire tumor. Some parts of the tumor have poorly vascularized area with resultant necrosis, while other parts are richly vascularized. Tumor vessels with abnormal and aberrant branching blind loops and tortuosity are leaky because of abnormal basement membrane and decreased numbers of pericytes lining rapidly proliferating endothelial cells, which results in enhanced permeability for substance passage from the vessel wall to the interstitium [29, 30]. The enhance permeability is believed to be regulated by vascular endothelium growth factor (VEGF), nitric oxide, bradykinin, prostaglandins, and matrix metalloproteinases [31]. The open gap size between the leaky endothelial cells ranges from 100 to 780 nm, much larger than that of 5–10 nm between normal vessels [32, 33]. The collagen network and the elastic fiber network in tumor interstitium induce high interstitial pressure resisting the inward flux of molecules. Therefore, the balanced force between the outward interstitial pressure and the drug properties, such as nanoparticle size, hydrophilicity, and surface charges, governs the delivery of drugs into the interstitium [28]. Due to the fact that the interstitial pressure is higher in the tumor center than in the periphery, the drug diffusion to the tumor center is resisted, which forms a barrier for drug delivery. Consequently, drugs inside interstitium theoretically have extended retention time, which is called the enhanced permeability and retention (EPR) effect favoring drug accumulation in tumor interstitium [31, 34]. Cellular mechanisms contribute a lot to drug resistance, which include altered activity of specific enzyme systems (topoisomerase activity), altered apoptosis regulation, and transport-based mechanisms (P-glycoprotein efflux system), responsible for the multidrug resistance (MDR) and the multidrug resistance-associated protein (MRP) [35, 36]. In addition to cellular resistance, noncellular resistance mechanisms also exert remarkable influence on therapeutic efficacy. As discussed earlier in this section, in some parts of tumor, the vascular is poorly formed, which significantly limit the drug access to the tumor and protect cancerous cells from external toxic invasion. Moreover, the tumor itself can produce an acidic environment, which ionizes basic drug system and decreases the drug diffusion across the cellular membrane [36]. Hence, an advanced and excellent modality to deliver therapeutic drugs to wanted tumor cells in vivo should conquer drug resistance (both cellular and noncellular), have good circulation time to render drug accumulation in tumors, and easy clearance out of the body to avoid toxin accumulation. As loading vehicles, nanoparticles have many factors to influence the NP–tissue interaction, such as particle size, surface properties, and targeting ligands of nanoparticle therapeutics. In the following sections, we will put concentration on how these factors affect nanoparticle–tissue interaction in vivo.

3.1 Particle Pize

Size and size distribution are essential characteristics of nanoparticles, which closely affect not only drug loading and release, and particle stability, but also in vivo biological behavior, such as distribution, biological fate, toxic effects, and targeting ability including passive and active targeting. With advantages over microparticles, nanoparticles possess higher intracellular uptake and wider range of biological targets. The particles with average diameters ranging from 100 nm to 10 μm prepared from polylactic polyglycolic acid copolymer (PLGA) were infused into the segments of intestine to investigate the uptake of particles in rat in situ intestinal tissue loop model [37]. The result demonstrated that small nanoparticles had higher advantage to penetrate throughout the submucosal layers. Due to small size and relative mobility, nanoparticles have the superior ability to nonspecifically open the tight junctions between endothelial cells in the brain microvasculature and thus generate a paracellular pathway through the BBB, which might provide sustained delivery of drugs for difficult-to-treat diseases in brain [38]. Polysorbate-80 (Tween 80)-coated poly(butyl cyanoacrylate) nanoparticles with an average diameter of 300 nm have been shown to overcome the BBB effect [39].

The nanoparticle size has close correlation with drug release kinetics. Smaller nanoparticles with larger surface area render more drugs near or at the nanoparticle surface, which causes fast drug release [37]. On the other hand, nanoparticles with larger diameters can encapsulate more drugs and release them out more slowly. Therefore, the selection of nanoparticle size depends on the application purpose. However, the negative effect for smaller nanoparticles is the aggregation during storage, transport, and operation before disease treatment, which might induce blood vessel occlusion and make them susceptible to MPS clearance [40].

3.2 Surface Properties

Surface properties contribute to the nanoparticle's aggregation tendency, ability to traverse biological. As discussed in previous sections, to increase the likelihood of success in drug delivery for tissue engineering, it is highly necessary to minimize the opsonization and prolong the circulation time in blood stream once the nanoparticle is administered. The key point to solve this problem is to modify the surface properties to avoid the recognition of immune system. Currently, the main strategy to achieve this is to modify the nanoparticles with hydrophilic components, such as polyethylene glycol (PEG), poloxamer, poloxamine, and polysorbate-80 [41]. Hydrophobicity directly influences the level of blood components which form the bio–nano interface. Different types of nanoparticles including linear polymer, dendrimer, and PEGylated liposome were employed as LHRH receptor-based targeting delivery on nude mice bearing A549 xenograft tumors [5, 42]. The results indicated that PEGylated liposome induced the most effective suppression of tumor growth in mice model, which might result from reduced opsonization in vivo by PEGylation. Polyvinylpyrrolidone nanoparticles (50–60 nm) loaded with taxol were used to treat B16F10 murine melanoma subcutaneously transplanted in mice model and showed higher advantage in inducing tumor regression and higher survival rates than free taxol through repeated intravenous injections [43, 44]. Similarly, chitosan nanoparticles (100 nm) loaded with dextran–doxorubicin conjugates also showed higher efficiency than free dextran–doxorubicin conjugates in a murine tumor model [45]. PIBCA nanospheres coated or uncoated with poloxamine loaded with mitoxantrone were intravenously injected into B16 melanoma-bearing mice [46]. However, the results did not strongly indicate the effect of hydrophilic coating, poloxamine, on the biodistribution and pharmacokinetics because of the important standard deviations. Similarly, polysorbate-80-coated PIBCA nanospheres were intravenously injected into tail vein to evaluate the possibility of delivery of anticancer drugs, doxorubicin, into the brain via overcoming BBB [47, 48]. After sacrifice of the rats, the biodistribution and pharmacokinetics were studied with HPLC, and the polysorbate-80 coating did not show significant influence on both biodistribution and pharmacokinetic parameters compared with uncoated PIBCA nanospheres. However, interestingly the PIBCA nanospheres with polysorbate-80 coating transport more doxorubicin (up to 6 μg/g) into the brain at 2–4 h post intravenous administration, whereas the doxorubicin concentration in plasma was only around 0.1 μg/g.

With development of engineered chemotherapeutic nanoparticles, recently poly(methyl methacrylate) (PMMA) nanoparticles modified with hydrophilic components, such as polysorbate-80, poloxamer 407, and poloxamine 908, were investigated in mice in terms of biodistribution for various types of tumor models, such as murine B16-melanoma, human breast cancer MaTu, and U-373 glioblastoma. A prolonged circulation time in blood stream and an accumulation and retention of coated PMMA nanoparticles in tumors were observed due to the surface hydrophilicity [49].

Even though these hydrophilic coatings improved the biological function and therapeutic efficacy of nanoparticles, most of them have been linked with nanoparticles via weak interactions, such as van der Waals and might cause rapid desorption upon contact with blood components or dilution. More encouraging strategy to formulate more stable linkage between nanoparticles and hydrophilic components is to employ covalent bonding. Unfortunately, even though poly(lactic acid) (PLA), polycaprolactone, and polycyanoacrylate covalently coupled with nanoparticles have been studied in vitro, the in vivo investigation for cancer themotherapy is expected to be performed in the near future [50–52].

Another property of importance is the surface charge, namely, represented by zeta potential. Zeta potential is the electrical potential influenced by the material and the dispersion medium. Nanoparticles with high zeta potential have less chance to form aggregation. Cationic polymers, e.g., polyethylenimine (PEI) and its derivatives, polylysine, polyamidoamine dendrimers, poly(beta-amino esters), and chitosan, which are water soluble, can induce sufficient levels of in vivo gene transfection [5]. However, nanoparticles bearing surface charge, cationic or anionic, are more attractive to phagocytes than neutral nanoparticles with similar other properties and might increase nonspecific uptake and clearance by the MPS, lowering the therapeutic efficacy [53].

3.3 Targeting Ligands

Targeting includes passive targeting and active targeting [54]. Passive targeting is driven by minimal renal clearance and the EPR effect in tumor sites. As mentioned earlier in this section, due to rapid angiogenesis or vascularization to supply large need of nutrients and oxygen, the blood vessel walls in tumors are full of defective vascular architecture compared with healthy blood vessel walls, which results in enhanced vascular permeability of tumor tissues. Thus, polymeric micelles, liposomes, and dendrimers in small size (50–500 nm) can penetrate and reach tumor tissues. Anticancer therapeutics can be easily delivered to tumor sites by incorporating into these particles. However, the interstitial pressure is higher in the tumor center than in the periphery, so the drug diffusion to the tumor center is resisted, which forms a barrier for drug delivery. This kind of resistant effect by diffusion can be more prominent when the nanoparticle size is smaller (<30 nm) [5].

More specific drug targeting has been achieved by binding ligands to the nanoparticle surface, namely, active targeting. The typical binding ligands include peptides, growth factors, antibodies or antibody fragments, transferring, and small compounds, such as folic acid (Table 3) [5, 55]. The binding ligand can specifically recognize receptors which are generated by cancer cells. LHRH

Table 3
Categories of ligands binding on nanoparticles in active targeting application

Ligand type	Ligand (target, reference)
Antibody or antibody fragment	Herceptin (Her2/neu [82]) Mabthera (CD20 [82]) F19 monoclonal antibodies (fibroblast activation protein [83]) Anti-CD19 scFv (CD19 [84])
Peptide	RGD peptide (integrin $\alpha v\beta 3$ [85, 86]) Fibronectin-mimetic peptide (integrin $\alpha 5\beta 1$ [87]) APRPG peptide (neovasculature [88]) CREKA peptide (fibrin–fibronectin complexes [89]) Transferrin (transferrin receptor [90])
Growth factor	EGF (EGF receptor [91, 92])
Hormone	Testosterone (androgen receptor [93]) LHRH agonist (LHRH receptor [94])
Small compound	Folate (folate receptor [95])

receptor-based targeting delivery was investigated on nude mice bearing subcutaneous grown xenografts of human lung cancer cells and prominently enhanced the anticancer activity of drugs [42]. More interestingly, the adverse effects of the treatment in normal tissues were, meanwhile, reduced.

4 Strategies for Curing Malignant Tissues

With development of nanotechnology, there are variety of methods to apply nanoparticles for curing malignant tissues, which can be exemplified as conventional delivery in which the nanoparticle only deliver one drug, co-delivery in which the nanoparticle can delivery multiple cargos, photodynamic therapy in which the photosensitizer accumulates in tumor sites and mediates the cancerous cellular death, and widely investigated magnetic nanoparticles.

4.1 Conventional Delivery

In conventional delivery, only single therapeutic drug is loaded into or onto nanoparticles and delivered into malignant tissues. It is classical and also the most widely investigated drug delivery system, including nontargeting and targeting nanoparticles. For conventional delivery, readers can refer to previous section or other reports for more information.

4.2 Co-delivery

Advanced nanotechnology enables the fabrication of multifunctional nanoparticles to load multiple therapeutic agents, such as small molecules, peptides, and proteins, in a single nanoparticle. Co-delivery of paclitaxel with an interleukin-12-encoded plasmid using core-shell nanoparticles suppressed cancer growth rate remarkably compared with the delivery of either paclitaxel or the interleukin-12-encoded plasmid in a 4T1 mouse breast cancer model [56]. Generally, in preclinical studies and phase II or phase III clinical trials, Herceptin and paclitaxel have been administered through separate injections to achieve synergistic antitumor effects [5]. However, Herceptin and paclitaxel have been loaded in a cationic P(MDS-co-CES) micelle, and this co-delivery approach shows advantages over the separated injections due to the reduction of injection times and achievement of synergistic effect. Paclitaxel-loaded nanoparticle/Herceptin complexes containing 200 nM of Herceptin and 6.7 mM of paclitaxel were used to treat BT474 cells with high-level Her2-expression [57]. The cytotoxicity data indicated that the cell viability with these complexes was only 60.2 %, while it was 92 % and 83 % for 200 nM Herceptin alone and paclitaxel-loaded nanoparticles, respectively. Apparently, this co-delivery system demonstrated a synergistic effect. PLGA nanoparticles were also used as a co-delivery vehicle for a vaccine [58]. In this co-delivery system, Toll-like receptor (TLR) ligand (7-acyl lipid A), poorly immunogenic melanoma antigen, and tyrosinase-related protein 2(TRP2) were co-encapsulated into the PLGA nanoparticles. Results clearly showed that activated TRP2-specific CD8 T cells could secret interferon (IFN)-γ at lymph nodes and spleen of the vaccinated mice. In addition, compared with control group, reduced levels of VEGF and increased levels of IL-2, IL-6, IL-12, IFN-γ, and TNF-α were found at the tumor microenvironment influenced by this co-delivery system, indicating immunostimulation.

4.3 Photodynamic Therapy (PDT)

Photodynamic therapy is a well-established clinical treatment modality for cancer and superficial tumors, such as bladder, melanoma, and esophagus [59]. Once the photosensitizer is administered with a predefined time interval and accumulates in tumor sites, the irradiation of the tumor tissues with nonthermal light (635–760 nm) induces the excited photosensitizer and molecular oxygen, which causes the formation of singlet oxygen ($^1O_2$), a vital factor mediating cellular death [60]. An ideal photosensitizer should possess some characteristics, such as stable composition, easy synthesis and good availability, minimal self-aggregation tendency, low hydrophobicity, non-toxicity in the absence of light exposure, photostability, absorbance in the red region of spectrum with high extinction molar coefficient, target specificity, and quick clearance from the body [61]. Unfortunately, none of commercially available photosensitizers have all the properties of an ideal photosensitizer. Most photosensitizers have poor hydrophilicity and easily form aggregation in aqueous media, which decreases the formation of singlet oxygen and solubility and inhibits biological properties [61]. The application of nanoparticles as carriers for photosensitizer can overcome most of those shortcomings for classic photosensitizers. According to the manner in which singlet oxygen is produced, the strategies applying nanoparticles to deliver photosensitizers have two categories. Either non-biodegradable nanoparticles, in which photosensitizers are not released from nanoparticles, but the oxygen can diffuse in and out of nanoparticles freely, or biodegradable nanoparticles (mainly polymer-based materials), from which the photosensitizers are released and generate singlet oxygen. The lipophilicity plays an important role in modulating photothrombic efficiency, and chick chorioallantoic membrane (CAM) is generally employed as in vivo model duo to the fact that destruction of the neovasculature is of importance in eradication of some vascularized tumors by PDT and the well-vascularized membrane of CAM is readily accessible for photosensitizer administration, light irradiation, optical examination, and fluorescence analysis of PDT-induced vascular damage [62, 63]. Additionally, detecting the fluorescence of the vascularized and non-vascularized tissues renders convenient monitoring of biodistribution of photosensitizer in the CAM and the extent of its leakage. More importantly, the photodynamic activity can be evaluated by observing the vascular occlusion. Poly(D,L-lactic acid) (PDLA) nanoparticles were used to deliver porphyrins *meso*-tetraphenylporphyrin (TPP), *meso*-tetra-(4-carboxyphenyl)-porphyrin (TCPP), chlorines pheophorbide-a (Pheo-a), and chlorine e_6 (Ce_6) to perform a preclinical intercomparison study using CAM as in vivo model [64]. The results indicated that the dye was more effectively entrapped in the PDLA nanoparticles with increasing the degree of lipophilicity. The more lipophilic dyes (TPP and Pheo-a) tended to remain inside the blood vessels, whereas less lipophilic compounds (TCPP and Ce_6) extravasated more easily. Once exposed to irradiation with light doses from 5 to 20 J/cm^2, the PDLA nanoparticle loaded with the most lipophilic molecule (TPP) showed the highest photothrombic efficiency, and the vascular damage was more highly induced as well, meanwhile causing the minimal leakage from blood vessels. The nanoparticle size also plays an essential role in photosensitizer circulation in the blood stream as discussed in Sect. 3.1. Consequently, the extravasation of photosensitizer could be governed by the nanoparticle size. PLGA nanoparticles with various particle sizes were studied using CAM as in vivo model [65]. It was found that smaller nanoparticle size showed stronger photodynamic activity.

4.4 Magnetic Nanoparticles

Magnetic nanoparticles with a diameter ranging from a few nanometers to tens of nanometers, one of the most widely investigated category of nanoparticles, provide many attractive advantages over other nanoparticles. Due to the property of magnetic, magnetic nanoparticles obey Coulomb's law and can be manipulated by an external magnetic field. This characteristic enables them to gain wide application in magnetic resonance imaging (MRI) and targeting drug delivery, in which the intrinsic penetrability of magnetic fields into tissues works with the external magnetic field. In addition, the magnetic nanoparticles can be prepared to resonantly respond to a time-varying magnetic field, in which the energy of the exciting field can be transferred to the magnetic nanoparticle. This special function renders them a wide application in hyperthermia. So, this section will focus on the in vivo application of magnetic nanoparticles, including MRI, magnetic drug targeting (MDT), and hyperthermia with magnetic ferrofluids.

MRI: MRI-based clinical diagnostics is a popular noninvasive modality for diagnosing soft tissues and recent cartilage pathologies due to the difference in the relaxation times of hydrogen atoms [66]. Dextran-stabilized magnetic nanoparticles with an overall size of ~45 nm and the iron oxide core of ~5 nm, after functionalized with HIV-Tat proteins, were able to be introduced into different cell types, such as human hematopoietic $CD34^+$ cells, mouse neural progenitor cells, mouse splenocytes, and human $CD4^+$ lymphocytes [67]. These cells could be administered *i.v.* into mice and monitored via MRI in bone marrow, liver, and spleen. More importantly, these cells had high MRI sensitivity, and even single cell could be detected. Magnetic nanoparticles can also be used as oral contrast agents for diagnosing gastrointestinal tumors and the detection of other tumors [68].

MDT: Previously we discussed the nanoparticle-based targeting drug delivery, employing binding ligands (peptides, growth factors, antibodies or antibody fragments, transferring, and small compounds). As an important advantage of magnetic nanoparticles, they can deliver drugs to a specific site in a unique manner compared with binding ligand-based targeting delivery, in which magnetic nanoparticles can be guided by means of external magnetic field to a specific location [66]. The other advantage of magnetic nanoparticle-based drug delivery is the maintenance of its location for the expected time length. Many factors can influence MDT modality, such as the physical properties, concentration, the amount of applied nanoparticles, and the nature of binded drugs. In addition, the external magnetic field, such as the geometry, size, and duration, and the vascular supply of the targeted tissues can also influence their effect. Complete remission of experimentally induced VX-2 squamous cell carcinomas after intra-arterial injection of starch-coated magnetic nanoparticles functionalized with methotrexate in the hind limbs of rabbits was successfully achieved [69]. In another study, magnetic nanoparticles functionalized with epirubicin and coated with polymeric anhydroglucose were administered into the femoral vein of rats under the influence of an external magnetic field [70]. Compared with controls (no magnetic field applied), an irreversible thrombus was formed in the capillary bed of the muscle at 10 min post magnet application, which strongly suggested that this modality could be used to induce microembolization of tumors.

Hyperthermia with magnetic ferrofluids: When magnetic nanoparticles are exposed to an alternating magnetic field, the induced oscillation of the magnetic moment inside the magnetic nanoparticles converts the magnetic field energy into the form of heat. Smaller magnetic nanoparticles generally have higher rate of specific absorption than larger ones [71]. Consequently, superparamagnetic iron oxide nanoparticles (SPION) with a core size less than 10 nm are widely used for hyperthermia, heating up tissues to 41–46 °C [68]. In general, necrosis and coagulation or carbonization of the tissue will be observed when the temperature exceeds 56 °C, which is called "thermoablation" [71]. Apparently, hyperthermia is a suitable strategy to treat cancers due to that tumor cells are extremely susceptible to elevated temperatures. When hyperthermia is applied to heat up to 41–45 °C, the tumors are irreversibly damaged, while healthy tissues are permanently damaged. Compared with conventional hyperthermia methods, such as microwaves, radio-frequency, ultrasound, and infrared, which show inability to selectively induce heat formation in specific abnormal tissue, the magnetic nanoparticle-based hyperthermia shows encouraging advantage in heating at specific tumor sites, especially when combined with chemotherapy, they can improve the cell surface receptor molecules and enhance the recognition of immune system. Many in vivo studies were performed (mostly using mice model) on experimentally induced tumors. The results demonstrated that homogenous cell–tissue inactivation was correlated well with the biodistribution of magnetic nanoparticles in the targeted tumor sites [71].

4.5 Multifunctional Platforms

Multifunctional nanoparticles open a door for possibly combining diagnosis and treatment of cancers at the same time, the functions of which depend on the design. Multifunctional nanoparticles conquer many limits of conventional nanoparticles to meet the requirements of an ideal delivery system. A polyacrylamide multifunctional platform was synthesized to diagnose brain cancer due to the presence of a magnetic resonance imaging (MRI) contrast enhancer. In addition, this multifunctional platform also contained a photosensitizer, Photofrin®, a polyethylene surface coating to increase circulation in blood stream, and a molecular targeting ligand, RGD peptide [72]. Therefore, this multifunctional platform was capable of diagnosis, enhancing nanoparticle residence time, and the recognition of the tumor neovasculature. Rats bearing intracerebral 9L tumors were employed as in vivo model to evaluate the therapeutic activity of this multifunctional platform [61]. Compared with untreated tumor-bearing rats and those only having laser treatment, this multifunctional nanoparticle could induce massive regional necrosis, in addition to the successful monitoring of changes in tumor diffusion, tumor growth, and tumor load. In a similar study, polyacrylamide nanoparticles encapsulating Photofrin®, imaging agents, such as fluorescent dye and iron oxide, and F3 peptide as a targeting ligand for surface-localized vasculature, were administered into 9L-glioma-bearing rats, followed by PDT treatment. The results showed that the survival rate was significantly higher compared with those rats receiving nontargeted nanoparticles or systemic Photofrin®. More encouragingly, 40 % of rats treated with F3-targeted Photofrin®nanoparticles were found to be tumor-free 60 days posttreatment [61].

5 Achievements and Future Challenges

Nanoparticles, undoubtedly, provide opportunities for designing and modulating properties that are not possible for non-nanoparticle types of therapeutics. More and more clinical trials will be performed with more advanced nanoparticle-based systems, and the nanoparticle system should be improved further as the optimal nanoparticle properties are elucidated. As discussed above, most of the nanoparticle-based therapy strategies are encouraging with promising application potentials and were demonstrated to be non-toxic both in vitro and in vivo. However, there are also issues of concern.

First, nanoparticles have also been found to be toxic for healthy tissues. The in vivo nanotoxicity is induced by oxidative stress via free radicals, generated by phagocytic cell response to foreign materials. Due to free radicals, oxidation of lipids, proteins, and DNA strongly causes damage to biological components. Oxidative stress can also induce or enhance inflammation through regulating redox-sensitive transcription factors, kinases, and activator protein-1. A single and repeated intravenous administration of poly-isobutyl cyanoacrylate (PIBCA) or polystyrene (PS) nanoparticles induced a depletion of reduced glutathione (GSH) and oxidized glutathione (GSSG) levels in the liver, inhibition of superoxide dismutase (SOD) activity, and a slight increase in catalase activity [73]. The results indicated that nanoparticles were not distributed in the hepatocytes, and oxidative species most probably were generated by activated hepatic macrophages after nanoparticle phagocytosis. Consequently, it needs to be emphasized that long-term studies are needed to prove the safe use of nanoparticles, which is also our challenge to advance the clinical application of nanoparticle-based therapeutics.

Second, while the particle size in nanoscale can provide positive features, such as high payloads and great accommodation of multiple targeting ligands, it can also be detrimental [74]. Presently, it remains unknown how nanoparticles move through malignant tissues after they arrive at the tumor area. It is of importance to perform more studies to understand how nanoparticles function in humans as early claims of some nanoparticle function are now being called into question. For example, evidence has shown that the proposed Abraxane nanoparticle delivery might not be the true mechanism causing the enhanced amounts of drug in tumors.

Last but not least, important commercial and regulatory challenges need to be tackled with the emerging generation of more advanced nanoparticles due to the multicomponent nature. Apparently, it will be more difficult and expensive to manufacture these nanoparticles at large scale with appropriate quality. Even though the challenge remains, some complex nanoparticles have already gone to clinic. For example, CALAA-01 consisting of four components with targeting function and siRNA is now in clinic studies, which strongly shows that complex nanoparticles can be manufactured and satisfy regulatory requirements, at least for the initiation of phase I trials. However, it does not reach the market yet. In addition, the high cost for intellectual properties and lack of sufficient financial support can be another two more challenging issues before commercialization of complex nanoparticles.

Even though some challenges put big barrier on the way that more therapeutic nanoparticles reach market, the prospective of nanoparticle-based system is still encouraging, and we believe that more and more advanced nanoparticle-based therapeutic modalities will be available on the huge market.

References

1. Safra T et al (2000) Pegylated liposomal doxorubicin (doxil): reduced clinical cardiotoxicity in patients reaching or exceeding cumulative doses of 500 mg/m2. Ann Oncol 11:1029–1033
2. Kukowska-Latallo JF et al (2005) Nanoparticle targeting of anticancer drug improves therapeutic response in animal model of human epithelial cancer. Cancer Res 65:5317–5324
3. Rifkin RM et al (2006) Pegylated liposomal doxorubicin, vincristine, and dexamethasone provide significant reduction in toxicity compared with doxorubicin, vincristine, and dexamethasone in patients with newly diagnosed multiple myeloma: a phase III multicenter randomized trial. Cancer 106:848–858
4. Kim S et al (2009) Engineered polymers for advanced drug delivery. Eur J Pharm Biopharm 71:420–430
5. Wang J, Sui M, Fan W (2010) Nanoparticles for tumor targeted therapies and their pharmacokinetics. Curr Drug Metab 11:129–141
6. Doshi N, Mitragotri S (2009) Designer biomaterials for nanomedicine. Adv Funct Mater 19:3843–3854
7. Mitragotri S, Lahann J (2009) Physical approaches to biomaterial design. Nat Mater 8:15–23
8. Sutton D et al (2007) Functionalized micellar systems for cancer targeted drug delivery. Pharm Res 24:1029–1046
9. Bellocq NC et al (2003) Transferrin-containing, cyclodextrin polymer-based particles for tumor-targeted gene delivery. Bioconjug Chem 14: 1122–1132
10. Tada H et al (2007) In vivo real-time tracking of single quantum dots conjugated with monoclonal anti-HER2 antibody in tumors of mice. Cancer Res 67:1138–1144
11. Sharma P et al (2006) Nanoparticles for bioimaging. Adv Colloid Interface Sci 123–126:471–485
12. Gupta AK, Gupta M (2005) Synthesis and surface engineering of iron oxide nanoparticles for biomedical applications. Biomaterials 26: 3995–4021
13. Gupta AK et al (2007) Recent advances on surface engineering of magnetic iron oxide nanoparticles and their biomedical applications. Nanomedicine (Lond) 2:23–39
14. McCarthy JR et al (2007) Targeted delivery of multifunctional magnetic nanoparticles. Nanomedicine (Lond) 2:153–167
15. Duguet E et al (2006) Magnetic nanoparticles and their applications in medicine. Nanomedicine (Lond) 1:157–168
16. Hillyer JF, Albrecht RM (2001) Gastrointestinal persorption and tissue distribution of differently sized colloidal gold nanoparticles. J Pharm Sci 90:1927–1936
17. Hirsch LR et al (2003) A whole blood immunoassay using gold nanoshells. Anal Chem 75:2377–2381
18. Lu J et al (2010) Biocompatibility, biodistribution, and drug-delivery efficiency of mesoporous silica nanoparticles for cancer therapy in animals. Small 6:1794–1805
19. Nel A et al (2006) Toxic potential of materials at the nanolevel. Science 311:622–627
20. Oberdorster G et al (2005) Principles for characterizing the potential human health effects from exposure to nanomaterials: elements of a screening strategy. Part Fibre Toxicol 2:8
21. Vertegel AA, Siegel RW, Dordick JS (2004) Silica nanoparticle size influences the structure and enzymatic activity of adsorbed lysozyme. Langmuir 20:6800–6807
22. Gilbert B et al (2004) Nanoparticles: strained and stiff. Science 305:651–654
23. Min Y et al (2008) The role of interparticle and external forces in nanoparticle assembly. Nat Mater 7:527–538
24. Velegol D (2007) Assembling colloidal devices by controlling interparticle forces. J Nanophoton 1:012502-012502-25
25. Nel AE et al (2009) Understanding biophysicochemical interactions at the nano-bio interface. Nat Mater 8:543–557
26. Zolnik BS et al (2010) Nanoparticles and the immune system. Endocrinology 151: 458–465
27. Shubayev VI, Pisanic TR 2nd, Jin S (2009) Magnetic nanoparticles for theragnostics. Adv Drug Deliv Rev 61:467–477

28. Jain RK (1987) Transport of molecules in the tumor interstitium: a review. Cancer Res 47:3039–3051
29. Baban DF, Seymour LW (1998) Control of tumour vascular permeability. Adv Drug Deliv Rev 34:109–119
30. Seymour LW (1992) Passive tumor targeting of soluble macromolecules and drug conjugates. Crit Rev Ther Drug Carrier Syst 9:135–187
31. Maeda H (2001) The enhanced permeability and retention (EPR) effect in tumor vasculature: the key role of tumor-selective macromolecular drug targeting. Adv Enzyme Regul 41:189–207
32. Hobbs SK et al (1998) Regulation of transport pathways in tumor vessels: role of tumor type and microenvironment. Proc Natl Acad Sci U S A 95:4607–4612
33. Rubin P, Casarett G (1966) Microcirculation of tumors part I: anatomy, function, and necrosis. Clin Radiol 17:220–229
34. Maeda H et al (2000) Tumor vascular permeability and the EPR effect in macromolecular therapeutics: a review. J Control Release 65:271–284
35. Links M, Brown R (1999) Clinical relevance of the molecular mechanisms of resistance to anti-cancer drugs. Expert Rev Mol Med 1999: 1–21
36. Krishna R, Mayer LD (2000) Multidrug resistance (MDR) in cancer: mechanisms, reversal using modulators of MDR and the role of MDR modulators in influencing the pharmacokinetics of anticancer drugs. Eur J Pharm Sci 11:265–283
37. Redhead HM, Davis SS, Illum L (2001) Drug delivery in poly(lactide-co-glycolide) nanoparticles surface modified with poloxamer 407 and poloxamine 908: in vitro characterisation and in vivo evaluation. J Control Release 70:353–363
38. Kroll RA et al (1998) Improving drug delivery to intracerebral tumor and surrounding brain in a rodent model: a comparison of osmotic versus bradykinin modification of the blood-brain and/or blood-tumor barriers. Neurosurgery 43:879–886, discussion 886–889
39. Kreuter J et al (2003) Direct evidence that polysorbate-80-coatedpoly(butylcyanoacrylate) nanoparticles deliver drugs to the CNS via specific mechanisms requiring prior binding of drug to the nanoparticles. Pharm Res 20: 409–416
40. Muller RH et al (1996) Phagocytic uptake and cytotoxicity of solid lipid nanoparticles (SLN) sterically stabilized with poloxamine 908 and poloxamer 407. J Drug Target 4:161–170
41. Singh R, Lillard JW Jr (2009) Nanoparticle-based targeted drug delivery. Exp Mol Pathol 86:215–223
42. Saad M et al (2008) Receptor targeted polymers, dendrimers, liposomes: which nanocarrier is the most efficient for tumor-specific treatment and imaging? J Control Release 130: 107–114
43. Brigger I, Dubernet C, Couvreur P (2002) Nanoparticles in cancer therapy and diagnosis. Adv Drug Deliv Rev 54:631–651
44. Sharma D et al (1996) Novel Taxol formulation: polyvinylpyrrolidone nanoparticle-encapsulated Taxol for drug delivery in cancer therapy. Oncol Res 8:281–286
45. Mitra S et al (2001) Tumour targeted delivery of encapsulated dextran-doxorubicin conjugate using chitosan nanoparticles as carrier. J Control Release 74:317–323
46. Reszka R et al (1997) Body distribution of free, liposomal and nanoparticle-associated mitoxantrone in B16-melanoma-bearing mice. J Pharmacol Exp Ther 280:232–237
47. Gulyaev A et al (1999) Significant transport of doxorubicin into the brain with polysorbate 80-coated nanoparticles. Pharm Res 16: 1564–1569
48. Kreuter J (2001) Nanoparticulate systems for brain delivery of drugs. Adv Drug Deliv Rev 47:65–81
49. Lode J et al (2001) Influence of surface-modifying surfactants on the pharmacokinetic behavior of 14C-poly (methylmethacrylate) nanoparticles in experimental tumor models. Pharm Res 18:1613–1619
50. Gref R et al (1994) Biodegradable long-circulating polymeric nanospheres. Science 263:1600–1603
51. Peracchia MT et al (1997) Development of sterically stabilized poly(isobutyl 2-cyanoacrylate) nanoparticles by chemical coupling of poly(ethylene glycol). J Biomed Mater Res 34: 317–326
52. Peracchia MT et al (1998) Pegylated nanoparticles from a novel methoxypolyethylene glycol cyanoacrylate-hexadecyl cyanoacrylate amphiphilic copolymer. Pharm Res 15:550–556
53. Zahr AS, Davis CA, Pishko MV (2006) Macrophage uptake of core-shell nanoparticles surface modified with poly(ethylene glycol). Langmuir 22:8178–8185
54. Cho K et al (2008) Therapeutic nanoparticles for drug delivery in cancer. Clin Cancer Res 14:1310–1316
55. Angst MS, Drover DR (2006) Pharmacology of drugs formulated with DepoFoam: a sustained release drug delivery system for paren-

teral administration using multivesicular liposome technology. Clin Pharmacokinet 45:1153–1176
56. Wang Y et al (2006) Co-delivery of drugs and DNA from cationic core-shell nanoparticles self-assembled from a biodegradable copolymer. Nat Mater 5:791–796
57. Lee AL et al (2009) The co-delivery of paclitaxel and Herceptin using cationic micellar nanoparticles. Biomaterials 30:919–927
58. Hamdy S et al (2008) Co-delivery of cancer-associated antigen and Toll-like receptor 4 ligand in PLGA nanoparticles induces potent CD8+ T cell-mediated anti-tumor immunity. Vaccine 26:5046–5057
59. Triesscheijn M et al (2006) Photodynamic therapy in oncology. Oncologist 11:1034–1044
60. Dougherty TJ et al (1998) Photodynamic therapy. J Natl Cancer Inst 90:889–905
61. Bechet D et al (2008) Nanoparticles as vehicles for delivery of photodynamic therapy agents. Trends Biotechnol 26:612–621
62. Vargas A et al (2007) The chick embryo and its chorioallantoic membrane (CAM) for the in vivo evaluation of drug delivery systems. Adv Drug Deliv Rev 59:1162–1176
63. Lange N et al (2001) A new drug-screening procedure for photosensitizing agents used in photodynamic therapy for CNV. Invest Ophthalmol Vis Sci 42:38–46
64. Pegaz B et al (2005) Encapsulation of porphyrins and chlorins in biodegradable nanoparticles: the effect of dye lipophilicity on the extravasation and the photothrombic activity. A comparative study. J Photochem Photobiol B 80:19–27
65. Vargas A et al (2008) In vivo photodynamic activity of photosensitizer-loaded nanoparticles: formulation properties, administration parameters and biological issues involved in PDT outcome. Eur J Pharm Biopharm 69: 43–53
66. Schutt W et al (1997) Applications of magnetic targeting in diagnosis and therapy – possibilities and limitations: a mini-review. Hybridoma 16:109–117
67. Lewin M et al (2000) Tat peptide-derivatized magnetic nanoparticles allow in vivo tracking and recovery of progenitor cells. Nat Biotechnol 18:410–414
68. Neuberger T et al (2005) Superparamagnetic nanoparticles for biomedical applications: possibilities and limitations of a new drug delivery system. J Magn Magn Mater 293:483–496
69. Alexiou C et al (2000) Locoregional cancer treatment with magnetic drug targeting. Cancer Res 60:6641–6648
70. Lübbe AS et al (1999) Physiological aspects in magnetic drug-targeting. J Magn Magn Mater 194:149–155
71. Jordan A et al (2001) Presentation of a new magnetic field therapy system for the treatment of human solid tumors with magnetic fluid hyperthermia. J Magn Magn Mater 225: 118–126
72. Kopelman R et al (2005) Multifunctional nanoparticle platforms for in vivo MRI enhancement and photodynamic therapy of a rat brain cancer. J Magn Magn Mater 293: 404–410
73. Hoet PH, Bruske-Hohlfeld I, Salata OV (2004) Nanoparticles – known and unknown health risks. J Nanobiotechnol 2:12
74. Davis ME, Chen Z, Shin DM (2008) Nanoparticle therapeutics: an emerging treatment modality for cancer. Nat Rev Drug Discov 7:771–782
75. Petros RA, DeSimone JM (2010) Strategies in the design of nanoparticles for therapeutic applications. Nat Rev Drug Discov 9:615–627
76. Ettinger AR (1995) Pegaspargase (Oncaspar). J Pediatr Oncol Nurs 12:46–48
77. Dinndorf PA et al (2007) FDA drug approval summary: pegaspargase (oncaspar) for the first-line treatment of children with acute lymphoblastic leukemia (ALL). Oncologist 12: 991–998
78. Tejada-Berges T et al (2002) Caelyx/Doxil for the treatment of metastatic ovarian and breast cancer. Expert Rev Anticancer Ther 2: 143–150
79. Girard PM et al (1996) Phase II study of liposomal encapsulated daunorubicin in the treatment of AIDS-associated mucocutaneous Kaposi's sarcoma. Aids 10:753–757
80. Batist G et al (2002) Myocet (liposome-encapsulated doxorubicin citrate): a new approach in breast cancer therapy. Expert Opin Pharmacother 3:1739–1751
81. Gradishar WJ (2006) Albumin-bound paclitaxel: a next-generation taxane. Expert Opin Pharmacother 7:1041–1053
82. Cirstoiu-Hapca A et al (2007) Differential tumor cell targeting of anti-HER2 (Herceptin) and anti-CD20 (Mabthera) coupled nanoparticles. Int J Pharm 331:190–196
83. Eck W et al (2008) PEGylated gold nanoparticles conjugated to monoclonal F19 antibodies as targeted labeling agents for human pancreatic carcinoma tissue. ACS Nano 2:2263–2272
84. Zhou Y et al (2007) Impact of single-chain Fv antibody fragment affinity on nanoparticle targeting of epidermal growth factor receptor-

expressing tumor cells. J Mol Biol 371: 934–947

85. Garanger E, Boturyn D, Dumy P (2007) Tumor targeting with RGD peptide ligands-design of new molecular conjugates for imaging and therapy of cancers. Anticancer Agents Med Chem 7:552–558
86. Danhier F et al (2009) Targeting of tumor endothelium by RGD-grafted PLGA-nanoparticles loaded with paclitaxel. J Control Release 140:166–173
87. Demirgoz D, Garg A, Kokkoli E (2008) PR_b--targeted PEGylated liposomes for prostate cancer therapy. Langmuir 24:13518–13524
88. Katanasaka Y et al (2008) Antiangiogenic cancer therapy using tumor vasculature-targeted liposomes encapsulating 3-(3,5-dimethyl-1H-pyrrol-2-ylmethylene)-1,3-dihydro-indol-2-one, SU5416. Cancer Lett 270:260–268
89. Ruoslahti E, Bhatia SN, Sailor MJ (2010) Targeting of drugs and nanoparticles to tumors. J Cell Biol 188:759–768
90. Jin Y et al (2010) Targeted delivery of antisense oligodeoxynucleotide by transferrin conjugated pH-sensitive lipopolyplex nanoparticles: a novel oligonucleotide-based therapeutic strategy in acute myeloid leukemia. Mol Pharm 7: 196–206
91. Fonge H et al (2010) Multifunctional block copolymer micelles for the delivery of 111In to EGFR-positive breast cancer cells for targeted Auger electron radiotherapy. Mol Pharm 7:177–186
92. Tseng CL et al (2008) Targeting efficiency and biodistribution of biotinylated-EGF-conjugated gelatin nanoparticles administered via aerosol delivery in nude mice with lung cancer. Biomaterials 29:3014–3022
93. Mishra PK et al (2009) Targeted delivery of an anti-cancer agent via steroid coupled liposomes. Drug Deliv 16:437–447
94. Sundaram S et al (2009) Targeted drug and gene delivery systems for lung cancer therapy. Clin Cancer Res 15:7299–7308
95. Seow WY, Xue JM, Yang YY (2007) Targeted and intracellular delivery of paclitaxel using multi-functional polymeric micelles. Biomaterials 28:1730–1740

Chapter 11

Pharmaceutics of Nanoparticles

Masami Ukawa, Hidenori Ando, Taro Shimizu, and Tatsuhiro Ishida

Abstract

Drug-incorporating nanoparticles (nanodrugs) have been approved for clinical use. Incorporating water-insoluble drugs such as anticancer agents, antimycotics, and photosensitizers into nanoparticles improves their bioavailability. Moreover, the essential advantage of nanodrugs is a reduction in adverse effects. This leads to an improvement in the quality of life (QOL) of patients. In this chapter, we focus on the pharmacokinetics and toxicity of clinically approved nanodrugs and of nanodrugs that are currently undergoing clinical trials. In addition, the preparation methods and structural features of nanodrugs are introduced.

Key words PEGylated liposome, Albumin-based nanoparticle technology (nab-technology), Antitumor drugs, Amphotericin B, Photodynamic therapy (PDT)

1 Introduction

Targeted, site-specific drug delivery using nanoparticles is one of the most promising applications of nanomaterials. By incorporating drugs within nanoparticles, it is possible to improve the biodistribution of the drugs depending on the properties of a particular nanoparticle. Such an alteration in drug distribution often affects desirable medicinal features. Actually, numerous traditional cytotoxic drugs, such as anticancer drugs, antimycotics, and photosensitizers, have been encapsulated in liposomes, and some of them have been approved for clinical use, as shown in Table 1.

In clinical use, drug-loaded nanoparticles are mainly categorized into assembled macromolecules and liposomes. Assembled macromolecules were formed by self-assembly of macromolecule possessing both of hydrophilic group and hydrophobic group. Abraxane® is an example of assembled macromolecules (Fig. 1a). Abraxane® was formed by self-assembly of paclitaxel (hydrophobic drug) bound to albumin (hydrophilic protein). Liposomes were assemblage of lipids which have hydrophilic head group and hydrophobic hydrocarbon chain. Therefore, liposomes are suitable for incorporating either water-soluble or lipid-soluble drugs.

Zheng-Rong Lu and Shinji Sakuma (eds.), *Nanomaterials in Pharmacology*, Methods in Pharmacology and Toxicology,
DOI 10.1007/978-1-4939-3121-7_11, © Springer Science+Business Media New York 2016

Table 1
Clinically approved nanoparticles

Ingredient	Proprietary name	Indication	Approval	Reference
Doxorubicin	Doxil® (US) Caelyx® (EU)	AIDS-related Kaposi's sarcoma	1995 (USA), 2007 (Japan)	[72–74]
		Ovarian cancer (after failure of platinum-based chemotherapy)	1999 (USA), 2009 (Japan)	[75–77]
		Multiple myeloma	2007 (USA)	[78, 79]
	Myocet®	Metastatic breast cancer	2004 (EU, Canada)	[80, 81]
Daunorubicin	Daunoxome®	AIDS-related Kaposi's sarcoma	1996 (USA)	[82, 83]
Cytarabine	Depocyt®	Lymphomatous meningitis	1999 (USA)	[84]
Vincristine	Marqibo®	Acute lymphoblastic leukemia	2012 (US)	[85]
Paclitaxel	Abraxane®	Breast cancer	2005 (USA), 2010 (Japan)	[86, 87]
		Non-small cell lung carcinoma	2012 (USA), 2013 (Japan)	[88, 89]
		Gastric cancer	2013 (Japan)	[88]
		Metastatic pancreatic cancer	2013 (USA)	[90]
Verteporfin	Visudyne®	Age-related macular degeneration	2000 (USA), 2003 (Japan)	[58, 91]
Amphotericin B	AmBisome®	Fungal infection	1997 (USA), 2006 (Japan)	[92, 93]

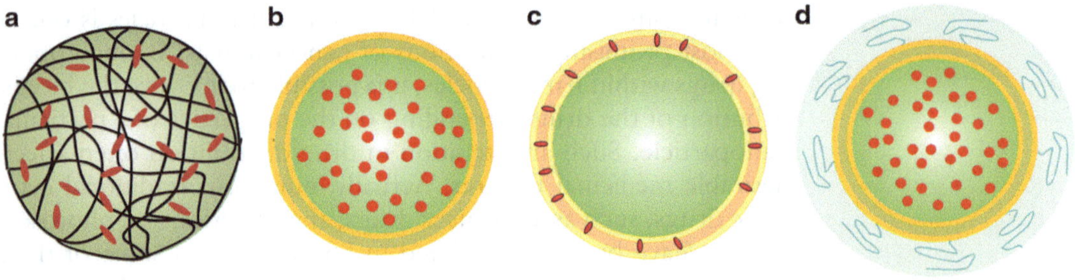

Fig. 1 Schematic representation of drug-loaded nanoparticles. (**a**) Assembled macromolecules. (**b**) Liposomes entrapping drugs in an aqueous interior. (**c**) Liposomes incorporating drugs in a hydrophobic lipid bilayer. (**d**) PEGylated liposomes

Hydrophilic drugs (vincristine and cytarabine) can be entrapped in the aqueous interior of liposomes (Fig. 1b), and lipid-soluble drugs (verteporfin) can be incorporated into the hydrophobic phospholipid bilayer (Fig. 1c). Even drugs without satisfactory solubility in either water or lipid (daunorubicin, doxorubicin, and amphotericin B) can be stably encapsulated into the liposomes by adequate preparation methods. Some liposomes encapsulating anticancer drugs are PEGylated (Doxil®) to promote long circulation and high stability (Fig. 1d).

This chapter introduces clinically used nanodrugs as well as nanodrugs currently undergoing clinical trials and preclinical studies.

2 Abraxane®

Albumin is emerging as a versatile protein carrier for improving the pharmacokinetic profile of the drugs it is associated with. Albumin is the most abundant plasma protein (35–50 g/L human serum) with a molecular weight of 66.5 kDa. Like most plasma proteins, albumin is synthesized in the liver where it is produced at a rate of approximately 0.7 mg/h for every gram of liver (i.e., 10–15 g daily); human serum albumin (HSA) exhibits an average half-life of 19 days.

Abraxane® (paclitaxel protein-bound particles for injectable suspension (albumin bound), also known as nab®-paclitaxel or ABI-007 (Abraxis BioScience/Celgene)) was the first albumin-based drug delivery system. It was approved at the beginning of 2005 for the treatment of metastatic breast cancer in the USA as well as in Europe, China, Russia, Japan, and several other countries. Abraxane® was also approved by the FDA for non-small lung cancer (2012) and pancreatic cancer (2013). Clinical trials for the treatment of bladder [1] and ovarian [2] cancer are currently being performed.

2.1 Preparation Method

Historically, the first drug albumin conjugates were synthesized by direct coupling methods followed by the development of albumin-binding peptides and prodrugs that bind rapidly and selectively to the cysteine-34 position of exogenous and endogenous albumin [3].

A unique albumin-based nanoparticle technology (nab-technology) has been developed that is ideal for encapsulating lipophilic drugs into nanoparticles. This technology appears to be simple: the drug is mixed with human serum albumin in an aqueous solvent and passed under high pressure through a jet to form drug albumin nanoparticles in sizes ranging between 100 and 200 nm, which is comparable to the size of small liposomes. Nab-paclitaxel (Abraxane®) has an approximate diameter of 130 nm.

2.2 Pharmacokinetical Advantages

Albumin has a number of characteristics that make it an attractive drug vehicle. It is a natural carrier of endogenous hydrophobic molecules (vitamins, hormones, and other water-insoluble plasma substances) that are bound in a reversible noncovalent manner. Moreover, albumin seems to help endothelial transcytosis of plasma constituents principally through binding to cell surface receptors (albondin) such as 60-kDa glycoprotein (gp60), which bind to caveolin-1 (an intracellular protein) with a subsequent formation of transcytotic vesicles (caveolae) (Fig. 2) [4–7].

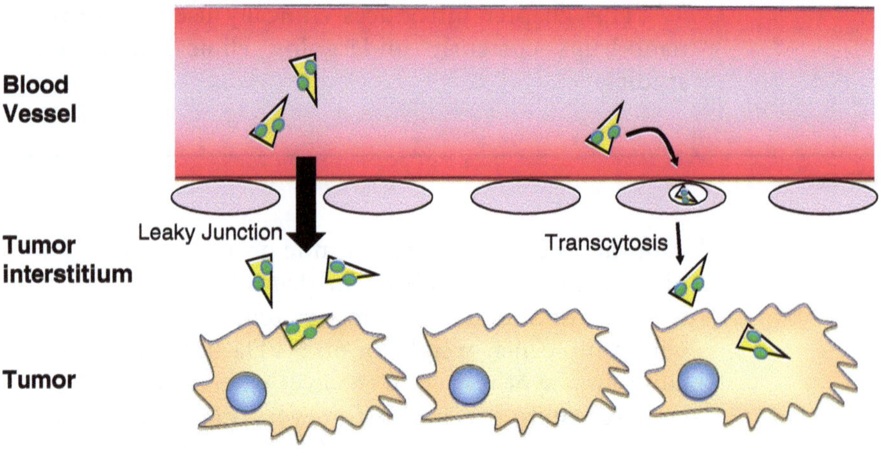

Fig. 2 Two routes of albumin-bound drugs to reach tumor cells

Circulating albumin must extravasate from blood vessels or cross endothelial cells to reach tumors, and albumin reportedly accomplishes this in at least two ways (Fig. 2): receptor-mediated transcytosis and the enhanced permeation and retention (EPR) effect [4, 8–10]. According to one hypothesis, nab-paclitaxel/Abraxane® may take advantage of each of these mechanisms to reach the tumor microenvironment [11, 12].

Additionally, cancer cells are believed to consume albumin from the tumor microenvironment and then metabolize it, possibly enhancing tumor growth [13, 14]. Desai et al. conducted experiments in tumor xenograft mouse models to determine whether albumin modification played a role in the tumor uptake of paclitaxel [11]. In these experiments, paclitaxel dissolved in Cremophor EL (solvent-based paclitaxel, sb-paclitaxel) and nanoparticle albumin-bound paclitaxel (nab-paclitaxel/Abraxane®) was radioactively labeled, and the amount of labeled paclitaxel that eventually reached tumors could then be quantified. When equal amounts were injected, researchers found that a third more paclitaxel from the nab-paclitaxel formulation (Abraxane®) was taken up by tumors. The researchers suggested that nab-paclitaxel/Abraxane® reached a higher tumor accumulation vs. sb-paclitaxel due to both the lack of drug-sequestering Cremophor EL micelles and enhanced albumin-mediated transcytosis. A subsequent report of similar experiments suggested that nab-paclitaxel/Abraxane® may achieve some degree of tumor selectivity relative to sb-paclitaxel, although the mechanisms responsible for this possibility were not characterized [15].

2.3 Advantages in Toxicity

A notable advantage of Abraxane® is Cremophor- and ethanol-free preparation. Cremophor was used as the solvent for sb-paclitaxel. Cremophor EL may add to paclitaxel's toxic effects by producing or contributing to the well-described hypersensitivity reactions that commonly occur during infusion, affecting 25–30 % of treated patients [16, 17]. To minimize the incidence and severity of these reactions, premedication with histamine 1 and 2 blockers, as well as glucocorticoids (usually dexamethasone), has become standard practice [18]. The cumulative side effects of dexamethasone used as a premedication may add to treatment-related morbidity and, in some instances, result in an early discontinuation of therapy. Cremophor EL may also contribute to chronic paclitaxel toxic effects, such as peripheral neuropathy [19]. An additional problem arising from the use of Cremophor and ethanol solvent is the leaching of plasticizers from PVC (polyvinyl chloride) bags and infusion sets in routine clinical use [20]. Consequently, Taxol containing Cremophor EL and ethanol must be prepared and administered in either glass bottles or non-PVC infusion systems with in-line filtration. These problematic issues have spurred interest in the development of taxanes with improved solubility in aqueous solutions [21]. Indeed, in phase I study, no hypersensitivity reactions were observed among patients who received infusions of Abraxane®.

2.4 Future Perspectives

Abraxane® has been approved for the treatment of breast cancer, non-small lung cancer, metastatic pancreatic cancer, and metastatic melanoma. As mentioned above, the clinical trials for expanding the application are ongoing.

On the other hand, another albumin-utilized approach that carries drugs by binding to serum albumin has been developed. For example, aldoxorubicin is based on a small molecule approach, in which thiol-binding prodrugs bind covalently to circulating albumin after intravenous administration. In a phase I study, aldoxorubicin showed a good safety profile at doses up to 260 mg/m^2 doxorubicin equivalents [22]. Although not the primary endpoint of the phase I study, aldoxorubicin induced tumor regressions in breast cancer, small cell lung cancer, and sarcoma. Aldoxorubicin is available in the form of commercially viable vials, is reconstituted with lactated Ringer's solution, and can be administered as an intravenous infusion over 30 min. Several clinical trials have been completed, are ongoing, or are being initiated.

3 Nanoparticles Carrying Antitumor Drugs

The clinical use of liposomes delivering antitumor drugs has been developed over the past 20 years. Doxil®, the first liposomal antitumor drug, was marketed in 1995. Liposomal drugs loading other antitumor drugs such as daunorubicin, cytarabine, and vincristine were subsequently approved. In the following paragraphs, we describe liposomal doxorubicin as a representative of liposomal antitumor drugs.

3.1 Pharmacokinetic Differences Between PEGylated and Non-PEGylated Liposomes

Intriguingly, two types of liposomal doxorubicin have been clinically used to treat distinct forms of cancer. Doxil® is the first FDA-approved nano-drug formulation of doxorubicin [23]. Due to an enhanced permeability and retention (EPR) effect, Doxil® is "passively targeted" to tumors, and its doxorubicin is released and then becomes available to tumor cells [23]. Higher drug levels in tumor tissue have been observed with Doxil® than with free doxorubicin in multiple cancer models [24, 25]. Liposomalization has clinically reduced cardiotoxicity, a hallmark side effect of free doxorubicin treatment [26, 27].

On the other hand, another formulation liposome encapsulating doxorubicin, Myocet™, has also been used in the clinical setting. Myocet™ is doxorubicin encapsulated in a non-PEGylated liposome composed of phosphatidylcholine and cholesterol. In combination with cyclophosphamide, Myocet™ has been approved as a first-line treatment of metastatic breast cancer (MBC) in both Europe and Canada.

The pharmacokinetics of non-PEGylated liposomal doxorubicin differs from both conventional doxorubicin and PEGylated liposomal doxorubicin [28]. Plasma levels of total doxorubicin are substantially higher with non-PEGylated liposomal doxorubicin than with conventional doxorubicin, while the peak plasma levels of free doxorubicin are lower with non-PEGylated liposomal doxorubicin. The clearance (5.1 ± 4.8 L/h) is much slower than that of conventional doxorubicin (46.7 ± 9.6 L/h) [29], but not as slow as with PEGylated liposomal doxorubicin. Palmar–plantar erythrodysesthesia (PPE) is known as a distinctive adverse effect of Doxil®, but it occurs rarely, with an incidence of <0.5 % in MBC patients who have been treated in phase III trials. In contrast with PEGylated liposomal doxorubicin, non-PEGylated liposomal doxorubicin is phagocytosed by mononuclear phagocytes [29, 30].

3.2 Preparation Using a Remote Loading Method

The remote loading of anticancer drugs into liposomes by transmembrane gradients is one of the best approaches for achieving a drug level per liposome that is sufficient for liposomal drugs to be therapeutically efficacious. A number of methods for the loading of ions and drugs into liposomes, based on pH and ammonium salt gradients, have been developed to optimize drug loading into vesicles [31, 32]. A remote loading procedure is available for encapsulating weak bases such as anthracyclines into liposomes. A mechanism for the remote loading of doxorubicin into an intraliposomal aqueous phase via an ammonium sulfate gradient is illustrated in Fig. 3.

3.3 Advantages in Reducing Toxicity

Cardiotoxicity, which is a typical adverse effect for doxorubicin, was suppressed in liposomal formulation. However, despite the overall tolerability and superiority of Doxil® over doxorubicin, two side effects that are not typical with free doxorubicin were observed for Doxil®.

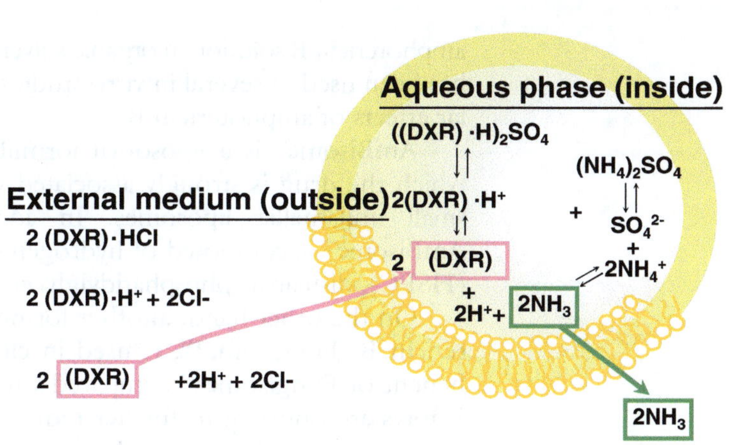

Fig. 3 Schematic diagram for liposomal encapsulation of doxorubicin (DXR) using a remote loading method

The first and most dominant one can result in a grade 2 or 3 of desquamating dermatitis and is referred to as PPE, or "foot and hand syndrome." The PPE was first demonstrated in a study involving humans by Barenholz's group [33] and was reviewed by Solomon and Gabizon [34]. The symptoms include redness, tenderness, and peeling of the skin. The prevalence of this side effect limits the Doxil® dose that can be given as compared with doxorubicin in the same treatment regimen. Of note, it was reported in phase III clinical trials of Myocet® that severe (grade 3 or 4) PPE was not observed. The second side effect is an infusion-related reaction that shows up as flushing and a shortness of breath; it is a unique adverse immune phenomenon that Doxil®, like many other nano-systems, can provoke. A complement activation-related pseudo-allergy (CARPA) has also been reported [35, 36]. CARPA is referred to as an acute hypersensitivity, or infusion reaction, because of the causal role in its patho-mechanism of complement activation instead of IgE binding. CARPA can be reduced by slowing the infusion rate and by premedication with corticosteroids and antihistamines [37].

4 Liposomal Amphotericin B

Amphotericin B is insoluble in aqueous solution. Thus, a vehicle (carrier) must be added to form a dispersion before it can be used clinically as an antifungal agent to treat systemic mycosis. The commercial preparation of amphotericin B, Fungizone®, is a mixture of amphotericin B, a detergent deoxycholate, and a buffer. When suspended in a glucose solution, Fungizone® forms a colloidal dispersion suitable for intravenous injection. Amphotericin B can also be obtained as a dispersion by the addition of a concentrated amphotericin B solution in organic solvents and water; this preparation has been used in several in vitro studies on the cellular and molecular effects of amphotericin B.

AmBisome® is a liposomal formulation of amphotericin B in which the drug is strongly associated with the bilayer structure of small unilamellar liposomes. In addition to amphotericin B, AmBisome® is composed of hydrogenated soy phosphatidylcholine (HSPC), distearoyl phosphatidylglycerol (DSPG), and cholesterol.

On the other hand, another formulation of liposomal amphotericin B, Fungisome™, is used in clinical settings in India. The benefit of Fungisome™ compared with AmBisome® is a low cost. Efforts are ongoing to further reduce the cost by pharmaceutical manufacture. Compared with the acquisition cost of the marketed liposomal preparations in India, the cost of Fungisome™ is 8–10 times less. Thus, Fungisome™ may be a safe and cost-effective option for Indian physicians.

4.1 Structural Features and Formulation

In AmBisome®, amphotericin B is integrated tightly within the liposomal membrane through formation of a noncovalent charge complex between the positively charged mycosamine in amphotericin B and the negatively charged distearoyl phosphatidylglycerol (DSPG) and hydrophobic interactions with the cholesterol components of the membrane. The lipid bilayer is made up of HSPC, cholesterol, DSPG, and amphotericin B in a 2:1:0.8:0.4 molar ratio [38]. These components have a high phase-transition temperature and are used to make a formulation that is stable at 37 °C. AmBisome® was designed as very rigid, small, unilamellar liposomes with mean diameters of 45–80 nm. Such small, rigid unilamellar liposomes are known to have long circulation times in the bloodstream following intravenous injection and may be sterilized by filtration through 0.2 μm pore membrane filters. AmBisome® was packed in the vial as freeze-dried powder similar to most liposomal drugs.

Fungisome™ is made of soy lecithin and cholesterol. Bottled Fungisome™ is sonicated using a bath sonicator with a thermostat, to maintain an ambient temperature for 45 min in order to convert multilamellar vesicles (MLV) into unilamellar vesicles (ULV). The sonicated drug, as per the manufacturer's instructions, must be used within 24 h after sonication. The particle size of MLV (tested using laser light scattering technique) is reported to be 1.53 ± 0.329 μm [39].

4.2 Pharmacokinetic Advantages

The rigid surface of AmBisome® has important clinical implications. Conventional amphotericin B is believed to produce toxicity by binding to cholesterol in mammalian cell membranes, followed by membrane damage/breakage. In vitro studies have demonstrated that Fungizone® at concentrations 200 μg/mL caused an approximate 60 % red blood cell lysis when incubated with red

Table 2
Amphotericin B concentrations in rodent tissues after administration of AmBisome and conventional Amphotericin B

		Tissue concentration (μg/mL)					
Product	**Dose (mg/kg)**	**Kidney**	**Liver**	**Spleen**	**Lung**	**Brain**	**Reference**
AmBisome	5	9.1 ± 0.5	374.7 ± 31.4	215.1 ± 62.3	8.2 ± 2.9	<0.5	[94]
Amphotericin B	1	1.5 ± 0.1	2.4 ± 0.9	5.7 ± 1.7	3.0 ± 1.4	NA	[95]

NA not available

blood cells for 24 h [40]. In contrast, red blood cell lysis caused by AmBisome® at the same concentration was as low as 6 % [40].

Administration of lipid formulations of amphotericin B generally results in higher tissue concentrations compared with conventional amphotericin B. The highest levels of amphotericin B are present in the organs of elimination: liver, spleen, and kidney (Table 2). An evaluation of the toxicokinetics (plasma concentration-time profiles and tissue concentrations) relative to the toxicological profiles leads to a conclusion that AmBisome administration results in less toxicity than conventional amphotericin B.

With conventional amphotericin B therapy, nephrotoxicity is the principal dose-limiting factor. In dogs, administration of conventional amphotericin B resulted in large increases in urea nitrogen and serum creatinine concentrations. These values remained within normal limits or were only slightly elevated after an administration of comparable doses of AmBisome® (1 and 4 mg/kg, respectively), even though systemic amphotericin B exposure with AmBisome® administration was 56 and 93 times higher, respectively, than with conventional amphotericin B. Hepatotoxicity is also a concern with amphotericin B administration. Although the indicators of hepatic toxicity were greatly elevated in dogs given conventional amphotericin B, these values remain within normal limits with AmBisome® administration (1 and 4 mg/kg), despite the large increase in systemic exposure to amphotericin B.

4.3 Challenges to the Oral Delivery of Amphotericin B

As mentioned above, injectable liposomal amphotericin B has achieved favorable pharmacokinetics. On the other hand, an oral formulation of amphotericin B has also been clinically used. For example, Halizon® and Fungizone® are available as tablets and syrups and can be applied to gastrointestinal fungal infections. However, conventional oral drugs also have problems. One of the main problems is poor bioavailability. Owing to its amphipathic nature, amphotericin B forms aggregates in water at concentrations around 2×10^{-7} M. These aggregates were formed well below critical micellar concentrations (ca. 3 μM) by the interaction between neighboring polyene chains (chromophores). This may be the reason for a low water solubility that leads to poor gastrointestinal absorption. Thus, amphotericin B has shown minimal bioavailability when given per os [41].

Several attempts have been made to enhance the oral bioavailability of amphotericin B. A lipid-based self-emulsifying drug delivery system was developed and showed significant antifungal activity in *Aspergillus fumigatus*-infected rats [42]. Amphotericin B was incorporated in Peceol® (mixture of mono- and diglycerides of oleic acid), which predominantly led to an increased absorption of the drug via the lymphatic transport mechanism. Additionally, the existence of amphotericin B in its native monomeric form in the lipidic environment, in contrast to the aggregated form in a conventional micellar solution, has been attributed to a significantly lesser degree of toxicity in lipid-based formulations.

Apart from lipid-based drug delivery systems, various other drug delivery systems, such as polymeric nanoparticles and nanosuspension approaches, have also been utilized for the oral delivery of amphotericin B [43–45].

Of note, a cochelate complex of amphotericin B, prepared by precipitation of a drug with phosphatidylserine and calcium cations, was under clinical trial for its oral delivery [46]. In 2009, BioDelivery Sciences International, Inc., announced initial results of a phase I study assessing the tolerability, safety, and pharmacokinetics of Bioral™ amphotericin B. The study identified doses that were well tolerated with no meaningful changes in laboratory safety values including those associated with renal function. The preliminary pharmacokinetic evaluation also revealed that plasma concentrations were comparable to those seen in prior animal toxicology studies using the same formulation. Recently, Aquarius Biotechonologies Inc. presented phase I results of their encochleated amphotericin B.

5 Liposomal Drugs for Photodynamic Therapy

5.1 Development of Photodynamic Therapy

Porphyrinoids form a large group of macrocyclic compounds with significant photochemical potential for application in photodynamic therapy (PDT)—a medical treatment that utilizes light to activate photosensitizers in the presence of oxygen, leading to localized photodamage by formed reactive oxygen species [47, 48]. Many of the porphyrinoid photosensitizers investigated in preclinical and clinical studies exhibit high lipophilicity. This feature is considered desirable because the solubilization of a photosensitizer in the lipid bilayer of the cell membrane has been noted as one of the main factors of photosensitizer efficacy. On the other hand, a hydrophobic nature and a lack of solubility in aqueous media were found to hamper the development of pharmaceutical formulations and are

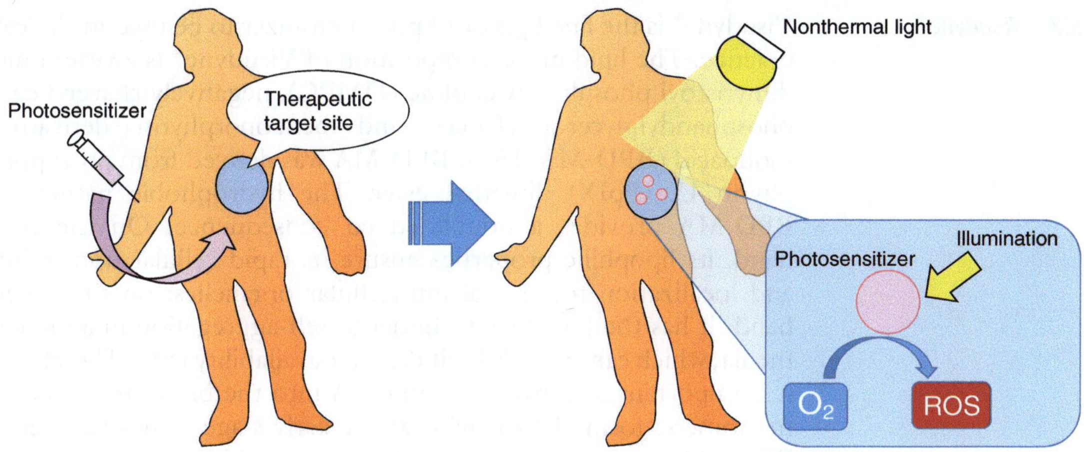

Fig. 4 Two-step process for photodynamic therapy

reasons for the aggregation of these compounds, which impedes photochemical properties and the bioavailability of the photosensitizer. Moreover, the specific delivery of photosensitizers to target cells remains a crucial challenge in photodynamic therapy.

The treatment of age-related macular degeneration with a photodynamic therapy (TAP) study group reported that photodynamic therapy with liposomal verteporfin (Visudyne) can reduce the risk of vision loss in patients with subfoveal choroidal neovascularization (CNV) due to age-related macular degeneration.

Photodynamic therapy is a two-step process. The first step requires the intravenous infusion of a photosensitive drug—in this case, verteporfin. The second step is activation of the drug by nonthermal light at the wavelength absorbed by a photosensitizer used and in the presence of oxygen [49] (Fig. 4). The activation probably results in the formation of cytotoxic oxygen species such as singlet oxygen and free radicals, which can damage cellular structures. This damage may lead to platelet activation and subsequent thrombosis and occlusion of choroidal neovasculature within the treated area. After studies reported that photosensitizers could be retained preferentially in tumors [50] and that photodynamic therapy could lead to tumor death by occlusion of the tumor vasculature and direct cytotoxic effects [51], investigators hypothesized that photodynamic therapy may be particularly useful in the selective destruction of CNV to confine the lesion from growing and thereby reduce the risk of progressive visual damage without causing significant destruction to viable neurosensory retina overlying the CNV [52, 53]. Verteporfin was believed to be a good photosensitizer for treatment of CNV, not only because of its potential selectivity for neovasculature lesions, but also because of its pharmacokinetics, which include rapid clearance within the first 24 h after infusion to reduce the chances of generalized photosensitivity of patients after treatment.

5.2 Visudyne®

Visudyne® is the first liposomal photosensitizer to be used in clinical practice. The lipid phase composition of Visudyne® is zwitterionic dimyristoyl phosphatidylcholine (DMPC), negatively charged egg phosphatidylglycerol (EPG), and benzoporphyrin derivative monoacid (BPD-MA) [54]. BPD-MA was derived from protoporphyrin IX (PpIX) dimethyl ester. The hydrophobic nature of BPD-MA provides a double-edged consequence. On the one hand, its lipophilic properties ensure its rapid cellular uptake by, and localization to, crucial intracellular organelles; on the other hand, it has the tendency to undergo self-aggregation in aqueous media, which can severely limit drug bioavailability [55]. Therefore, it is important to introduce BPD-MA into the bloodstream in its monomeric form. This is why, at the early stage of development, BPD-MA was incorporated into liposomes, which provided a vehicle for intravenous delivery of the hydrophobic photosensitizer.

Based on preclinical studies [53, 56, 57], a phase I and II investigation was designed to evaluate the safety of verteporfin therapy for the treatment of patients with CNV and to determine the effects of this therapy on fluorescein leakage from CNV [58–60]. This investigation showed that an initial treatment of photodynamic therapy with verteporfin could cause short-term cessation of fluorescein leakage from CNV without damage to retinal blood vessels or loss of vision [58]. In most cases, fluorescein leakage from CNV became apparent by 12 weeks after this initial treatment, even in subjects who had received the maximum tolerated light dose (in which nonselective damage to sensory retinal blood vessels with visual loss had occurred). The investigators suspected that this reappearance of leakage probably would be accompanied by subsequent growth of the neovascular lesion with progressive vision loss. Therefore, they considered evaluating a treatment strategy that could confine the neovascular lesion and reduce the risk of vision loss by periodically applying photodynamic therapy with verteporfin to an eye with subfoveal CNV.

5.3 Application of Liposomal Photosensitizers to Cancer Therapy

Photodynamic therapy (PDT) has also shown promise in the treatment of early and superficial tumors. There are three main mechanisms by which PDT mediates tumor destruction [61]. In the first, the reactive oxygen species (ROS) that is generated by PDT can kill tumor cells directly. In the second, PDT damages the tumor-associated vasculature, leading to tumor infarction. Finally, PDT can activate an immune response against tumor cells. These three mechanisms can also influence each other. The relative importance of each for the overall tumor response is yet to be defined. It is clear, however, that the combination of all these components is required for long-term tumor control.

To avoid reticuloendothelial system (RES) trapping of conventional DPPC/DPPG liposomes, a long-circulating moiety,

PEGylated distearoylphosphatidylethanolamine (DSPE), was incorporated at about 2 % of the total lipid, thus leading to the Fospeg® formulation [62, 63]. As shown by Reddi's group [63], the PEG layer coating can influence cytotoxicity and cellular uptake by liposomes.

Fospeg® performed better than Foscan® (nonliposomal photosensitizer formulation), presenting superior pharmacokinetic properties such as a higher tumor-to-skin ratio, higher bioavailability, higher plasma concentrations, and earlier maximal tumor accumulation in the PDT treatment of feline squamous cell carcinoma in vivo [64]. Fospeg® also showed a significant decrease in vascularity and blood volume in the same animal model [65].

Meanwhile, a major, and well-known, drawback of photosensitizers is prolonged photosensitivity. In order to prevent photosensitivity, combination therapy with antioxidants has been reported. *P. halepensis* bark extract is a natural product that is rich in antioxidant agents and can be injected into a tumor prior to Fospeg-interstitial PDT. In a concentration of 100 μg/mL, it totally eliminates the remaining photosensitivity and leaves the Fospeg-interstitial PDT efficacy unaffected.

6 Future Perspective

As described in this chapter, many liposomal drugs have already been clinically approved. On the other hand, polymeric micelles are still undergoing clinical trials (Table 3).

Micelles have a significant feature in terms of particle size. The diameter of polymeric micelles resembles that of natural viruses, and they can be tuned from 10 to 100 nm [66, 67], which reduces their accumulation in the organs of the RES and helps them overcome physiological barriers such as lymphatic transport to lymph nodes after intradermal injection [68], extravasation, deep penetration, and high accumulation in solid tumors after systemic injection [69]. Clinical trials have revealed that anticancer drug-loaded polymeric micelles enhanced efficacy and reduced side effects. The recent progress of NK105 and NC-6004 in phase III studies allows the envisioning of an imminent translation of polymeric micelles in the clinical setting.

Meanwhile, it is also noteworthy that various combination therapies were tried in liposomal and micellar anticancer drugs. Multidrug regimens have been developed to enhance anticancer efficacy and suppress the emergence of drug resistance. However, patients receiving such multidrug regimens sometimes experience additional and stronger adverse effects to drugs that could necessitate a discontinuation of the treatment. The utilization of nanoparticles selective to tumor tissue appears to be a good solution

Table 3
Micellar formulations under clinical or preclinical trials

Name	Drug	Block copolymer	Size (nm)	Company	Development phase	Indication	References
NK105	Paclitaxel	PEG-*b*-poly (α,β-aspartic acid)	85	Nippon Kayaku, Co.	Phase III (started July 2012; breast cancer)	Gastric cancer/ breast cancer	[96]
NK012	SN-38	PEG-*b*-poly (L-glutamic acid)	20	Nippon Kayaku, Co.	Phase II	Triple negative breast cancer	[97]
NK911	Doxorubicin	PEG-*b*-poly (α,β-aspartic acid)	40	Nippon Kayaku, Co.	Phase II	Various solid tumors	[98]
NC-6004	Cisplatin	PEG-*b*-poly (L-GLUTAMIC acid)	20	Nanocarrier, Co.	Phase III (started 2013)	Pancreatic cancer	[99]
NC-4016	Oxaliplatin	PEG-*b*-poly (L-glutamic acid)	30	Nanocarrier, Co.	Phase I	Various solid tumors	[70]
NC-6300	Epirubicin	PEG-*b*-poly (aspartate-hydrazone)	60	Nanocarrier, Co.	Phase I	Various solid tumors	[70, 100]
siRNA micelles	siRNA	PEG-*b*-polycations	40–60	Nanocarrier, Co.	Preclinical	–	[101, 102]

for this problem. For example, the following therapeutic combinations of polymeric micelles and anticancer drugs exerted prominent therapeutic effect and low toxicity: oxaliplatin parent complex and epirubicin [70] or rapamycin and paclitaxel [71].

Nanocarriers have improved the distribution of drugs and achieved improvements in therapeutic effects and in the suppression of adverse effects. Novel and pharmacologically active compounds are difficult to discover. By altering the pharmacokinetics and pharmacodynamics of conventional drugs, however, it is possible to enhance their therapeutic effect and safety and apply these effects to other diseases. This is a worthwhile pursuit for pharmaceutical companies that require life cycle management of drug products, as well as for patients who are unsatisfied with conventional treatments. Nanoparticulation of conventional drugs and exploitation of new clinical applications of nanodrugs, mostly in combination with other drugs, will remain an essential strategy for pharmaceutical development.

Acknowledgment

This work was partially supported by a research program for development of intelligent Tokushima artificial exosome (iTEX) from Tokushima University.

References

1. McKiernan JM, Barlow LJ, Laudano MA, Mann MJ, Petrylak DP, Benson MC (2011) A phase I trial of intravesical nanoparticle albumin-bound paclitaxel in the treatment of bacillus Calmette-Guerin refractory nonmuscle invasive bladder cancer. J Urol 186(2): 448–451
2. Tillmanns TD, Lowe MP, Walker MS, Stepanski EJ, Schwartzberg LS (2013) Phase II clinical trial of bevacizumab with albumin-bound paclitaxel in patients with recurrent, platinum-resistant primary epithelial ovarian or primary peritoneal carcinoma. Gynecol Oncol 128(2):221–228
3. Kratz F, Muller-Driver R, Hofmann I, Drevs J, Unger C (2000) A novel macromolecular prodrug concept exploiting endogenous serum albumin as a drug carrier for cancer chemotherapy. J Med Chem 43(7):1253–1256
4. John TA, Vogel SM, Tiruppathi C, Malik AB, Minshall RD (2003) Quantitative analysis of albumin uptake and transport in the rat microvessel endothelial monolayer. Am J Physiol Lung Cell Mol Physiol 284(1): L187–L196
5. Minshall RD, Sessa WC, Stan RV, Anderson RG, Malik AB (2003) Caveolin regulation of endothelial function. Am J Physiol Lung Cell Mol Physiol 285(6):L1179–L1183
6. Vogel SM, Minshall RD, Pilipovic M, Tiruppathi C, Malik AB (2001) Albumin uptake and transcytosis in endothelial cells in vivo induced by albumin-binding protein. Am J Physiol Lung Cell Mol Physiol 281(6):L1512–L1522
7. Tiruppathi C, Song W, Bergenfeldt M, Sass P, Malik AB (1997) Gp60 activation mediates albumin transcytosis in endothelial cells by tyrosine kinase-dependent pathway. J Biol Chem 272(41):25968–25975
8. Simionescu M, Gafencu A, Antohe F (2002) Transcytosis of plasma macromolecules in endothelial cells: a cell biological survey. Microsc Res Tech 57(5):269–288
9. Matsumura Y, Maeda H (1986) A new concept for macromolecular therapeutics in cancer chemotherapy: mechanism of tumoritropic accumulation of proteins and the antitumor agent smancs. Cancer Res 46(12 Pt 1): 6387–6392
10. Maeda H, Wu J, Sawa T, Matsumura Y, Hori K (2000) Tumor vascular permeability and the EPR effect in macromolecular therapeutics: a review. J Control Release 65(1-2):271–284
11. Desai N, Trieu V, Yao Z, Louie L, Ci S, Yang A et al (2006) Increased antitumor activity, intratumor paclitaxel concentrations, and endothelial cell transport of cremophor-free, albumin-bound paclitaxel, ABI-007, compared with cremophor-based paclitaxel. Clin Cancer Res 12(4):1317–1324
12. Desai N, Trieu V, Damascelli B, Soon-Shiong P (2009) SPARC expression correlates with tumor response to albumin-bound paclitaxel in head and neck cancer patients. Transl Oncol 2(2):59–64
13. Kratz F (2008) Albumin as a drug carrier: design of prodrugs, drug conjugates and nanoparticles. J Control Release 132(3): 171–183
14. Stehle G, Sinn H, Wunder A, Schrenk HH, Stewart JC, Hartung G et al (1997) Plasma protein (albumin) catabolism by the tumor itself – implications for tumor metabolism and the genesis of cachexia. Crit Rev Oncol Hematol 26(2):77–100
15. Scheff RJ (2008) Breast cancer and the new taxanes: focus on nab-paclitaxel. Commun Oncol 5(7 Suppl 8):7–13
16. Weiss RB, Donehower RC, Wiernik PH, Ohnuma T, Gralla RJ, Trump DL et al (1990) Hypersensitivity reactions from taxol. J Clin Oncol 8(7):1263–1268
17. Rowinsky EK, Donehower RC (1995) Paclitaxel (taxol). N Engl J Med 332(15):1004–1014
18. Finley RS, Rowinsky EK (1994) Patient care issues: the management of paclitaxel-related toxicities. Ann Pharmacother 28(5 Suppl):S27–S30
19. Windebank AJ, Blexrud MD, de Groen PC (1994) Potential neurotoxicity of the solvent

vehicle for cyclosporine. J Pharmacol Exp Ther 268(2):1051–1056
20. Waugh WN, Trissel LA, Stella VJ (1991) Stability, compatibility, and plasticizer extraction of taxol (NSC-125973) injection diluted in infusion solutions and stored in various containers. Am J Hosp Pharm 48(7): 1520–1524
21. Hidalgo M, Aylesworth C, Hammond LA, Britten CD, Weiss G, Stephenson J Jr et al (2001) Phase I and pharmacokinetic study of BMS-184476, a taxane with greater potency and solubility than paclitaxel. J Clin Oncol 19(9):2493–2503
22. Unger C, Haring B, Medinger M, Drevs J, Steinbild S, Kratz F et al (2007) Phase I and pharmacokinetic study of the (6-maleimidocaproyl)hydrazone derivative of doxorubicin. Clin Cancer Res 13(16): 4858–4866
23. Barenholz Y (2012) Doxil(R) – the first FDA-approved nano-drug: lessons learned. J Control Release 160(2):117–134
24. Hau P, Fabel K, Baumgart U, Rummele P, Grauer O, Bock A et al (2004) Pegylated liposomal doxorubicin-efficacy in patients with recurrent high-grade glioma. Cancer 100(6):1199–1207
25. Anders CK, Adamo B, Karginova O, Deal AM, Rawal S, Darr D et al (2013) Pharmacokinetics and efficacy of PEGylated liposomal doxorubicin in an intracranial model of breast cancer. PLoS One 8(5), e61359
26. Gill SE, Savage K, Wysham WZ, Blackhurst DW, Winter WE, Puls LE (2013) Continuing routine cardiac surveillance in long-term use of pegylated liposomal doxorubicin: is it necessary? Gynecol Oncol 129(3):544–547
27. Rahman AM, Yusuf SW, Ewer MS (2007) Anthracycline-induced cardiotoxicity and the cardiac-sparing effect of liposomal formulation. Int J Nanomedicine 2(4):567–583
28. Batist G, Ramakrishnan G, Rao CS, Chandrasekharan A, Gutheil J, Guthrie T et al (2001) Reduced cardiotoxicity and preserved antitumor efficacy of liposome-encapsulated doxorubicin and cyclophosphamide compared with conventional doxorubicin and cyclophosphamide in a randomized, multicenter trial of metastatic breast cancer. J Clin Oncol 19(5):1444–1454
29. Swenson CE, Perkins WR, Roberts P, Janoff AS (2001) Liposome technology and the development of Myocet™ (liposomal doxorubicin citrate). Breast 10(Suppl 2(0)):1–7
30. Sparano JA, Winer EP (2001) Liposomal anthracyclines for breast cancer. Semin Oncol 28(4 Suppl 12):32–40
31. Clerc S, Barenholz Y (1995) Loading of amphipathic weak acids into liposomes in response to transmembrane calcium acetate gradients. Biochim Biophys Acta 1240(2): 257–265
32. Haran G, Cohen R, Bar LK, Barenholz Y (1993) Transmembrane ammonium sulfate gradients in liposomes produce efficient and stable entrapment of amphipathic weak bases. Biochim Biophys Acta 1151(2):201–215
33. Gabizon A, Catane R, Uziely B, Kaufman B, Safra T, Cohen R et al (1994) Prolonged circulation time and enhanced accumulation in malignant exudates of doxorubicin encapsulated in polyethylene-glycol coated liposomes. Cancer Res 54(4):987–992
34. Soloman R, Gabizon AA (2008) Clinical pharmacology of liposomal anthracyclines: focus on pegylated liposomal Doxorubicin. Clin Lymphoma Myeloma 8(1):21–32
35. Szebeni J, Muggia F, Gabizon A, Barenholz Y (2011) Activation of complement by therapeutic liposomes and other lipid excipient-based therapeutic products: prediction and prevention. Adv Drug Deliv Rev 63(12):1020–1030
36. Szebeni J, Bedocs P, Rozsnyay Z, Weiszhar Z, Urbanics R, Rosivall L et al (2012) Liposome-induced complement activation and related cardiopulmonary distress in pigs: factors promoting reactogenicity of Doxil and Am Bisome. Nanomedicine 8(2):176–184
37. Chanan-Khan A, Szebeni J, Savay S, Liebes L, Rafique NM, Alving CR et al (2003) Complement activation following first exposure to pegylated liposomal doxorubicin (Doxil): possible role in hypersensitivity reactions. Ann Oncol 14(9):1430–1437
38. Proffitt JPA-M, Richard T (2008) Development, characterization, efficacy and mode of action of ambisome, a unilamellar liposomal formulation of amphotericin B. http://dxdoi org/103109/08982109309150729
39. Kshirsagar NA, Pandya SK, Kirodian GB, Sanath S (2005) Liposomal drug delivery system from laboratory to clinic. J Postgrad Med 51(Suppl 1):S5–S15
40. Serrano DR, Hernandez L, Fleire L, Gonzalez-Alvarez I, Montoya A, Ballesteros MP et al (2013) Hemolytic and pharmacokinetic studies of liposomal and particulate amphotericin B formulations. Int J Pharm 447(1–2):38–46
41. Lemke A, Kiderlen AF, Kayser O (2005) Amphotericin B. Appl Microbiol Biotechnol 68(2):151–162
42. Risovic V, Rosland M, Sivak O, Wasan KM, Bartlett K (2007) Assessing the antifungal

activity of a new oral lipid-based amphotericin B formulation following administration to rats infected with Aspergillus fumigatus. Drug Dev Ind Pharm 33(7):703–707

43. Italia JL, Yahya MM, Singh D, Ravi Kumar MN (2009) Biodegradable nanoparticles improve oral bioavailability of amphotericin B and show reduced nephrotoxicity compared to intravenous Fungizone. Pharm Res 26(6):1324–1331
44. Golenser J, Domb A (2006) New formulations and derivatives of amphotericin B for treatment of leishmaniasis. Mini Rev Med Chem 6(2):153–162
45. Kayser O, Olbrich C, Yardley V, Kiderlen AF, Croft SL (2003) Formulation of amphotericin B as nanosuspension for oral administration. Int J Pharm 254(1):73–75
46. Delmas G, Park S, Chen ZW, Tan F, Kashiwazaki R, Zarif L et al (2002) Efficacy of orally delivered cochleates containing amphotericin B in a murine model of aspergillosis. Antimicrob Agents Chemother 46(8): 2704–2707
47. Allison RR, Sibata CH (2010) Oncologic photodynamic therapy photosensitizers: a clinical review. Photodiagnosis Photodyn Ther 7(2):61–75
48. Shigenobu Yano, Shiho Hirohara, Makoto Obata, Yuichiro Hagiya, Shun-ichiro Ogura, Atsushi Ikeda, Hiromi Kataoka, Mamoru Tanaka, Takashi Joh et al (2011) Current states and future views in photodynamic therapy. J Photochem. Photobiol. C: Photochemistry Res 12(1):46–67
49. Manyak MJ, Russo A, Smith PD, Glatstein E (1988) Photodynamic therapy. J Clin Oncol 6(2):380–391
50. Roberts WG, Hasan T (1992) Role of neovasculature and vascular permeability on the tumor retention of photodynamic agents. Cancer Res 52(4):924–930
51. Zhou CN (1989) Mechanisms of tumor necrosis induced by photodynamic therapy. J Photochem Photobiol B Biol 3(3):299–318
52. Schmidt-Erfurth U, Hasan T, Gragoudas E, Michaud N, Flotte TJ, Birngruber R (1994) Vascular targeting in photodynamic occlusion of subretinal vessels. Ophthalmology 101(12):1953–1961
53. Miller JW, Walsh AW, Kramer M, Hasan T, Michaud N, Flotte TJ et al (1995) Photodynamic therapy of experimental choroidal neovascularization using lipoprotein-delivered benzoporphyrin. Arch Ophthalmol 113(6):810–818
54. Chowdhary RK, Shariff I, Dolphin D (2003) Drug release characteristics of lipid based benzoporphyrin derivative. J Pharm Pharm Sci 6(1):13–19
55. Aveline BM, Hasan T, Redmond RW (1995) The effects of aggregation, protein binding and cellular incorporation on the photophysical properties of benzoporphyrin derivative monoacid ring A (BPDMA). J Photochem Photobiol B Biol 30(2-3):161–169
56. Kramer M, Miller JW, Michaud N, Moulton RS, Hasan T, Flotte TJ et al (1996) Liposomal benzoporphyrin derivative verteporfin photodynamic therapy. Selective treatment of choroidal neovascularization in monkeys. Ophthalmology 103(3):427–438
57. Husain D, Miller JW, Michaud N, Connolly E, Flotte TJ, Gragoudas ES (1996) Intravenous infusion of liposomal benzoporphyrin derivative for photodynamic therapy of experimental choroidal neovascularization. Arch Ophthalmol 114(8):978–985
58. Miller JW, Schmidt-Erfurth U, Sickenberg M, Pournaras CJ, Laqua H, Barbazetto I et al (1999) Photodynamic therapy with verteporfin for choroidal neovascularization caused by age-related macular degeneration: results of a single treatment in a phase 1 and 2 study. Arch Ophthalmol 117(9):1161–1173
59. Schmidt-Erfurth U, Miller JW, Sickenberg M, Laqua H, Barbazetto I, Gragoudas ES et al (1999) Photodynamic therapy with verteporfin for choroidal neovascularization caused by age-related macular degeneration: results of retreatments in a phase 1 and 2 study. Arch Ophthalmol 117(9):1177–1187
60. Sickenberg M, Schmidt-Erfurth U, Miller JW, Pournaras CJ, Zografos L, Piguet B et al (2000) A preliminary study of photodynamic therapy using verteporfin for choroidal neovascularization in pathologic myopia, ocular histoplasmosis syndrome, angioid streaks, and idiopathic causes. Arch Ophthalmol 118(3): 327–336
61. Dougherty TJ, Gomer CJ, Henderson BW, Jori G, Kessel D, Korbelik M et al (1998) Photodynamic therapy. J Natl Cancer Inst 90(12):889–905
62. Kuntsche J, Freisleben I, Steiniger F, Fahr A (2010) Temoporfin-loaded liposomes: physicochemical characterization. Eur J Pharm Sci 40(4):305–315
63. Compagnin C, Moret F, Celotti L, Miotto G, Woodhams JH, MacRobert AJ et al (2011) Meta-tetra(hydroxyphenyl)chlorin-loaded liposomes sterically stabilised with poly(ethylene glycol) of different length and density: characterisation, in vitro cellular uptake and phototoxicity. Photochem Photobiol Sci 10(11):1751–1759

64. Buchholz J, Kaser-Hotz B, Khan T, Rohrer Bley C, Melzer K, Schwendener RA et al (2005) Optimizing photodynamic therapy: in vivo pharmacokinetics of liposomal meta-(tetrahydroxyphenyl)chlorin in feline squamous cell carcinoma. Clin Cancer Res 11(20):7538–7544
65. Ohlerth S, Laluhova D, Buchholz J, Roos M, Walt H, Kaser-Hotz B (2006) Changes in vascularity and blood volume as a result of photodynamic therapy can be assessed with power Doppler ultrasonography. Lasers Surg Med 38(3):229–234
66. Kataoka K, Harada A, Nagasaki Y (2001) Block copolymer micelles for drug delivery: design, characterization and biological significance. Adv Drug Deliv Rev 47(1): 113–131
67. Nishiyama N, Kataoka K (2006) Current state, achievements, and future prospects of polymeric micelles as nanocarriers for drug and gene delivery. Pharmacol Ther 112(3):630–648
68. Reddy ST, van der Vlies AJ, Simeoni E, Angeli V, Randolph GJ, O'Neil CP et al (2007) Exploiting lymphatic transport and complement activation in nanoparticle vaccines. Nat Biotechnol 25(10):1159–1164
69. Cabral H, Matsumoto Y, Mizuno K, Chen Q, Murakami M, Kimura M et al (2011) Accumulation of sub-100 nm polymeric micelles in poorly permeable tumours depends on size. Nat Nanotechnol 6(12):815–823
70. Yamamoto Y, Hyodo I, Takigahira M, Koga Y, Yasunaga M, Harada M et al (2014) Effect of combined treatment with the epirubicin-incorporating micelles (NC-6300) and 1,2-diaminocyclohexane platinum (II)-incorporating micelles (NC-4016) on a human gastric cancer model. Int J Cancer 135(1):214–223
71. Mishra GP, Nguyen D, Alani AW (2013) Inhibitory effect of paclitaxel and rapamycin individual and dual drug-loaded polymeric micelles in the angiogenic cascade. Mol Pharm 10(5):2071–2078
72. Stewart S, Jablonowski H, Goebel FD, Arasteh K, Spittle M, Rios A et al (1998) Randomized comparative trial of pegylated liposomal doxorubicin versus bleomycin and vincristine in the treatment of AIDS-related Kaposi's sarcoma. International Pegylated Liposomal Doxorubicin Study Group. J Clin Oncol 16(2):683–691
73. Northfelt DW, Dezube BJ, Thommes JA, Miller BJ, Fischl MA, Friedman-Kien A et al (1998) Pegylated-liposomal doxorubicin versus doxorubicin, bleomycin, and vincristine in the treatment of AIDS-related Kaposi's sarcoma: results of a randomized phase III clinical trial. J Clin Oncol 16(7):2445–2451
74. Cianfrocca M, Lee S, Von Roenn J, Tulpule A, Dezube BJ, Aboulafia DM et al (2010) Randomized trial of paclitaxel versus pegylated liposomal doxorubicin for advanced human immunodeficiency virus-associated Kaposi sarcoma: evidence of symptom palliation from chemotherapy. Cancer 116(16): 3969–3977
75. Gordon AN, Fleagle JT, Guthrie D, Parkin DE, Gore ME, Lacave AJ (2001) Recurrent epithelial ovarian carcinoma: a randomized phase III study of pegylated liposomal doxorubicin versus topotecan. J Clin Oncol 19(14):3312–3322
76. Fujisaka Y, Tamura T, Ohe Y, Kunitoh H, Sekine I, Yamamoto N et al (2006) Pharmacokinetics and pharmacodynamics of weekly epoetin beta in lung cancer patients. Jpn J Clin Oncol 36(8):477–482
77. Katsumata N, Fujiwara Y, Kamura T, Nakanishi T, Hatae M, Aoki D et al (2008) Phase II clinical trial of pegylated liposomal doxorubicin (JNS002) in Japanese patients with mullerian carcinoma (epithelial ovarian carcinoma, primary carcinoma of fallopian tube, peritoneal carcinoma) having a therapeutic history of platinum-based chemotherapy: a Phase II Study of the Japanese Gynecologic Oncology Group. Jpn J Clin Oncol 38(11):777–785
78. Orlowski RZ, Nagler A, Sonneveld P, Blade J, Hajek R, Spencer A et al (2007) Randomized phase III study of pegylated liposomal doxorubicin plus bortezomib compared with bortezomib alone in relapsed or refractory multiple myeloma: combination therapy improves time to progression. J Clin Oncol 25(25):3892–3901
79. Sonneveld P, Hajek R, Nagler A, Spencer A, Blade J, Robak T et al (2008) Combined pegylated liposomal doxorubicin and bortezomib is highly effective in patients with recurrent or refractory multiple myeloma who received prior thalidomide/lenalidomide therapy. Cancer 112(7):1529–1537
80. Swenson CE, Bolcsak LE, Batist G, Guthrie TH Jr, Tkaczuk KH, Boxenbaum H et al (2003) Pharmacokinetics of doxorubicin administered i.v. as Myocet (TLC D-99; liposome-encapsulated doxorubicin citrate) compared with conventional doxorubicin when given in combination with cyclophosphamide in patients with metastatic breast cancer. Anticancer Drugs 14(3):239–246
81. Mross K, Niemann B, Massing U, Drevs J, Unger C, Bhamra R et al (2004) Pharmacokinetics of liposomal doxorubicin

(TLC-D99; Myocet) in patients with solid tumors: an open-label, single-dose study. Cancer Chemother Pharmacol 54(6):514–524
82. Gill PS, Wernz J, Scadden DT, Cohen P, Mukwaya GM, von Roenn JH et al (1996) Randomized phase III trial of liposomal daunorubicin versus doxorubicin, bleomycin, and vincristine in AIDS-related Kaposi's sarcoma. J Clin Oncol 14(8):2353–2364
83. Latagliata R, Breccia M, Fazi P, Iacobelli S, Martinelli G, Di Raimondo F et al (2008) Liposomal daunorubicin versus standard daunorubicin: long term follow-up of the GIMEMA GSI 103 AMLE randomized trial in patients older than 60 years with acute myelogenous leukaemia. Br J Haematol 143(5):681–689
84. Glantz MJ, LaFollette S, Jaeckle KA, Shapiro W, Swinnen L, Rozental JR et al (1999) Randomized trial of a slow-release versus a standard formulation of cytarabine for the intrathecal treatment of lymphomatous meningitis. J Clin Oncol 17(10):3110–3116
85. Rodriguez MA, Pytlik R, Kozak T, Chhanabhai M, Gascoyne R, Lu B et al (2009) Vincristine sulfate liposomes injection (Marqibo) in heavily pretreated patients with refractory aggressive non-Hodgkin lymphoma: report of the pivotal phase 2 study. Cancer 115(15):3475–3482
86. Yamamoto Y, Kawano I, Iwase H (2011) Nab-paclitaxel for the treatment of breast cancer: efficacy, safety, and approval. Onco Targets Ther 4:123–136
87. Gradishar WJ, Tjulandin S, Davidson N, Shaw H, Desai N, Bhar P et al (2005) Phase III trial of nanoparticle albumin-bound paclitaxel compared with polyethylated castor oil-based paclitaxel in women with breast cancer. J Clin Oncol 23(31):7794–7803
88. Taiho Pharmaceutical Co., Ltd. (2013) Antitumor agent "ABRAXANE® I.V. Infusion 100 mg" approved for additional indications of gastric cancer and non-small cell lung cancer. http://www.taiho.co.jp/english/news/20130221.html
89. Socinski MA, Okamoto I, Hon JK, Hirsh V, Dakhil SR, Page RD et al (2013) Safety and efficacy analysis by histology of weekly nab-paclitaxel in combination with carboplatin as first-line therapy in patients with advanced non-small-cell lung cancer. Ann Oncol 24(9):2390–2396
90. Von Hoff DD, Ramanathan RK, Borad MJ, Laheru DA, Smith LS, Wood TE et al (2011) Gemcitabine plus nab-paclitaxel is an active regimen in patients with advanced pancreatic cancer: a phase I/II trial. J Clin Oncol 29(34):4548–4554
91. Azab M, Boyer DS, Bressler NM, Bressler SB, Cihelkova I, Hao Y et al (2005) Verteporfin therapy of subfoveal minimally classic choroidal neovascularization in age-related macular degeneration: 2-year results of a randomized clinical trial. Arch Ophthalmol 123(4): 448–457
92. Ringden O, Meunier F, Tollemar J, Ricci P, Tura S, Kuse E et al (1991) Efficacy of amphotericin B encapsulated in liposomes (AmBisome) in the treatment of invasive fungal infections in immunocompromised patients. J Antimicrob Chemother 28(Suppl B):73–82
93. Meunier F, Prentice HG, Ringden O (1991) Liposomal amphotericin B (AmBisome): safety data from a phase II/III clinical trial. J Antimicrob Chemother 28(Suppl B):83–91
94. Boswell GW, Bekersky I, Buell D, Hiles R, Walsh TJ (1998) Toxicological profile and pharmacokinetics of a unilamellar liposomal vesicle formulation of amphotericin B in rats. Antimicrob Agents Chemother 42(2): 263–268
95. van Etten EW, van den Heuvel-de Groot C, Bakker-Woudenberg IA (1993) Efficacies of amphotericin B-desoxycholate (Fungizone), liposomal amphotericin B (AmBisome) and fluconazole in the treatment of systemic candidosis in immunocompetent and leucopenic mice. J Antimicrob Chemother 32(5): 723–739
96. Kato K, Chin K, Yoshikawa T, Yamaguchi K, Tsuji Y, Esaki T et al (2012) Phase II study of NK105, a paclitaxel-incorporating micellar nanoparticle, for previously treated advanced or recurrent gastric cancer. Invest New Drugs 30(4):1621–1627
97. Matsumura TH, Toshihiko D, Takako E-N, Ken K, Yasuhide Y, Yasuhiro S et al (2010) Phase I study of NK012, a novel SN-38-incorporating micellar nanoparticle, in adult patients with solid tumors. Clin Cancer Res 16(20):5058–5066.
98. Nakanishi T, Fukushima S, Okamoto K, Suzuki M, Matsumura Y, Yokoyama M et al (2001) Development of the polymer micelle carrier system for doxorubicin. J Control Release 74(1–3):295–302
99. Plummer R, Wilson RH, Calvert H, Boddy AV, Griffin M, Sludden J et al (2011) A phase I clinical study of cisplatin-incorporated polymeric micelles (NC-6004) in patients with solid tumours. Br J Cancer 104(4):593–598

100. Takahashi A, Yamamoto Y, Yasunaga M, Koga Y, Kuroda J, Takigahira M et al (2013) NC-6300, an epirubicin-incorporating micelle, extends the antitumor effect and reduces the cardiotoxicity of epirubicin. Cancer Sci 104(7):920–925
101. Pittella F, Cabral H, Maeda Y, Mi P, Watanabe S, Takemoto H et al (2014) Systemic siRNA delivery to a spontaneous pancreatic tumor model in transgenic mice by PEGylated calcium phosphate hybrid micelles. J Control Release 178:18–24
102. Pittella F, Miyata K, Maeda Y, Suma T, Watanabe S, Chen Q et al (2012) Pancreatic cancer therapy by systemic administration of VEGF siRNA contained in calcium phosphate/charge-conversional polymer hybrid nanoparticles. J Control Release 161(3):868–874

Chapter 12

Pharmacokinetic Properties of Nanomaterials

Makiya Nishikawa

Abstract

Nanomaterials are a class of materials with unique properties owing to their submicron size. Their possible application as delivery systems for bioactive compounds has been extensively studied for decades. Successful use depends on how well their pharmacokinetics can be controlled after administration into the body. There is plenty of experimental data on the tissue distribution of nanomaterials, but it is still premature to design nanomaterials optimally for the delivery of bioactive compounds. In this chapter, the basic pharmacokinetic properties of nanomaterials, including their interactions with the body, are summarized, followed by a description of some of the challenges for their targeted delivery.

Key words Pharmacokinetics, Tissue distribution, Size, Mononuclear phagocyte system, Glomerular filtration

1 Background

Low-molecular-weight drugs including aspirin, atorvastatin (Lipitor®), and oseltamivir (Tamiflu®) are molecules with a molecular weight from several hundreds to less than a thousand AMU. These molecules are in the sub-nanometer range and are generally not categorized as nanomaterials. Molecules with a diameter of about one nanometer vary in molecular weight, owing to their different shapes. For instance, a linear molecule and a globular molecule with an identical size have quite different molecular weights: 10 base pairs of B-form double-stranded DNA has a molecular weight of about 6200 AMU and is 3.4 nm in length, whereas serum albumin at a molecular weight of about 67,000 AMU has a Stokes radius of about 3.5 nm. In addition, most amino acid polymers (e.g., peptides and proteins), sugars (polysaccharides), nucleic acids (DNA and RNA), and synthetic compounds (e.g., polyethylene glycol [PEG]) are within the nanometer range and materials that will be covered in this chapter.

Nanoparticles in the nanosize range can also be categorized as nanomaterials. They include liposomes, lipid emulsions, polymeric

Zheng-Rong Lu and Shinji Sakuma (eds.), *Nanomaterials in Pharmacology*, Methods in Pharmacology and Toxicology, DOI 10.1007/978-1-4939-3121-7_12,

micelles, and polymeric nanoparticles. These nanoparticles have been used as delivery systems for anticancer agents and other bioactive compounds [1–3]. Recently, exosomes, cell-derived particles of about 100 nm in diameter that contain proteins, RNA, and other cell-derived molecules [4], have also been recognized as nanoparticles [5–7]. The reason why these nanoparticles are frequently used as drug delivery system is due to the fact that the tissue distribution of nanoparticles, especially ones with a diameter of less than 150 nm, is partially controllable, as described below.

Micron-sized particles are also used in drug delivery, especially perorally [8]. Such relatively large particles are not frequently used in parenteral drug delivery because of their limited distribution after administration. An exception is Lupron Depot®, a microcapsule formulation of leuprorelin acetate with a diameter of about 20 μm [9]. Leuprorelin acetate is slowly released from poly(lactide-co-glycolide) microparticles, and thus the plasma concentration of the gonadotropin-releasing hormone agonist can be maintained for up to 6 months [10]. These microparticles, however, are not discussed here since they are not considered nanomaterials.

2 Mechanisms and Biological Processes That Determine the Pharmacokinetics of Nanomaterials

Pharmacokinetics is the science of the rate of absorption, distribution, metabolism, and excretion of a drug after administration into the body. Since the intestinal absorption of nanomaterials, such as polymers and nanoparticles, is highly limited, nanomaterials are generally administered to patients via the parenteral route. Distribution and excretion are then the major processes that determine their pharmacodynamics.

From a theoretical point of view, the pharmacokinetics of a nanomaterial is determined by the summation of the numerous interactions it has with various biological components after administration to the body (Fig. 1). Factors affecting this process are the physicochemical properties of nanomaterials, such as molecular/particulate size, electric charge, and tertiary structure, and the anatomical and physiological properties of the body, such as organ size, blood flow rate, and vascular permeability [11]. For example, interactions between a nanomaterial and blood components, such as serum proteins and blood cells, would alter the physicochemical property of the nanomaterial, which would then result in significant changes to its pharmacokinetics.

Nanomaterials are distributed throughout the body mainly through the blood. They then pass through the endothelial cell layer of an organ in order to access the parenchymal cells in a process called extravasation [12]. Table 1 summarizes the type of vascular endothelium found in various organs [13–15]. The presence

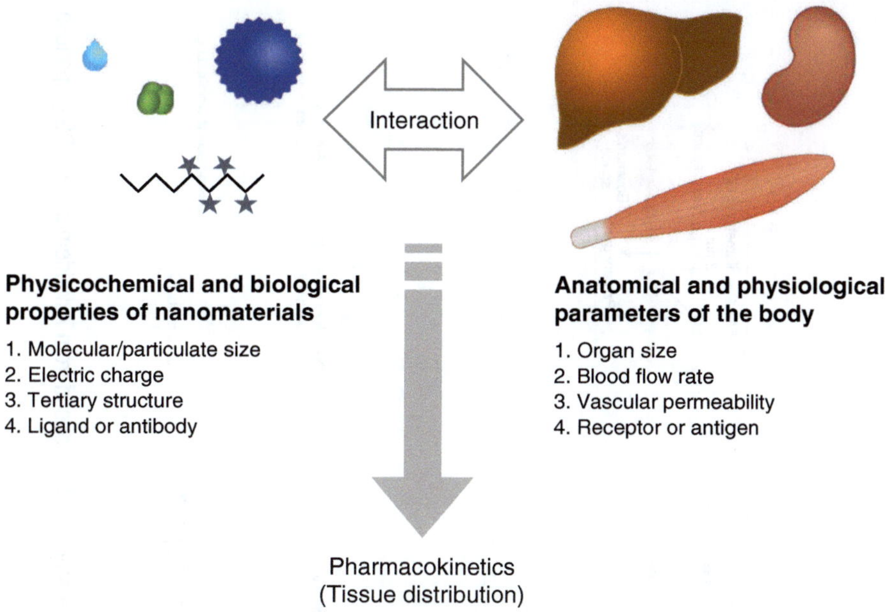

Fig. 1 Factors that determine the pharmacokinetics of nanomaterials (Reproduced from Zukaidemanabu DDS (Japanese, 2010) with permission from Jiho Inc.)

Table 1
Structural classifications of vascular endothelium

Type	Organs	Characteristics
Continuous	Muscle, skin, lung, central nervous system (brain)	Basement membrane is continuous and cells are connected by tight junctions
Fenestrated	Exocrine glands, renal glomeruli, intestinal mucosa	Fenestrae in endothelium result in relatively high permeability
Discontinuous	Liver, spleen, bone marrow	Intracellular gaps and discontinuous basal lamina result in extremely high permeability

of a specific receptor or antigen that is involved in the interaction with a nanomaterial will increase its binding or uptake. The physicochemical and biological properties of the nanomaterial, including the molecular/particular size, electric charge, tertiary structure, and ligand or antibody, determine the rate and extent of its interaction with the body [11]. In this section, the mechanisms and processes that determine their pharmacokinetics are reviewed and discussed, with particular focus on their interaction with body components.

2.1 Size-Dependent Tissue Distribution of Nanomaterials

The passage of nanomaterials through capillaries depends both on their size/diameter and on the characteristics of the capillaries [16, 17]. Figure 2 summarizes the anatomical sizes of capillaries,

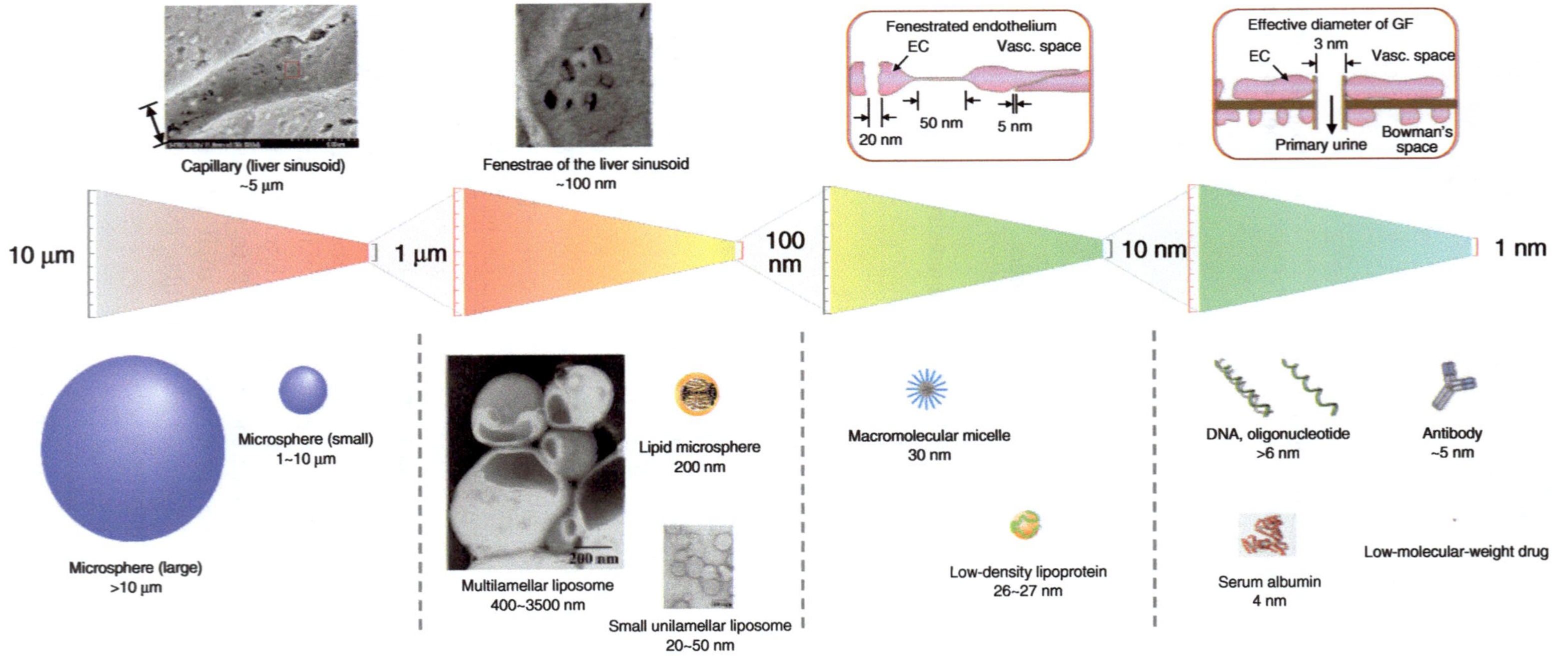

Fig. 2 Anatomical size of capillaries, pores, and junctions and the size of micro-, nano-, and sub-nanomaterials (Reproduced from Zukaidemanabu DDS (Japanese, 2010) with permission from Jiho Inc.)

pores, and junctions, along with several micro-, nano-, and sub-nanomaterials of varying sizes.

Microparticles with a diameter greater than the diameter of capillaries (generally about 5 μm) are trapped in the capillaries of first-pass organs after administration [18]. Since nanomaterials are much smaller than the diameter of capillaries, if they do not form aggregates, nanomaterials can thus then be distributed to the whole body through the blood. Extravasation of nanomaterials occurs in tissues with discontinuous or fenestrated endothelium (Table 1). Nanomaterials with a diameter of about 100 nm or smaller can pass through the discontinuous endothelium of the liver and then access hepatocytes, the parenchymal cells. It is well accepted that solid tumors also have leaky vasculature [19, 20] and nanomaterials with diameter of 100–200 nm can extravasate into the interstitial space of tumor tissues. Therefore, long-circulating nanomaterials could be delivered to solid tumors via the enhanced permeability and retention (EPR) effect [20–22].

Nanomaterials with a diameter greater than the threshold of glomerular filtration of the kidneys are rarely excreted into urine [12, 23]. These include serum proteins, such as serum albumin, transferrin, and immunoglobulins (Igs), as well as polymers with molecular weights 40,000 AMU and above. These macromolecules remain in the systemic circulation for a long period of time if they are not rapidly captured by macrophages and other cells of the mononuclear phagocyte system. Macromolecules smaller than the glomerular filtration threshold are filtered in the glomerulus at a rate depending on their molecular size [24, 25].

Organs with continuous endothelium, such as the heart, lung, skeletal muscle, and skin, are rarely reached by nanomaterials via the blood, because the cells of the continuous endothelium are joined by tight junctions and supported by an underlying basement membrane [14, 15]. The tightest endothelium can be found in the brain, called as blood-brain barrier [26, 27]. Therefore, the delivery of nanomaterials to brain parenchyma requires further modification in order to increase transport [28]. Attempts have been made to widen the tight junctions of endothelial cells by infusing a hypertonic solution of arabinose or mannitol; the estimated size of the opening is up to 20 nm [29].

2.2 Interaction of Nanomaterials with Blood Components

Interaction of nanomaterials with the components of blood, such as serum proteins and circulating blood cells, significantly alter their physicochemical and biological properties, which then result in changes to tissue distribution [30]. Nanoparticles, such as liposomes and emulsions, are typical examples of nanomaterials whose distribution would be greatly affected. Generally speaking, the binding of serum proteins to the surface of nanoparticles increases the chance they will be recognized by professional phagocytic cells, such as macrophages. This process, called opsonization, is responsible for increased clearance of nanoparticles from the blood. It was reported that the amount of large unilamellar liposomes with diameters of about 100 nm cleared from the blood depended on the total amount of proteins bound their surfaces following injection [31, 32]. In addition, the amount of proteins bound to the surface of liposomes was dependent on their lipid composition [31, 33].

Cationic compounds, such as cationic polymers and cationic liposomes, can electrostatically interact with negatively charged components, including serum albumin and red blood cells [34, 35]. Such interactions can reduce the positive charge of the nanoparticles and, possibly, increase their size. The tissue distribution of cationic nanoparticles would then be determined by the size and electric charge of the resulting cationic compound/blood component complex.

Various cationic polymers and nanoparticles have been developed and used for the in vivo delivery of nucleic acid drugs, including antisense oligonucleotides, aptamer, siRNA, and plasmid DNA [36–39]. These cationic compounds form complexes with nucleic acid drugs via electrostatic interactions. This complex formation is designed to deliver nucleic acid drugs into the cytoplasm or the nucleus of cells. In most cases, they are positively charged to interact with the negatively charged cell surface. Therefore, these complexes, most of which are also nanomaterials with a diameter of about several hundred nm, interact with negatively charged serum proteins as well as blood cells. Sakurai et al. reported that several types of plasmid DNA/cationic liposome complexes were bound to red blood cells and this interaction greatly affected their transgenic expression after in vivo administration [35].

Igs, or antibodies, are proteins used to identify foreign materials. Materials marked with Ig are recognized by immune cells and then cleared from the blood. Igs, such as IgG and IgM, are responsible for the rapid clearance of nanomaterials that have triggered their production. Recent studies on PEGylated liposomes (PEG-liposomes) have shown that the first injection of PEG-liposomes induces the production of PEG-specific IgM, which then triggers the rapid clearance of the second dose of PEG-liposomes by splenic macrophages [40, 41]. A key factor for this rapid clearance has been reported to be the dose of PEG-liposomes for the initial injection, and the medium-to-high doses that are used clinically rarely lead to the rapid clearance of repeated injections of PEG-liposomes.

2.3 Recognition of Nanomaterials by the Mononuclear Phagocyte System

Cells of the mononuclear phagocyte system are the major cells that remove foreign materials, including bacteria and viruses, from the blood. Therefore, as described above, nanomaterials marked with opsonins are cleared by these professional phagocytes [42]. Major cells responsible for their removal include Kupffer cells in the liver, as well as splenic macrophages. It has been reported that the physicochemical properties of the nanoparticles are important for recognition by these cells.

2.4 Uptake of Nanomaterials by Hepatocytes

The discontinuous endothelium and high blood flow rate of the liver provide nanomaterials with great opportunity to interact with hepatocytes, the parenchymal cells of the liver. Hepatocytes are highly active and take up a variety of nanomaterials, depending on their physicochemical and/or biological properties [43, 44]. Long-circulating nanomaterials are gradually taken up by hepatocytes by fluid-phase endocytosis. For example, serum albumin labeled with indium-111 was mainly delivered to hepatocytes after intravenous injection into mice [45].

Hepatocytes express many receptors on their surfaces, and some of these receptors are specific to certain cells. Thus, some nanomaterials are selectively recognized by hepatocytes and quickly taken up. A typical example is the rapid removal of asialoglycoproteins by hepatocytes from the blood [46, 47], based on the recognition of galactose on the nonreducing terminal of the sugar chains of asialoglycoproteins by asialoglycoprotein receptors. Another example is the transport of cholesterol to hepatocytes. High-density lipoproteins (HDLs) carrying cholesterol are taken up by hepatocytes through HDL receptors [48, 49].

Cationic macromolecules, including poly-L-lysine, diethylaminoethyl-dextran, and cationized bovine serum albumin, are efficiently delivered to the liver after intravenous injection into mice (*see* Fig. 3 in Sect. 3). This rapid uptake is mainly mediated by hepatocytes and the electrostatic interaction between cationic macromolecules and the negatively charged surface of hepatocytes [45, 50].

3 Approaches to Control the Tissue Distribution of Nanomaterials

As summarized in Sect. 2, the physicochemical and biological properties of nanomaterials are major determinants for their tissue distribution. Two major processes are important for their clearance from systemic circulation. One is urinary excretion, in which nanomaterials smaller than the threshold of the glomerular filtration of the kidney are filtered. The other is hepatic uptake, i.e., the uptake by hepatocytes, Kupffer cells, and sinusoidal endothelial cells of the liver. Figure 3 summarizes the relationship between the physicochemical properties and the tissue distribution of nanomaterials (macromolecules) after intravenous injection in mice, the latter of which is expressed using hepatic uptake (the vertical axis) and urinary excretion clearance (the horizontal axis) [11]. These relationships provide a reasonable framework by which to adjust the tissue distribution of nanomaterials by modifying their physicochemical and biological properties [51, 52].

3.1 Size Control

An increase in the size of a nanomaterial to a value greater than the threshold of the glomerular filtration of the kidney is a useful way to increase its retention time in the blood. There are several products that are used in clinical practice, for example, PEGylated bioactive

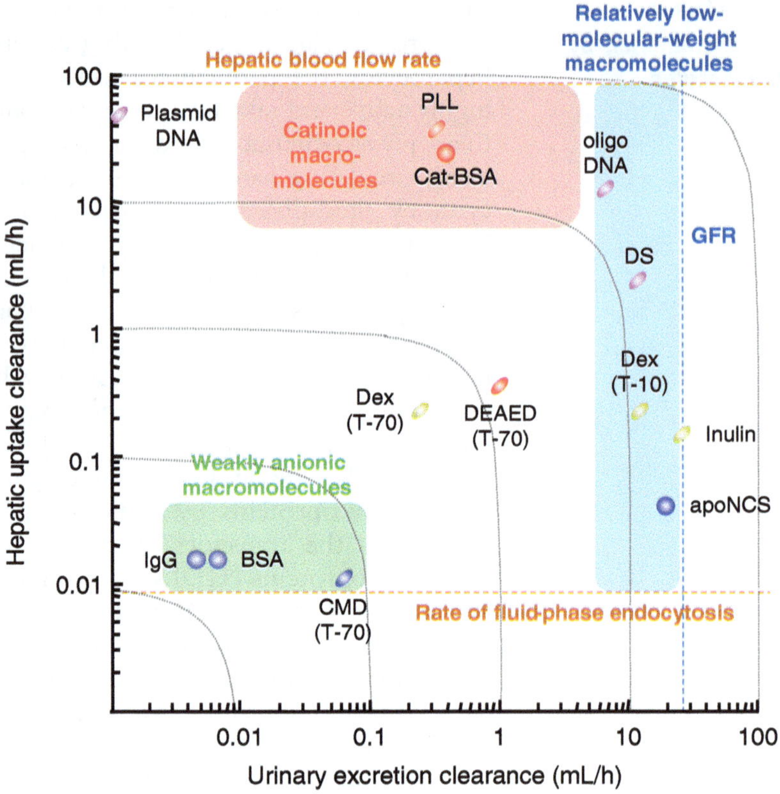

Fig. 3 Relationship between the physicochemical properties and the tissue distribution of macromolecules after intravenous injection in mice. apoNCS, apoprotein of neocarzinostatin (molecular weight 12,000); BSA, bovine serum albumin (67,000); Cat-BSA, cationized bovine serum albumin (70,000); CMD(T-70); carboxymethyl-dextran derived from Dex(T-70); DEAED(T-70), diethylaminoethyl-dextran derived from Dex(T-70); Dex(T-10), dextran (10,000); Dex(T-70), dextran (70,000); DS, dextran sulfate (5000); IgG, bovine immunoglobulin G (150,000); inulin (5000); oligoDNA, single-stranded DNA (3000); plasmid DNA (4,000,000); PLL, poly-L-lysine (4000); GFR, glomerular filtration rate of the kidney (Reproduced from Zukaidemanabu DDS (Japanese, 2010) with permission from Jiho Inc.)

proteins [53, 54]. PEG-interferon α-2a and -2b are derivatives of human interferon α, which are used in the treatment of patients with hepatitis virus C infection. PEG molecules with a molecular weight of several thousand or greater are generally used for modification [55]. Other polymers, such as polyvinylpyrrolidine, dextran, and N-(2-hydroxypropyl) methacrylamide, exhibit similar effects on the tissue distribution of nanomaterials [56–58].

3.2 Blocking Recognition of Nanomaterials by the Cells of the Mononuclear Phagocyte System

Shielding the surface of nanomaterials that are recognized by the cells of the mononuclear phagocyte system has long been used to increase the circulation time of drug delivery systems, including liposomes, after systemic administration [59, 60]. Again, PEG is the most frequently used molecule for this purpose. Doxil® is a PEGylated liposomal formulation of doxorubicin used for patients with ovarian cancer, multiple myeloma, and Kaposi's sarcoma [61]. PEG inhibits serum components that might attach onto the nanoparticles.

Polymeric micelles have relatively long circulation times after intravenous administration, indicating that they are not efficiently recognized by the cells of the mononuclear phagocyte system [62]. They consist of block copolymers with hydrophilic and hydrophobic units; the most commonly used polymer used for the hydrophilic unit is PEG. Other polymers have been also extensively examined, including poloxamer, polyvinyl alcohol, polyamino acids, and polysaccharide [63–66]. However, no polymer has been discovered that is better than PEG as far as nanomaterial retention in the blood, especially nanoparticles, is concerned.

3.3 Cell-Specific Delivery of Nanomaterials

Targeted delivery of nanomaterials occurs by using antibodies or ligands that are involved in specific intermolecular interactions. Monoclonal antibodies are nanomaterials that have a high affinity to a specific antigen, and many are now in clinical use. They recognize specific antigens and thus have been used to deliver therapeutic compounds to specific types of cells. Yttrium-90 ibritumomab tiuxetan (Zevalin®) is a radiolabeled monoclonal antibody directed to the B-lymphocyte antigen CD20, which is used in the treatment of patients with relapsed lymphoma [67].

Receptor-mediated endocytosis is another mechanism that has been used to deliver bioactive compounds to specific cells. Since asialoglycoprotein receptors recognize galactose and are expressed only on hepatocytes, galactose modification has been used to deliver drugs to hepatocytes. A variety of molecules, including enzymes, genes, and small interfering RNA, have been delivered using galactose as a targeting ligand [68–73]. Since the asialoglycoprotein receptor consists of three polypeptide subunits, each of which contains one carbohydrate recognition domain, the binding affinity of galactose-containing nanomaterials is greatly affected by the number, location, and/or density of galactose moieties on the nanomaterials [74, 75]. Pharmacokinetic studies on the galactosylated proteins showed that the surface density of galactose on the protein is an important parameter that determines the uptake of galactosylated proteins by hepatocytes [68]. Recently, a triantennary *N*-acetyl galactosamine ligand has been used to deliver siRNA to hepatocytes [76].

4 Conclusion and Perspective

Blockbuster drugs have shifted from low molecular weight drugs like Lipitol® to monoclonal antibodies and other protein-based drugs, like Etanercept (Enbrel®), a fusion protein consisting of the extracellular binding domains of tumor necrosis factor receptor and the Fc portion of a human IgG1 antibody. In addition, the number of liposomal drugs has increased since the first liposomal drug Doxil® was approved by the FDA in 1995. Nanomaterials will become more important as therapeutic agents or drug delivery systems as time goes on. Therefore, further comprehensive understanding of their tissue distribution, as well as how to control it, will greatly increase the importance of nanomaterials in therapeutic treatment of patients.

References

1. Allen TM, Cullis PR (2004) Drug delivery systems: entering the mainstream. Science 303: 1818–1822
2. Samad A, Sultana Y, Aqil M (2007) Liposomal drug delivery systems: an update review. Curr Drug Deliv 4:297–305
3. Zhang L, Gu FX, Chan JM et al (2008) Nanoparticles in medicine: therapeutic applications and developments. Clin Pharmacol Ther 83:761–769
4. Théry C, Zitvogel L, Amigorena S (2002) Exosomes: composition, biogenesis and function. Nat Rev Immunol 2:569–579
5. Iero M, Valenti R, Huber V et al (2008) Tumour-released exosomes and their implications in cancer immunity. Cell Death Differ 15:80–88
6. Pegtel DM, Cosmopoulos K, Thorley-Lawson DA et al (2010) Functional delivery of viral miRNAs via exosomes. Proc Natl Acad Sci U S A 107:6328–6333
7. Takahashi Y, Nishikawa M, Shinotsuka H et al (2013) Visualization and in vivo tracking of the exosomes of murine melanoma B16-BL6 cells in mice after intravenous injection. J Biotechnol 165:77–84
8. Desai MP, Labhasetwar V, Amidon GL et al (1996) Gastrointestinal uptake of biodegradable microparticles: effect of particle size. Pharm Res 13:1838–1845
9. Okada H (1997) One- and three-month release injectable microspheres of the LH-RH superagonist leuprorelin acetate. Adv Drug Deliv Rev 28:43–70
10. Sethi R, Sanfilippo N (2009) Six-month depot formulation of leuprorelin acetate in the treatment of prostate cancer. Clin Interv Aging 4:259–267
11. Nishikawa M, Takakura Y, Hashida M (2005) Theoretical considerations involving the pharmacokinetics of plasmid DNA. Adv Drug Deliv Rev 57:675–688
12. Takakura Y, Mahato RI, Hashida M (1998) Extravasation of macromolecules. Adv Drug Deliv Rev 34:93–108
13. Cleaver O, Melton DA (2003) Endothelial signaling during development. Nat Med 9: 661–668
14. Aird WC (2007) Phenotypic heterogeneity of the endothelium: I. Structure, function, and mechanisms. Circ Res 100:158–173
15. Aird WC (2007) Phenotypic heterogeneity of the endothelium: II. Representative vascular beds. Circ Res 100:174–190
16. Rippe B, Rosengren BI, Carlsson O et al (2002) Transendothelial transport: the vesicle controversy. J Vasc Res 39:375–390
17. Mehta D, Malik AB (2006) Signaling mechanisms regulating endothelial permeability. Physiol Rev 86:279–367
18. Bae YH, Park K (2011) Targeted drug delivery to tumors: myths, reality and possibility. J Control Release 153:198–205
19. Hobbs SK, Monsky WL, Yuan F et al (1998) Regulation of transport pathways in tumor vessels: role of tumor type and microenvironment. Proc Natl Acad Sci U S A 95:4607–4612
20. Maeda H, Wu J, Sawa T, Matsumura Y et al (2000) Tumor vascular permeability and the EPR effect in macromolecular therapeutics: a review. J Control Release 65:271–284
21. Matsumura Y, Maeda H (1986) A new concept for macromolecular therapeutics in cancer chemotherapy: mechanism of tumoritropic accumulation of proteins and the antitumor agent smancs. Cancer Res 46:6387–6392
22. Brannon-Peppas L, Blanchette JO (2004) Nanoparticle and targeted systems for cancer therapy. Adv Drug Deliv Rev 56:1649–1659
23. Brenner BM, Hostetter TH, Humes HD (1978) Glomerular permselectivity: barrier function based on discrimination of molecular size and charge. Am J Physiol 234:F455–F460
24. Maack T, Johnson V, Kau ST et al (1979) Renal filtration, transport, and metabolism of low-molecular-weight proteins: a review. Kidney Int 16:251–270
25. Stevens LA, Coresh J, Greene T et al (2006) Assessing kidney function – measured and esti-

mated glomerular filtration rate. N Engl J Med 354:2473–2483
26. Wolburg H, Lippoldt A (2002) Tight junctions of the blood-brain barrier: development, composition and regulation. Vascul Pharmacol 38:323–337
27. Abbott NJ, Patabendige AA, Dolman DE et al (2010) Structure and function of the blood-brain barrier. Neurobiol Dis 37:13–25
28. Lockman PR, Mumper RJ, Khan MA et al (2002) Nanoparticle technology for drug delivery across the blood-brain barrier. Drug Dev Ind Pharm 28:1–13
29. Rapoport SI (2000) Osmotic opening of the blood-brain barrier: principles, mechanism, and therapeutic applications. Cell Mol Neurobiol 20:217–230
30. Opanasopit P, Nishikawa M, Hashida M (2002) Factors affecting drug and gene delivery: effects of interaction with blood components. Crit Rev Ther Drug Carrier Syst 19:191–233
31. Chonn A, Semple SC, Cullis PR (1982) Association of blood proteins with large unilamellar liposomes in vivo. Relation to circulation lifetimes. J Biol Chem 267: 18759–18765
32. Cullis PR, Chonn A, Semple SC (1998) Interactions of liposomes and lipid-based carrier systems with blood proteins: Relation to clearance behaviour in vivo. Adv Drug Deliv Rev 32:3–17
33. Devine DV, Wong K, Serrano K et al (1994) Liposome-complement interactions in rat serum: implications for liposome survival studies. Biochim Biophys Acta 1191:43–51
34. Zelphati O, Uyechi LS, Barron LG et al (1998) Effect of serum components on the physicochemical properties of cationic lipid/oligonucleotide complexes and on their interactions with cells. Biochim Biophys Acta 1390: 119–133
35. Sakurai F, Nishioka T, Saito H et al (2001) Interaction between DNA-cationic liposome complexes and erythrocytes is an important factor in systemic gene transfer via the intravenous route in mice: the role of the neutral helper lipid. Gene Ther 8:677–686
36. De Smedt SC, Demeester J, Hennink WE (2000) Cationic polymer based gene delivery systems. Pharm Res 17:113–126
37. Zhang S, Zhao B, Jiang H et al (2007) Cationic lipids and polymers mediated vectors for delivery of siRNA. J Control Release 123:1–10
38. Morille M, Passirani C, Vonarbourg A et al (2008) Progress in developing cationic vectors for non-viral systemic gene therapy against cancer. Biomaterials 29:3477–3496
39. Semple SC, Akinc A, Chen J et al (2010) Rational design of cationic lipids for siRNA delivery. Nat Biotechnol 28:172–176
40. Dams ET, Laverman P, Oyen WJ et al (2000) Accelerated blood clearance and altered biodistribution of repeated injections of sterically stabilized liposomes. J Pharmacol Exp Ther 292:1071–1079
41. Ishida T, Kiwada H (2008) Accelerated blood clearance (ABC) phenomenon upon repeated injection of PEGylated liposomes. Int J Pharm 354:56–62
42. Owens DE 3rd, Peppas NA (2006) Opsonization, biodistribution, and pharmacokinetics of polymeric nanoparticles. Int J Pharm 307:93–102
43. Wu J, Nantz MH, Zern MA (2002) Targeting hepatocytes for drug and gene delivery: emerging novel approaches and applications. Front Biosci 7:d717–d725
44. Nishikawa M (2005) Development of cell-specific targeting systems for drugs and genes. Biol Pharm Bull 28:195–200
45. Takakura Y, Fujita T, Hashida M et al (1990) Disposition characteristics of macromolecules in tumor-bearing mice. Pharm Res 7:339–346
46. Ashwell G, Morell AG (1974) The role of surface carbohydrates in the hepatic recognition and transport of circulating glycoproteins. Adv Enzymol Relat Areas Mol Biol 41:99–128
47. Hashida M, Nishikawa M, Yamashita F et al (2001) Cell-specific delivery of genes with glycosylated carriers. Adv Drug Deliv Rev 52:187–196
48. Kozarsky KF, Donahee MH, Rigotti A et al (1997) Overexpression of the HDL receptor SR-BI alters plasma HDL and bile cholesterol levels. Nature 387:414–417
49. Kingwell BA, Chapman MJ, Kontush A et al (2014) HDL-targeted therapies: progress, failures and future. Nat Rev Drug Discov 13: 445–464
50. Nishida K, Mihara K, Takino T et al (1991) Hepatic disposition characteristics of electrically charged macromolecules in rat in vivo and in the perfused liver. Pharm Res 8:437–444
51. Nishikawa M, Takakura Y, Hashida M (1996) Pharmacokinetic evaluation of polymeric carriers. Adv Drug Delivery Rev 21:135–155
52. Takakura Y, Hashida M (1996) Macromolecular carrier systems for targeted drug delivery: pharmacokinetic considerations on biodistribution. Pharm Res 13:820–831
53. Berenguer M (2008) Systematic review of the treatment of established recurrent hepatitis C with pegylated interferon in combination with ribavirin. J Hepatol 49:274–287

54. Jevsevar S, Kunstelj M, Porekar VG (2010) PEGylation of therapeutic proteins. Biotechnol J 5:113–128
55. Caliceti P, Veronese FM (2003) Pharmacokinetic and biodistribution properties of poly(ethylene glycol)-protein conjugates. Adv Drug Deliv Rev 55(10):1261–1277
56. Fujita T, Nishikawa M, Tamaki C et al (1992) Targeted delivery of human recombinant superoxide dismutase by chemical modification with mono- and polysaccharide derivatives. J Pharmacol Exp Ther 263:971–978
57. Shiah JG, Dvorák M, Kopecková P et al (2001) Biodistribution and antitumour efficacy of long-circulating N-(2-hydroxypropyl)methacrylamide copolymer-doxorubicin conjugates in nude mice. Eur J Cancer 37:131–139
58. Kaneda Y, Tsutsumi Y, Yoshioka Y et al (2004) The use of PVP as a polymeric carrier to improve the plasma half-life of drugs. Biomaterials 25:3259–3266
59. Moghimi SM, Szebeni J (2003) Stealth liposomes and long circulating nanoparticles: critical issues in pharmacokinetics, opsonization and protein-binding properties. Prog Lipid Res 42:463–478
60. Alexis F, Pridgen E, Molnar LK et al (2008) Factors affecting the clearance and biodistribution of polymeric nanoparticles. Mol Pharm 5:505–515
61. Barenholz Y (2012) Doxil® – the first FDA-approved nano-drug: lessons learned. J Control Release 160:117–134
62. Nishiyama N, Kataoka K (2006) Current state, achievements, and future prospects of polymeric micelles as nanocarriers for drug and gene delivery. Pharmacol Ther 112(3): 630–648
63. Müller RH, Maassen S, Weyhers H et al (1996) Phagocytic uptake and cytotoxicity of solid lipid nanoparticles (SLN) sterically stabilized with poloxamine 908 and poloxamer 407. J Drug Target 4:161–170
64. Takeuchi H, Kojima H, Yamamoto H et al (2000) Polymer coating of liposomes with a modified polyvinyl alcohol and their systemic circulation and RES uptake in rats. J Control Release 68:195–205
65. Metselaar JM, Bruin P, de Boer LW et al (2003) A novel family of L-amino acid-based biodegradable polymer-lipid conjugates for the development of long-circulating liposomes with effective drug-targeting capacity. Bioconjug Chem 14:1156–1164
66. Peer D, Park EJ, Morishita Y et al (2008) Systemic leukocyte-directed siRNA delivery revealing cyclin D1 as an anti-inflammatory target. Science 319:627–630
67. Morschhauser F, Illidge T, Huglo D et al (2007) Efficacy and safety of yttrium-90 ibritumomab tiuxetan in patients with relapsed or refractory diffuse large B-cell lymphoma not appropriate for autologous stem-cell transplantation. Blood 110:54–58
68. Nishikawa M, Miyazaki C, Yamashita F et al (1995) Galactosylated proteins are recognized by the liver according to the surface density of galactose moieties. Am J Physiol 268:G849–G856
69. Remy JS, Kichler A, Mordvinov V et al (1995) Targeted gene transfer into hepatoma cells with lipopolyamine-condensed DNA particles presenting galactose ligands: a stage toward artificial viruses. Proc Natl Acad Sci U S A 92:1744–1748
70. Zanta MA, Boussif O, Adib A et al (1997) In vitro gene delivery to hepatocytes with galactosylated polyethylenimine. Bioconjug Chem 8:839–844
71. Nishikawa M, Takemura S, Takakura Y et al (1998) Targeted delivery of plasmid DNA to hepatocytes in vivo: optimization of the pharmacokinetics of plasmid DNA/galactosylated poly(L-lysine) complexes by controlling their physicochemical properties. J Pharmacol Exp Ther 287:408–415
72. Yabe Y, Nishikawa M, Tamada A et al (1999) Targeted delivery and improved therapeutic potential of catalase by chemical modification: combination with superoxide dismutase derivatives. J Pharmacol Exp Ther 289:1176–1184
73. Sato A, Takagi M, Shimamoto A et al (2007) Small interfering RNA delivery to the liver by intravenous administration of galactosylated cationic liposomes in mice. Biomaterials 28: 1434–1442
74. Connolly DT, Townsend RR, Kawaguchi K et al (1982) Binding and endocytosis of cluster glycosides by rabbit hepatocytes. Evidence for a short-circuit pathway that does not lead to degradation. J Biol Chem 257:939–945
75. Rensen PC, van Leeuwen SH, Sliedregt LA et al (2004) Design and synthesis of novel N-acetylgalactosamine-terminated glycolipids for targeting of lipoproteins to the hepatic asialoglycoprotein receptor. J Med Chem 47:5798–5808
76. Akinc A, Querbes W, De S et al (2010) Targeted delivery of RNAi therapeutics with endogenous and exogenous ligand-based mechanisms. Mol Ther 18:1357–1364

Chapter 13

Cardiovascular Nanomedicine: Materials and Technologies

Anirban Sen Gupta

Abstract

The advent of nanotechnology in the medical arena has led to unique ways of biomaterials engineering and device modifications, disease detection and treatment. To this end, the two principal nanomedicine focus areas are cancer and cardiovascular pathologies. The current chapter is aimed at presenting a comprehensive review of nanotechnology-based strategies in cardiovascular diseases, with emphasis on targeted delivery of therapeutic payloads selectively at the disease site. The rationale for such strategies stem from the need of resolving the issues of (1) rapid drug clearance, (2) plasma-induced drug deactivation, (3) suboptimal drug availability at the disease site, and (4) indiscriminate biodistribution of the drugs leading to harmful systemic side effects, all of which arise when drugs are administered directly in systemic circulation. The most significant application of nanotechnology in resolving these issues is by packaging the drugs within plasma stable nanovehicles that can preferentially accumulate at the vascular disease site via passive uptake or bind actively to the site via antigen-specific ligands decorated on the vehicle surface. During past three decades, significant advancements in understanding vascular disease-associated genomics and proteomics, cellular and molecular mechanisms as well as nanoscale and microscale strategies of biomaterials engineering have led to several exciting nanomedicine approaches in vascular disease treatment. The chapter will describe these approaches in terms of materials engineering, payload release mechanisms, biochemical and biophysical design parameters of the delivery platforms, and integration of multiple design parameters and functionalities on single vehicle platform, along with discussing the promises and limitations of such vascular nanomedicine approaches.

Key words Nanotechnology, Cardiovascular, Targeting, Drug delivery, Nanomedicine

1 Introduction

Vascular diseases continue to be the number one cause of tissue morbidities and mortalities in the USA and globally [1, 2]. According to the recent statistical data reported by the American Heart Association, ~40 % of adult American adults suffer from vascular diseases and the number is over 80 % in the aging (80+ years) population. Mortalities from vascular diseases in the USA were reported to be close to 800,000 (male + female) in a recent statistical report in 2010 [1]. Consequently, significant research and

Zheng-Rong Lu and Shinji Sakuma (eds.), *Nanomaterials in Pharmacology*, Methods in Pharmacology and Toxicology,
DOI 10.1007/978-1-4939-3121-7_13,

clinical efforts are directed in prevention and treatment of these diseases. Vascular diseases can fall into many categories, for example, coronary heart disease leading to unstable angina and myocardial infarction, cerebrovascular disease leading to ischemia and stroke, atherosclerosis and peripheral arterial diseases, deep vein thrombosis, pulmonary and distal embolisms, restenosis following catheterized interventions, and congenital or acquired heart diseases or hemostatic dysfunctions. Many of these disease conditions have common spatiotemporal cellular and molecular mechanisms, the most predominant of which is the formation of intravascular occlusive clots (thrombi) that reduce antegrade blood flow to vital tissues and organs, often leading to tissue morbidities and mortalities. Therefore, many clinical strategies are focused on prophylactic, emergent and sustained prevention of thrombo-occlusive events to maintain normal blood flow to tissues and organs. The prophylactic strategies mainly involve oral or systemic administration of anticoagulant (e.g., heparin) and antiplatelet (e.g., Aspirin and Clopidogrel) agents, the emergent strategies mainly involve mechanical (e.g., catheter-mediated or aspiration-based thrombectomy, balloon angioplasty), surgical (e.g., aortic or coronary thrombus removal, bypass grafting) and fibrinolytic pharmacotherapy (e.g., intravascular bolus administration or infusion of plasminogen activators like streptokinase (SK) and tissue plasminogen activator (tPA)) procedures, while the sustained strategies mostly involve post-procedural prolonged oral administration of anticoagulant and antiplatelet drugs as well as drug-eluting stent (DES, releasing anticoagulant or antiproliferative drugs) placement during catheter-based interventional procedures like balloon angioplasty. As evident from these descriptions, systemic (oral and intravascular) administration of drug molecules that prevent platelet activation and aggregation (antiplatelet agents), block coagulation pathways (anticoagulant agents), degrade clot proteins (fibrinolytic agents), or downregulate unwanted cellular proliferation (antiproliferative agents) remain a major component of clinical regimen in treating occlusive vascular disease conditions. Systemic administration of these drugs presents several harmful issues [3–6]:

(a) Rapid drug washout and clearance from the target site due to dynamic blood flow

(b) Plasma-induced inactivation of the drugs and reduced circulation half-life

(c) Systemic nonspecific distribution of the drugs resulting in suboptimal availability at target

(d) Systemic nonspecific action of the drugs leading to harmful side effects like coagulopathy, neurotoxicity and nephrotoxicity, and hemorrhage

These issues can be potentially resolved by localizing the delivery (and action) of the drugs at the target clot sites. One way to achieve such site-selective delivery is by implanted devices like trans-arterial infusion catheters and DES. Implantation procedures like these are expensive, require specific expertise in terms personnel and facilities, and are not accessible by or amenable to many patients within required treatment windows [7–10]. Another way is to manufacture drug molecules that possess some target-specificity of binding (and action) by virtue of bioconjugation of antibodies and other ligands directly to the drug molecules or by recombinant modifications of the drug itself to impart target-specificity [11–15]. Direct antibody conjugation to drugs may affect drug activity and recombinant technologies make the resultant products quite expensive for global use especially in developing countries. Therefore, in recent years, alternative drug delivery strategies utilizing the "nanomedicine" approach have raised significant clinical interest [16]. The ideal "nanomedicine" design for site-selective delivery of drugs in vascular diseases should consist of a "carrier vehicle" that can encapsulate the drug in its core or embed it on the vehicle surface, protect the drug from plasma-induced inactivation while increasing its circulation half-life, localize via passive uptake and/or active molecular mechanisms to the vascular disease site to ensure site-specific delivery of the drug payload, enable controlled release of the payload via diffusion, dispersion, or stimuli-triggered mechanisms to allow site-selective therapeutic action while reducing systemic harmful side-effects, and biodegrade or get cleared from the body safely within a reasonable time frame so as to not render long term effects. The "payload" in such vehicles can not only be drug molecules, but also imaging probes that can allow detection and diagnosis of disease sites, and the combination of therapeutic and diagnostic payloads can potentially lead to "theranostic" nanomedicine systems targeted to vascular disease sites. The following sections review the various "nanomedicine" technologies that have been developed and are undergoing research currently in the context of the above-described design, followed by a discussion of the pros and cons and future endeavors.

2 Nanomedicine Systems Without Ligand-Based Site-Specific Active Binding Mechanisms

Direct systemic delivery of therapeutic (and diagnostic) agents often leads to inactivation of the agents by various plasma components, rapid washout from target site, and rapid clearance from circulation via organs like liver and kidney. Resolving these issues require increasing the circulation residence time of the agents in active form. This is where "packaging" of the agents within carrier vehicles can provide a solution. The concept is derived originally from the "Ringsdorf Model" in the application of macromolecular modifications of cancer drugs (Fig. 1), where the drug molecules are conjugated to polymers that prevent rapid plasma clearance of the small drug molecules due to enhancement of overall hydrodynamic radius by virtue of the drug–polymer conjugates [17–19]. The conjugation of the drugs to the various polymers are mediated

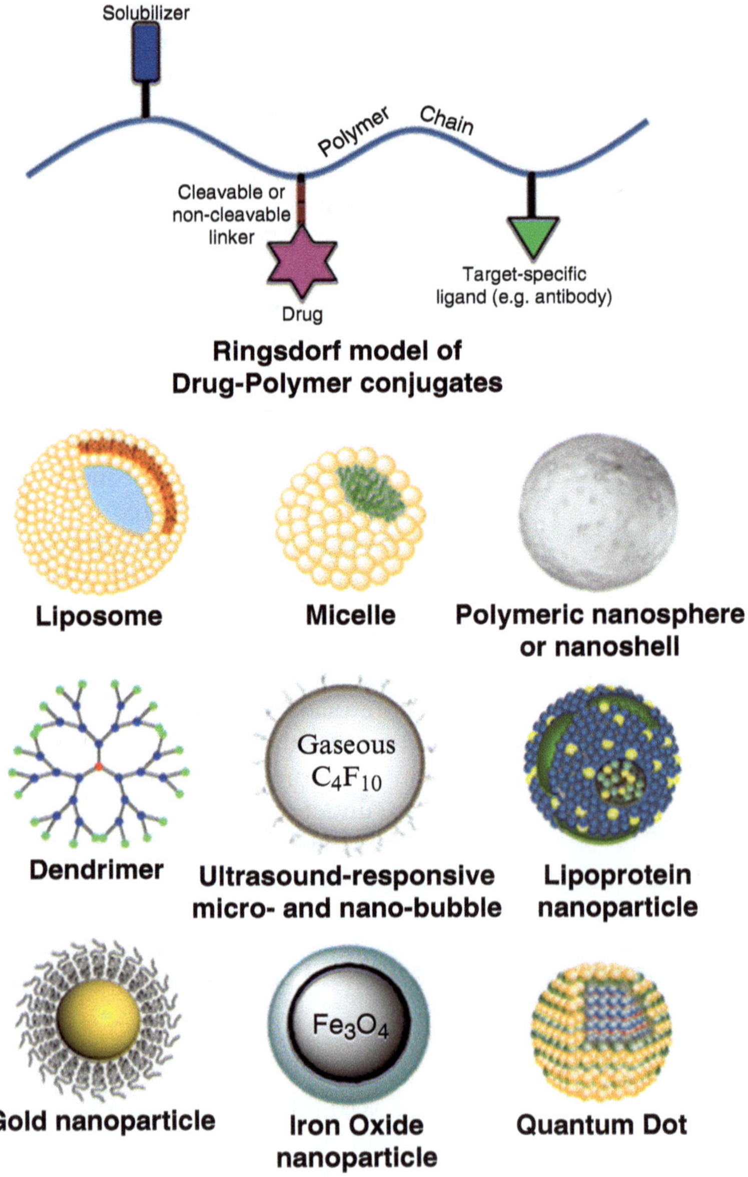

Fig. 1 The Ringsdorf Model of drug–macromolecule conjugates and some common nanoparticle systems utilized for vascular nanomedicine technologies

by chemical bonds like amide, orthoester, ester, anhydride, carbonate, and urethane that can be cleaved by enzymatic and/or pH-sensitive reaction mechanisms to release the active drug for subsequent action. For cardiovascular drugs, this design has been tried by polyethylene glycol (PEG)-based modification (PEGylation) of fibrinolytic agents like tPA, SK, urokinase (uPA), and staphylokinase (Sak) [20–24]. The antiproliferative drug Paclitaxel (clinicaly used in DES for treatment of restenosis and intimal hyperplasia) has also been conjugated to polymers like polyglutamic acid (PGA) to result in products like Xyotax that are undergoing clinical study for cancer treatment but may also find cardiovascular applications. Besides drug–polymer conjugates, the other strategy to protect the drugs and increase circulation stability and residence time, is to package them in microparticulate and nanoparticulate vehicles. To this end, extensive research has been carried out using vehicles like liposomes, polymeric particles, lipoprotein particles, micelles, engineered red blood cells (RBCs), quantum dots, gold particles, dendrimers, ultrasound-sensitive bubbles and iron oxide particles (Fig. 1).

Vesicular liposomal structures, originally reported by Sir Alec Bangham [25, 26], have a lipidic (hydrophobic) shell and an aqueous core, thereby providing potential volume fractions for encapsulating both hydrophobic and hydrophilic drugs. Liposomes are formed by thermodynamically driven self-assembly of lipid-based amphiphilic molecules when exposed to an aqueous environment. Specifically, these molecules would need to have a *packing fraction* ($v \times a^{-1} \times l^{-1}$ where "v" is the hydrophobic volume, "a" is the hydrophilic surface area, "l" is hydrophobic length) equal to 1, such that when exposed in an aqueous environment, they would form planar lamellar bilayer structures that ultimately fold into spherical vesicles with a bilayer lipidic shell and aqueous core. This kind of self-assembled vesicular structure can be unilamellar (single lamellar shell) or multilamellar (multiple concentric bilayer shells), and their size can range from about 50 nm to a few microns in diameter. Usually by extrusion through nanoporous polycarbonate membranes or by exposing to high frequency ultrasound, larger multilamellar vesicles can be reduced to nanoscale (50–200 nm diameter) unilamellar vesicles. Furthermore, modification of the liposome lamella outer surface with hydrophilic polymers like PEG imparts a steric hindrance to opsonization (blood protein adsorption) and macrophagic uptake, and thereby renders a "stealth" property to avoid rapid clearance from circulation [27], that in effect enhances the circulation residence time of the encapsulated drug payload. The most significant clinical application of liposomes is in the formulation of cancer drugs like Doxil®, Daunosome®, and Myocet® [28], which have made this class of vehicles a popular choice in studying encapsulation and delivery of drugs to other diseases including cardiovascular diseases. To this end, various antithrombotic agents have been encapsulated in liposomes and these formulations have shown enhanced circulation half-life of the drugs and increased therapeutic efficacy in vitro as well as in vivo in small animal models [29–33]. Liposomes, especially with cationic lipid shells, have been also used to complex DNA for gene delivery in cardiovascular diseases [34–39]. Besides drugs and DNA, liposomes have also been reported to encapsulate imaging agents like the MRI contrast agent gadolinium (Gd), either by direct loading of Gd salts or by lipid conjugation of Gd chelates, for imaging of vascular diseases [40–43]. Instead of lipidic systems, amphiphilic block co-polymeric systems with *packing fraction* equal to 1 can also be used to assemble similar vesicular structures called polymersomes [44–46]. Potentially such structures can also be used to package and deliver a wide variety of therapeutic agents in cardiovascular pathologies. Similar to liposomes, micelles are also self-assembled colloidal nanostructures with a hydrophobic core and a hydrophilic shell formed from amphiphilic molecules with packing parameter of ~1/3 when exposed to aqueous environment, and can be formed from lipid-based or polymer-based amphiphilic systems. These vehicles also have been extensively investigated in formulation of cancer drugs, but only a limited number of reports are available regarding their drug delivery applications in the cardiovascular area. PEG-polycation micelles have been utilized for gene delivery to arterial disease lesions in rabbit models [47]. Potential micelle-based strategies that could be directed toward diseased or dysregulated endothelial components of atherosclerotic and thrombotic sites in vascular diseases have been recently reviewed [48, 49]. To this end, several micelle-based strategies have been studied by incorporating ligand-based active targeting, which will be discussed in the next section.

Polymer based microparticles and nanoparticles have been of great interest in vascular drug delivery for past two decades [7, 8, 50]. Polymer-based drug-carrier particles can be formed by a wide variety of methods like oil/water or water/oil/water emulsion based solvent evaporation technique, solvent diffusion technique, solvent displacement technique, salting out technique, interfacial polymerization technique, and supercritical fluid technologies [51]. Polymeric nanoparticle carriers based on co-polymerized systems of biocompatible polymers like poly-lactic-*co*-glycolic acid (PLGA), polyethylene glycol (PEG), polyvinyl alcohol (PVA), etc. have been utilized to encapsulate and deliver anticoagulant agents like heparin [52], fibrinolytic agents like tPA and SK for clot dissolution [31, 53], and antiproliferative agents like probucol, rapamycin and paclitaxel for reducing restenosis [54–61]. Some polymer nanoparticle-based anti-restenotic formulations have also been evaluated in clinical studies [62]. Ultrasound imaging modalities are well established in diagnosis of physiological and pathological tissues, and ultrasound contrast agent bubbles like Definity (Bristol Meyers Squibb), a perfluoropropane/air filled lipid-shelled microbubble, have been approved in the clinic for cardiac imaging [63]. Consequently, such bubble systems have also been investigated for vascular therapeutic and diagnostic applications, where the bubble not only acts as a carrier for drugs but also allows focused ultrasound-mediated cavitation for site-selective release of the drugs. For example, poly(vinyl alcohol) (PVA)-based bubble structures were reported that can be loaded with the vasodilatory and antithrombotic bioactive gas nitric oxide (NO), for simultaneous imaging and NO delivery to vascular disease tissues [64]. Ultrasound-sensitive bubbles that allow cavitation-induced payload release have been reported for delivery of DNA, double stranded RNA and oligonucleotides, recombinant proteins, growth factors and thrombolytic agents (e.g., SK, tPA, etc.) [65–69]. Terminologies like "sonothrombolysis" has been coined to emphasize the combined effect of ultrasound-induced mechanical cavitation and site-specific thrombolytic drug release to enhance clot dissolution properties. Dendrimers are another important class of highly branched polymeric globular nanosystems originally developed in the 1980s by "convergent" or "divergent" chemical techniques [70, 71], that have undergone extensive studies in the delivery of genes, drugs and imaging agents utilizing the dendrimer core, the branching zone and the branch extremities [72]. Most dendrimeric applications in vascular drug delivery have involved ligand-based active targeting and will be discussed in the next section.

Among inorganic nanovehicle systems, carrier particles made from gold and iron oxide have been extensively studied in delivery of therapeutic and imaging agents in cancer [73–78]. Colloidal gold nanoparticles can be prepared by an array of methods that are mainly based on reduction of chloroauric acid in presence of a colloidal suspension stabilizing agent, and the methods vary mostly in terms of the reducing agents and reaction conditions [79–82]. Galvanic replacement methods have also been utilized to synthesize hollow gold nanostructures from gold salts [83, 84]. Gold nanoparticles and nanostructures have been studied not only as carrier vehicles for drug delivery and imaging, but also because of their plasmonic activity and near infra-red (NIR) wavelength sensitivity, they have been used to render NIR-induced targeted photothermal phenomena and photoacoustic imaging. To this end, gold nanoparticles have been recently reported in the context of cell-specific imaging as well as image-guided targeted drug delivery in the cardiovascular disease area [85, 86]. In a recent report, novel Au-based lipoprotein-coated nanoparticles (Au core coated with Apolipoprotein A-1 and phospholipids) were shown to be taken up by atherosclerosis-relevant macrophages in ApoE−/− mice in vivo and hence provided a way for enhanced multispectral and multimodality imaging of the lesions for characterization of macrophage burden, calcification and stenosis [87]. In another report, NIR-fluorescence-quenched gold nanoparticle based imaging probes were used where the particles were surface-modified by a peptide sequence that can be specifically degraded by matrix metalloproteases (MMPs) and also surface-modified with an NIR fluorescence dye, Cy5.5 [88]. MMP activity is prevalent in matrix remodeling and lesion progression processes in atherosclerosis, and therefore such nanosystems may become useful in detection and evaluation of vascular lesion progression. In another interesting work, the photothermal ablative effects of gold nanoparticles were used to render disruption and recanalization of atherosclerotic plaques in coronary arteries in human postmortem ex vivo specimens [89]. Iron oxide particles are usually prepared by co-precipitation methods involving addition of alkali to iron salts [90]. Superparamagnetic iron oxide (SPIO) particles are categorized mostly by their hydrodynamic diameter, e.g., Oral-SPIO (300 nm–3.5 μm), Standard-SPIO (SSPIO, 60–150 nm), Ultrasmall-SPIO (USPIO, 5–40 nm), and a subset of USPIO called monocrystalline iron oxide NPs (MION). Furthermore, MIONs with a chemically cross-linked polysaccharide shell are termed Cross Linked Iron Oxide (CLIO) [91, 92]. Iron oxide nanoparticles have been extensively reported in magnetic resonance based cellular and molecular imaging of cardiovascular diseases [93–102]. Incorporating therapeutic molecules in such iron oxide systems can provide efficient theranostic systems for cardiovascular therapies, as has been recently demonstrated regarding delivery of antithrombotic and anticoagulant agents using such particles [103, 104]. In another interesting work, iron oxide nanoparticles were incorporated within PLGA particles and co-loaded with paclitaxel to form drug-loaded magnetic nanoconstructs, which were guided by an induced magnetic field to carotid artery sites in vivo in animal models for sustained-release vascular antiproliferative therapy [105]. In recent years, there has been significant interest in engineering of multicomponent nanoparticle systems for theranostic use or multimodal targeted imaging applications, by combining different types of imaging probes and therapeutic agents on an iron oxide nanoparticle platform [106–109]. Another class of inorganic nanostructures that have been extensively researched in targeted drug delivery and imaging is Quantum dots (QDs), that are semiconductor nanocrystals (e.g., QD with a cadmium selenide core with a zinc sulfide shell) with unique size- and composition-dependent fluorescent properties and are also sufficiently electron dense to facilitate electron microscopy [110]. The in vivo distribution, residence, and safety of QDs remain a matter of debate [111–114].

Nonetheless, QDs have been investigated in vascular delivery and imaging applications, for example, by incorporating them in high density lipoprotein (HDL)-based plaque-targeting for optical imaging of plaques [115]. The same HDL particles, incorporated with MRI probes, have been further investigated for targeted imaging of atherosclerotic plaques [115–117]. Several QD-based nanosystems have also been investigated in ligand-mediated active targeting to vascular lesions, which will be discussed in the next section.

3 Nanomedicine Systems with Ligand-Based Site-Specific Active Binding Mechanisms

Many of the nanovehicle systems described in the previous section have also been utilized to developed "actively targeted" delivery devices where the particles can bind to disease sites and diseased cells by virtue of specific ligand–receptor interactions. The ligands in such cases can be antibodies, antibody fragments, proteins and peptides, while, the receptors are antigens and proteins either uniquely expressed or quantitatively upregulated at the disease site cells and matrix. Such active targeting is thought to help with selectivity and specificity of targeting as well as with receptor-mediated internalization of the vehicles within diseased cells for intracellular delivery in some cases [118–120]. The ligands can be decorated on the nanoparticulate vehicles via non-covalent methods as well as a variety of covalent bioconjugation techniques.

Non-covalent adsorption methods to surface-decorate nanovehicles with ligands mostly involve physical (e.g., hydrophobic, affinity-based, charge-based) interactions of ligand molecules with the surface material of the particles. For example, polystyrene particles have been reported to be coated with P-selectin and E-selectin targeting antibodies using adsorbed bacterial protein A molecules as spacers [121]. These selectins are often expressed on activated platelets, stimulated endothelial cells and monocytes at the site of vascular injuries and lesions, and therefore are relevant systems for active targeting of drug delivery systems to such vascular disease sites. Similar techniques have also been reported for coating chitosan particles with anti-amyloid monoclonal antibodies to target amyloid beta-protein deposits in cerebral vasculature of mice [122]. In other work, liposomes, latex beads and albumin particles have been non-covalently surface-modified with recombinant glycoprotein Ib-alpha (rGPIbα) and recombinant glycoprotein Ia-IIa (rGPIa-IIa) to actively bind to von Willebrand Factor (vWF) and collagen respectively [123–125]. vWF is secreted and deposited from injured endothelial cells and activated platelets, while collagen is often exposed as the major sub-endothelial matrix protein at vascular injury sites due to endothelial denudation. Therefore such vWF- and collagen-targeting systems can have potential application in targeted delivery to vascular injury sites. Another interesting non-covalent approach to decorate nanoparticles with targeting motifs is the use of avidin-biotin affinity interaction. Avidin (and analogous Streptavidin) is a highly glycosylated positively charged protein that is uniquely stable against heat, denaturants, pH and proteolytic enzymes, and has high affinity towards Biotin (Vitamin B6) with a dissociation constant (K_d) of 10^{-15} M [126, 127]. Consequently particles can be surface-modified with avidin and incubated with biotinylated ligand motifs, or vice versa, to create ligand-decorated actively targeted delivery systems. This approach has been used extensively in decorating particle surfaces with antibodies and antibody fragments for targeting to cancer. In the area of targeting cardiovascular diseases, this technique has been employed to surface-decorate RBCs with antithrombotic molecules (e.g., tPA) as well as to decorate various nanovehicle systems with antibodies directed to a variety of vascularly relevant cell adhesion molecules (CAMs) [128–131]. Covalent bioconjugation techniques involve specific chemical reactions of reactive groups on ligand motifs to complimentary reactive groups on the nanovehicle surface. The most common chemical bioconjugation methods are amide linkages (reaction between amine and carboxyl termini), hydrazine-based linkages (reaction between hydrazide and aldehyde termini), sulfhydryl-mediated linkages (reaction between sulfhydryl group and maleimide, sulfone, acetamide or pyridyl groups) and alkyne-azide based "click" chemistry [132]. Figure 2 shows schematic of some common bioconjugation strategies for

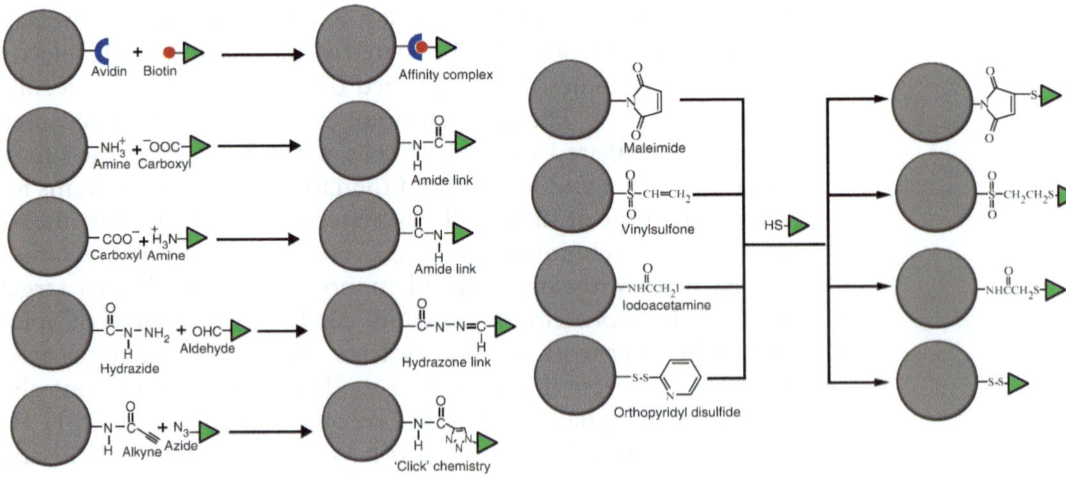

Fig. 2 Common bioconjugation strategies for decorating nanoparticle surfaces with targeting motifs; the targeting motifs can be antibodies, antibody fragments, peptides, aptamers, etc.

decorating nanoparticle surfaces with targeting motifs. These methods can be utilized to conjugate antibodies, antibody fragments, aptamers, proteins, and peptides to a wide variety of nanovehicle systems either by reacting to appropriate functional groups on the surface of preformed particles (solid polymer particles, QDs, dendrimers, etc.), or by reacting to the termini of constituent molecules first and then assembling the modified molecules into particles (e.g., liposomes, micelles). Figure 3 shows the commonly studied cellular and noncellular targets for vascular nanomedicine technologies.

By utilizing the various non-covalent or covalent surface-modification techniques stated above, a large number of actively targeted nanoparticle systems have been reported for site-specific delivery of drugs and imaging probes in vascular diseases. To this end, echogenic liposomes have been reported that can target fibrinogen, fibrin or intercellular adhesion molecule-1 (ICAM-1)

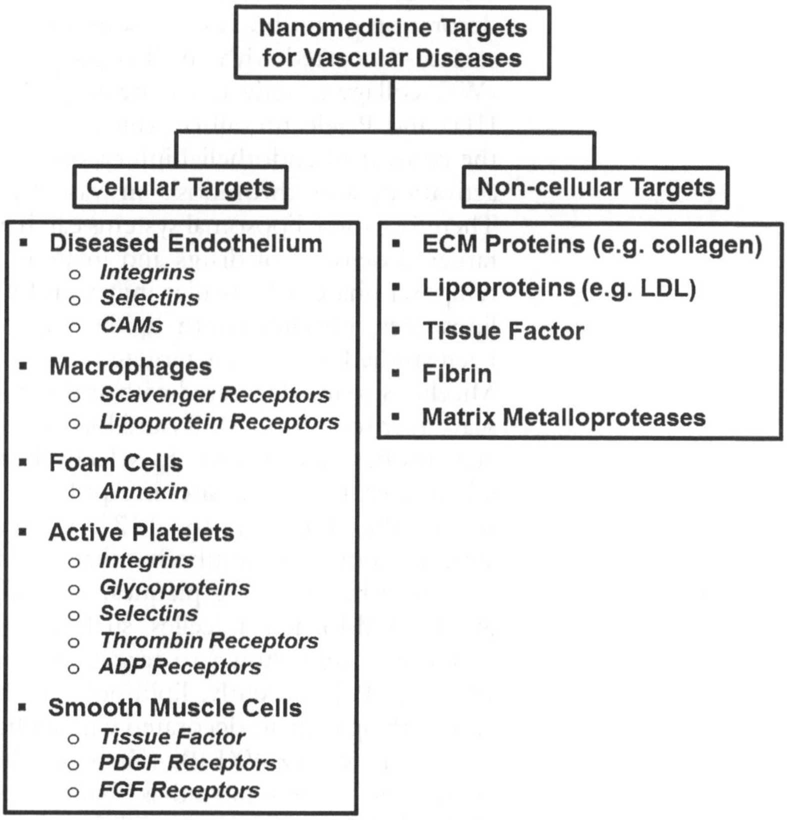

Fig. 3 Relevant cellular and noncellular targets utilized for active targeting of vascular nanomedicine systems. The targets can be cell-surface antigens as well as a variety of substrate proteins relevant to the vascular disease site. *CAMs* cell adhesion molecules, *ADP* adenosine diphosphate, *PDGF* platelet derived growth factor, *FGF* fibroblast growth factor, *LDL* low density lipoproteins

by virtue of anti-fibrinogen, anti-fibrin, and anti-ICAM-1 antibodies and allow ultrasound-induced cavitation mediated delivery of thrombolytic agents [133–135]. In another work, Gadolinium (Gd)-based MRI contrast agent delivery to atherosclerotic tissue was demonstrated by using liposomes modified with Gd-lipid conjugates and phosphatidylserine (PS) to enable preferential uptake by atherosclerotic site-relevant macrophages [41]. Similar strategy in macrophage-targeting of liposomes was also demonstrated with liposomes modified by the ligand decadeoxyguanine, which has high affinity to macrophagic scavenger receptor class A (SRA) [42]. Liposomes surface-decorated with antibodies directed to low density lipoprotein receptors LOX-1 have been reported to enable atherosclerotic lesion-targeted delivery of radioimaging and MR imaging agents [136]. Another liposomal formulation, named LipoCardium, was reported for targeted delivery of anti-inflammatory prostaglandins to atheroslecrotic sites using liposomes surface decorated with antibodies directed to Vascular Cell Adhesion Molecule-1 (VCAM-1) [137]. Besides surface-decoration of antibodies, liposomes have also been reported to be surface-decorated with small peptides having targeting ability to vWF, collagen, activated platelet glycoprotein IIb-IIIa (GPIIb-IIIa) and P-selectin, all of which are suitable target molecules in the context of endothelial injury, endothelial denudation, platelet activation, and thrombosis in vascular pathologies [138–145]. Therefore these liposomal systems can have potential application in targeted delivery of drugs and imaging agents to various spatio-temporal phases of vascular injury and vascular disease. Similar to liposomes, micelles (both lipidic and block co-polymeric) have been studied for actively targeted delivery to vascular disease sites. Micelles surface-decorated with antibodies specific for macrophage scavenger receptors (MSR) and loaded with Gd chelates or fluorescent probes were shown to selectively target and accumulate at atherosclerotic arterial sites in ApoE−/− mice for molecular imaging of the disease [146, 147]. Gd-loaded PEG-lipid micelles surface-modified by antibodies that bind to oxidized LDL lipoproteins in atherosclerotic plaques, have also been reported [148]. Similar Gd-loaded micelles surface-decorated with anti-CD36 antibodies were shown to target macrophages in atherosclerotic vessels [149]. Recently, lipid-polymer hybrid particles (polymer core with lipid shell) decorated with a phage library-identified peptide sequence KZWXLPX (Z: hydrophobic amino acid, X: any amino acid) were reported as "nanoburrs" that can actively target exposed collagen IV at arterial injury (i.e., endothelial denudation) sites and deliver antiproliferative agents to modulate smooth muscle cell activity [150, 151]. In another recent work, micelles were surface decorated with a 9-amino acid sequence CGNKRTRGC (also known as Lyp-1) that binds to p32 receptors in atherosclerotic plaques as well as with CREKA peptides that bind to fibrin-fibronectin clots, and these micelles showed enhanced homing to atherosclerotic plaques in vivo [152, 153].

Similar to liposomes and micelles, solid polymeric particles have also been studied for surface-modification with ligands to enable targeted binding to vascular injury or vascular disease sites. For example, PLGAnanoparticles have been loaded with thrombolytic drugs like tPA and coated with Arginine-Glycine-Aspartic Acid (RGD)-peptide modified chitosan to render targeted binding to clots for enhanced thrombolytic efficacy [53]. PLGA nanoparticles have also been reported to be surface-modified with anti-ICAM-1 antibodies for specific immunotargeting to inflamed vascular endothelium in vitro and in vivo, which has relevance to targeting atherosclerotic plaques [154]. Similarly, poly(sebacic acid)-co-PEG (PSAPEG) microparticles and nanoparticles surface-modified with anti-VCAM-1 antibodies have been reported to undergo enhanced adhesion, binding and accumulation at atherosclerotic lesion sites in ApoE−/− mice [155]. Nanoparticles made from poly-l-lysine-co-poly-lactic acid copolymer (PLL-PLA), surface-decorated with RGD peptides have been reported to be able to aggregate with active platelets at the site of traumatic vascular injury [156]. Similar designs of RGD-decorated or the fibrinogen-derived peptide sequence HHLGGAKQAGDV-decorated particles have also been reported using RBCs, latex beads or albumin particles as the carrier vehicle [157–162]. The HDL nanoparticles described in the previous section were designed to be naturally taken up into atherosclerotic lesions via lipoprotein transport mechanisms; however these same particles have also been reported to be modified with RGD peptides to enable active targeting ability to vasculature [163]. Ligand-based active targeting strategies have also been reported for ultrasound-sensitive bubbles where the bubbles were surface-decorated with antibodies directed against inflammation and atherosclerosis relevant upregulated cell-surface markers like various CAMs and integrins (e.g., $\alpha V\beta 3$), on leukocytes and injured endothelium, in vitro and in vivo, for targeted drug delivery to and molecular imaging of vascular disease [164–166]. In similar work, ultrasound-sensitive bubbles were developed with shells bearing maleimido-4(p-phenylbutyrate)-phospholipid, which were then surface-conjugated with platelet integrin GPIIb-IIIa-specific therapeutic antibody Abciximab (ReoPro by Eli Lilly, Indianapolis, Indiana), that enabled enhanced targeting to activated platelet-rich thrombi for molecular imaging applications in vitro and in vivo [167]. Dendrimers have also been studied for active targeting to vascular pathology sites, where biodegradable dendritic structures surface-modified with endothelial $\alpha V\beta 3$ integrin-targeting cyclic RGD peptides and loaded with radioactive Bromine (^{76}Br) for positron emission tomography

(PET), were capable of targeted molecular imaging of hindlimb ischemia in a mouse model [168]. Similar targeted molecular imaging of vascular disease-specific biomolecules and cellular phenotypes have also been demonstrated with dendrimers modified by a variety of other ligands [169–171].

The inorganic nanosystems described in the previous section have also undergone extensive investigation for actively targeted delivery to vascular disease and injury sites. Cross-linked dextran-coated iron oxide (CLIO) nanoparticles have also been surface-decorated with peptides and small molecules that can target CAMs and clot-associated fibrin to enable active targeting of the particles to inflammatory, angiogenic and thrombotic cellular phenotypes and biomarkers of atherosclerosis for contrast enhanced targeted molecular imaging [92]. Iron oxide particles have also been reported to be surface-decorated with ligands directed towards VCAM-1, P-selectin and platelet integrin GPIIb-IIIa for targeted contrast-enhanced MR imaging of atherosclerosis and thrombosis in animal models [172]. In another interesting work, SPIOs were surface-modified by Annexin V that can specifically interact with lipoproteins on the outer membrane leaflet of apoptotic cells and hence enabled interaction and selective targeting of "foam cells" in atheromatous plaque in rabbit models for T2-weighted MR imaging [173]. QDs have also been utilized to actively bind a variety of CAMs (e.g., VCAM, ICAM, PECAM) using QD surface-decoration with anti-CAM antibodies [174, 175] and these facilitated in vivo optical imaging of atherosclerotic lesions. Other approaches to ligand-directed vascular disease-specific targeting of QDs for optical imaging include targeting to oxidized LDL receptor CD36, phosphatidylserine-exposing cells, and plaque-relevant MMPs [176, 177]. Instead of directly targeting QDs to the vascular disease site, they have also been used as "payloads" in other actively targeted nanosystems to allow for concurrent optical imaging modality for vascular diseases. This strategy has been utilized by loading QDs within paramagnetic micelles immunotargeted to macrophagic scavenger receptors [178] as well as within HDL nanoparticles [115]. In an interesting work, gold nanoparticles were conjugated to QDs via a proetolytically degradable peptide sequence such that in the "bound" state the QD luminescence was non-radiatively suppressed, and enzymatic cleavage of the conjugate links significantly restored luminescence [179]. Such unique strategies can be envisioned to be applicable in probing proteolytic activities (e.g., MMP activity) in atherosclerotic lesions.

4 Other Miscellaneous Applications of Nanomaterials in Cardiovascular Disease Treatment

As evident from the descriptions and examples provided in the previous sections, "nanotechnology" has provided an efficient way to render localized or site-selective delivery of various therapeutic agents and imaging probes in vascular diseases and injuries. Such localized delivery can potentially overcome the issues of potency and narrow therapeutic window of many drug molecules by achieving greater local concentrations with lower overall dose, to maximize the effects in target tissue while avoiding systemic indiscriminate distribution and harmful side-effects. The idea of local delivery in the cardiovascular arena emerged about two decades ago in the context of using perivascular delivery systems successfully in animal models [180, 181]. In these systems, heparin-releasing polymeric matrix devices were placed around rat carotid arteries at the time of balloon angioplasty, to allow continuous local release of the drug for predetermined periods of time. These approaches were found to reduce post-procedural arterial occlusion more effectively compared to systemic heparin infusion from pumps or from drug-releasing polymer matrices placed subcutaneously distant from the target artery site. Similar local polymeric systems bearing endothelial cells as a source of endogenous vasoregulatory agents were also shown to have enhanced efficiency in reducing neointimal hyperplasia in rat and pig models of vascular injury [182, 183]. Over the past two decades, other "local delivery" systems have been developed for cardiovascular applications, including intraluminal, intramural and stent-based systems [184], all of which have proved to be much more efficient in rendering therapeutic effect at the target tissue while avoiding poor distribution and harmful side-effect issues of systemic delivery. Nanotechnology has contributed to refinement such devices. For example, silver nanoparticles have been used to modify implantable and intravascular devices to prevent bacterial adhesion, growth and biofilm development [185]. Carbon nanotubes have been incorporated in catheters to provide mechanical versatility as well as impart antithrombotic and drug delivery functions [186]. Such carbon nanotubes have also been incorporated in stents [187]. Other application of nanotechnology in stents include refined nanofabrication and nanomorphological texturing techniques to allow for enhanced drug loading, tissue-material interactions and drug release [188], as well as incorporating drug- or gene-loaded nanoparticles within stent coatings for sustained local delivery following angiopalstic procedures and stent placement [189, 190]. Nanotechnology has also been used in fabrication of artificial arterial grafts and conduits [191], although it is too early to conclude on long-term success of these designs. In the context of artificial vascular grafts, chemical nanocomposites have also been incorporated to release nitric oxide and to impart infection resistance [192].

In recent years, another facet of nanotechnology that is raising significant interest, especially in the context of drug delivery vehicles in the vascular compartment, is the role of "physical" design parameters like shape, size, modulus, etc. Several recent reports have established that particles of anisotropic shapes (spheroids, rods, disks, etc.) have a higher probability of margination from flowing blood volume towards the vascular wall [193–195]. Parallel studies have also shown that size of particles play an important role in their extent of margination to the vascular wall [196–198]. In fact a natural example of this is seen in blood platelets which can marginate better to the vascular wall through the RBC volume of flowing blood owing to their biconvex discoid shape and their quiescent ~2 μm size [199–201]. Based on such studies, recent research has focused on development of particles with tailored shapes and sizes to facilitate margination to the vascular wall [202–207]. Such margination-facilitating geometric parameters can be potentially integrated with ligand-based active targeting functionalities on particle platforms to create drug delivery and nanomedicine systems with increased site-selective localization and delivery efficiency in the vascular compartment. Another important design parameter for drug delivery systems is the mechanism of drug release. Traditionally most particulate delivery systems depend upon diffusion and degradation/dissolution mediated mechanisms for payload release [208–210]. Beyond such mechanisms, certain stimuli-triggered mechanisms have been investigated for drug delivery systems, where the payload release is induced by chemical and/or physical changes in the drug delivery system in response to internal stimuli like pH, enzyme action, temperature, etc., or, external triggers like NIR irradiation (e.g., for gold nanoparticles), electromagnetic wave (e.g., for iron oxide particles), high frequency focused ultrasound (e.g., for ultrasound bubbles), etc. [211–216]. A few recent studies have utilized "shear forces" as a physical release trigger because of its relevance to vascular thrombo-occlusive sites. In these studies using polymeric or lipidic particles, the increased shear forces caused by thrombo-occlusion have resulted in the disintegration of the carrier particles to release drugs like thrombolytic agents, site-selectively [217, 218]. Furthermore, an interesting aspect in the context of ligand-mediated active targeting of drug delivery vehicles is the utilization of concurrent binding to multiple receptor/antigen types pertinent to the disease site (also known as heteromultivalent binding) instead of targeting to only one type of receptor. Such targeting approaches have shown enhanced efficacy of anchorage of the vehicles to the target site under hemodynamic flow environment [142, 219], and this can potentially allow for increased target specificity as well as retention for enhanced therapeutic release. These newer design parameters are continuing to add exciting properties to vascular nanomedicine systems, that can be tailored to act selectively at disease sites by virtue of enhanced margination, enhanced anchorage, and enhanced drug release.

5 Discussion

Localized delivery of therapeutic molecules and imaging probes at the sites of vascular disease results in enhanced treatment and detection efficacy. Nanotechnology provides an efficient way to achieve such localized delivery in the context of packaging therapeutic payloads within nanoparticulate vehicles that can be intravenously injected and can accumulate passively or bind actively at the target vascular sites. The success of such approaches depend upon efficient encapsulation of the payload within the nanoparticles to protect from plasma-induced deactivation, minimize pre-target leakage or release of the payload, maintain circulation for sufficient periods of time to reach the target site, render efficient passive or active binding to the target site under hemodynamic flow, and enable efficient release of the payload by internal or external triggers. Because of the need to stay retained at the target site under hemodynamic flow environment, active binding strategies may be more effective in vascular drug delivery, compared to passive accumulation mechanisms. The delivery systems must be biocompatible, in terms of minimal immunogenicity, minimal complement activation, minimal toxicity, and minimal carcinogenicity. The drug delivery systems must also be either easily cleared from the body within a reasonable period of time, or easily biodegradable to resorbable or metabolizable products in the body. Additional design parameters to consider for the particulate vehicles are their margination-influencing shape, size, and morphology, their active targeting and anchorage-influencing ligand decoration chemistry and density, and their response to internal and external triggers. For efficient clinical translation, research should also be focused on cost and convenience of manufacture and quality control of vascular nanomedicine technologies.

References

1. Go AS, Mozaffarian D, Roger VL, Benjamin EJ, Berry JD, Blaha MJ et al. (2014) On behalf of the American Heart Association Statistics Committee and Stroke Statistics Subcommitte. Heart disease and stroke statistics – 2014 update: a report from the American Heart Association. Circulation 129: e28
2. WHO (2011) Global atlas on cardiovascular disease prevention and control. World Health Organization, Geneva

3. Phillips DR, Conley PB, Sinha U, Andre P (2005) Therapeutic approaches in arterial thrombosis. J Thromb Haemost 3:1577–1589
4. Gurbel PA, Serebruany VL (2000) Oral Platelet IIb/IIIa inhibitors: from attractive theory to clinical failures. J Thromb Thrombolysis 10:217–220
5. Marzilli M (1995) From the experimental myocardial infarction to the clinical acute myocardial infarction: limitations of thrombolytic therapy. Int J Cardiol 49:S71–S75
6. Rebeiz AG, Granger CB, Simoons ML (2005) Incidence and management of complications of fibrinolytic, antiplatelet, and anticoagulant therapy. Fundam Clin Cardiol 52:375–395
7. Brieger D, Topol E (1997) Local drug delivery systems and prevention of restenosis. Cardiovasc Res 35:405–413
8. Eccleston DS, Lincoff AM (1997) Catheter-based drug delivery for restenosis. Adv Drug Deliv Rev 24:31–43
9. Fattori R, Piva T (2003) Drug-eluting stents in vascular intervention. Lancet 361:247–249
10. Torchilin VP (1995) Targeting of drugs and drug carriers within the cardiovascular system. Adv Drug Deliv Rev 17:75–101
11. Zolot RS, Basu S, Million RP (2013) Antibody–drug conjugates. Nat Rev Drug Discov 12:259–260
12. Wang X, Palasubramaniam J, Gkanatsas Y, Hohmann JD, Westein E, Kanojia R, Alt K, Huang D, Jia F, Ahrens I, Medcalf RL, Peter K, Hagemeyer CE (2014) Towards effective and safe thrombolysis and thromboprophylaxis: preclinical testing of a novel antibody-targeted recombinant plasminogen activator directed against activated platelets. Circ Res 114:1083–1093
13. Dong N, Da Cunha V, Citkowicz A, Wu F, Vincelette J, Larsen B, Wang YX, Ruan C, Dole WP, Morser J, Wu Q, Pan J (2004) P-selectin-targeting of the fibrin selective thrombolytic Desmodus rotundus salivary plasminogen activator alpha1. Thromb Haemost 92:956–965
14. Diamond SL (1999) Engineering design of optimal strategies for blood clot dissolution. Annu Rev Biomed Eng 1:427–461
15. Thomas AC, Campbell JH (2004) Targeted delivery of heparin and LMWH using a fibrin antibody prevents restenosis. Atherosclerosis 176:73–81
16. Sen Gupta A (2011) Nanomedicine approaches in vascular disease: a review. Nanomedicine 7:763–779
17. Ringsdorf H (1975) Structure and properties of pharmacologically active polymers. J Poly Sci Symp 51:135–153
18. Elvira C, Gallardo A, Roman JS, Cifuentes A (2005) Covalent polymer-drug conjugates. Molecules 10:114–125
19. Duncan R (2006) Polymer conjugates as anticancer nanomedicines. Nat Rev Cancer 6:688–701
20. Berger HJ Jr, Pizzo SV (1988) Preparation of polyethylene glycol-tissue plasminogen activator adducts that retain functional activity: characteristics and behavior in three animal species. Blood 71:1641–1647
21. Rajagopalan S, Gonias SL, Pizzo SV (1985) A nonantigenic covalent streptokinasepolyethylene glycol complex with plasminogen activator function. J Clin Invest 75:413–419
22. Sakuragawa N, Shimizu K, Kondo K, Kondo S, Niwa M (1986) Studies on the effect of PEG-modified urokinase on coagulation-fibrinolysis using beagles. Thromb Res 41:627–635
23. Moreadith RW, Collen D (2003) Clinical development of PEGylated recombinant staphylokinase (PEGSak) for bolus thrombolytic treatment of patients with acute myocardial infarction. Adv Drug Deliv Rev 55:1337–1345
24. Collen D, Sinnaeve P, Demarsin E, Moreau H, De Maeyer M, Jespers L, Laroche Y, Van de Werf F (2000) Polyethylene glycol-derivatized cysteine substitution variants of recombinant staphylokinase for single-bolus treatment of acute myocardial infarction. Circulation 102:1766–1772
25. Lasic DD, Papahadjopaulos D (eds) (1998) Medical applications of liposomes. Elsevier, Amsterdam
26. Torchilin VP (2005) Recent advances with liposomes as pharmaceutical carriers. Nat Rev Drug Discov 4:145–160
27. Cˇeh B, Winterhalter M, Frederik PM, Vallner JJ, Lasic DD (1997) Stealth® liposomes: from theory to product. Adv Drug Deliv Rev 24:165–177
28. Wang AZ, Langer R, Farokhzad OC (2012) Nanoparticle delivery of cancer drugs. Annu Rev Med 63:185–198
29. Nguyen PD, O'Rear EA, Johnson AE, Patterson E, Whitsett TL, Bhakta R (1990) Accelerated thrombolysis and reperfusion in a canine model of myocardial infarction by liposomal encapsulation of streptokinase. Circ Res 66:875–878
30. Heeremans JLM, Prevost R, Bekkers MEA, Los P, Emeis JJ, Kluft C, Crommelin DJ (1995) Thrombolytic treatment with tissue-type plasminogen activators (t-PA) containing liposomes in rabbit: a comparison with free t-PA. Thromb Haemost 73:488–494
31. Leach JK, O'Rear EA, Patterson E, Miao Y, Johnson AE (2003) Accelerated thrombolysis

in a rabbit model of carotid artery thrombosis with liposome-encapsulated and microencapsulated streptokinase. Thromb Haemost 90:64–70
32. Perkins WR, Vaughan DE, Plavin SR, Daley WL, Rauch J, Lee L, Janoff AS (1997) Streptokinase entrapment in interdigitation-fusion liposomes improves thrombolysis in an experimental rabbit model. Thromb Haemost 77:1174–1178
33. Kim I-S, Choi H-G, Choi H-S, Kim B-K, Kim C-K (1998) Prolonged systemic delivery of streptokinase using liposome. Arch Pharm Res 21:248–252
34. Dzau VJ, Mann MJ, Morishita R, Kaneda Y (1996) Fusigenic viral liposome for gene therapy in cardiovascular diseases. Proc Natl Acad Sci U S A 93:11421–11425
35. Nabel EG (1995) Gene therapy for cardiovascular disease. Circulation 91:541–548
36. Morishita R, Gibbons GH, Kaneda Y, Ogihara T, Dzau VJ (1993) Novel and effective gene transfer technique for study of vascular renin angiotensin system. J Clin Invest 91:2580–2585
37. Leclerc G, Gal D, Takeshita S, Nikol S, Weir L, Isner JM (1992) Percutaneous arterial gene transfer in a rabbit model: efficiency in normal and balloon-dilated atherosclerotic arteries. J Clin Invest 90:936–944
38. Lim CS, Chapman GD, Gammon RS, Muhlestein JB, Bauman RP, Stack RS, Swain JL (1991) Direct in vivo gene transfer into the coronary and peripheral vasculatures of the intact dog. Circulation 83:2007–2011
39. Chapman GD, Lim CS, Gammon RS, Culp SC, Desper S, Bauman RP, Swain JL, Stack RS (1992) Gene transfer into coronary arteries of intact animals with a percutaneous balloon catheter. Circ Res 71:27–33
40. Zheng J, Liu J, Dunne M, Jaffray DA, Allen C (2007) In vivo performance of a liposomal vascular contrast agent for CT and MR-based image guidance applications. Pharm Res 24:1193–1201
41. Maiseyeu A, Mihai G, Kampfrath T, Simonetti OP, Sen CK, Roy S, Rajagopalan S, Parthasarathy S (2009) Gadolinium-containing phosphatidylserine liposomes for molecular imaging of atherosclerosis. J Lipid Res 50:2157–2163
42. Rensen PC, Gras JC, Lindfors EK, van Dijk KW, Jukema JW, van Berkel TJ, Biessen EA (2006) Selective targeting of liposomes to macrophages using a ligand with high affinity for the macrophage scavenger receptor class A. Curr Drug Discov Technol 3:135–144
43. Mulder WJM, Douma K, Koning GA, van Zandvoort MA, Lutgens E, Daemen MJ, Nikolay K, Strijkers GJ (2006) Liposome-enhanced MRI of neointimal lesions in the ApoE-KO mouse. Magn Reson Med 55:1170–1174
44. Discher DE, Ahmed F (2006) Polymersomes. Annu Rev Biomed Eng 8:323–341
45. Lee JS, Feijen J (2012) Polymersomes for drug delivery: design, formation and characterization. J Control Release 161:473–483
46. Massignani M, Lomas H, Battaglia G (2010) Polymersomes: a synthetic biological approach to encapsulation and delivery. Adv Polym Sci 229:115–154
47. Akagi D, Oba M, Koyama H, Nishiyama N, Fukushima S, Miyata T, Nagawa H, Kataoka K (2007) Biocompatible micellar nanovectors achieve efficient gene transfer to vascular lesions without cytotoxicity and thrombus formation. Gene Ther 14:1029–1038
48. Ding B-S, Dziubla T, Shuvaev VV, Muro S, Muzykantov VR (2006) Advanced drug delivery systems that target the vascular endothelium. Mol Interv 6:98–112
49. Torchilin VP (2007) Micellar nanocarriers: pharmaceutical perspectives. Pharm Res 24:1–16
50. Lincoff MA, Topol EJ, Ellis SG (1994) Local drug delivery for the prevention of restenosis: facts, fancy and future. Circulation 90:2070–2084
51. Soppimath KS, Aminabhavi TM, Kulkarni AR, Rudzinski WE (2001) Biodegradable polymeric nanoparticles as drug delivery devices. J Control Release 70:1–20
52. Yang Z, Birkenhauer P, Julmy F, Chickering D, Ranieri JP, Merkle HP, Lüscher TF, Gander B (1999) Sustained release of heparin from polymeric particles for inhibition of human vascular smooth muscle cell proliferation. J Control Release 60:269–277
53. Chung T-W, Wang SS, Tsai W-J (2008) Accelerating thrombolysis with chitosan-coated plasminogen activators encapsulated in poly-(lactide-co-glycolide) (PLGA) nanoparticles. Biomaterials 29:228–237
54. Klugherz BD, Meneveau N, Chen W, Wade-Whittaker F, Papandreou G, Levy R, Wilensky RL (1999) Sustained intramural retention and regional redistribution following local vascular delivery of Polylactic-co-glycolic acid and liposomal nanoparticulate formulations containing probucol. J Cardiovasc Pharmacol Ther 4:167–174
55. Kolodgie FD, John M, Khurana C, Farb A, Wilson PS, Acampado E, Desai N, Soon-Shiong P, Virmani R (2002) Sustained reduction of in-stent neointimal growth with the use of a novel systemic nanoparticle paclitaxel. Circulation 106:1195–1198

56. Westedt U, Kalinowski M, Wittmer M, Merdan T, Unger F, Fuchs J, Schaller S, Bakowsky U, Kissel T (2007) Poly (vinyl alcohol)-graft-poly (lactide-co-glycolide) nanoparticles for local delivery of paclitaxel for restenosis treatment. J Control Release 119:41–51
57. Deshpande D, Devalapally H, Amiji M (2008) Enhancement in anti-proliferative effects of paclitaxel in aortic smooth muscle cells upon coadministration with ceramide using biodegradable polymeric nanoparticles. Pharm Res 25:1936–1947
58. Zou W, Cao G, Xi Y, Zhang N (2009) New approach for local delivery of rapamycin by bioadhesive PLGA-carbopol nanoparticles. Drug Deliv 16:15–23
59. Zweers ML, Engbers GH, Grijpma DW, Feijen J (2006) Release of anti-restenosis drugs from poly (ethylene oxide)-poly(DL-lactic-co-glycolic acid) nanoparticles. J Control Release 114:317–324
60. Luderer F, Lobler M, Rohm HW, Gocke C, Kunna K, Kock K, Kroemer HK, Westschies W, Shmitz KP, Sternberg K (2011) Biodegradable sirolimus loaded poly(lactide) nanoparticles as drug delivery systems for the prevention of in-stent restenosis in coronary stent application. J Biomater Appl 25:851–875
61. Nakano K, Egashira K, Masuda S, Funakoshi K, Zhao G, Kimura S, Matoba T, Sueishi K, Endo Y, Kawashima Y, Hara K, Tsujimoto H, Tominagu R, Sunagawa K (2009) Formulation of nanoparticle eluting stents by a cationic electrodesposition coating technology: efficient nano-drug delivery via bioabsorbable polymeric nanoparticle eluting stents in porcine coronary arteries. JACC Cardiovasc Interv 2:277–283
62. Margolis J, McDonald J, Heuser R, Klkinke P, Waksman R, Virmani R, Desai N, Hilton D (2007) Systemic nanoparticle paclitaxel (nab-paclitaxel) for in-stent restenosis-I (SNAPIST-I): a first in human safety and dose finding study. Clin Cardiol 30:165–170
63. Unger E, Matsunaga TO, Schumann PA, Zutshi R (2003) Microbubbles in molecular imaging and therapy. Medicamundi 47:58–65
64. Cavalieri F, Finelli I, Tortora M, Mozetic P, Chiessi E, Polizio F, Brismar TB, Paradossi G (2008) Polymer microbubbles as diagnostic and therapeutic gas delivery device. Chem Mater 20:3254–3258
65. Tsivgoulis G, Culp WC, Alexandrov AV (2008) Ultrasound enhanced thrombolysis in acute arterial ischemia. Ultrasonics 48:303–311
66. Marta R, Alexandrov AV (2010) Sonothrombolysis in the management of acute ischemic stroke. Am J Cardiovasc Drugs 10:5–10
67. Mayer CR, Bekeredjian R (2008) Ultrasonic gene and drug delivery to cardiovascular system. Adv Drug Deliv Rev 60:1177–1192
68. Shaw GJ, Meunier JM, Huang SL, Lindsell CJ, McPherson DD, Holland CK (2009) Ultrasound-enhanced thrombolysis with tPA-loaded echogenic liposomes. Thromb Res 124:306–310
69. Tiukinhoy-Laing SD, Buchanan K, Parikh D, Huang S, MacDonald RC, McPherson DD, Klegerman ME (2007) Fibrin targeting of tissue plasminogen activator-loaded echogenic liposomes. J Drug Target 15:109–114
70. Tomalia DA (1996) Starburst dendrimers—nanoscopic supermolecules according to dendritic rules and principles. Macromol Symp 101:243–255
71. Hawker CJ, Fréchet JMJ (1990) Preparation of polymers with controlled molecular architecture. A new convergent approach to dendritic macromolecules. J Am Chem Soc 112:7638–7647
72. Svenson S, Tomalia DA (2005) Dendrimers in biomedical applications - reflections on the field. Adv Drug Deliv Rev 57:2106–2129
73. Chen PC, Mwakwari SC, Oyelere AK (2008) Gold nanoparticles: from nanomedicine to nanosensing. Nanotechnol Sci Appl 1:45–66
74. Sperling RA, Gil PR, Zhang F, Zanella M, Parak WJ (2008) Biological applications of gold nanoparticles. Chem Soc Rev 37:1896–1908
75. Huang X, Jain PK, El-Sayed IH, El-Sayed MA (2008) Lasers Med Sci 23:217–228
76. Rosen JE, Chan L, Shieh DB, Gu FX (2012) Iron oxide nanoparticles for targeted cancer imaging and diagnostics. Nanomedicine 8:275–290
77. Tassa C, Shaw SY, Weissleder R (2011) Dextran-coated iron oxide nanoparticles: a versatile platform for targeted molecular imaging, molecular diagnostics, and therapy. Acc Chem Res 44:842–852
78. Yen SK, Padmanabhan P, Selvan ST (2013) Multifunctional iron oxide nanoparticles for diagnostics, therapy and macromolecule delivery. Theranostics 3:986–1003
79. Turkevitch J, Stevenson PC, Hillier J (1951) A study of the nucleation and growth process in the synthesis of colloidal gold. Discuss Faraday Soc 11:55–75
80. Brust M, Walker M, Bethell D, Schiffrin DJ, Whyman RJ (1994) Synthesis of thiol derivatized gold nanoparticles in a two phase liquid-liquid system. J Chem Soc Chem Commun 7:801–802
81. Sun Y, Xia Y (2002) Shape-controlled synthesis of gold and silver nanoparticles. Science 298:2176–2179

82. Vekilov PG (2011) Gold nanoparticles: grown in a crystal. Nat Nanotechnol 6:82–83
83. Au L, Lu X, Xia Y (2008) A comparative study of galvanic replacement reactions involving Ag nanocubes and $AuCl^{2-}$ or $AuCl^{4-}$. Adv Mater 20:2517–2522
84. Choi Y, Hong S, Liu L, Kim SK, Park S (2012) Galvanically replaced hollow Au-Ag nanospheres: study of their surface plasmon resonance. Langmuir 28:6670–6676
85. Spivak MY, Bubnov RV, Yemets IM, Lazarenko LM, Tymoshok NO, Ulberg ZR (2013) Gold nanoparticles - the theranostic challenge for PPPM: nanocardiology application. EPMA J 4:18. doi:10.1186/1878-5085-4-18
86. Wang B, Yantsen E, Larson T, Karpiouk AB, Sethuraman S, Su JL, Sokolov K, Emelianov SY (2009) Plasmonic intravascular photoacoustic imaging for detection of macrophages in atherosclerotic plaques. Nano Lett 9:2212–2217
87. Cormode DP, Roessl E, Thran A, Skajaa T, Gordon RE, Schlomka JP, Fuster V, Fisher EA, Mulder WJ, Proksa R, Fayad ZA (2010) Atherosclerotic plaque composition: analysis with multicolor CT and targeted gold nanoparticles. Radiology 256:774–782
88. Lee S, Cha EJ, Park K, Lee SY, Hong JK, Sun IC, Kim SY, Choi K, Kwon IC, Kim K, Ahn CH (2008) A near-infrared fluorescence-quenched gold-nanoparticle imaging probe for in vivo drug screening and protease activity determination. Angew Chem Int Ed 47:2804–2807
89. Lukianova-Hleb EY, Mrochek AG, Lapotko DO (2009) Method for disruption and recanalization of atherosclerotic plaques in coronary vessels with photothermal bubbles generated around gold nanoparticles. Lasers Surg Med 41:240–247
90. Karaagac O, Kockar H, Beyaz S, Tanrisever T (2010) A simple way to synthesize superparamagnetic Iron Oxide nanoparticles in air atmosphere: iron ion concentration effect. IEEE Trans Magn 46:3978–3983
91. Weissleder R, Elizondo G, Wittenberg J, Rabito CA, Bengele HH, Josephson L (1990) Ultrasmall superparamagnetic iron oxide: characterization of a new class of contrast agents for MR imaging. Radiology 175:489–493
92. McCarthy JR, Weissleder R (2008) Multifunctional magnetic nanoparticles for targeted imaging and therapy. Adv Drug Deliv Rev 60:1241–1251
93. Sosnovik DE, Nahrendorf M, Weissleder R (2008) Magnetic nanoparticles for MR imaging: agents, techniques and cardiovascular applications. Basic Res Cardiol 103:122–130
94. Bjørnerud A, Johansson L (2004) The utility of superparamagnetic contrast agents in MRI: theoretical consideration and applications in the cardiovascular system. NMR Biomed 17:465–477
95. Yilmaz A, Dengler MA, van der Kuip H, Yildiz H, Rösch S, Klumpp S, Klingel K, Kandolf R, Helluy X, Hiller KH, Jakob PM, Sechtem U (2013) Imaging of myocardial infarction using ultrasmall superparamagnetic iron oxide nanoparticles: a human study using a multi-parametric cardiovascular magnetic resonance imaging approach. Eur Heart J 34:462–475
96. Jaffer FA, Nahrendorf M, Sosnovik D, Kelly KA, Aikawa E, Weissleder R (2006) Cellular imaging of inflammation in atherosclerosis using magnetofluorescent nanomaterials. Mol Imaging 5:85–92
97. Trivedi RA, U-King-Im JM, Graves MJ, Cross JJ, Horsley J, Goddard MJ, Skepper JN, Quartey G, Warburton E, Joubert I, Wang L, Kirkpatrick PJ, Brown J, Gillard JH (2004) In vivo detection of macrophages in human carotid atheroma: temporal dependence of ultrasmall superparamagnetic particles of iron oxide-enhanced MRI. Stroke 35:1631–1635
98. Tang TY, Muller KH, Graves MJ, Li ZY, Walsh SR, Young V, Sadat U, Howarth SP, Gillard JH (2009) Iron oxide particles for atheroma imaging. Arterioscler Thromb Vasc Biol 29:1001–1008
99. Schmitz SA, Taupitz M, Wagner S, Wol KJ, Beyersdorff D, Hamm B (2001) Magnetic resonance imaging of atherosclerotic plaques using superparamagenetic iron oxide particles. J Magn Reson Imaging 14:355–361
100. Morishige K, Kacher DF, Libby P, Josephson L, Ganz P, Weissleder R, Aikawa M (2010) High- resolution magnetic resonance imaging enhanced with superparamagnetic nanoparticles measures macrophage burden in atherosclerosis. Circulation 122:1707–1715
101. Sigovan M, Boussel L, Sulaiman A, Sappet-Marinier D, Alsaid H, Desbled-Mansard C, Ibarrola D, Gamondès D, Corot C, Lancelot E, Raynaud JS, Vives V, Laclédère C, Violas X, Douek PC, Canet-Soulas E (2009) Rapid clearance iron nanoparticles for inflammation imaging of atherosclerotic plaque: initial experience in animal model. Radiology 252:401–409
102. Kawahara I, Nakamoto M, Kitagawa N, Tsutsumi K, Nagata I, Morikawa M, Hayashi T (2008) Potential of magnetic resonance plaque imaging using superparamagnetic particles of iron oxide for the detection of carotid plaque. Neurol Med Chir 48: 157–162
103. Erdem SS, Sazonova IY, Hara T, Jaffer FA, McCarthy JR (2012) Detection and treatment of intravascular thrombi with magneto-

fluorescent nanoparticles. Methods Enzymol 508:191–209
104. Wuang SC, Neoh KG, Kang E-T, Pack DW, Leckband DE (2006) Heparinized magnertic nanoparticles: in vitro assessment for biomedical applications. Adv Funct Mater 16:1723–1730
105. Chorny M, Fishbein I, Yellen BB, Alferiev IS, Bakay M, Ganta S, Adamo R, Amiji M, Friedman G, Levy RJ (2010) Targeting stents with local delivery of paclitaxel-loaded magnetic nanoparticles using uniform fields. Proc Natl Acad Sci U S A 107:8346–8651
106. Sharma R, Kwon S (2007) New applications of nanoparticles in cardiovascular imaging. J Exp Nanosci 2:115–126
107. Cormode DP, Skajaa T, Fayad ZA, Mulder WJM (2009) Nanotechnology in medical imaging. Probe design and applications. Arterioscler Thromb Vasc Biol 29:992–1000
108. Sinusas AJ, Bengel F, Nahrendorf M, Epstein FH, Wu JC, Villanueva FS, Fayad ZA, Gropler RJ (2008) Multimodality cardiovascular molecular imaging, Part I. Circ Cardiovasc Imaging 1:244–256
109. Nahrendorf M, Sosnovik DE, French BA, Swirski FK, Bengel F, Sadeghi MM, Lindner JR, Wu JC, Kraitchman DL, Fayad ZA, Sinusas AJ (2009) Multimodality cardiovascular molecular imaging, Part II. Circ Cardiovasc Imaging 2:56–70
110. Smith AM, Gao X, Nie S (2004) Quantum dot nanocrystals for in vivo molecular and cellular imaging. Photochem Photobiol 80:377–385
111. Douma K, Prinzen L, Slaaf DW, Reutelingsperger CPM, Biessen EA, Hackeng TM, Post MJ, van Zandvoort MA (2009) Nanoparticles for optical molecular imaging of atherosclerosis. Small 5:544–557
112. Choi HS, Ipe BI, Misra P, Lee JH, Bawendi MG, Frangioni JV (2009) Tissue and organ-selective biodistribution of NIR-fluorescent quantum dots. Nano Lett 9:2354–2359
113. Tang Y, Han S, Liu H, Chen X, Huang L, Li X, Zhang J (2013) The role of surface chemistry in determining in vivo biodistribution and toxicity of CdSe/ZnS core-shell quantum dots. Biomaterials 34:8741–8755
114. Hauck TS, Anderson RE, Fischer HC, Newbigging S, Chan WC (2010) In vivo quantum-dot toxicity assessment. Small 6:138–144
115. Skajaa T, Cormode DP, Falk E, Mulder WJM, Fisher EA, Fayad ZA (2010) High-density lipoprotein based contrast agents for multimodal imaging of atherosclerosis. Arterioscler Thromb Vasc Biol 30:169–176
116. Frias JC, Williams KJ, Fisher EA, Fayad ZA (2004) Recombinant HDL-like nanoparticles: a specific contrast agent for MRI of atherosclerotic plaques. J Am Chem Soc 126:16316–16317
117. Frias JC, Ma Y, Williams KJ, Fayad ZA, Fisher EA (2006) Properties of a versatile nanoparticle platform contrast agent to image and characterize atherosclerotic plaques by magnetic resonance imaging. Nano Lett 6:2220–2224
118. Danhier F, Feron O, Préat V (2010) To exploit the tumor microenvironment: passive and active tumor targeting of nanocarriers for anti-cancer drug delivery. J Control Release 148:135–146
119. Hirsjärvi S, Passirani C, Benoit JP (2011) Passive and active tumour targeting with nanocarriers. Curr Drug Discov Technol 8:188–196
120. Huynh NT, Roger E, Lautram N, Benoît JP, Passirani C (2010) The rise and rise of stealth nanocarriers for cancer therapy: passive versus active targeting. Nanomedicine (Lond) 5:1415–1433
121. Blackwell JE, Dagia NM, Dickerson JB, Berg EL, Goetz DJ (2001) Ligand coated nanosphere adhesion to E- and P-selectin under static and flow conditions. Ann Biomed Eng 29:523–533
122. Jancsó G, Domoki F, Sántha P, Varga J, Fischer J, Orosz K, Penke B, Becskei A, Dux M, Tóth L (1998) Beta-amyloid (1-42) peptide impairs blood-brain barrier function after intracarotid infusion in rats. Neurosci Lett 253:139–141
123. Nishiya T, Kainoh M, Murata M, Handa M, Ikeda Y (2002) Reconstitution of adhesive properties of human platelets in liposomes carrying both recombinant glycoproteins Ia/IIa and Ib alpha under flow conditions: specific synergy of receptor-ligand interactions. Blood 100:136–142
124. Wada T, Okamura Y, Takeoka S, Sudo R, Ikeda Y, Tanishita K (2009) Deformability and adhesive force of artificial platelets measured by atomic force microscopy. J Biorheol 23:35–40
125. Nishiya T, Kainoh M, Murata M, Handa M, Ikeda Y (2001) Platelet interactions with liposomes carrying recombinant platelet membrane glycoproteins or fibrinogen: approach to platelet substitutes. Artif Cells Blood Substit Immobil Biotechnol 29:453–464
126. Wilchek M, Bayer EA, Livnah O (2006) Essentials of biorecognition: the (strept) avidin-biotin system as a model for protein-protein and protein-ligand interaction. Immunol Lett 103:27–32
127. Lesch HP, Kaikkonen MU, Pikkarainen JT, Ylä-Herttuala S (2010) Avidin-biotin tech-

nology in targeted therapy. Expert Opin Drug Deliv 7:551–564
128. Ganguly K, Krasik T, Medinilla S, Bdeir K, Cines DB, Muzykantov VR, Murciano JC (2005) Blood clearance and activity of erythrocyte-coupled fibrinolytics. J Pharmacol Exp Ther 312:1106–1113
129. Gersh KC, Zaitsev S, Cines DB, Muzykantov V, Weisel JW (2011) Flow-dependent channel formation in clots by an erythrocyte-bound fibrinolytic agent. Blood 117:4964–4967
130. Murciano JC, Medinilla S, Eslin D, Atochina E, Cines DB, Muzykantov VR (2003) Prophylactic fibrinolysis through selective dissolution of nascent clots by tPA-carrying erythrocytes. Nat Biotechnol 21:891–896
131. Muzykantov V (2013) Targeted drug delivery to endothelial adhesion molecules. ISRN Vasc Med 2013, 916254, http://dx.doi.org/10.1155/2013/916254
132. Sen Gupta A, von Recum HA (2014) Bioconjugation strategies: lipids, liposomes, polymersomes, and microbubbles. Chapter 6. In: Narain R (ed) Chemistry of bioconjugates: synthesis, characterization, and biomedical applications. Wiley, New York, NY
133. Demos MS, Alkan-Onyuksel H, Kane BJ, Ramani K, Nagaraj A, Greene R, Klegerman M, McPherson DD (1999) In vivo targeting of acoustically reflective liposomes for intravascular and transvascular ultrasonic enhancement. J Am Coll Cardiol 33:867–875
134. Klegerman ME, Zou Y, McPherson DD (2008) Fibrin targeting of echogenic liposomes with inactivated tissue plasminogen activator. J Liposome Res 18:95–112
135. Huang S-L (2008) Liposomes in ultrasonic drug and gene delivery. Adv Drug Deliv Rev 60:1167–1176
136. Li D, Patel AR, Klibanov AL, Kramer CM, Ruiz M, Kang BY, Mehta JL, Beller GA, Glover DK, Meyer CH (2010) Molecular imaging of atherosclerotic plaques targeted to oxidized LDL receptor LOX-1by SPECT/CT and Magnetic Resonance. Circ Cardiovasc Imaging 3:464–472
137. De Bittencourt PIH Jr, Lagranha DJ, Maslinkiewicz A, Senna SM, Tavares AMV, Baldissera LP, Janner DR, Peralta JS, Bock PM, Gutierrez LL, Scola G, Heck TG, Krause MS, Cruz LA, Abdalla DS, Lagranha CJ, Lima T, Curi R (2007) LipoCardium: endotheliumdirected cyclopentanone prostaglandin-based liposome formulation that completely reverses atherosclerotic lesions. Atherosclerosis 193:245–258
138. Haji-Valizadeh H, Modery-Pawlowski CL, Sen Gupta A (2014) An FVIII-derived peptide enables VWF-binding of a synthetic platelet surrogate without interfering with natural platelet adhesion to VWF. Nanoscale 6:4765–4773
139. Modery-Pawlowski CL, Tian LL, Ravikumar M, Wong TL, Sen Gupta A (2013) In vitro and in vivo hemostatic capabilities of a functionally integrated platelet-mimetic liposomal nanoconstruct. Biomaterials 34:3031–3041
140. Ravikumar M, Modery CL, Wong TL, Dzuricky M, Sen Gupta A (2012) Mimicking adhesive functionalities of blood platelets using ligand-decorated liposomes. Bioconjug Chem 23:1266–1275
141. Ravikumar M, Modery CL, Wong TL, Sen Gupta A (2012) Peptide-decorated liposomes promote arrest and aggregation of activated platelets under flow on vascular injury relevant protein surfaces in vitro. Biomacromolecules 13:1495–1502
142. Modery CL, Ravikumar M, Wong T, Dzuricky M, Durongkaveroj N, Sen Gupta A (2011) Heteromultivalent liposomal nanoconstructs for enhanced targeting and shear-stable binding to active platelets for site-selective vascular drug delivery. Biomaterials 32:9504–9514
143. Srinivasan R, Marchant RE, Sen Gupta A (2010) In vitro and in vivo platelet targeting by cyclic RGD-modified liposomes. J Biomed Mater Res A 93:1004–1015
144. Huang G, Zhou Z, Srinivasan R, Penn MS, Kottke-Marchant K, Marchant RE, Sen Gupta A (2008) Affinity manipulation of surface-conjugated RGD peptide to modulate binding of liposomes to activated platelets. Biomaterials 29:1676–1685
145. Sen Gupta A, Huang G, Lestini BJ, Sagnella S, Kottke-Marchant K, Marchant RE (2005) RGD-modified liposomes targeted to activated platelets as a potential vascular drug delivery system. Thromb Haemost 93:106–114
146. Mulder WJM, Strijkers GJ, Briley-Saboe KC, Frias JC, Aguinaldo JGS, Vucic E, Amirbekian V, Tang C, Chin PT, Nicolay K, Fayad ZA (2007) Molecular imaging of macrophages in atherosclerotic plaques using biomodal PEG-micelles. Magn Reson Med 58:1164–1170
147. Lipinski MJ, Amirbekian V, Frias JC, Aguinaldo JGS, Mani V, Briley-Saebo KC, Fuster V, Fallon JT, Fisher EA, Fayad ZA (2006) MRI to detect atherosclerosis with Gadoliniumcontaining immunomicelles targeting the macrophage scavenger receptor. Magn Reson Med 56:601–610
148. Briley-Saebo KC, Shaw PX, Mulder WJM, Choi SH, Vucic E, Aguinaldo JGS, Witztum JL, Fuster V, Tsimikas S, Fayad ZA (2008) Targeted molecular probes for imaging atherosclerotic lesions with magnetic resonance

using antibodies that recognize oxidation-specific epitopes. Circulation 117:3206–3215

149. Amirbekian V, Lipinski MJ, Frias JC, Amirbekian S, Briley-Saebo KC, Mani V, Samber D, Abbate A, Aguinaldo JGS, Masey D, Fuster V, Vetrovec G, Fayad ZA (2009) MR imaging of human atherosclerosis using immunomicelles molecularly targeted to macrophages. J Cardiovasc Magn Reson 11(Suppl 1):83
150. Chan JM, Zhang L, Tong R, Ghosh D, Gao W, Liao G, Yuet KP, Gray D, Rhee JW, Cheng J, Golomb G, Libby P, Langer R, Farokhzad OC (2010) Spatiotemporal controlled delivery of nanoparticles to injured vasculature. Proc Natl Acad Sci U S A 107:2213–2218
151. Chan JM, Rhee JW, Drum CL, Bronson RT, Golomb G, Langer R, Farokhzad OC (2011) In vivo prevention of arterial restenosis with paclitaxel-encapsulated targeted lipid-polymeric nanoparticles. Proc Natl Acad Sci U S A 108:19347–19352
152. Peters D, Kastantin M, Kotamraju VR, Karmali PP, Gujraty K, Tirrell M, Ruoslahti E (2009) Targeting atherosclerosis by using modular, multifunctional micelles. Proc Natl Acad Sci U S A 106:9815–9819
153. Hamzah J, Kotamraju VR, Seo JW, Agemy L, Fogal V, Mahakian LM, Peters D, Roth L, Gagnon MK, Ferrara KW, Ruoslahti E (2011) Specific penetration and accumulation of a homing peptide within atherosclerotic plaques of apolipoprotein E-deficient mice. Proc Natl Acad Sci U S A 108:7154–7159
154. Muro S, Dziubla T, Qiu W, Leferovich J, Cui X, Berk E, Muzykantov VR (2006) Endothelial targeting of high-affinity multivalent polymer nanocarriers directed to intracellular adhesion molecule. J Pharmacol Exp Ther 317:1161–1169
155. Deosarkar SP, Malgor R, Fu J, Kohn LD, Hanes J, Goetz DJ (2008) Polymeric particles conjugated with a ligandto VCAM-1 exhibit selective avid and focal adhesion to sites of atherosclerosis. Biotechnol Bioeng 101:400–407
156. Bertram JP, Williams CA, Robinson R, Segal SS, Flynn NT, Lavik EB (2009) Intravenous hemostat: nanotechnology to halt bleeding. Sci Transl Med 1:11–22
157. Coller BS, Springer KT, Beer JH, Mohandas N, Scudder LE, Norton KJ, West SM (1992) Thromboerythrocytes. In vitro studies of a potential autologous, semiartificial alternative to platelet transfusions. J Clin Invest 89:546–555
158. Levi M, Friederich PW, Middleton S, de Groot PG, Wu YP, Harris R, Biemond BJ, Heijnen HF, Levin J, ten Cate JW (1999) Fibrinogen-coated albumin microcapsules reduce bleeding in severely thrombocytopenic rabbits. Nat Med 5:107–111
159. Okamura Y, Takeoka S, Teramura Y, Maruyama H, Tsuchida E, Handa M, Ikeda Y (2005) Hemostatic effects of fibrinogen gamma-chain dodecapeptide-conjugated polymerized albumin particles in vitro and in vivo. Transfusion 45:1221–1228
160. Okamura Y, Fujie T, Nogawa M, Maruyama H, Handa M, Ikeda Y, Takeoka S (2008) Haemostatic effects of polymerized albumin particles carrying fibrinogen gamma-chain dodecapeptide as platelet substitutes in severely thrombocytopenic rabbits. Transfus Med 18:158–166
161. Takeoka S, Okamura Y, Teramura Y, Watanabe N, Suzuki H, Tsuchida E, Handa M, Ikeda Y (2003) Function of fibrinogen gamma-chain dodecapeptide-conjugated latex beads under flow. Biochem Biophys Res Commun 312:773–779
162. Okamura Y, Handa M, Suzuki H, Ikeda Y, Takeoka S (2006) New strategy of platelet substitutes for enhancing platelet aggregation at high shear rates: cooperative effects of a mixed system of fibrinogen gamma-chain dodecapeptide- or glycoprotein Ibalpha-conjugated latex beads under flow conditions. J Artif Organs 9:251–258
163. Chen W, Jarzyna PA, van Tilborg GA, Nguyen VA, Cormode DP, Klink A, Griffioen AW, Randolph GJ, Fisher EA, Mulder WJ, Fayad ZA (2010) RGD peptide functionalized and reconstituted high-density lipoprotein nanoparticles as a versatile and multimodal tumor targeting molecular imaging probe. FASEB J 24:1689–9169
164. Kaufmann BA, Sanders JM, Davis C, Xie A, Aldred P, Sarembock IJ, Lindner JR (2007) Molecular imaging of inflammation in atherosclerosis with targeted ultrasound detection of vascular cell adhesion molecule-1. Circulation 116:276–284
165. Lindner JR (2009) Molecular imaging of cardiovascular disease with contrastenhanced ultrasonography. Nat Rev Cardiol 6:475–481
166. Villanueva FS, Wagner W (2006) Ultrasound molecular imaging of cardiovascular disease. Nat Clin Pract Cardiovasc Med 5:S26–S32
167. Alonso A, Della Martina A, Stroick M, Fatar M, Griebe M, Pochon S, Schneider M, Hennerici M, Allémann E, Meairs S (2007) Molecular imaging of human thrombus with novel abciximab immunobubbles and ultrasound. Stroke 38:1508–1514
168. Hagooly A, Almutairi A, Rossin R, Shokeen M, Ananth A, Anderson C, Abendschein D,

Fréchet J, Welch M (2008) Evaluation of a RGD-dendrimer labeled with 76Br in hindlimb ischemia mouse model. J Nucl Med 49(Suppl 1):184
169. Taite LJ, West JL (2006) Poly(ethylene glycol)-lysine dendrimers for targeted delivery of nitric oxide. J Biomat Sci Polym Ed 17:1159–1172
170. Makowski M, Jansen C, Botnar R, Kim WY, Maintz D, Spuentrup E (2010) Molecular MRI of atherosclerosis: from mouse to man. Medicamundi 54:14
171. Thukkani AK, Glaus C, Welch MJ (2010) Molecular imaging of vascular inflammation with nanoparticles. Curr Cardiovasc Imaging Rep 3:151–161
172. McAteer MA, Akhtar AM, von Zuhr Muhlen C, Choudhury RP (2010) An approach to molecular imaging of atherosclerosis, thrombosis, and vascular inflammation using microparticles of iron oxide. Atherosclerosis 209:18–27
173. Smith BR, Heverhagen J, Knopp M, Schmalbrock P, Shapiro J, Shiomi M, Moldovan NI, Ferrari M, Lee SC (2007) Localization to atherosclerotic plaque and biodistribution of biochemically derivatized superparamagnetic iron oxide nanoparticles (SPIONs) contrast particles for magnetic resonance imaging (MRI). Biomed Microdevices 9:719–727
174. Ferrara DE, Glaus C, Taylor WR (2008) Targeting vascular epitopes using quantum dots. Nanoparticles in biomedical imaging. Fundam Biomed Tech 102:443–461
175. Jayagopal A, Russ PK, Haselton FR (2007) Surface engineering of quantum dots for in vivo vascular imaging. Bioconjug Chem 18:1424–1433
176. Kahn E, Vejux A, Menetrier F, Maiza C, Hammann A, Sequeira-Le GA, Frouin F, Tourneur Y, Brau F, Riedinger JM, Steinmetz E, Todd-Pokropek A, Lizard G (2006) Analysis of CD36 expression on human monocytic cells and atherosclerotic tissue sections with quantum dots: investigation by flow cytometry and spectral imaging microscopy. Anal Quant Cytol Histol 28:14–26
177. Prinzen L, Miserus RJHM, Dirksen A, Hackend TM, Deckers N, Bitsch NJ, Megens RT, Douma K, Heemskerk JW, Kooi ME, Frederik PM, Slaaf DW, van Zandvoort MA, Reutelingsperger CP (2007) Optical and magnetic resonance imaging of cell death and platelet activation using Annexin A5-functionalized quantum dot. Nano Lett 7:93–100
178. Mulder WJM, Koole R, Brandwijk RJ, Storm G, Chin PTK, Strijkers GJ (2006) Quantum dots with a paramagnetic coating as a bimodal molecular imaging probe. Nano Lett 6:1–6
179. Chang E, Miller JS, Sun J, Yu WW, Colvin VL, Drezek R, West JL (2005) Protease-activated quantum dot probes. Biochem Biophys Res Commun 334:1317–1321
180. Edelman ER, Adams DA, Karnovsky MJ (1990) Effect of controlled adventitial heparin delivery on smooth muscle cell proliferation following endothelial injury. Proc Natl Acad Sci U S A 87:3773–3777
181. Villa AE, Guzman LA, Chen W, Golomb G, Levy RJ, Topol EJ (1994) Local delivery of dexamethasone for prevention of neointimal proliferation in a rat model of balloon angioplasty. J Clin Invest 93:1243–1249
182. Nathan A, Nugent MA, Edelman ER (1995) Tissue engineered perivascular endothelial cell implants regulate vascular injury. Proc Natl Acad Sci U S A 92:8130–8134
183. Nugent HM, Rogers C, Edelman ER (1999) Endothelial implants inhibit intimal hyperplasia after porcine angioplasty. Circ Res 84:384–391
184. Wilensky RL, March KL, Gradus-Pizlo I et al (1995) Regional and arterial localization of radioactive microparticles after local delivery by unsupported or supported porous balloon catheters. Am Heart J 129:852–859
185. Zhang L, Keogh S, Rickard CM (2013) Reducing the risk of infection associated with vascular access devices through nanotechnology: a perspective. Int J Nanomed 8:4453–4466
186. Harris DL, Graffagnini MJ (2007) Nanomaterials in medical devices: a snapshot of markets, technologies and companies. Nanotechnol Law Business 4:415–422
187. Martinez AW, Chaikof EL (2011) Microfabrication and nanotechnology in stent design. Wiley Interdiscip Rev Nanomed Nanobiotechnol 3:256–268
188. McDowell G, Slevin M, Krupinski J (2011) Nanotechnology for the treatment of coronary in stent restenosis: a clinical perspective. Vasc Cell 3:8, http://www.vascularcell.com
189. Yin R-X, Yang D-Z, Wu J-Z (2014) Nanoparticle drug- and gene-eluting stents for the prevention and treatment of coronary restenosis. Theranostics 4:175–200
190. Goh D, Tan A, Farhatnia Y, Rajadas J, Alavijeh MS, Seifalian AM (2013) Nanotechnology-based gene-eluting stents. Mol Pharm 10:1279–1298
191. Sarkar S, Schmitz-Rixen T, Hamilton G, Seifalian AM (2007) Achieving the ideal properties for vascular bypass grafts using a tissue engineered approach: a review. Med Biol Eng Comput 45:327–336

192. de Mel A, Naghavi N, Cousins BG, Clatworthy I, Hamilton G, Darbyshire A, Seifalian AM (2014) Nitric oxide-eluting nanocomposite for cardiovascular implants. J Mater Sci Mater Med 25:917–929
193. Tao L, Hu W, Liu Y, Huang G, Sumer BD, Gao J (2011) Shape-specific polymeric nanomedicine: emerging opportunities and challenges. Exp Biol Med 236:20–29
194. Champion JA, Katare YK, Mitragotri S (2007) Particle shape: a new design parameter for micro- and nanoscale drug delivery carriers. J Control Release 121:3–9
195. Shah S, Liu Y, Hu W, Gao J (2011) Modeling particle shape-dependent dynamics in nanomedicine. J Nanosci Nanotechnol 11:919–928
196. Charoenphol P, Huang RB, Eniola-Adefeso O (2010) Potential role of size and hemodynamics in the efficacy of vascular-targeted spherical drug carriers. Biomaterials 31:1392–1402
197. Toy R, Hayden E, Shoup C, Baskaran H, Karathanasis E (2011) The effects of particle size, density and shape on margination of nanoparticles in microcirculation. Nanotechnology 22:1–9
198. Decuzzi P, Lee S, Bhushan B, Ferrari M (2005) A theoretical model for the margination of particles within blood vessels. Ann Biomed Eng 33:179–190
199. Skorczewski T, Erickson LC, Fogelson AL (2013) Platelet motion near a vessel wall or thrombus surface in two-dimensional whole blood simulations. Biophys J 104:1764–1772
200. Tokarev AA, Butylin AA, Ermakova EA, Shnol EE, Panasenko GP, Ataullakhanov FI (2011) Finite platelet size could be responsible for platelet margination effect. Biophys J 101:1835–1843
201. Aarts PA, van den Broek SA, Prins GW, Kuiken GD, Sixma JJ, Heethaar RM (1988) Blood platelets are concentrated near the wall and red blood cells, in the center in flowing blood. Arterioscler Thromb Vasc Biol 8:819–824
202. Perry JL, Herlihy KP, Napier ME, Desimone JM (2011) PRINT: a novel platform toward shape and size specific nanoparticle theranostics. Acc Chem Res 44:990–998
203. Daum N, Tscheka C, Neumeyer A, Schneider M (2012) Novel approaches for drug delivery systems in nanomedicine: effects of particle design and shape. Wiley Interdiscip Rev Nanomed Nanobiotechnol 4:52–65
204. Caldorera-Moore M, Guimard N, Shi L, Roy K (2010) Designer nanoparticles: incorporating size, shape, and triggered release into nanoscale drug carriers. Expert Opin Drug Deliv 7:479–495
205. Mitragotri S, Lahann J (2009) Physical approaches to biomaterial design. Nat Mater 8:15–23
206. Champion JA, Katare YK, Mitragotri S (2007) Making polymeric micro- and nanoparticles of complex shapes. Proc Natl Acad Sci U S A 104:11901–11904
207. Doshi N, Orje JN, Molins B, Smith JW, Mitragorti S, Ruggeri ZM (2012) Platelet mimetic particles for targeting thrombi inflowing blood. Adv Mater 24:3864–3869
208. Siepmann J, Siepmann F (2012) Modeling of diffusion controlled drug delivery. J Control Release 161:351–362
209. Siepmann J, Siepmann F (2013) Mathematical model of drug dissolution. Int J Pharm 453:12–24
210. Peppas NA, Narasimhan B (2014) Mathematical models in drug delivery: how modeling has shaped the way we design new drug delivery systems. J Control Release 190:75
211. Schmaljohann D (2006) Thermo- and pH-responsive polymers in drug delivery. Adv Drug Deliv Rev 58:1655–1670
212. Meng F, Zhong Z, Feijen J (2009) Stimuli-responsive polymersomes for programmed drug delivery. Biomacromolecules 10:197–209
213. Shum P, Kim JM, Thompson DH (2001) Phototriggering of liposomal drug delivery systems. Adv Drug Deliv Rev 53:273–284
214. Paasonen L, Sipilä T, Subrizi A, Laurinmäki P, Butcher SJ, Rappolt M, Yaghmur A, Urtti A, Yliperttula M (2010) Gold-embedded photosensitive liposomes for drug delivery: triggering mechanism and intracellular release. J Control Release 147:136–143
215. Peiris PM, Toy R, Abramowski A, Vicente P, Tucci S, Bauer L, Mayer A, Tam M, Doolittle E, Pansky J, Tran E, Lin D, Schiemann WP, Ghaghada KB, Griswold MA, Karathanasis E (2014) Treatment of cancer micrometastasis using a multicomponent chain-like nanoparticle. J Control Release 173:51–58
216. Marsh JN, Senpan A, Hu G, Scott MJ, Gaffney PJ, Wickline SA, Lanza GM (2007) Fibrin-targeted perfluorocarbon nanoparticles for targeted thrombolysis. Nanomedicine (Lond) 2:533–543
217. Korin N, Kanapathipillai M, Matthews BD, Crescente M, Brill A, Mammoto T, Ghosh K, Jurek S, Bencherif SA, Bhatta D, Coskun AU, Feldman CL, Wagner DD, Ingber DE (2012) Shear-activated nanotherapeutics for drug tar-

geting to obstructed blood vessels. Science 337:738–742
218. Holme MN, Fedotenko IA, Abegg D, Althaus J, Babel L, Favarger F, Reiter R, Tanasescu R, Zaffalon PL, Ziegler A, Müller B, Saxer T, Zumbuehl A (2012) Shear-stress sensitive lenticular vesicles for targeted drug delivery. Nat Nanotechnol 7:536–543
219. Modery-Pawlowski CL, Sen Gupta A (2014) Heteromultivalent ligand-decoration for actively targeted nanomedicine. Biomaterials 35:2568–2579

Chapter 14

Gastrointestinal System

Yoshimine Fujii and Shinji Sakuma

Abstract

Nanotechnologies are currently an undoubted driving force for innovative progress in science. Particularly, successful development of nano-/micromaterials has largely contributed to medical innovation. Here, the potential of nano-/micromaterials used for the treatment and diagnosis of gastrointestinal diseases is described. Furthermore, the gastrointestinal system is most commonly utilized as the route of drug administration. We also discuss the potential of nano-/micromaterials as carriers that enhance oral absorption of drugs from the perspective of improvement of solubility and permeability.

Key words Gastrointestinal disease, *Helicobacter pylori* infection, Inflammatory bowel disease, Ulcerative colitis, Colorectal cancer, Intestinal transporter, Gut-associated lymphoid tissue, Oral absorption enhancement, Solubility improvement, Permeability improvement

1 Introduction

The gastrointestinal system possesses diverse functions that are indispensable for the maintenance of life. The primal function is the absorption of nutrients in the diet. For instance, carbohydrates, which are one of the three major nutrients, are hydrolyzed by digestive enzymes in the gastrointestinal tract, and the resultant monosaccharides are delivered to the systemic circulation via influx hexose transporters expressed in the apical membranes of intestinal epithelial cells [1]. The gastrointestinal system has another function that protects the body from unfavorable substances. Such substances taken up into intestinal epithelial cells are often excreted to the intestinal lumen via efflux transporters such as P-glycoprotein [2]. Unfavorable substances may be inactivated inside the cells by cytosolic enzymes such as CYP3A4 [3]. These protective functions sometimes induce drug–drug and drug–food interactions. The gastrointestinal system also contributes to homeostasis through immune response and hormone control [4, 5].

Zheng-Rong Lu and Shinji Sakuma (eds.), *Nanomaterials in Pharmacology*, Methods in Pharmacology and Toxicology, DOI 10.1007/978-1-4939-3121-7_14, © Springer Science+Business Media New York 2016

Nanomaterials have been investigated with the aim of treating local and systemic diseases related to the gastrointestinal system. The local diseases mainly include infection, inflammation, and cancer. Nanomaterials are also studied as diagnostic tools for these diseases. Researchers have separately taken up the challenge for the treatment of the systemic diseases through interactions between nanomaterials and functional molecules at the gastrointestinal mucosa. Nanomaterials are also expected to act as drug carriers that enhance pharmacological activities of oral medicines through solubility improvement, absorption enhancement, etc. This chapter describes a potential of nano-/micromaterials in the gastrointestinal system from the abovementioned three perspectives.

2 Nano-/Micromaterials for the Treatment of Local Diseases

Nano-/micromaterials for the treatment and diagnosis of local diseases in the gastrointestinal system are described in this section. We focused on *Helicobacter pylori (H. pylori)* infection in the stomach, ulcerative colitis, and colorectal cancer diagnosis.

2.1 Treatment of H. pylori Infection

H. pylori, which is one of the gram-negative bacteria, is regarded as a major pathogen that causes chronic gastritis, peptic ulcers, and gastric cancer in humans [6]. Current drug therapy is a combination of antibiotics and proton pump inhibitors. As the former drug, clarithromycin is orally administered with either amoxicillin or metronidazole [7]. These antibiotics are usually given twice a day for 1 week. However, the standard regimen does not always provide successful treatment of *H. pylori* infection due to resistance against the antibiotics and poor adherence of patients. It seems that an extension of the dose period and an increase in the number of antibiotics improve the success rate of the treatment.

Nano-/micromaterials have been investigated with the aim of improving drug therapeutics for *H. pylori* infection. The scientific basis is prolonged gastric retention of nano-/micromaterials containing antibiotics and sustained drug release in the stomach [8–10]. Since a couple of the abovementioned functions lead to a significant exposure of antibiotics for *H. pylori*, the pathogen is effectively eradicated from the stomach. On the other hand, when conventional pharmaceutical products, which are rapidly emptied from the stomach and from which antibiotics are immediately released, are used, the performance of antibiotics in the stomach is not maximized. Hao et al. evaluated a potential of metronidazole-loaded porous Eudragit® RS microparticles as a drug candidate used for the treatment of *H. pylori* infection [8]. Eudragit® RS, which is a water-insoluble polymer, was dissolved in dichloromethane with metronidazole, and the electrospray was conducted to prepare drug-loaded microparticles. The mean particle size was about 1 μm and a porous structure was observed. When Eudragit® RS concentration in the organic solvent was set to 1 %, the resulting microparticles floated in the simulated gastric fluid of pH 1.2 for more than 10 h. The concentration ratio of metronidazole to the polymer largely affected drug dissolution from microparticles. When the ratio was set to 3 (drug/polymer = 0.35 %/1 %), 12-h sustained release of metronidazole was observed in the simulated gastric fluid. Gamma scintigraphy demonstrated that ^{131}I-labeled microparticles remained in the stomach of fasted New Zealand white rabbits even at 8 h after oral administration. Figure 1 shows in vitro and in vivo activities of metronidazole and metronidazole-loaded microparticles. An immediate reduction of *H. pylori* count (colony-forming unit (CFU)/mL) was observed, irrespective of

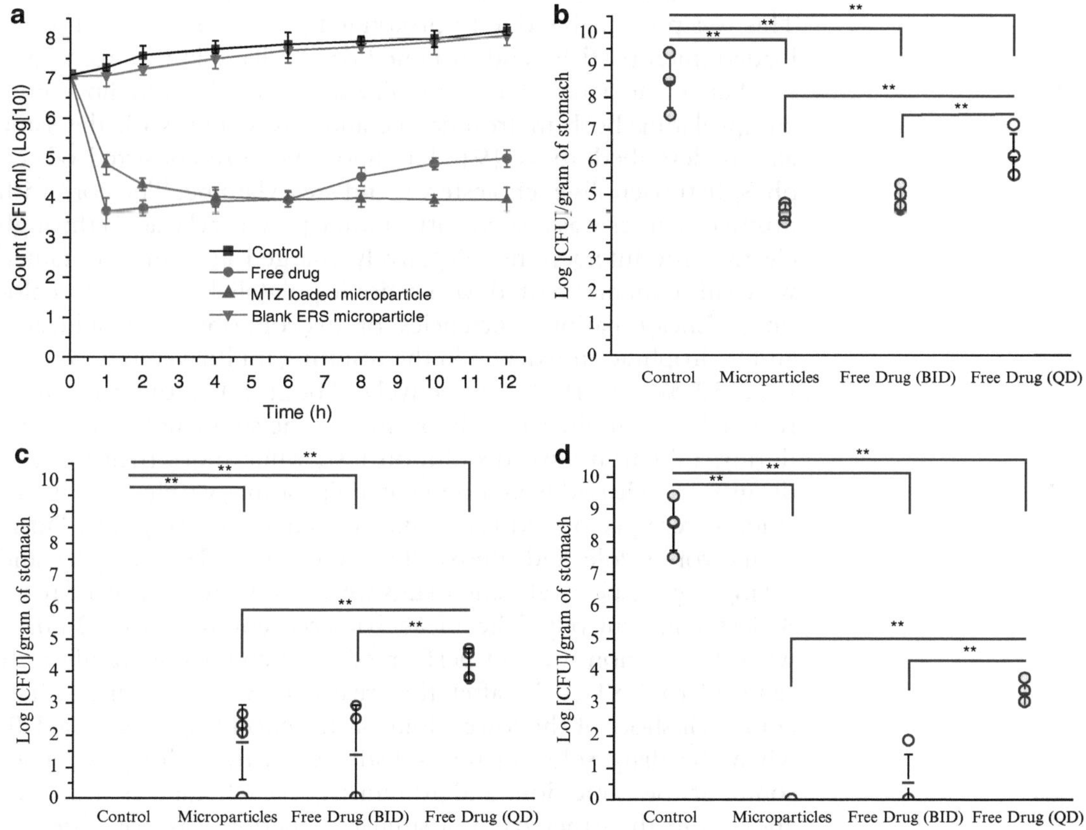

Fig. 1 (**a**) In vitro antibacterial effect of free metronidazole (MTZ) and Eudragit RS (ERS) microparticles with or without metronidazole. Drug concentration in media was adjusted to 40 μg/mL. (**b–d**) Mice infected with *H. pylori* were treated with either free MTZ or MTZ-loaded microparticles for 3 days. Free drug was consecutively administered once (QD) or twice (BID) a day, while microparticles were administered once a day. Each dose was set to 5 mg/kg/time (**b**), 15 mg/kg/time (**c**), and 25 mg/kg/time (**d**). Each figure represents bacterial counts of *H. pylori* in the stomach after the treatment (**$p < 0.01$, *$p < 0.05$, compared with the control group)

the drug type; however, the antibacterial effect of metronidazole loaded in microparticles seemed to be more sustainable than that of free drug. Mouse experiments revealed that the antibacterial effect of metronidazole depended on the dose and frequency of administration. The mean bacterial count (log of CFU per gram of stomach) was 8.49 ± 0.79 when medication was not performed. The count was significantly reduced to 6.15 ± 0.73 when metronidazole was orally given once a day at a dose of 5 mg/kg/time. A further reduction was observed as the dose was escalated. In vivo antibacterial effects strengthened when the number of administration was doubled, indicating that the daily dose was also doubled. The best regimen of free metronidazole was to be given twice a day at a dose of 25 mg/kg/time (the daily dose was 50 mg/kg). On the other hand, an equivalent antibacterial effect was observed when metronidazole-loaded microparticles were orally given once a day at a dose of 25 mg/kg/time (the daily dose was 25 mg/kg). This was presumably due to prolonged gastric retention of drug-loaded microparticles and sustained drug release in the stomach.

Jain et al. studied the usefulness of multilayered liposomes encapsulating both metronidazole and amoxicillin with the same aim as described above [9]. The liposome core consisted of egg phosphatidylcholine, cholesterol, and stearylamine. The core with positive charges was coated with anionic poly(acrylic acid) through electrostatic interactions. Negatively charged liposomes obtained were subsequently coated with cationic poly(allylamine hydrochloride). Encapsulation efficiencies of hydrophobic metronidazole and hydrophilic amoxicillin in the resulting multilayered liposomes were 52 % and 48 %, respectively. About 50 % of drugs were released from multilayered liposomes in the simulated gastric fluid during a 24-h in vitro dissolution test, while more than 95 % of drugs were released from non-coated liposomes within 6 h. In vivo studies were performed using mice infected with *H. pylori.* Doses of metronidazole and amoxicillin were set to 16.5 mg/kg and 30 mg/kg, respectively, and drugs were orally given once a day for 3 days consecutively. The mean bacterial count was 6.82 ± 0.13 when medication was not performed. The count was significantly reduced to 1.84 ± 0.24 after the treatment with free drugs. The count fell short of the lower limit of detection (log of CFU < 1.0) when the drug solution was substituted with multilayered liposomes at the same dose and administration schedule as described above. On the other hand, a similar reduction was not observed when non-coated liposomes were administered. Electrostatic interactions between cationic multilayered liposomes and anionic gastric mucosa protected the mucosa from *H. pylori* attachment. It appeared that an increase in the antibacterial effect was due to the protection and sustained drug release.

2.2 Treatment of Ulcerative Colitis

Chronic inflammatory bowel disease (IBD), such as ulcerative colitis, causes severe digestive organ symptoms such as diarrhea, bloody stool, and abdominal pain [11]. Anti-inflammatory drugs and immunosuppressive agents are currently used for the treatment of IBD. The most common anti-inflammatory drugs are sulfasalazine, mesalamine, olsalazine, and balsalazide [12]. These anti-inflammatory drugs, which are suitable for the treatment of mild and moderate IBD, act directly in inflamed sites of the large intestine. However, since orally administered drugs are absorbed from the small intestine, a limited amount of drugs reaches the inflamed sites. Therefore, nano-/micromaterials used for the treatment of IBD are primarily required to possess the targeting ability to inflamed sites, which is accompanied by high safety, because the systemic exposure of drugs is reduced and the disease is locally treated with a small amount of drugs.

Lamprecht et al. found that there was a tendency for small particles to accumulate on inflamed sites of the large intestine [13]. Fluorescent polystyrene particles with negative charges were orally administered to rats with or without trinitrobenzene sulfonic acid (TNBS)-induced ulcerative colitis. Three days after administration, fluorescence in the large intestine of rats with ulcerative colitis was compared with that of normal rats. The former fluorescence was 6.5 times that of the latter fluorescence when fluorescent particles with a mean diameter of 0.1 μm were used. The fluorescence ratio (rat with ulcerative colitis/colitis-free normal rat) was reduced to 5 and 4 when the mean particle size was escalated to 1 μm and 10 μm, respectively. Deposition of the fluorescent particles in the colonic mucosa of the same individual with ulcerative colitis was subsequently evaluated. Approximately 15 % of administered particles with a mean diameter of 0.1 μm accumulated in inflamed sites; however, the percentage decreased with an increase in the particle size (approximately 9 % of particles with a diameter of 1 μm and 5 % of particles with a diameter of 10 μm). An extreme increase in mucosal production in inflamed sites was observed when compared with normal sites. It appeared that this change resulted in high accumulation of particulate substances in inflamed sites. Nano-sized particles might easily reach the mucus layers because they are relatively small.

The same research group also evaluated a potential of poly(lactic acid-co-glycolic acid) (PLGA) nanoparticles incorporating rolipram, which is a phosphodiesterase IV inhibitor with anti-inflammatory activities, as a drug candidate used for the treatment of ulcerative colitis [14]. One-week sustained release of rolipram was observed after about 30 % of the drug was initially released within 2 h. Figure 2 shows the change in the mean clinical activity score after oral administration of each formulation containing rolipram to rats with or without ulcerative colitis. This score increases as the disease becomes worse. The score exceeded 2 when

Fig. 2 Change in the mean clinical activity score after oral administration of each formulation containing rolipram to rats with or without trinitrobenzene sulfonic acid (TNBS)-induced ulcerative colitis ($n=6$). The intrarectal administration of TNBS (150 mg/kg) was followed by drug administration with a 3-day interval. Each formulation was orally given once a day for 5 days consecutively at a dose of 10 mg/kg as a rolipram equivalent (*filled square*, normal rats; *filled circle*, non-treated rats with colitis (saline administered); *filled triangle*, rats with colitis treated with rolipram solution; *filled inverted triangle*, rats with colitis treated with rolipram-containing PLGA nanoparticles (an average molecular weight of PLGA, 20,000); *filled diamond*, rats with colitis treated with rolipram-containing PLGA nanoparticles (an average molecular weight of PLGA, 5000)). *$p<0.05$ (compared with non-treated rats with colitis)

rats were maintained for 3 days after TNBS administration. A significant reduction of the mean clinical activity was observed when medication was performed, irrespective of the formulation type. However, at 5 days after discontinuance of medication, the score for rats treated with drug solution returned to the high value observed before the drug treatment. On the other hand, the score was constantly low when rats were treated with nanoparticles incorporating rolipram. Unfavorable neurotropic actions, caused by the systemic exposure of rolipram (forepaw shaking and grooming), were also observed when rats were treated with drug solution. The adverse effects were reduced when PLGA nanoparticles incorporating rolipram were used. An advantage of nanoparticles to solution was presumably due to the specific delivery of anti-inflammatory drugs to inflamed sites and sustained drug release in the target area.

2.3 Diagnosis of Colorectal Cancer

Colorectal cancer is a major cause of mortality and morbidity in developed countries [15]. Currently, surgical removal is the primary treatment of choice, and early detection and resection are indispensable for curing colorectal cancer [16]. Colonoscopy has been effectively used for screening colorectal cancer due to its ability to provide a definitive diagnosis [17]. Colorectal cancer initially develops in the mucous membrane of the large intestine. The cancer, which remains in the mucous membrane or only minimally invades the submucosal tissues without vessel invasion, is often removed through a colonoscopy procedure. Alternatively, when the cancer is detected in the early stage, it can be treated by a minimally invasive operation, known as endoscopic mucosal resection [18].

Magnifying endoscopy and novel imaging strategies for endoscopy have enabled physicians to detect small changes on the mucosal surface of the large intestine [19]. Most colorectal cancer can be prevented through the detection and removal of premalignant polypoid lesions [20]. However, conventional endoscopy is not suitable for flat and depressed neoplasms [21]. Patients with chronic IBD face increased risk of developing malignancy due to undetected dysplastic lesions [22]. The limitation of current endoscopic screening is due to lack of diagnosis at the molecular level as it is based on morphological changes visualized through a macroscopic view of the mucosal surface. Improved methods for detecting early changes in high-risk individuals are strongly required [23]. Furthermore, accurate detection of neoplastic mucosal changes in real time still remains a significant challenge. Tissues that look abnormal are sampled under endoscopic observation. Subsequent histological evaluation of the samples is a prerequisite for a definitive diagnosis of the cancer. There is also a requirement for a new method that allows physicians to diagnose early-stage primary colon carcinoma on the mucosal surface in real time.

The imaging agent can become a useful diagnostic tool for minute tumors that are currently undetectable or difficult to detect under endoscopic observation. Sakuma et al. designed a nonabsorbable imaging agent capable of being administered intracolonically for the purpose of colonoscopy [24–26]. The imaging agent consists of peanut agglutinin (PNA)-immobilized polystyrene nanospheres with surface poly(N-vinylacetamide) (PNVA) chains encapsulating coumarin 6 (Fig. 3). The Thomsen–Friedenreich (TF) antigen is specifically expressed on the mucosal side of colorectal cancer cells [27]. Its terminal sugar is β-D-galactosyl-(1-3)-N-acetyl-D-galactosamine (Gal-β(1-3)GalNAc), and this sugar is masked by an oligosaccharide side chain extension or sialylation in normal cells [27]. Lectins are proteins that recognize and bind reversibly to specific carbohydrate residues expressed on the cell surface [28]. PNA, which is a typical lectin that recognizes Gal-β(1-3)GalNAc, is immobilized on the nanosphere surface as a targeting moiety that binds to the TF antigen through sugar recognition. Sakuma et al. has separately found that PNVA rarely adhered to the intestinal mucosa due to its strong hydrophilicity [29]. This polymer chain is localized on the nanosphere surface to

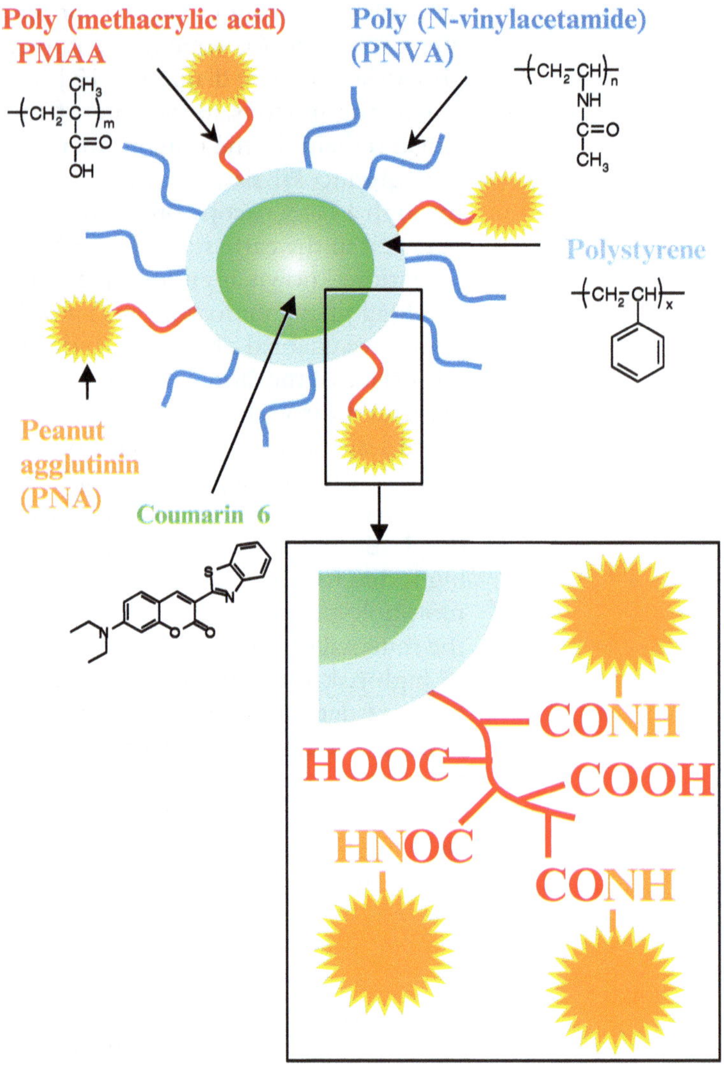

Fig. 3 Schematic representation of PNA-immobilized polystyrene nanospheres with surface PNVA chains encapsulating coumarin 6 (PMAA chains are used as a linker for the PNA immobilization)

enhance the specificity of PNA by reducing nonspecific interactions between the nanospheres and normal tissues. Coumarin 6 is encapsulated into the nanosphere core as the fluorescent dye that produces an endoscopically detectable fluorescence intensity. The research group has successfully demonstrated that the imaging agent recognized millimeter-sized colorectal tumors on the mucosal surface with high affinity and specificity in human colorectal cancer orthotopic mouse models [24]. Furthermore, as shown in Fig. 4, the imaging agent, which was named nanobeacon, detected dynamic changes of the TF antigen in human colonic tissues from

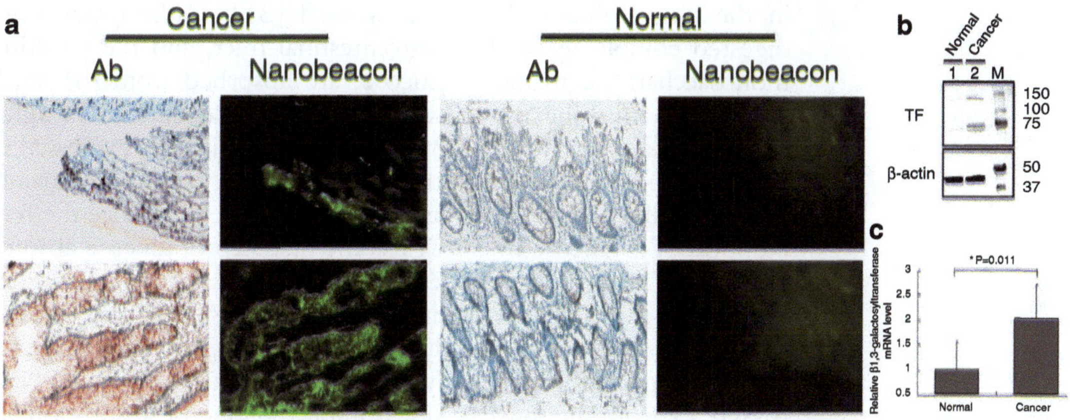

Fig. 4 (**a**) The expression of TF antigen on human colonic tissues from normal controls and cancer patients was detected using PNA molecules immobilized on the surface of the nanobeacon and confirmed by immunohistochemistry. Strong fluorescence from the cancer section was correlated to a positive signal in IHC staining of the consecutive slide. Exposure time in fluorescence observation was 400 ms with magnification at ×200 each. (**b**) Representative results of Western blot (immunoblot) analysis of TF antigen expression in clinical human tissues with and without colorectal cancer. β-Actin was shown as a loading control. Molecular weights of TF antigen detected in human colorectal tissue samples were approximately 147, 84, and 77 kDa, respectively. (**c**) A relative mRNA expression level of β1,3-galactosyltransferase in clinical human colorectal tissues with and without cancer was analyzed by qPCR ($n = 3$, *$p = 0.011$)

patients with colorectal tumors; however, the nanobeacon did not bind to human colonic tissues from normal controls [26]. Data strongly supported the potential use of the nanobeacon for imaging the TF antigen as a biomarker for the early detection and prediction of the progression of colorectal cancer at a molecular level.

3 Nano-/Micromaterials for the Treatment of Systemic Diseases

Generally speaking, nano-/micromaterials are not absorbed through the gastrointestinal tract. Therefore, interactions of these materials with functional molecules on the gastrointestinal mucosa are expected to trigger off the treatment of systemic diseases. Here, a couple of attempts are focused: the treatment of diabetes through inhibition of hexose transporters and oral vaccination through association with the gut-associated lymphoid tissue (GALT).

3.1 Treatment of Diabetes

Diabetes is a metabolic disease caused by either the deficiency of insulin secretion or cellular resistance to insulin, which results in hyperglycemia. The disease is classified as insulin-dependent type I diabetes mellitus and non-insulin-dependent type II diabetes mellitus; over 90 % of diabetic patients suffer from the latter type. The aim of most diabetes treatments is to maintain an appropriate blood glucose level [30]. It is also important to suppress the rapid increase in the blood glucose level after a meal [31]. Carbohydrates are digested completely in the gastrointestinal tract, and the resulting monosaccharides, mainly D-glucose, are absorbed from the small intestine via influx hexose transporters. Sodium-dependent Na^+/glucose cotransporter 1 (SGLT1), which is predominantly expressed in the apical membranes of intestinal epithelial cells, contributes mainly to the apical membrane permeation of D-glucose (1). Since the recognition of D-glucose by SGLT1 is the first step of glucose absorption, SGLT1 inhibition can be one of the most effective approaches to suppress the rapid increase in the blood glucose level after a meal.

Ikumi et al. designed polymeric conjugates bearing glucosides with the expectation that orally administered conjugates would bind to SGLT1 from the mucosal side, inhibit the glucose absorption via SGLT1, and consequently suppress an increase in the blood glucose level without systemic exposure of the conjugates [32, 33]. Phloridzin is a glucoside that inhibits D-glucose transport competitively through the binding of intramolecular glucose moieties to SGLT1 [34]. Strong inhibition was observed through in vitro experiments; however, phloridzin rarely inhibits D-glucose transport when it was orally given to animals, due to removal of the glucose moieties through the hydrolysis of the glucoside bond by β-glucosidase located on the apical membranes of the intestine. Steric hindrance of the polymer chain often contributes to the stability of enzyme-susceptible chemical bonds [35]. As shown in Fig. 5, phloridzin was grafted onto the polymer backbone of poly(γ-glutamic acid)

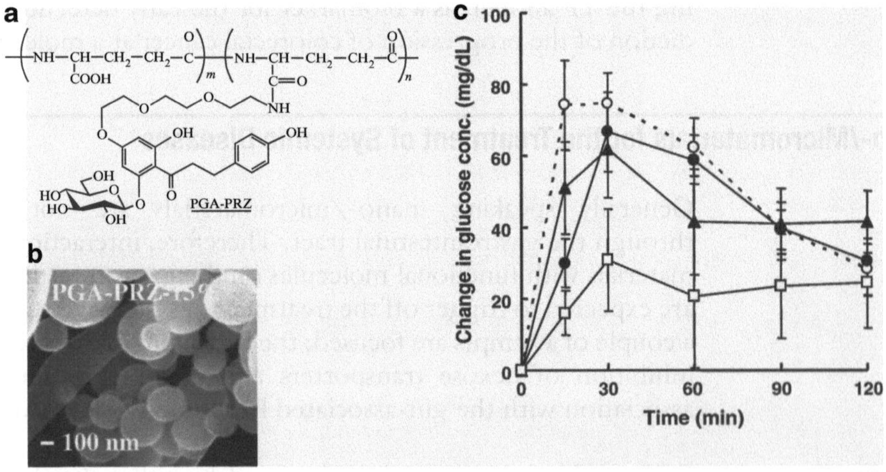

Fig. 5 (**a**) Chemical structure of poly(γ-glutamic acid) bearing phloridzin (PGA-PRZ). (**b**) Scanning electron microscope image of PGA-PRZ with a phloridzin content of 15 %. (**c**) Concentration–time profiles of glucose in blood after oral administration of glucose. Water (*open circle*), phloridzin (*filled circle*, 0.125 mmol/kg; *filled triangle*, 0.25 mmol/kg), or PGA-PRZ with a phloridzin content of 15 % (*open square*, 0.125 mmol/kg as a phloridzin equivalent) were given orally at 10 min before glucose administration. Data were represented as the change in glucose concentration from before to after glucose administration ($n=6$, mean ± s.e.)

(γ-PGA). In vitro stability studies indicated that γ-PGA bearing phloridzin remained unchanged in the gastrointestinal tract. The stabilization of the glucoside bond was presumably due to the spontaneous self-assembly of the conjugate. This nanostructure prevented the glucoside bond from being hydrolyzed by β-glucosidase. The conjugate significantly suppressed an increase in the blood glucose level after oral administration of D-glucose in rats through inhibition of SGLT1-mediated D-glucose transport. The research group has also demonstrated that phloridzin conjugates whose polymeric platform was composed of dendrimers, which are nanometer-sized starburst macromolecules, possessed a similar inhibitory effect [33].

3.2 Oral Vaccination

The gastrointestinal membranes are always exposed to foreign antigens and pathogens present in the lumen. The GALT, dotted in the small intestine, is the largest lymphoid organ, and the GALT protects the bodies against invading antigens and pathogens through mucosal immunization. The GALT consists of both isolated and aggregated lymphoid follicles [36]. Of these, Peyer's patches, which are composed of aggregated lymphoid follicles surrounded by the follicle-associated epithelium (FAE), form the interface between the GALT and the luminal microenvironment. Microfold (M) cells, which are specific epithelial cells present in the FAE, play an important role in the immunization at the mucosa. Antigens and pathogens taken up into M cells are delivered to antigen-presenting cells such as dendritic cells in Peyer's patches. This delivery triggers off immune reactions, and the mucosal immunization, which is mainly composed of secreted immunoglobulin A (sIgA), is finally established. It appears that the GALT is related to immune tolerance.

Oral vaccination using nano-/micromaterials as antigen carriers has been investigated for the past two decades [37–45]. Jain et al. prepared block copolymers composed of poly(ethylene glycol) (PEG) and poly(lactic acid) (PLA) and evaluated a potential of polymeric nanoparticles as carriers for hepatitis B surface antigens [41]. Nanoparticles prevented the antigen from being degraded by gastric acid and digestive enzymes. Fluorescence microphotographs suggested that nanoparticles were taken up by the GALT at the intestinal mucosa. Not only did hepatitis B surface antigens encapsulated into nanoparticles increase IgA secretion at the nasal, salivary, intestinal, and vaginal mucosa, but they induced humoral immunity in systemic circulation (production of serum IgG1 and IgG2a), when orally administered to mice, irrespective of the chemical structure of block copolymers. However, low production of antibodies was observed when the antigen carrier was substituted with PLA nanoparticles. The observation was presumably due to less stability of the antigens encapsulated into PLA nanoparticles in the gastrointestinal tract. Free PEG chains on the nanoparticle surface possibly contributed to the stabilization.

Particulate carriers incorporating antigen-encoded DNA vaccines have also been studied as oral vaccinations [42–45]. It appears that such system enables the DNA to deliver efficiently to lymphoid organs in the intestinal membranes. He et al. reported that PLGA microparticles encapsulating hepatitis B virus antigen-encoded plasmid DNA was capable of inducing both humoral and cellular immunities when administered orally to mice [45]. Recent studies demonstrated that transcytotic receptors, such as the complement 5a receptor, glycoprotein 2, toll-like receptor-2/toll-like receptor-4, and platelet-activating factor receptor, were expressed on the apical surface of M cells [46–48]. Several previous reports revealed that these receptors seemed to contribute to the cellular uptake of antigens. Nano-/micromaterials that recognize the receptors with high affinity and specificity may induce mucosal immunity more effectively.

4 Nano-/Micromaterials as Drug Carriers

Most oral medicines are absorbed passively from the intestine, although drugs whose chemical structures are analogous to those of nutrients are sometimes absorbed actively via influx transporters [1, 2, 49, 50]. Table 1 summarizes factors that affect drug absorption from the gastrointestinal tract. Water solubility and intestinal membrane permeability mainly influence oral absorption of drugs [51]. Drugs with high solubility and high permeability are highly absorbed from the intestine [52]. Interactions between drugs and components in the gastrointestinal tract such as digestive enzymes/fluids and foods often attribute to an elevation or reduction of drug absorption [53, 54]. Here, nano-/micromaterials as carriers that enhance oral absorption of drugs are discussed.

Table 1
Factors that affect drug absorption from the gastrointestinal tract

Solubility	Solubility Dissolution rate
Permeability	Membrane permeability on the basis of lipophilicity Influx transporter-mediated uptake Efflux transporter-mediated excretion Metabolism in intestinal epithelial cells
Interactions with components in the gastrointestinal tract	Increase/decrease in solubility induced by interactions with the components Degradation by gastric acid/digestive enzymes

4.1 Improvement of Solubility

Oral absorption of drugs with low solubility and high permeability can be enhanced by pharmaceutical approaches that increase their solubility and/or the dissolution rate. The available approaches include a reduction of the particle size of drugs [56, 57], lipid-based formulations [58, 59], and solid dispersions containing amorphous drugs [60]. A combination of these pharmaceutical technologies has also been studied [61, 62].

An increase in the dissolution rate of drugs is observed when their particle size is reduced. This is due to an increase in the surface area, while the solubility remains unchanged. Elan Pharmaceuticals has developed NanoCrystal® technology, which is based on wet milling. Submicron-sized particles are obtained when drugs are milled by this technology [56, 57]. Such particles easily aggregate; however, NanoCrystal® technology prevents the particles from aggregating through their coating with adequate dispersants such as surfactants and hydrophilic polymers. Commercial products to which this technology is applied are listed in Table 2. Wu et al. reported that oral absorption of aprepitant (MK-0869), whose solubility is 3–7 μg/mL in the pH range that corresponded to the gastrointestinal tract, was improved by NanoCrystal® technology [57]. Aprepitant with a mean diameter of 0.12 μm was prepared by this technology, and its oral absorption was compared with that of conventional powders with a mean diameter of 5.5 μm. The dissolution rate of aprepitant from the former was extremely higher than that from the latter because there was a 40-fold increase in the surface area through the treatment of the drug by NanoCrystal® technology. As shown in Fig. 6, when submicron-sized aprepitant was used, a clear elevation of drug absorption was observed in fasted dogs. It is also known that drug absorption via the gastrointestinal tract is often affected by the timing of drug administration in relation to meals [53, 54]. NanoCrystal® technology also reduced food–drug interactions (Fig. 6).

The self-micro-/nano-emulsifying drug delivery system (SMEDDS/SNEDDS) improves both solubility and dissolution rates. In this system, drugs are formulated with oil, surfactants, and cosurfactants [58]. The components filled into capsules are self-assembled when they are mixed with water. SMEDDS and SNEDDS form thermodynamically stable microemulsions and nano-sized emulsions with good dispersibility, respectively. Table 2 summarizes commercial products to which SMEDDS/SNEDDS is applied. Neoral® has been developed to improve inter- and intraindividual variation of oral absorption of cyclosporine from Sandimmune®, which has been clinically used prior to the launch of Neoral®. Micro-sized mixed micelles are formed when oily Sandimmune® is mixed with water containing bile acids and pancreatic enzymes. However, the micelles are too unstable to obtain stable bioavailability because the amount of the intestinal components is not constant. As shown in Table 3, less variation

Table 2
Commercial products to which technologies for solubility improvement are applied

Product name	Drug	Dosage form	Company
NanoCrystal Technologies			
Rapamune	Sirolimus	Tablet	Wyeth Pharmaceuticals
Tricor	Fenofibrate	Tablet	Abbott Laboratories
Triglide	Fenofibrate	Tablet	Sciele Pharma
Emend	Aprepitant	Capsule	Merck & Company
Zanaflex	Tizanidine HCl	Capsule	Acorda
Megace ES	Megestrol acetate	Suspension	Par Pharmaceutical
Self-micro-/nano-emulsifying drug delivery system (SMEDDS/SNEDDS)			
Neoral	Cyclosporine A	Soft gelatin capsule	Novartis
Norvir	Ritonavir	Soft gelatin capsule	Abbott
Fortovase	Saquinavir	Soft gelatin capsule	Roche
Agenerase	Amprenavir	Soft gelatin capsule	GlaxoSmithKline
Convulex	Valproic acid	Soft gelatin capsule	Pharmacia
Rocaltrol	Calcitriol	Soft gelatin capsule	Roche
Targretin	Bexarotene	Soft gelatin capsule	Novartis
Vesanoid	Tretinoin	Soft gelatin capsule	Roche
Accutane	Isotretionin	Soft gelatin capsule	Roche
Aptivus	Tipranavir	Soft gelatin capsule	Boehringer Ingelheim
Gengraf	Cyclosporine A	Hard gelatin capsule	Abbott
Lipirex	Fenofibrate	Hard gelatin capsule	Sanofi-Aventis
Kaletra	Lopinavir/ritonavir	Solution	Abbott

of pharmacokinetic parameters was observed when Neoral® was administered to humans when compared with Sandimmune®. Food effects on cyclosporine absorption were also improved through substitution of Neoral® to Sandimmune® [59].

4.2 Improvement of Permeability

Generally, there are few risks associated with the administration of drugs with high membrane permeability via the oral route. To the contrary, invasive routes such as injections are essential to obtain therapeutic effects of drugs with low membrane permeability. A large number of drugs, mainly peptides, proteins, antibodies, and nucleic acids, which are called bio-drugs, belong to this category. Many researchers have taken up the challenge using medicinal chemistry-based and pharmaceutical technology-based approaches

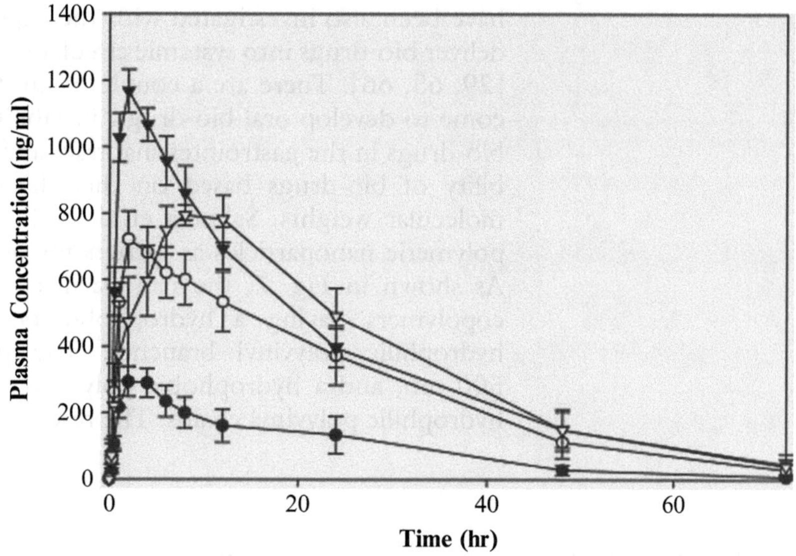

Fig. 6 Plasma concentration–time profiles of MK-0869 after oral administrations of a conventional suspension (***filled circle***, fasted; ***open circle***, fed) and a NanoCrystal® dispersion formulation (***filled inverted triangle***, fasted; ***open inverted triangle***, fed) at a dose of 2 mg/kg in beagle dogs (***n*** = 5, mean ± s.e.)

Table 3
Pharmacokinetic parameters after oral administration of Neoral® (180 mg/man) and Sandimmune® (300 mg/man)

	Sandimmune®	**Neoral®**
AUC (ng·h/mL)	3076 ± 1099	3514 ± 878
C_{max} (ng·mL)	645 ± 248	1011 ± 192
t_{max} (h)	2.5 ± 0.9	1.5 ± 0.4

with the aim of improving the oral absorption of poorly membrane-permeable drugs. Prodrug, which is the typical former approach, is currently the most practical strategy. Drugs with increased lipophilicity, such as bacampicillin which is a prodrug of ampicillin [63], and drugs absorbed via the H^+/peptide cotransporter, such as valacyclovir which is a prodrug of aciclovir (2), are typically successful cases.

Prodrug is effective for organic compounds with low molecular weight; however, there has been no success with bio-drugs. Conjugation with cell-penetrating peptides, which are taken up into cells via macropinocytosis, is one of the most promising approaches that enhance membrane permeation of bio-drugs applied to the mucosa [64]. Nano-/micromaterials, which are categorized into the pharmaceutical technology-based approaches, have been also investigated with the expectation that they would deliver bio-drugs into systemic circulation after oral administration [29, 65, 66]. There are a couple of hurdles that should be overcome to develop oral bio-drugs: instability of enzyme-susceptible bio-drugs in the gastrointestinal tract and low membrane permeability of bio-drugs based on their hydrophilicity and/or high molecular weights. Sakuma et al. evaluated a potential of novel polymeric nanoparticles as carriers for oral peptide delivery [29]. As shown in Fig. 7, the nanoparticles were composed of graft copolymers having a hydrophobic polystyrene backbone and hydrophilic polyvinyl branches. The particle size was about 500 nm, and a hydrophobic polystyrene core was covered with hydrophilic polyvinyl chains. The research group studied effects of

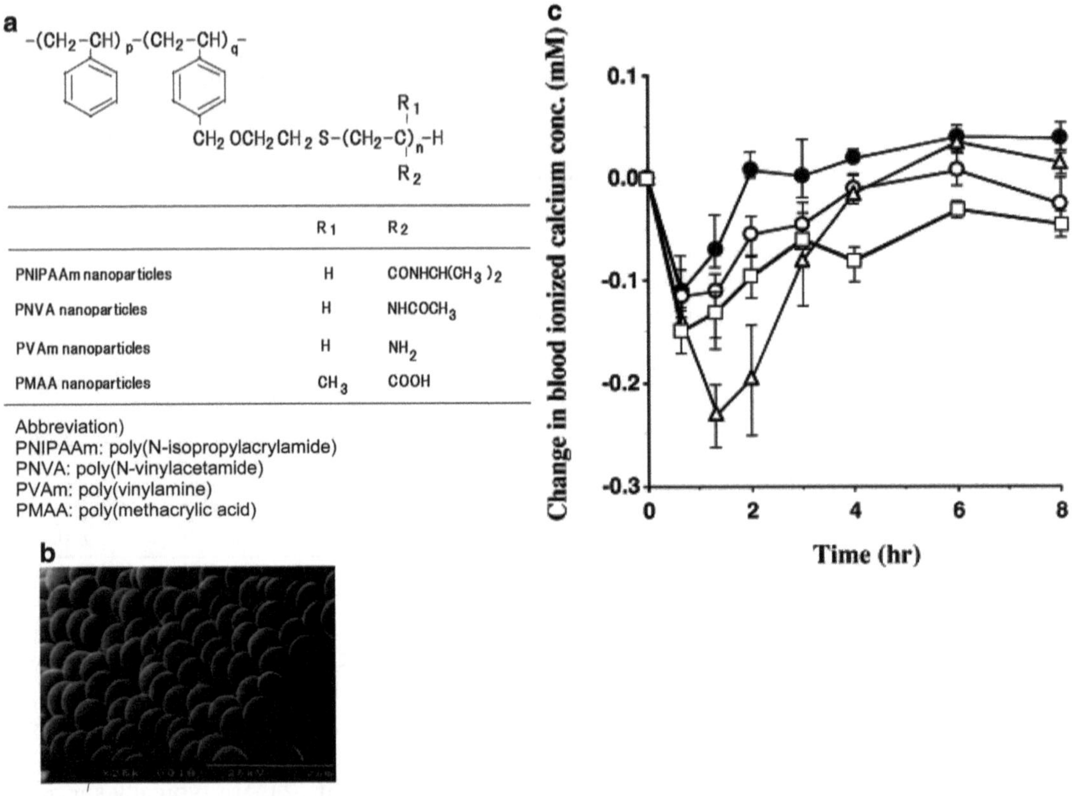

Fig. 7 (**a**) Chemical structure of nanoparticles composed of graft copolymers having a polystyrene backbone and various polyvinyl branches. (**b**) Scanning electron microscope image of nanoparticles having poly(N-isopropylacrylamide) (PNIPAAm) chains on their surface. (**c**) Concentration–time profiles of ionized calcium in blood after oral administration of sCT aqueous solution (*filled circle*), a mixture of sCT and poly(methacrylic acid) (PMAA) nanoparticles (*open circle*), a mixture of sCT and PNIPAAm nanoparticles (*open triangle*), and a mixture of sCT and poly(vinylamine) (PVAm) nanoparticles (*open square*) in rats (0.25 mg sCT/2.5 mL dosing solution/kg rat). The nanoparticle concentration in the dosing solution was 10 mg/mL. Each value represents the mean ± s.e

the surface structure of nanoparticles on oral absorption of salmon calcitonin (sCT) in rats and found that sCT absorption was enhanced most strongly by nanoparticles having poly(N-isopropylacrylamide) (PNIPAAm) chains on their surface [29]. Various in vitro/in vivo studies indicated that the absorption enhancement of sCT by nanoparticles resulted from both mucoadhesion of nanoparticles incorporating sCT to the intestinal mucosa and an increase in stability of sCT against digestive enzymes [26, 67]. A large amount of sCT was accumulated in the vicinity of the intestinal mucosa, and membrane permeation of sCT was enhanced on the basis of Fick's diffusion law [26, 67, 68]. Their successive research on absorption enhancement demonstrated that nanoparticles having surface PNIPAAm and cationic poly(vinylamine) (PVAm) chains at a ratio of 3:1 as a unit equivalent were superior to those having each chain solely [69].

Tight junctions are established between intestinal epithelial cells. The average size of aqueous pores made by tight junctions is approximately 7–9 Å at the jejunum, 3–4 Å at the ileum, and 8–9 Å at the colon in humans [70]. The aqueous pores have been studied as one of the pathways that would deliver bio-drugs into systemic circulation. However, the pore size is so narrow that the membrane permeation of bio-drugs is rate limited by their diffusion through the aqueous pores. Furthermore, since only less than 1 % of the mucosal surface is occupied with the pores, the systemic delivery of bio-drugs through this pathway is severely limited. Rekha et al. evaluated a potential of nanoparticles composed of either native chitosan or lauryl succinyl chitosan as carriers for oral peptide delivery [71]. Native chitosan nanoparticles were positively charged in neutral solution, and their mean particle size was 270 nm, while the charge and size of lauryl succinyl chitosan nanoparticles were negative and 650 nm, respectively. Insulin loaded into the respective nanoparticles was orally administered to diabetic rats, and the blood glucose level was monitored (Fig. 8). The glucose level was clearly reduced when insulin-loaded native chitosan nanoparticles were given orally. Further reduction was observed when the nanoparticles were replaced with insulin-loaded lauryl succinyl chitosan nanoparticles. No glucose reduction was observed after oral administration of either insulin solution or insulin-free nanoparticles. In vitro cell studies demonstrated that the integrity of tight junctions (TEER) was reduced to 70 % and 54 % of the initial value in the presence of native chitosan nanoparticles and lauryl succinyl chitosan nanoparticles, respectively. In vitro dissolution revealed that less than 10 % of insulin was released from drug-loaded lauryl succinyl chitosan nanoparticles in acidic solution of pH 1.2 during 2 h, while more than 60 % of insulin was released from drug-loaded native chitosan nanoparticles under the same conditions. It seemed that a difference in pharmacological effects of insulin in animal studies was mainly due to stabilization

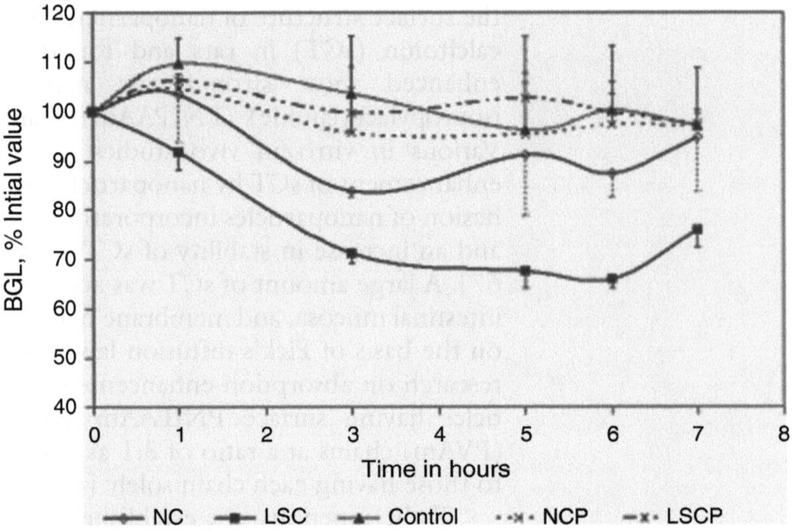

Fig. 8 Change in the blood glucose level after oral administration of insulin solution (control), insulin-free native chitosan particles (NCP), insulin-free lauryl succinyl chitosan particles (LSCP), insulin-loaded native chitosan particles (NC), and insulin-loaded lauryl succinyl chitosan particles (LSC) in streptozotocin-induced diabetic rat at a dose of 60 IU as an insulin equivalent/kg (***n*** = 4)

of insulin in the stomach through loading into lauryl succinyl chitosan nanoparticles. The stability possibly resulted from a difference in the surface charge of each of nanoparticles.

4.3 Reduction of Interactions Between Drugs and Components in the Gastrointestinal Tract

Drug absorption is often increased when patients take a drug after a meal (positive food effect), but in other cases, drugs show poor absorption when they are administered after a meal (negative food effect) [54, 55]. One of the typical drugs in the latter case is bisphosphonates used for the treatment of osteoporosis such as risedronate sodium hydrate and alendronate sodium hydrate [72]. Since oral bioavailability of them in the fed state is less than one-tenth of that in the fasted state, they must be taken about 1 h before the first food or beverage in the day. Digestive enzymes such as bile acids also affect the drug absorption. DX-9065, which Daiichi Pharmaceuticals has found to be an inhibitor of factor Xa, is one of the compounds whose oral bioavailability is reduced through interactions with bile acids [73]. The factor Xa accelerates the conversion of prothrombin to thrombin. Electrostatic interactions between the amidino group of this compound and the carboxyl group of bile acids result in insoluble complex. Fujii et al. hypothesized that DX-9065 absorption would be enhanced when this cationic drug candidate was free from the complex through its replacement with other cationic substances [74]. Cholestyramine, which is clinically used as a cholesterol-lowering agent, is a microparticle with a positive charge. In vitro studies revealed that cholestyramine dramatically prevented DX-9065 from interacting with chenodeoxycholic acid, which is a typical bile acid. Animal studies showed that bioavailability of DX-9065 administered with cholestyramine was 2–3 times that of DX-9065 administered solely. A cholestyramine-based dry syrup formulation was designed, and the clinical trial was performed. A 1.3-fold increase in bioavailability of DX-9065 was observed when the dry syrup was administered to fasted humans. The research group demonstrated that DX-9065 absorption was enhanced when the drug was administered with cationic additives; however, the absorption-enhancing function of cholestyramine largely depended on its dose. It appeared that the dose escalation of cholestyramine was a prerequisite for the significant improvement of DX-9065 absorption in humans.

5 Conclusions

In the field of the gastrointestinal system, many researchers have endeavored to develop nano-/micromaterials used for the treatment of gastrointestinal diseases and the materials as carriers that enhance oral absorption of drugs. However, successful cases are largely limited except for nano-/micromaterials with solubilization abilities. This chapter is closed with the expectation that innovative technologies are being developed in the near future.

References

1. Hediger MA, Coady MJ, Ikeda TS et al (1987) Expression cloning and cDNA sequencing of the Na+/glucose cotransporter. Nature 330:379–381
2. Sai Y, Tsuji A (2004) Transporter-mediated drug delivery: recent progress and experimental approaches. Drug Discov Today 9:712–720
3. Rendic S, Di Carlo FJ (1997) Human cytochrome P450 enzymes: a status report summarizing their reactions, substrates, inducers, and inhibitors. Drug Metab Rev 29:413–580
4. Rothenberg ME, Mishra A, Brandt EB et al (2001) Gastrointestinal eosinophils. Immunol Rev 179:139–155
5. Wideman RD, Kieffer TJ (2004) Glucose-dependent insulinotropic polypeptide as a regulator of beta cell function and fate. Horm Metab Res 36:782–786
6. Konturek PC, Bielański W, Konturek SJ (1999) *Helicobacter pylori* associated gastric pathology. J Physiol Pharmacol 50:695–710
7. Graham DY, Fischbach L (2010) *Helicobacter pylori* treatment in the era of increasing antibiotic resistance. Gut 59:1143–1153
8. Hao S, Wang Y, Wang B et al (2014) A novel gastroretentive porous microparticle for anti-Helicobacter pylori therapy: preparation, in vitro and *in vivo* evaluation. Int J Pharm 463:10–21
9. Jain P, Jain S, Prasad KN et al (2009) Polyelectrolyte coated multilayered liposomes (nanocapsules) for the treatment of Helicobacter pylori infection. Mol Pharm 6:593–603
10. Moogooee M, Ramezanzadeh H, Jasoori S et al (2011) Synthesis and *in vitro* studies of cross-linked hydrogel nanoparticles containing amoxicillin. J Pharm Sci 100:1057–1066
11. Cosnes J, Gower-Rousseau C, Seksik P et al (2011) Epidemiology and natural history of inflammatory bowel diseases. Gastroenterology 140:1785–1794
12. Podolsky DK (2002) Inflammatory bowel disease. N Engl J Med 347:417–429
13. Lamprecht A, Schafer U, Lehr CM (2001) Size-dependent bioadhesion of micro- and nanoparticulate carriers to the inflamed colonic mucosa. Pharm Res 18:788–793

14. Lamprecht A, Ubrich N, Yamamoto H et al (2001) Biodegradable nanoparticles for targeted drug delivery in treatment of inflammatory bowel disease. J Pharmacol Exp Ther 299:775–781
15. Siegel R, Naishadham D, Jamal A (2013) Cancer statistics 2013. CA Cancer J Clin 63:11–30
16. Balch GC, De Meo A, Guillem JG (2006) Modern management of rectal cancer: a 2006 update. World J Gastroenterol 12:3186–3195
17. Young PE, Womeldorph CM (2013) Colonoscopy for colorectal cancer screening. J Cancer Educ 4:217–226
18. Moss A, Bourke MJ, Williams SJ et al (2011) Endoscopic mucosal resection outcomes and prediction of submucosal cancer from advanced colonic mucosal neoplasia. Gastroenterology 140:1909–1918
19. Fukuzawa M, Saito Y, Matsuda T et al (2010) Effectiveness of narrow-band imaging magnification for invasion depth in early colorectal cancer. World J Gastroenterol 16:1727–1734
20. Winawer SJ, Zauber AG, Ho MN et al (1993) Prevention of colorectal cancer by colonoscopic polypectomy. The National Polyp Study Workgroup. N Engl J Med 329:1977–1981
21. Kudo S, Kashida H, Tamura T et al (2000) Colonoscopic diagnosis and management of nonpolypoid early colorectal cancer. World J Surg 24:1081–1090
22. Mayer R, Wong WD, Rothenberger DA et al (1999) Colorectal cancer in inflammatory bowel disease: a continuing problem. Dis Colon Rectum 42:343–347
23. Hsiung PL, Hardy J, Friedland S et al (2008) Detection of colonic dysplasia *in vivo* using a targeted heptapeptide and confocal microendoscopy. Nat Med 14:454–458
24. Sakuma S, Yamashita S, Hiwatari K et al (2011) Lectin-immobilized fluorescent nanospheres for targeting to colorectal cancer from a physicochemical perspective. Curr Drug Discov Technol 8:367–378
25. Sakuma S, Higashino H, Oshitani H et al (2011) Essence of affinity and specificity of peanut agglutinin-immobilized fluorescent nanospheres with surface poly(N-vinylacetamide) chains for colorectal cancer. Eur J Pharm Biopharm 79:537–543
26. Kumagai H, Pham W, Kataoka M et al (2013) Multifunctional nanobeacon for imaging Thomsen-Friedenreich antigen-associated colorectal cancer. Int J Cancer 132:2107–2117
27. Boland CR, Roberts JA (1988) Quantitation of lectin binding sites in human colon mucins by use of peanut and wheat germ agglutinin. J Histochem Cytochem 36:1305–1307
28. Rini JM (1995) Lectin structure. Annu Rev Biophys Biomol Struct 24:551–577
29. Sakuma S, Hayashi M, Akashi M (2001) Design of nanoparticles composed of graft copolymers for oral peptide delivery. Adv Drug Deliv Rev 47:21–37
30. Mertes G (2001) Safety and efficacy of acarbose in the treatment of type 2 diabetes: data from a 5-year surveillance study. Diabetes Res Clin Pract 52:193–204
31. Chiasson JL, Josse RG, Gomis R et al (2002) Acarbose for prevention of type 2 diabetes mellitus: the STOP-NIDDM randomized trial. Lancet 359:2072–2077
32. Ikumi Y, Kida T, Sakuma S et al (2008) Polymer-phloridzin conjugates as an anti-diabetic drug that inhibits glucose absorption through the Na+/glucose cotransporter (SGLT1) in the small intestine. J Control Release 125:42–49
33. Sakuma S, Teraoka Y, Sagawa T et al (2010) Carboxyl group-terminated polyamidoamine dendrimers bearing glucosides inhibit intestinal hexose transporter-mediated D-glucose uptake. Eur J Pharm Biopharm 75:366–374
34. Tyagi NK, Kumar A, Goyal P et al (2007) D-Glucose-recognition and phlorizin-binding sites in human sodium/D-glucose cotransporter 1 (hSGLT1): a tryptophan scanning study. Biochemistry 46:13616–13628
35. Kopeček J (2003) Smart and genetically engineered biomaterials and drug delivery systems. Eur J Pharm Sci 20:1–16
36. Neutra MR, Mantis NJ, Kraehenbuhl JP (2001) Collaboration of epithelial cells with organized mucosal lymphoid tissues. Nat Immunol 2:1004–1009
37. Rescia VC, Takata CS, de Araujo PS et al (2011) Dressing liposomal particles with chitosan and poly(vinylic alcohol) for oral vaccine delivery. J Liposome Res 21:38–45
38. Bharali DJ, Mousa SA, Thanavala Y (2007) Micro- and nanoparticle-based vaccines for hepatitis B. Adv Exp Med Biol 601:415–421
39. Eldridge JH, Staas JK, Meulbroek JA et al (1991) Biodegradable microspheres as a vaccine delivery system. Mol Immunol 28:287–294
40. Fujii Y, Aramaki Y, Hara T et al (1993) Enhancement of systemic and mucosal immune responses following oral administration of liposomes. Immunol Lett 36:65–69
41. Jain AK, Goyal AK, Gupta PN et al (2009) Synthesis, characterization and evaluation of novel triblock copolymer based nanoparticles for vaccine delivery against hepatitis B. J Control Release 136:161–169
42. Donnelly JJ, Wahren B, Liu MA (2005) DNA vaccines: progress and challenges. J Immunol 175:633–639

43. Horner AA, Van Uden JH, Zubeldia JM et al (2001) DNA-based immunotherapeutics for the treatment of allergic disease. Immunol Rev 179:102–118
44. Channarong S, Chaicumpa W, Sinchaipanid N et al (2011) Development and evaluation of chitosan-coated liposomes for oral DNA vaccine: the improvement of Peyer's patch targeting using a polyplex-loaded liposomes. AAPS PharmSciTech 12:192–200
45. He XW, Wang F, Jiang L et al (2005) Induction of mucosal and systemic immune response by single-dose oral immunization with biodegradable microparticles containing DNA encoding HBsAg. J Gen Virol 86:601–610
46. Kim SH, Yang IY, Jang SH et al (2013) C5a receptor-targeting ligand-mediated delivery of dengue virus antigen to M cells evokes antigen-specific systemic and mucosal immune responses in oral immunization. Microbes Infect 15:895–902
47. Hase K, Kawano K, Nochi T et al (2009) Uptake through glycoprotein 2 of FimH+ bacteria by M cells initiates mucosal immune response. Nature 462:226–230
48. Kyd JM, Cripps AW (2008) Functional differences between M cells and enterocytes in sampling luminal antigens. Vaccine 26:6221–6224
49. Fei YJ, Kanai Y, Nussberger S et al (1994) Expression cloning of a mammalian protein-coupled oligopeptide transporter. Nature 368:563–566
50. Altmann SW, Davis HR Jr, Zhu LJ et al (2004) Niemann-Pick C1 Like 1 protein is critical for intestinal cholesterol absorption. Science 303:1201–1204
51. Lipinski CA, Lombardo F, Dominy BW et al (2001) Experimental and computational approaches to estimate solubility and permeability in drug delivery and development setting. Adv Drug Deliv Rev 46:3–26
52. Amidon GL, Lennernäs H, Shah VP et al (1995) A theoretical basis for a biopharmaceutic drug classification: the correlation of *in vitro* drug product dissolution and *in vivo* bioavailability. Pharm Res 12:413–420
53. Schmidt LE, Dalhoff K (2002) Food–drug interactions. Drugs 62:1481–1502
54. Sakuma S, Tanno FK, Masaoka Y et al (2007) Effect of administration site in the gastrointestinal tract on bioavailability of poorly absorbed drugs taken after a meal. J Control Release 118:59–64
55. Kawai Y, Fujii Y, Tabata F et al (2011) Profiling and trend analysis of food effects on oral drug absorption considering micelle interaction and solubilization by bile micelles. Drug Metab Pharmacokinet 26:180–191
56. Merisko-Liversidge E, Liversidge GG, Cooper ER (2003) Nanosizing: a formulation approach for poorly-water-soluble compounds. Eur J Pharm Sci 18:113–120
57. Wu Y, Loper A, Landis E et al (2004) The role of biopharmaceutics in the development of a clinical nanoparticle formulation of MK-0869: a Beagle dog model predicts improved bioavailability and diminished food effect on absorption in human. Int J Pharm 285:135–146
58. Cerpnjak K, Zvonar A, Gašperlin M et al (2013) Lipid-based systems as a promising approach for enhancing the bioavailability of poorly water-soluble drugs. Acta Pharm 63:427–445
59. Mueller EA, Kovarik JM, van Bree JB et al (1994) Influence of a fat-rich meal on the pharmacokinetics of a new oral formulation of cyclosporine in a crossover comparison with the market formulation. Pharm Res 11:151–155
60. Vo CL, Park C, Lee BJ (2013) Current trends and future perspectives of solid dispersions containing poorly water-soluble drugs. Eur J Pharm Biopharm 85:799–813
61. Kawakami K, Zhang S, Chauhan RS et al (2013) Preparation of fenofibrate solid dispersion using electrospray deposition and improvement in oral absorption by instantaneous post-heating of the formulation. Int J Pharm 450:123–128
62. Zhang S, Kawakami K, Yamamoto M et al (2011) Coaxial electrospray formulations for improving oral absorption of a poorly water-soluble drug. Mol Pharm 8:807–813
63. Bodin NO, Ekström B, Forsgren U et al (1975) Bacampicillin: a new orally well-absorbed derivative of ampicillin. Antimicrob Agents Chemother 8:518–525
64. Futaki S (2005) Membrane-permeable arginine-rich peptides and the translocation mechanisms. Adv Drug Deliv Rev 57:547–558
65. Niu M, Lu Y, Hovgaard L et al (2011) Liposomes containing glycocholate as potential oral insulin delivery systems: preparation, *in vitro* characterization, and improved protection against enzymatic degradation. Int J Nanomedicine 6:1155–1166
66. Bayat A, Dorkoosh FA, Dehpour AR et al (2008) Nanoparticles of quaternized chitosan derivatives as a carrier for colon delivery of insulin: *ex vivo* and *in vivo* studies. Int J Pharm 356:259–266
67. Sakuma S, Sudo R, Suzuki N et al (2002) Behavior of mucoadhesive nanoparticles having hydrophilic polymeric chains in the intestine. J Control Release 81:281–290

68. Sakuma S, Matsumoto T, Yamashita S et al (2007) Conjugation of poorly absorptive drugs with mucoadhesive polymers for the improvement of oral absorption of drugs. J Control Release 123:195–202
69. Sakuma S, Suzuki N, Sudo R et al (2002) Optimized chemical structure of nanoparticles as carriers for oral delivery of salmon calcitonin. Int J Pharm 239:185–195
70. Tomita M, Shiga M, Hayashi M et al (1988) Enhancement of colonic drug absorption by the paracellular permeation route. Pharm Res 5:341–346
71. Rekha MR, Sharma CP (2009) Synthesis and evaluation of lauryl succinyl chitosan particles towards oral insulin delivery and absorption. J Control Release 135:144–151
72. Ogura Y, Gonsho A, Cyong JC et al (2004) Clinical trial of risedronate in Japanese volunteers: a study on the effect of timing of dosing on absorption. J Bone Miner Metab 22:120–126
73. Fujii Y, Takahashi M, Morita H et al (2007) Characteristics of gastrointestinal absorption of DX-9065a, a new synthetic anticoagulant. Drug Metab Pharmacokinet 22:26–32
74. Fujii Y, Kanamaru T, Kikuchi H et al (2011) Improvement of low bioavailability of a novel factor Xa through formulation of cationic additives in its oral dosage form. Int J Pharm 421:244–251

Chapter 15

Respiratory System

Kohsaku Kawakami

Abstract

The potential therapeutic benefits of drug molecules can be maximized by well-designed delivery technology. Improvements in nanotechnology have facilitated innovations in pulmonary drug delivery, because inhalation is a drug administration route for which the size of particles in the formulation has an extensive effect on the fate of the drug molecules after administration. Deposition site of the drug in the lung is determined by the aerodynamic size of the inhaled particles, and the absorption and clearance processes after deposition also are influenced by particle size. Inhalation of a nanoparticulate drug is the simplest idea to apply nanotechnology in this field, but it is not technically easy because nanoparticulate drugs are prone to aggregate. Thus, various efforts have been made to prevent aggregation for exerting advantages of nanoparticles. This chapter describes various efforts for utilizing nanotechnology for pulmonary drug delivery.

Key words Nanoparticles, Inhalation, Deposition site, Aerodynamic diameter, Mucociliary clearance, Poly(DL-lactide-co-glycolide) (PLGA)

1 Introduction

Inhalation is an effective method for systemic as well as local drug delivery [1–3]. Drugs can be administered either in the liquid or solid state, but much attention has been paid to dry powder inhalation because of the high stability and low administration volumes required for dry powder formulations. However, both inhalation devices and formulation technology still require development to achieve effective pulmonary drug delivery. Particle size is one of the most important factors in determining the deposition site of the formulation in the lung [4–8]. Several deposition models are available for predicting efficiency of delivery of the particles as a function of their aerodynamic diameter. The most famous one is the ICRP (International Commission on Radiological Protection) model [9], which was developed after experimental observations and model calculations that considered lung morphology. Figure 1 shows particle distribution after aspiration of the particles as a function of their aerodynamic size based on this model.

Zheng-Rong Lu and Shinji Sakuma (eds.), *Nanomaterials in Pharmacology*, Methods in Pharmacology and Toxicology, DOI 10.1007/978-1-4939-3121-7_15, © Springer Science+Business Media New York 2016

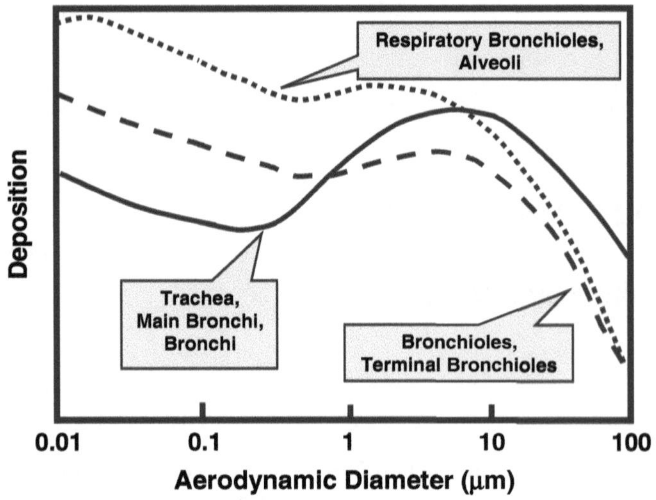

Fig. 1 Deposition of particles in each region of the respiratory tract based on the ICRP model

Particles smaller than 100 nm are effectively deposited in the alveolar region, from which the most effective systemic drug delivery can be expected. However, because particles smaller than 100 nm are difficult to manufacture and handle with current powder technology, micron-sized particles are regarded as the best practical option for pulmonary drug delivery.

Efficient deposition is not the only advantage of the nanoparticles. They can escape from mucociliary clearance after deposition [10]. Macrophage clearance has been shown to be minimized as well [11]. Rapid dissolution and/or permeation across biological membranes are also great advantages. Moreover, size reduction below 200 nm enables sterile filtration in the manufacturing process. Nanoparticles can be delivered in a mist when nebulizers are used, although this is not possible for microparticles [12].

This chapter examines various efforts to use nanotechnology for pulmonary drug delivery. "Nanomaterials" are usually defined as a material in which at least one dimension has the length below 100 nm. Although the US Food and Drug Administration (FDA) employs the same definition [13], exceptions are accepted if the material exerts size effect. Thus, this chapter also deals with particles with physical size exceeding 100 nm.

2 Nanosizing of Active Pharmaceutical Ingredients

Nanosizing of active pharmaceutical ingredients has various advantages. Notably, it may improve the oral bioavailability of poorly soluble drugs [14, 15]. An increase in the surface area plays a dominant role in increasing the dissolution rate, because they are inversely related. The solubility per se may increase, as shown by the Ostwald–Freundlich equation, although this advantage is usually marginal. Exposure of the highly energetic surface of the drug crystals may enhance the dissolution process. These advantages may also be applicable to the pulmonary delivery of poorly soluble drugs.

Nanoparticles for pulmonary drug delivery can be manufactured in the same manner as those intended for oral formulations. The top-down procedures that are commonly employed in industry include media milling and high-pressure homogenization [10]. Although reducing the particle size to the nanoscale is not difficult, it is challenging to prevent aggregation during the storage [15]. Bottom-up methods such as preparation via solvent evaporation and anti-solvent crystallization have also been actively investigated [10].

In oral formulations, excipients that increase dispersion efficiency can be added to promote the formulation's disintegration via mechanical stress in the gastrointestinal tract. However, dry powder formulations for pulmonary drug delivery must disintegrate following only the weak stress introduced during aspiration, which is challenging for nanoparticle formulations. To date, the number of reported in vivo inhalation studies of solid nanoparticles has been limited. Ali et al. employed a lactose carrier for administration of atropine sulfate nanoparticles to healthy volunteers using a dry powder inhaler [16]. The drug's rapid action due to its prompt absorption from the lung, followed by sustained action due to absorption from the gastrointestinal tract, indicated the potential of a nanoparticulate formulation as a replacement for the injectable formulation.

3 Nanosuspensions

Nebulizers usually produce micron-sized droplets that may accommodate nanoparticles. A frequently reported benefit of the nanosuspensions in clinical and animal studies has been a decrease in side effects. Shrewsbury et al. administered a budesonide nanosuspension to healthy volunteers using a jet nebulizer and observed more rapid absorption and a decrease in the absorbed amount relative to those from a commercially available suspension [17]. The time to maximum plasma concentration (T_{max}) for the commercial budesonide formulation was 9.1 min, but it decreased to 3.1–4.5 min for the nanosuspension. Although the maximum plasma concentration (C_{max}) also increased following administration of the nanosuspension, the area under the plasma drug concentration–time curve (AUC) decreased because of the rapid absorption. Consequently, higher efficacy and safety were expected for the nanosuspension formulation. Chiang et al. observed similar effects in a fluticasone propionate nanosuspension [18].

Encapsulation of drug molecules in polymeric nanoparticles has also been of great interest. Notably, poly(DL-lactide-co-glycolide) (PLGA) has been the most actively investigated material for encapsulation because of its biodegradable property [19]. Pandey et al. administered rifampicin, isoniazid, and pyrazinamide encapsulated in PLGA nanoparticles using a jet nebulizer to achieve increases in both the mean residence time (MRT) and bioavailability for all these drugs (Table 1) [20]. Decoration of the particle surface using lectin resulted in further increases in efficacy because lectin is recognized by epithelial cell receptors [21]. Yamamoto et al. decorated PLGA nanoparticles using chitosan to improve pulmonary absorption of the peptide drug, elcatonin [12]. The chitosan-decorated PLGA nanoparticles reduced blood calcium levels to 80 % of the initial concentration. Moreover, the pharmacological efficacy was maintained for 24 h, which was explained by mucoadhesive properties and the tight junction opening effect of chitosan. In addition, polymeric nanoparticles are also regarded as promising vehicles for gene delivery [22].

Liposomes have also been investigated as nanoparticulate carriers because of their advantages that include biocompatibility, good dispersion efficiency, ease of surface decoration, and suitability for both hydrophilic and lipophilic drugs. Liposomes may be formulated either as powders [23, 24] or suspensions [25, 26]. Although the former have advantages such as higher stability and portability (because nebulizers are required for administration of suspensions), majority of the researches have been on the latter use. Chono et al. administered insulin using liposome carriers and found that dipalmitoylphosphatidylcholine was effective as a constituent for improving absorption behavior, but similar effects were not observed for dilauroyl, dimyristoyl, distearoyl, and dioleoyl liposomes [25]. Hydrophilic drugs are usually entrapped into liposomes only with low entrapment efficiency. The efficiency is apparently improved if the free drug is removed. However, it makes the production process very complicated, which is not acceptable from an industrial viewpoint. In some cases, coexistence of free and liposome-encapsulated drugs offers an advantage. In the case of a fentanyl formulation, their coexistence provided rapid and prolonged action [26].

4 Nanoparticle Aggregates

If nanoparticles are spray-dried under optimized conditions, hollow particles may be obtained [27, 28]. The formation of the hollow structure can be explained by considering the mass transport of each component in the radial direction during the drying

Table 1
Effect of nanosuspension administered by nebulizer [20, 21]

	Rifampicin			Isoniazid			Pyrazinamide		
	Solution	PLGA nanoparticles	PLGA/lectin nanoparticles	Solution	PLGA nanoparticles	PLGA/lectin nanoparticles	Solution	PLGA nanoparticles	PLGA/lectin nanoparticles
C_{max} (mg/L)	–	1.29	1.07	–	5.06	5.79	–	25.6	22.5
T_{max} (h)	–	24	72	–	96	120	–	96	96
MRT (h)	2.5–4.0	60.3	–	2.5–4.0	98.6	–	2.5–4.0	101	–
AUC (mg h/L)	2.10	107	117	18.0	359	584	98.0	2720	4670
Ratio of bioavailability (pulmonary/oral)	0.13	6.5	13	0.96	19	53	0.48	13	22

Mean particle size of PLGA nanoparticles: 186–290 nm (droplet diameter, 1.9 μm)
Mean particle size of PLGA/lectin nanoparticles: 350–400 nm (droplet diameter, 2.8 μm)

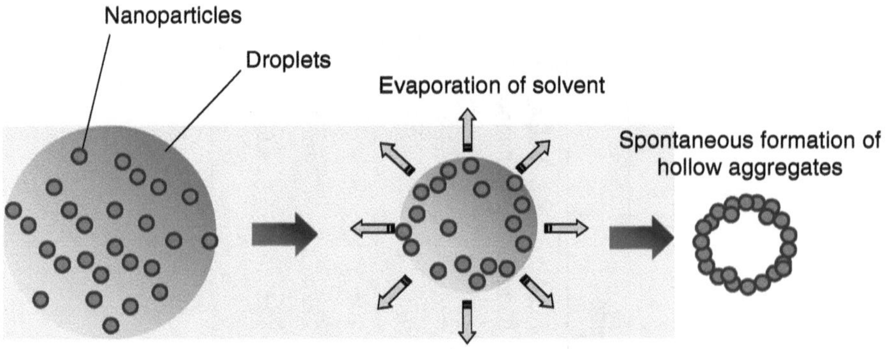

Fig. 2 The process of formation of hollow aggregates composed of nanoparticles

process [29, 30]. Peclet number, Pe, is a convenient parameter to describe this process and is described by the following equation:

$$\mathrm{Pe} = \frac{R_\mathrm{d}^{\ 2}}{\tau D_i} \tag{1}$$

where R_d, τ, and Di are the radius of the droplet, the drying time, and the diffusion coefficient of the component i, respectively. If the component cannot catch up with the shrinkage of the droplets, Pe has a large value (>>1), and the component is likely to accumulate on the surface of the spray-dried particle. This process is described in Fig. 2. In contrast, a small Pe (<<1) means that the diffusion of the component is sufficiently rapid to catch up with the shrinkage of the droplets, and one would expect homogeneous distribution of the component within the particle. The hollow aggregates, termed PNAPs (porous nanoparticle-aggregate particles) [31], may be suitable for pulmonary drug delivery because of their low density.

Sung et al. entrapped rifampicin in PLGA nanoparticles, followed by spray-drying to form PNAPs [32]. Although the pharmacokinetic parameters obtained after pulmonary administration of PNAPs were comparable with those of the solution, the drug concentrations in the lung tissue and bronchoalveolar lavage components were significantly higher than those after administration of the solution (Fig. 3). Yang et al. employed PNAPs for pulmonary delivery of a peptide drug, octreotide acetate [33]. Plasma aspartate aminotransferase levels for the PNAP formulation was significantly higher compared to the clinically used formulation injected subcutaneously.

Technosphere®, which is known as a formulation technology applied to an inhalable insulin formulation, uses aggregates of fumaryl diketopiperazine nanocrystals [34]. In the case of the insulin formulation (Afrezza®), insulin molecules are adsorbed on the aggregates to form microparticles that have an aerodynamic diameter of 2.5 μm. The insulin molecules are adsorbed in a monomeric form, and it offers more rapid action (T_{max}, 12–14 min) than that of the injectable formulation (T_{max}, 45–60 min), which contains insulin

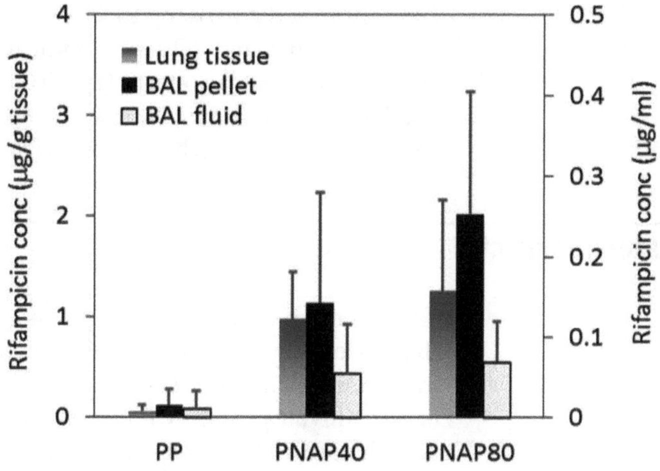

Fig. 3 Rifampicin concentration in homogenized lung tissue and the bronchoalveolar lavage (BAL) components in guinea pigs. BAL pellets were obtained by centrifuging BAL fluid. Dry powder formulations were administered via intratracheal insufflation at a dose of 2.5 mg/kg, and the drug concentrations were determined 8 h after administration. The formulations were prepared using L-leucine as an excipient. The nanoparticles were composed of rifampicin and PLGA. PP, spray-dried porous powder; PNAP40, the formulation containing 40 % nanoparticles; PNAP80, the formulation containing 80 % nanoparticles

in a hexameric form. This formulation was approved by FDA in June 2014. Although it is difficult to prevent aggregation of the nanoparticles, certain nanoparticle aggregates are also promising for pulmonary drug delivery as demonstrated by this example.

5 Nanoparticle-Containing Microparticles

Entrapment of nanoparticles in a microparticulate matrix eliminates the problem of aggregation. In this case, distribution of the particles in the lung after inhalation follows that of microparticles. Nevertheless, other effects specific for nanoparticles including avoidance of mucociliary clearance and efficient absorption after deposition should be maintained. Ohashi et al. entrapped rifampicin-containing PLGA nanoparticles in mannitol microspheres in one step using a 4-fluid nozzle spray drier [35]. Uptake of rifampicin by macrophages was increased by using the microspheres. Their imaging study revealed that PLGA nanoparticles administered in mannitol microparticles were effectively retained in the lung, although microparticulate PLGA was found to be eliminated rapidly from the lung. Ungaro et al. entrapped tobramycin in nanoparticles composed of PLGA and another polymer, which was included in the lactose microsphere, to investigate the effects of the composition of nanoparticles on the formulation performance [36]. Poly(vinyl alcohol) (PVA)-modified alginate/PLGA nanoparticles were found to reach deep in the lung, while

PVA-modified chitosan/PLGA nanoparticles were mainly found in the upper airways. Thus, modifications of the surface properties and sizes of the nanoparticles, although they were incorporated in the lactose microparticles, were shown to significantly influence the performance of the nanoparticles after deposition.

6 Future Prospects

This chapter focused on formulation technologies for pulmonary drug delivery based on nanotechnologies. However, another important challenging issue in the field of pulmonary drug delivery is the development of inhalation devices. In addition to the aerodynamic diameter of particles in the formulation, how the formulation is inhaled also influences its deposition site. Thus, attention is required as well on the development of an inhalation device that maximizes the efficacy of the formulation.

Future drug treatments will greatly depend on biopharmaceuticals, which are currently administered by injection. The lungs are a promising portal for systemic delivery of biopharmaceuticals, because the oral route is almost useless for high-molecular weight drugs. Withdrawal of Exubera®, the first inhalable product for systemic administration of a peptide drug, from the market indicated that significant effort is still required before the lung can be used for systemic drug delivery. Nanotechnology is still in development and may promote innovation in pulmonary drug delivery for more patient-friendly administration of biopharmaceuticals.

Acknowledgement

This work was in part supported by World Premier International Research Center (WPI) Initiative on Materials Nanoarchitectonics, MEXT, Japan.

References

1. Patton JS (1996) Mechanisms of macromolecule absorption by the lungs. Adv Drug Delivery Rev 19:3–36
2. Patton JS, Fishburn CS, Weers JG (2004) The lungs as a portal of entry for systemic drug delivery. Proc Am Thorac Soc 1:338–344
3. Shoyele SA, Slowey A (2006) Prospects of formulating proteins/peptides as aerosols for pulmonary drug delivery. Int J Pharm 314:1–8
4. Katz IM, Schroeter JD, Martonen TB (2001) Factor affecting the deposition of aerosolized insulin. Diabetes Technol Ther 3:387–397
5. Patton JS, Byron PR (2007) Inhaling medicines: delivering drugs to the body through the lungs. Nat Rev Drug Discov 6:67–74
6. Shekunov BY, Chattopadhyay P, Tong HHY, Chow AHL (2007) Particle size analysis in pharmaceutics: principles, methods and applications. Pharm Res 24:203–227
7. Glover W, Chan HK, Eberl S, Daviskas E, Verschuer J (2008) Effect of particle size of dry powder mannitol on the lung deposition in healthy volunteers. Int J Pharm 349:314–322

8. Park SS, Wexler AS (2008) Size-dependent deposition of particles in the human lung at steady-state breathing. J Aerosol Sci 39: 266–276
9. Smith H (1994) ICRP publication 66: human respiratory tract model for radiological protection. Pergamon, New York
10. Zhang J, Wu L, Chan HK, Watanabe W (2011) Formation, characterization, and fate of inhaled drug nanoparticles. Adv Drug Deliv Rev 63:441–455
11. Geiser M (2010) Update on macrophage clearance of inhaled micro- and nanoparticles. J Aerosol Med Pulmonary Drug Deliv 23: 207–217
12. Yamamoto H, Kuno Y, Sugimoto S, Takeuchi H, Kawashima Y (2005) Surface-modified PLGA nanosphere with chitosan improved pulmonary delivery of calcitonin by mucoadhesion and opening of the intercellular tight junctions. J Control Release 102:373–381
13. FDA Guidance for Industry (2014) Considering whether an FDA-regulated product involves the application of nanotechnology
14. Merisko-Liversidge E, Liversidge GG (2011) Nanosizing for oral and parenteral drug delivery: a perspective on formulating poorly water soluble compounds using wet media milling technology. Adv Drug Deliv Rev 63:427–440
15. Kawakami K (2012) Modification of physicochemical characteristics of active pharmaceutical ingredients and application of supersaturatable dosage forms for improving bioavailability of poorly absorbed drugs. Adv Drug Deliv Rev 64:480–495
16. Ali R, Jain GK, Iqbal Z, Talegaonkar S, Pandit P, Sule S, Malhotra G, Khar RK, Bhatnagar A, Ahmad FJ (2009) Development and clinical trial of nano-atropine sulfate dry powder inhaler as a novel organophosphorous poisoning antidote. Nanomedicine 5:55–63
17. Shrewsbury SB, Bosco AP, Uster PS (2009) Pharmacokinetics of a novel submicron budesonide dispersion for nebulized delivery in asthma. Int J Pharm 365:12–17
18. Chiang PC, Hu Y, Blom JD, Thompson DC (2010) Evaluating the suitability of using rat models for preclinical efficacy and side effects with inhaled corticosteroids nanosuspension formulations. Nanoscale Res Lett 5:1010–1019
19. Ungaro F, d'Angelo I, Miro A, La Rotonda MI, Quaglia F (2012) Engineered PLGA nano- and micro-carriers for pulmonary delivery: challenges and promises. J Pharm Pharmacol 64:1217–1235
20. Pandey R, Sharma A, Zahoor A, Sharma S, Khuller GK, Prasad B (2003) Poly (DL-lactide-co-glycolide) nanoparticle-based inhalable sustained drug delivery system for experimental tuberculosis. J Antimicrob Chemther 52: 981–986
21. Sharma A, Sharma S, Khuller GK (2004) Lectin-functionalized poly (lactide-co-glycolide) nanoparticles as oral/aerosolized antitubercular drug carriers for treatment of tuberculosis. J Antimicrob Chemther 54:761–766
22. Beck-Broichsitter M, Merkel OM, Kissel T (2012) Controlled pulmonary drug and gene delivery using polymeric nano-carriers. J Control Release 161:214–224
23. Lo Y, Tsai J, Kuo J (2004) Liposomes and saccharides as carriers in spray-dried powder formulations of superoxide dismutase. J Control Release 94:259–272
24. Lu D, Hickey AJ (2005) Liposomal dry powders as aerosols for pulmonary delivery of proteins. AAPS PharmSciTech 6:E641–E648
25. Chono S, Fukuchi R, Seki T, Morimoto K (2009) Aerosolized liposomes with dipalmitoyl phosphatidylcholine enhance pulmonary insulin delivery. J Control Release 137:104–109
26. Hung OR, Whynot SC, Varvel JR, Shafer SL, Mezei M (1995) Pharmacokinetics of inhaled liposome-encapsulated fentanyl. Anesthesiology 83:277–281
27. Tsapis N, Bennett D, Jackson B, Weitz DA, Edwards DA (2002) Trojan particles: large porous carriers of nanoparticles for drug delivery. Proc Natl Acad Sci U S A 99: 12001–12005
28. Hadinoto K, Phanapavudhikul P, Kewu Z, Tan RBH (2006) Novel formulation of large hollow nanoparticles aggregates as potential carriers in inhaled delivery of nanoparticulate drugs. Ind Eng Chem Res 45:3697–3706
29. Vehring R (2007) Pharmaceutical particle engineering via spray drying. Pharm Res 25:999–1022
30. Kawakami K, Hasegawa Y, Deguchi K, Ohki S, Shimizu T, Yoshihashi Y, Yonemochi E, Terada K (2013) Competition of thermodynamic and dynamic factors during formation of multicomponent particles via spray-drying. J Pharm Sci 102:518–529
31. Sung JC, Pulliam BL, Edwards DA (2007) Nanoparticles for drug delivery to the lungs. Trends Biotechnol 25:563–570
32. Sung JC, Padilla DJ, Garcia-Contreras L, VerBerkmoes JL, Durbin D, Peloquin CA, Elbert KJ, Hickey AJ, Edwards DA (2009) Formulation and pharmacokinetics of self-assembles rifampicin nanoparticle systems for pulmonary delivery. Pharm Res 26: 1847–1855
33. Yang L, Luo J, Shi S, Zhang Q, Sun X, Zhang Z, Gong T (2013) Development of a

pulmonary peptide delivery system using porous nanoparticle-aggregate particles for systemic application. Int J Pharm 451:104–111

34. Kraft KS, Grant M (2009) Preparation of macromolecule-containing dry powders for pulmonary delivery. In: Belting M (ed) Macromolecular drug delivery. Humana Press, New York, pp 165–174

35. Ohashi K, Kabasawa T, Ozeki T, Okada H (2009) One-step preparation of rifampicin/poly(lactic-co-glycolic acid) nanoparticle-containing mannitol microspheres using a four-fluid nozzle spray drier for inhalation therapy of tuberculosis. J Control Release 135:19–24

36. Ungaro F, d'Angelo I, Coletta C, d'Emmanuele di Villa Bianca R, Sorrentino R, Perfetto B, Tufano MA, Miro A, La Rotonda MI, Quaglia F (2012) Dry powders based on PLGA nanoparticles for pulmonary delivery of antibiotics: Modulation of encapsulation efficiency, release rate and lung deposition pattern by hydrophilic polymers. J Control Release 157:149–159

Chapter 16

Depot Microcapsules Containing Biologic Nanoparticles and Cytoplasm-Responsive Nanocarriers for Nucleotides

Hiroaki Okada

Abstract

Insulin is synthesized in the rough endoplasmic reticulum as proinsulin, converted and packed into secretory granules as 200-nm insulin nanoparticles after Golgi processing, and secreted from pancreatic β-cells followed by signaling of blood glucose elevation. Lupron Depot® injectable microcapsules containing nanoparticles of leuprorelin (a superagonist of luteinizing hormone-releasing hormone), encapsulated with a biodegradable polymer, can persistently release peptides for a long time (1, 3, and 6 months) for treating hormone-dependent diseases such as prostate cancer, breast cancer, and endometriosis. Arginine-rich cell-penetrating peptides (CPPs) involved in the uptake of large molecules such as proteins, nucleotides, and even nanoparticles are expected to be nonviral carriers for nucleotides. The cytoplasm-responsive CPP—$CH_2R_4H_2C$ (C, cysteine; H, histamine; R, arginine)—was synthesized and conjugated with stearic acid for local administration or with methoxy poly(ethylene glycol)-block-poly(ε-caprolactone) for systemic administration. Nucleotides were shielded rigidly on the surface of nanomicelles by the intramolecular and intermolecular disulfide linkages of 2 cysteine residues, and protected against nucleases in blood, and were definitely released in the reductive environment of the cytoplasm. In this chapter, leuprorelin depot microcapsules using biodegradable polymers for long-term release and cytoplasm-responsive nanocarriers using functional CPP for siRNA transfection are described.

Key words Leuprorelin-injectable microcapsules, Peptide nanocores, Chemical castration, siRNA silencing, Functional cell-penetrating peptides, Cytoplasm-responsive nanocarriers

1 Introduction

Two historic innovations in drug discovery were made in 2012, i.e., development of the gene therapy Glybera® [1] and stem cell therapy Prochymal® [2]. Glybera® (alipogene tiparvovec) is the first gene therapy for lipoprotein lipase deficiency (familial hyperchylomicronemia) and was developed by UniQure (Amsterdam, the Netherlands). In this agent, the unique adeno-associated virus (AAV) is used as a gene carrier. Prochymal is the first system using human mesenchymal stem cells for treating graft-versus-host disease and has been developed by Osiris Therapeutics (Columbia, MD, USA).

Zheng-Rong Lu and Shinji Sakuma (eds.), *Nanomaterials in Pharmacology*, Methods in Pharmacology and Toxicology, DOI 10.1007/978-1-4939-3121-7_16, © Springer Science+Business Media New York 2016

These epoch-making medicines could usher a new era for the development of biologic agents. Furthermore, several novel biologics and biological materials such as diabodies, functional peptide sequences of endogenous proteins, micro-ribonucleic acid (miRNA) molecules, short interfering RNA (siRNA) molecules, and DNA vaccines are under clinical study.

In the human body, there are many autocrine, paracrine, and endocrine factors. These include peptides, proteins, and nucleotides that constitute hormones and cytokines. Hormones and cytokines regulate numerous biological events and maintain circadian rhythm and homeostasis [3–6]. They also protect the body against foreign invaders (e.g., bacteria, viruses) to prevent many diseases [7, 8]. Most proteins in eukaryotic cells are synthesized and excreted from cells. They exert physiological activities on the surface and milieu of cells or target tissue after circulation in blood. For example, in healthy individuals, insulin is synthesized in the β-cells of pancreatic islets and secreted into blood after elevation of blood glucose level, and subsequently glucose metabolism is maintained at an appropriate level. Figure 1 shows the rapid synthesis of proinsulin in the rough endoplasmic reticulum, processing in the Golgi apparatus (conversion from proinsulin to insulin), as well as condensation and storage in secretory granules. Granule contents spill into the extracellular space via exocytosis from β-cells and diffuse into blood vessels. Surprisingly, insulin is released from β-cells as nanosized particles with a diameter of 200 nm (Fig. 1) [9].

Our research team developed a long-term sustained-release system for a superactive analog of luteinizing hormone-releasing hormone (LH-RH) to suppress the endocrine system to treat hormone-dependent diseases [10–20]. This preparation is not a stimulus-responsive system like a cell, but can persistently suppress the normal hormone response and achieve strong "chemical castration." Thereafter, we developed a microcapsule (mcp) system containing siRNA/polyethylenimine (PEI) nanolipoplexes for treating cancer via inhibition of neovascularization and induction of apoptosis and for treating peripheral arterial disease via induction of angiogenesis by sustained release of siRNA nanomaterials [21–23].

Recently, miRNAs and siRNAs have also been studied for clinical application. More than 20 projects for clinical study are underway for the treatment of cancer, infection, asthma, macular degeneration, and common metabolic diseases [24, 25]. However, half of these siRNA clinical studies have only limited local applications, while few others have been investigated for systemic delivery (mainly using liposomes), and the progress of these trials has been very slow. Outstanding drug delivery systems (DDSs) to safely achieve maximum therapeutic efficacy using siRNAs are required urgently.

Kim et al. actively investigated the development of bioreducible poly(disulfide amine)s for gene delivery with high efficiency and

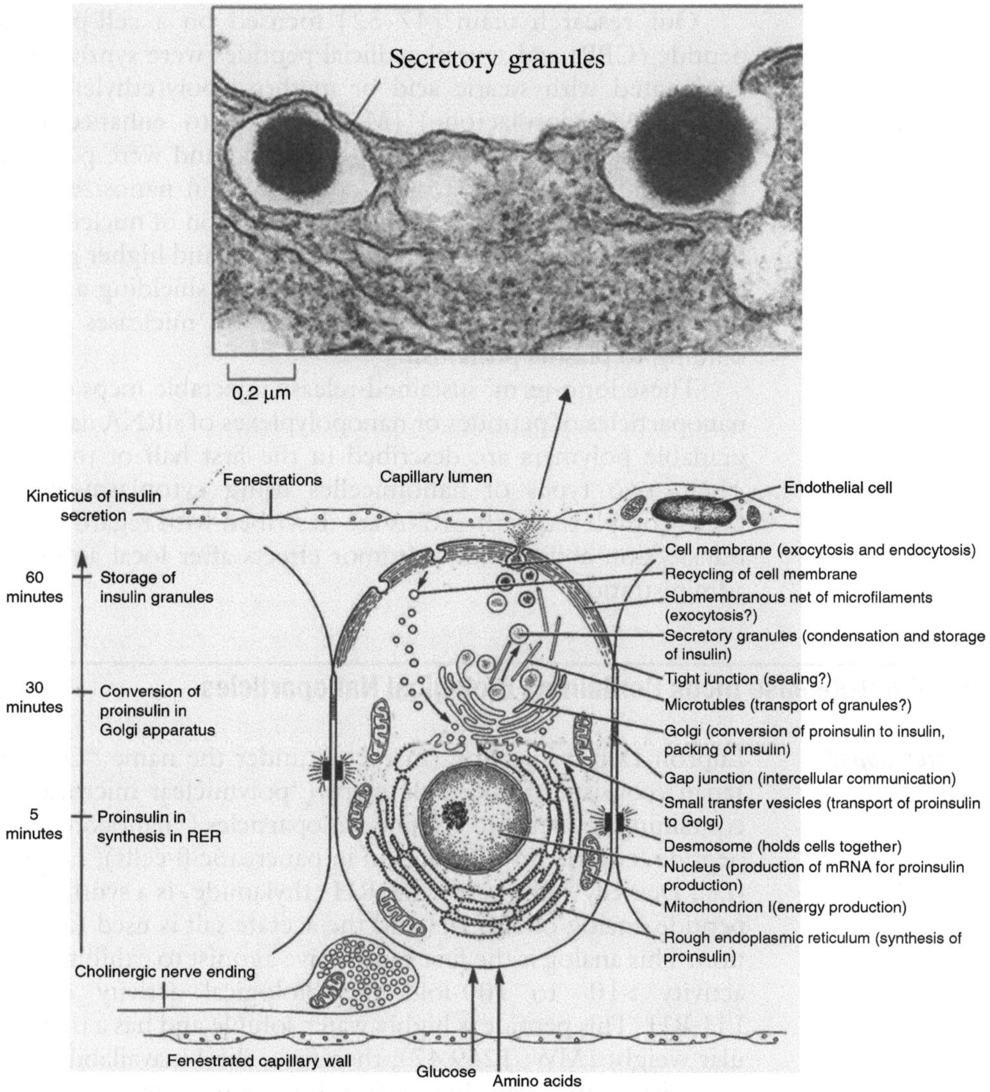

Fig. 1 Biosynthesis of insulin in β-cells of pancreatic islets and the stimuli-responsive exocytosis pathway of insulin nanoparticles from excretory granules

low cytotoxicity [26–38]. Cystamine bisacrylamide-based SS-poly(amido amine)s (PAAs) were developed, and Arg [30, 31, 37] as well as guanidine [33, 38] was grafted to PAA to enhance transfection efficiency. Self-assembly of DNA with template disulfide polymerization of peptides and di-Cys-nuclear localizing signals (CGYGPKKKRKVGGC) have been investigated as carriers for transfection with low cytotoxicity into cells [39]. Furthermore, other reducible polycationic peptides based on $CH_6K_3H_6C$ [40], fusion peptide KALA [41], $C(D\text{-}R)_9C$ [42–45], and CHR_6HC [46] have been developed as effective cytoplasm-responsive peptide carriers for nucleotides. In most of these studies, treatments have been also carried out after local administration of these agents.

Our research team [47–52] focused on a cell-penetrating peptide (CPP) and several artificial peptides were synthesized and conjugated with stearic acid or methoxy poly(ethylene glycol)-block-poly(ε-caprolactone) (MPEG-PCL) to enhance transfection. These peptide carriers self-assembled and were polymerized by disulfide bonding via oxidization in air in nanosized micelles after mixing with siRNAs. Complex formation of nucleotides with these nanocarriers afforded less cytotoxicity and higher gene transfection efficiency. This was because of high shielding and protection of nucleotides from degradation by nucleases and from binding to plasma proteins.

These long-term, sustained-release injectable mcps containing nanoparticles of peptides or nanopolyplexes of siRNA using biodegradable polymers are described in the first half of this chapter. Then, two types of nanomicelles using cytoplasm-responsive CPPs complexed with siRNA are described with regard to cellular transfection ability and antitumor effects after local and systemic administration.

2 Sustained-Release mcps Containing Biological Nanoparticles

2.1 Lupron Depot® Injection

Lupron Depot injection (marketed under the name "Leuplin" in Japan) consists of injectable mcps ("polynuclear microcapsules") containing numerous very fine nanoparticles ("nanocores") of the peptide leuprorelin (like insulin in pancreatic β-cells). Leuprorelin (i.e., Des-Gly^{10}-(D-Leu^{6})-LH-RH ethylamide) is a synthetic nonapeptide analog of LH-RH and the acetate salt is used for preparation. This analog is the first superactive agonist to exhibit biological activity >10- to 100-fold the biological activity of natural LH-RH. This peptide is highly water soluble and has a high molecular weight (MW; 1269.47); therefore, the bioavailability by oral administration is very low owing to poor membrane permeability and degradation by gastrointestinal enzymes. The peptide is extremely stable in water but is unstable in blood and body fluids owing to enzymatic degradation and is excreted rapidly from the body soon after injection. Therefore, daily injection over a prolonged period is needed for therapeutic efficacy. To overcome these disadvantages, we focused on developing a sustained-release depot injection using biodegradable polymers. Depot-injectable formulations were prepared using our in-water drying method (1983) [11]. A reconstituted mcp suspension was injected using a fine needle (23–26G), because the particles have an average diameter of <20 μm. The wall of 1-month depot mcp encapsulated nanoparticles of the peptide is comprised of the biodegradable polymer, PLGA (75/25)-14,000 [poly(DL-lactic and glycolic acid), and lactic/glycolic acid ratio of 75/25, MW of 14,000]. Three-month depot mcp wall is comprised of PLA-15,000 [poly(lactic acid) having a MW of 15,000]. The peptide are released continuously after dissolution and diffusion through the hydrated polymer following biodegradation in body fluids.

Leuprorelin acetate is an agonistic analog of LH-RH. It induces sexual maturation and ovulation by stimulating gonadotropin (LH and follicle-stimulating hormone [FSH]) secretion in the pituitary gland as well as steroidogenesis of estradiol (females) and testosterone (males) in the genital organs. However, if administered chronically at a relatively high dose, paradoxically it exerts antagonistic inhibitory effects on gonadotropin secretion from the pituitary gland and testicular/ovarian steroidogenesis: chemical castration. These effects are attributed to downregulation of the expression of LH-RH receptors in the pituitary gland owing to chronic stimulation by the stronger pharmacological potency of leuprorelin acetate as compared with native LH-RH.

Chronic administration of 1-month depot mcp has been shown to markedly inhibit blood levels of gonadotropin and sex hormones in rats and dogs over 4 weeks [12–16]. Persistent suppression of the growth of genital organs such as the testis, prostate gland, and seminal vesicles in male rats, as well as the ovary and uterus in female rats, was obtained even with a single injection of mcp. These inhibitory effects have been used to treat sex hormone-dependent diseases such as tumors in the prostate gland, breast tumors, endometriosis, uterine fibroids, and central precocious puberty without serious side effects or the need for surgical castration.

2.1.1 Preparation of Depot mcps

The in-water drying method is based on a novel $W_1/O/W_2$ dual-emulsion technique for water-soluble peptides devised originally by Okada et al. [11]. The method for preparing 1-month depot mcps on a laboratory scale is shown schematically in Fig. 2. In brief, the peptide and gelatin are dissolved in a small amount of distilled water (W_1) at about 60 °C. The peptide solution is homogenized vigorously with PLGA-dichloromethane (DCM) solution (O) by using a Polytron homogenizer (PT3100; Kinematica AG, Littau, Switzerland) and cooled to 15–18 °C to stabilize the W_1/O emulsion. Then, the emulsion is infused into a large volume of 0.25 % polyvinyl alcohol (PVA) solution using a glass injector with a long, narrow needle, just under the agitating blades, while homogenizing in a turbine-shaped homogenizer at >6000 rpm. The resulting dual emulsion is stirred gently for 3 h in a fume hood to remove the organic solvent. These semi-dried mcps are sieved through 74-μm apertures to remove larger particles and washed twice with water using gentle centrifugation. The sedimented mcp pellet is re-dispersed in mannitol solution and lyophilized to remove residual organic solvent and water. This procedure affords much higher trapping efficiency of a water-soluble compound in the mcps owing to the stability of the emulsion during the interaction between the nanosized-cationic drug cores and anionic polymer (Fig. 2).

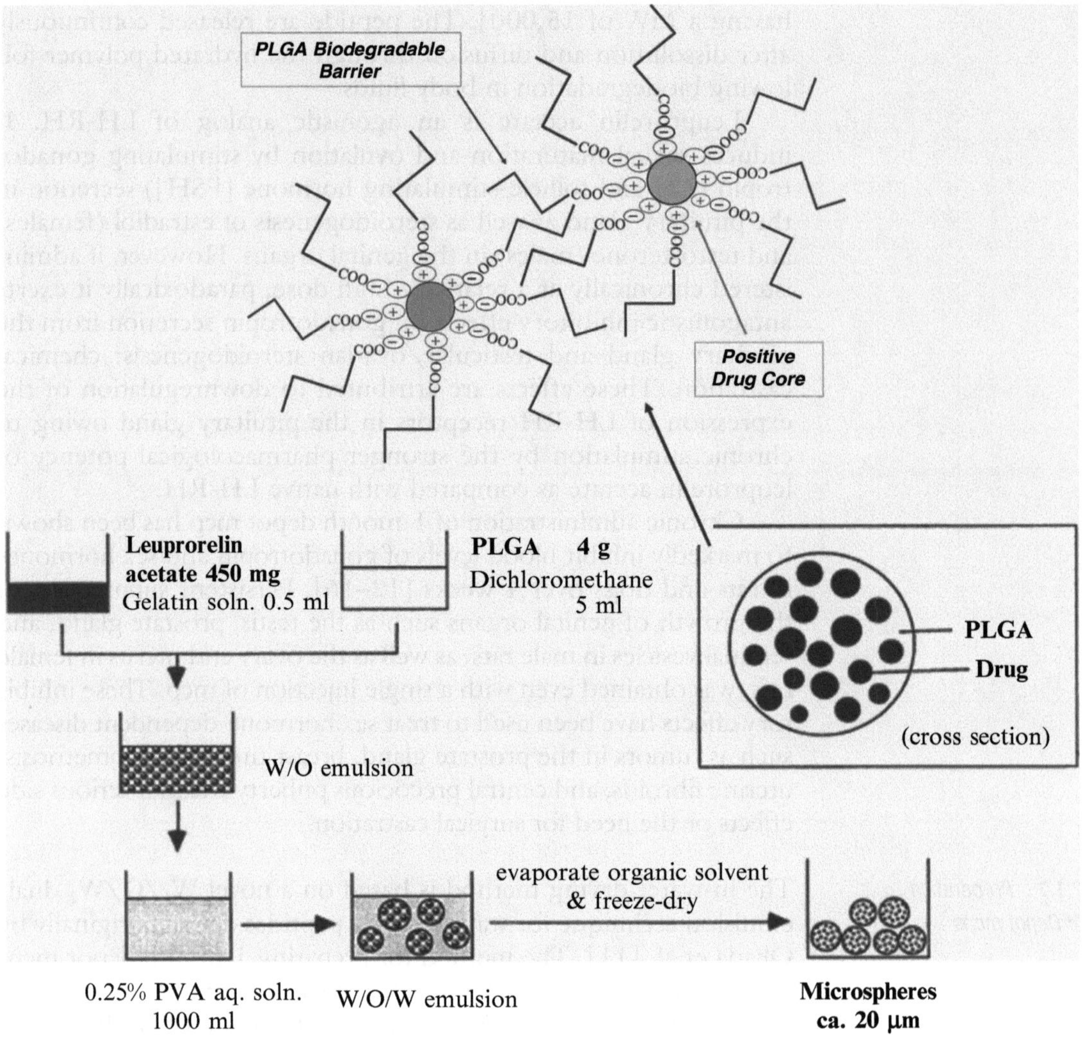

Fig. 2 Preparation procedure for 1-month depot PLGA microspheres of leuprorelin acetate using a W/O/W dual-emulsion-solvent evaporation method and schematic entrapment of micelle-like nanocores of the water-soluble peptide with polymer for sustained release

This procedure results in rigid micelle-like nanodomains of the drug surrounded by polymeric alkyl chains.

The rigid structure of mcps can also provide very long-term, continuous drug release in the body because of bioerosion of the polymer, which is attributed to its micelle-like nanostructure. The change in the remaining amount of the peptide at the injection site after subcutaneous injection in rats is dependent on bioerosion of the polymer in the mcp with different types of polymer (Fig. 3). Thus, release of peptides from the mcp prepared with a rapid-erosion polymer (PLGA[75/25]-15,800: around 1-month depot) was rapid and that with a slow-erosion polymer (PLA-18,200: around 3-month depot) was slow.

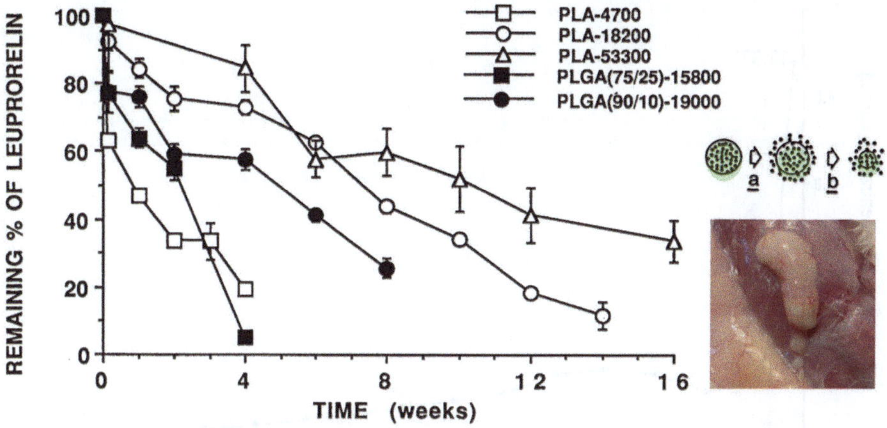

Fig. 3 Remaining amount of leuprorelin at the injection site in microcapsules prepared by several types of biodegradable polymer and a photograph of microcapsules wrapped by a thin film of collagen with neovascularization after subcutaneous injection in rats. Dose = 0.9 mg, mean ± SE, $n = 5$

Three-month release mcps of leuprorelin are prepared using a similar in-water drying method, with minor modifications to the volumes of solvent used [17, 18]. We have also achieved a 6-month depot preparation of leuprorelin using PLA-30,000, which was synthesized by a ring opening method and hydrolyzed by 1 N NaOH to reveal free carboxylic acids at the polymer ends. In the absence of these free anions, encapsulation efficiency was low and the initial burst large. This is the most important point of this methodology. Gelatin was eliminated from the inner drug solution in the 1-month depot preparation when bovine spongiform encephalopathy was prevalent worldwide.

2.1.2 Drug Release from mcps

Drug-release profiles during setting up of the final formulation were assessed by the peptide remaining at the injection site using high-performance liquid chromatography (HPLC) after subcutaneous injection in rats (Fig. 3). Serum drug levels were determined using our radioimmunoassay (RIA) system after injection of the mcp, which recently can be easily assayed by liquid chromatography-tandem mass spectrometry (LC/MS/MS). Serum levels of the peptide were maintained over 4 weeks in rats, dogs, and humans (Fig. 4) to similar extents after a single subcutaneous or intramuscular injection of the 1-month depot formulation [14]. Serum leuprorelin levels in rats and dogs after subcutaneous or intramuscular injection of the 3-month depot msp preparation were stable over 13 weeks after a short-lived initial elevation [19].

2.1.3 Pharmacological Activities in Animals

Suppression of Steroidogenesis

Strong suppression of serum levels of estradiol, testosterone, LH, and FSH for 6 weeks following initial elevation of levels of these hormones following an agonistic activity was induced in male and female rats as well as dogs by single injection of the 1-month depot

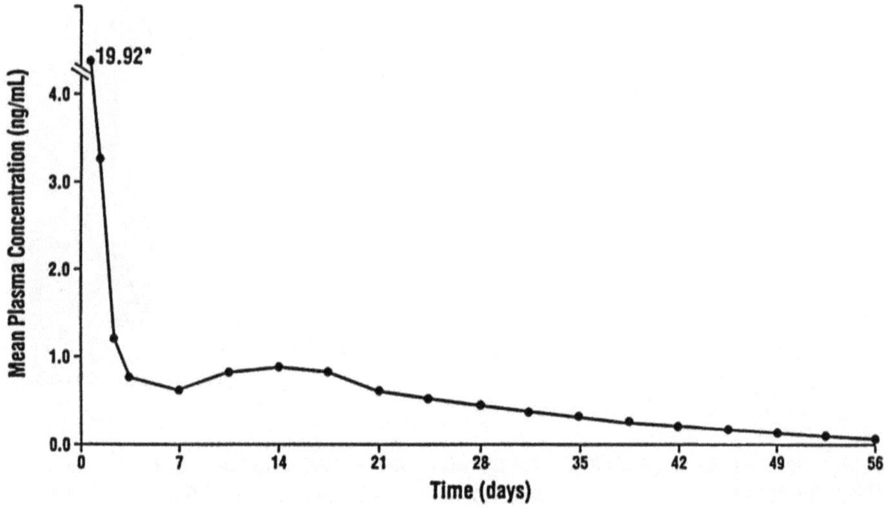

Fig. 4 Mean plasma concentration of leuprorelin in patients suffering from prostate cancer after intramuscular injection of 1-month sustained-release injection, Lupron Depot 7.5 mg

formulation [12–15]. The initial flare-up of serum testosterone disappeared completely after 3 days in rats and after 2 weeks in dogs and humans. With multiple injections, little flare-up was observed after the second and subsequent injections as long as chemical castration was maintained [15]. Growth of the genital organs was obviously inhibited in rats within 2 weeks and lasted for >6 weeks following a single injection at the dose of over 100 μg/kg/day [14]. Serum estradiol levels were suppressed for 6 weeks after injection without an initial flare-up.

Serum testosterone was strongly suppressed for >16 weeks after a single intramuscular injection of the 3-month depot in male rats at 1–100 μg/kg/day (Fig. 5) [19]. Strong suppression of growth of the genital organs (including the testis, seminal vesicles, and prostate gland) was observed. This suppression served as a indication of suppression of hormone-dependent tumors of the prostate gland. This growth suppression occurred at 100 μg/kg/day for >16 weeks.

A periodic challenge test with a peptide solution (100 μg) revealed that single injection of the mcp caused dramatic suppression of the ability of the pituitary-gonadal system to secrete gonadotropin and testosterone. This effect lasted for >5 weeks with the 1-month depot and for >15 weeks with the 3-month depot [15, 19]. Complete recovery of these functions was observed 10 weeks after injection of the 1-month depot, showing it to be a temporary form of chemical castration. Cytological examination of vaginal smears after injection of the mcp in female rats also showed reversible and sustained inhibition of the estrous cycle. The cycle was arrested in diestrus for 6 weeks after injection and recovered 8–10 weeks later

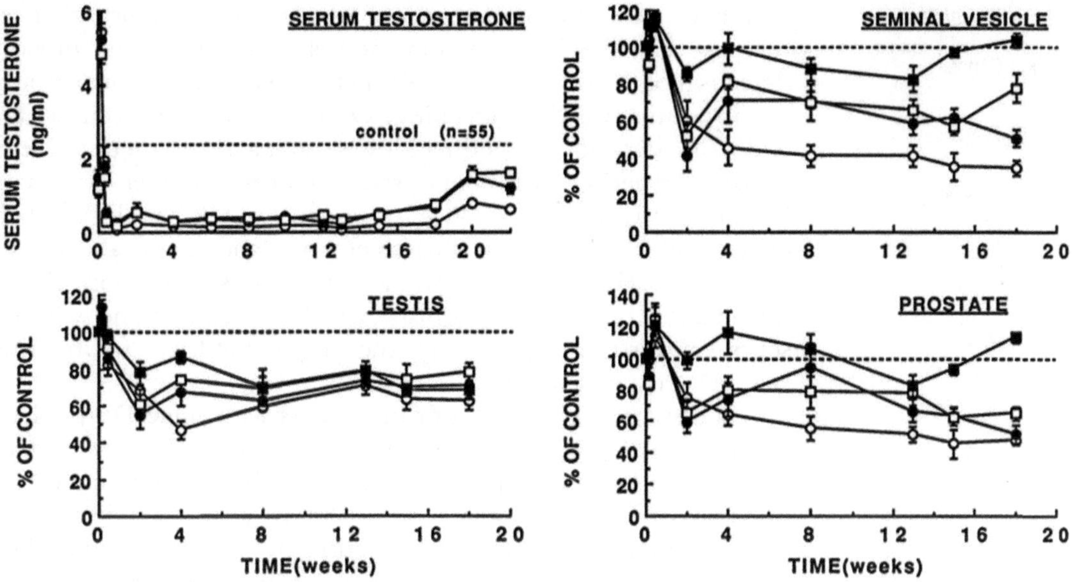

Fig. 5 Serum testosterone and weight change of genital organs in rats after intramuscular injection of a 3-month depot of leuprorelin. Dose: 100 (*open circle*), 30 (*filled circle*), 10 (*open square*), 1 (*filled square*) μg/kg/day (mean ± SE, *n* = 5)

[15]. This recovery of function of the ovary is desirable, resulting in the possible induction of fertility. It is very beneficial, especially for young women.

Inhibition in a Prostate Tumor Model

Ichikawa et al. [53] reported that single injection of a depot preparation of leuprorelin (10 mg/kg/month) suppressed tumor growth in the Dunning rat R3327 prostatic tumor model much more robustly than did daily injection of the peptide (333 μg/kg/day) solution at the same dose. Antitumor effects were potentiated if the dose was divided and administered twice a day. The depot formulation had the greatest effect of all the treatments and was almost equal to that of surgical castration. These results clearly indicated that the depot formulation could produce potent antitumor activity by providing persistent levels of the peptide in blood.

Treatment in a Model of Endometriosis

Endometriosis is caused by the growth of an aberrant or ectopic endometrium at various locations within the pelvic cavity, including the ovaries, uterine ligaments, rectovaginal septum, and pelvic peritoneum. We examined the effect of the 1-month depot on endometriosis in a Jones experimental endometriosis model in female rats [12]. Single injection of the mcp at 100 μg/kg/day significantly decreased endometrial explants (94 % regression and 54 % disappearance) 3 weeks after injection, which was comparable with that achieved by surgical ovariectomy. Daily intermittent subcutaneous injection of the peptide at 100 μg/kg significantly suppressed the growth of all explants (though they remained visible).

2.1.4 Clinical Studies

Prostate Cancer

Incidence rates of prostate cancer have increased significantly over the past 35 years. This phenomenon is probably a result of early detection of the tumor due to the increased availability of prostate-specific antigen (PSA) screening. Over 80 % of these cancers are endocrine dependent, tend to grow slowly, and can metastasize in >50 % of patients. Treatment of stage D prostate cancer focuses on hormonal therapies to reduce androgen levels or to block their effects and includes surgical (orchiectomy) and chemical (diethylstilbestrol, LH-RH agonist, and antiandrogens) castration. Depot formulation of LH-RH agonists, which is effective and without serious adverse effects, is now the "gold standard" for treating stage D prostate cancer.

In a study first carried out in patients with stage D2 prostate cancer in the USA, *plateau* serum levels of leuprorelin persisted for >4 weeks after single injection of the mcp (Fig. 4). Dramatic suppression of serum testosterone to below castration levels was achieved after 4-week repeated injection at 7.5 mg (corresponding to 1/4 the dose used with peptide solution). These results agree well with preclinical animal studies. In worldwide studies, a satisfactory objective response (no progression) in 88–98 % of patients treated with 3.75-mg and 7.5-mg depots was observed. Overall, 50–60 % of patients had complete or partial responses. Rapid relief from bone pain (80–90 % of patients), significant improvement of nocturnal problems (dysuria, 60–80 %), and general well-being were also reported. In clinical studies of the 3-month depot, safety and efficacy of Lupron Depot (3-month) (22.5 mg) similar to that of the original daily subcutaneous injection and monthly depot formulation were achieved during the initial 24 weeks of treatment. About 60 % of patients experienced hot flashes/sweats, and other mild side effects such as gynecomastia (16 %), nausea, vomiting (13 %), and diarrhea (2 %) were also observed.

Endometriosis

Endometriosis occurs in about 10 % of all women of reproductive age and is a common cause of chronic pelvic pain and/or infertility. In the USA, the safety and efficacy of Lupron Depot (3.75 mg) in patients with endometriosis was first assessed using six injections every 4 weeks. Estradiol levels decreased significantly to menopausal levels (<30 pg/mL) and menses were suppressed completely. In a double-blind randomized clinical trial of depot formulation versus danazol in 270 patients, Lupron Depot caused more rapid and profound suppression of estradiol than danazol and was similarly effective in decreasing the extent of endometriosis as assessed by laparoscopy. In addition, dysmenorrhea (99 %), pelvic pain (55 %), and tenderness (73 %) were improved by the end of treatment. Common side effects of the depot formulation were hot flashes (84 %) and vasomotor symptoms (91 %), headache (35 %), vaginitis (29 %), insomnia (17 %), emotional liability (16 %), nausea (13 %), weight gain (13 %), nervousness (13 %), decreased libido (13 %), acne (11 %), depression (11 %), and dizziness (10 %). The leuprorelin group showed a greater mean loss of bone mineral density than the danazol group. Most bone loss caused by treatment with LH-RH agonists was reversible, but strategic approaches to avoid such bone loss should be considered (especially for young women).

2.2 Mcps Containing Nanocomplexes of siRNAs

We are investigating rational delivery systems for siRNAs that inhibit expression of a specific DNA by cleaving the complementary sequence in mRNA ("gene silencing"). siRNAs are synthesized easily, and a small dose specifically inhibits the disease-related gene. siRNAs are expected to be major biomaterials for molecular-targeted medicines without serious side effects.

The focus for our siRNA studies is inhibition of gene expression of vascular endothelial growth factor (VEGF), which regulates tumor angiogenesis and is an important factor in tumor growth [21]. However, siRNAs are readily hydrolyzed by RNAse in body fluids and are poorly permeable in cells and organs. Therefore, an efficient transfection carrier for siRNAs within cells is required to achieve potency. siRNAs can inhibit translation of mRNA by repeatedly degrading mRNA enzymatically for 5–7 days by single transfection (which is more prolonged than that by antisense nucleotides). However, if sustained silencing for long-term therapy is required, a form that can produce sustained dose release is essential for disease suppression. Thus, we investigated preparation of depot PLGA(75/25)-14,000 mcp encapsulating anti-VEGF siRNA (siVEGF) complexes with branched PEI in an in-water drying method to attain continuous silencing and antitumor activities [21]. The encapsulation efficiency of siRNA increased if arginine or PEI was added to the inner water phase of the W_1/O emulsion. After single intratumoral injection, the siRNA PLGA mcp persistently inhibited VEGF secretion from tumor cells and suppressed tumor growth for >4 weeks in mice bearing S-180 tumors (Fig. 6). Antitumor activity was strongest upon combination therapy with anti-angiogenesis by siVEGF and induction of apoptosis by sicFLIP (anti-cFLIP [cellular FLICE-inhibitory protein] siRNA). FLICE is a FADD-like IL-1β-converting enzyme, and FADD is a Fas-associated protein with a death domain. These results indicate that long-term, controlled release of siRNA by a delivery system can be effective. They also serve as an example for potentiating the medical usefulness of a biomaterial by matching the drug and intensive DDS (e.g., long-term depot formulations).

We have also developed a depot-injectable mcp containing siRNA/PEI nanosized complexes (N/P ratio, 15) for treating arteriosclerosis obliterans (ASO) and intermittent claudication [22, 23]. Anti-Int6 RNA/DNA chimera siRNA (siInt6, Alphagen, Yokohama, Japan) was used for inducing neovascularization around the avascular zone by ASO. Integration site 6 (Int6) is an

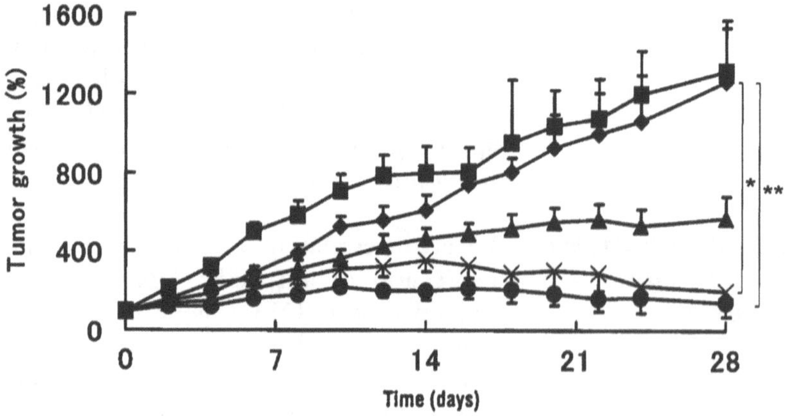

Fig. 6 Antitumor effects of siRNA microcapsules after single intratumoral injection in mice bearing S-180 sarcoma cells. PBS (*diamond*), PLGA msp (*filled square*), siVEGF mcp (12.6 μg, *filled triangle*), sicFLIP mcp (12.6 μg, ×), and combination mcp (sicFLIP 18.5 μg, siVEGF 9.0 μg, *filled circle*) (mean ± SE, $n = 5$, * $p < 0.05$; ** $p < 0.01$, Student's t-test)

inhibitor of hypoxia-inducible factor (HIF)-2α, which is an angiogenesis factor to increase levels of erythropoietin (EPO) and VEGF. The mcp containing siInt6/PEI nanocomplexes had a diameter of 34 μm, could release nanosized complexes from PLGA(75/25)-14,000 mcp for 2 weeks, and induced neovascularization by single injection of 10.5 μg siInt6 at the avascular zone on femoral muscle developed following ligation of the femoral arterial vein. The neovascular capillaries observed by microscopy were comparable with daily injection of a siInt6 (1.5 μg)/PEI complex solution and could detect many neocapillaries at the injection site after immunostaining endothelial cells with anti-rat CD31 (cluster of differentiation 31, a marker of endothelial cells) antibody 2 weeks after surgery and treatment. Hence, sustained release of siRNAs can achieve continuous silencing and promote the pharmacological effect of siRNAs.

3 Cytoplasm-Responsive CPP Nanocarriers

3.1 Mechanism of Cytoplasm-Responsive Gene Carriers

Glutathione tripeptide (GSH; γ-glutamyl-cysteinyl-glycine) is the most abundant biological thiol, and GSH/glutathione disulfide (GSSG) is the major redox couple in animal cells [54]. In body fluids, blood, and the extracellular matrix, proteins are rich in stabilizing disulfides due to a low concentration of GSH (2–20 μM) (Fig. 7). Within cells, the GSH concentration is about 1000-times higher (0.5–10 mM), which is kept reduced by NADPH and glutathione reductase, thereby maintaining a highly reducing environment inside cells. The large difference in reducing potential

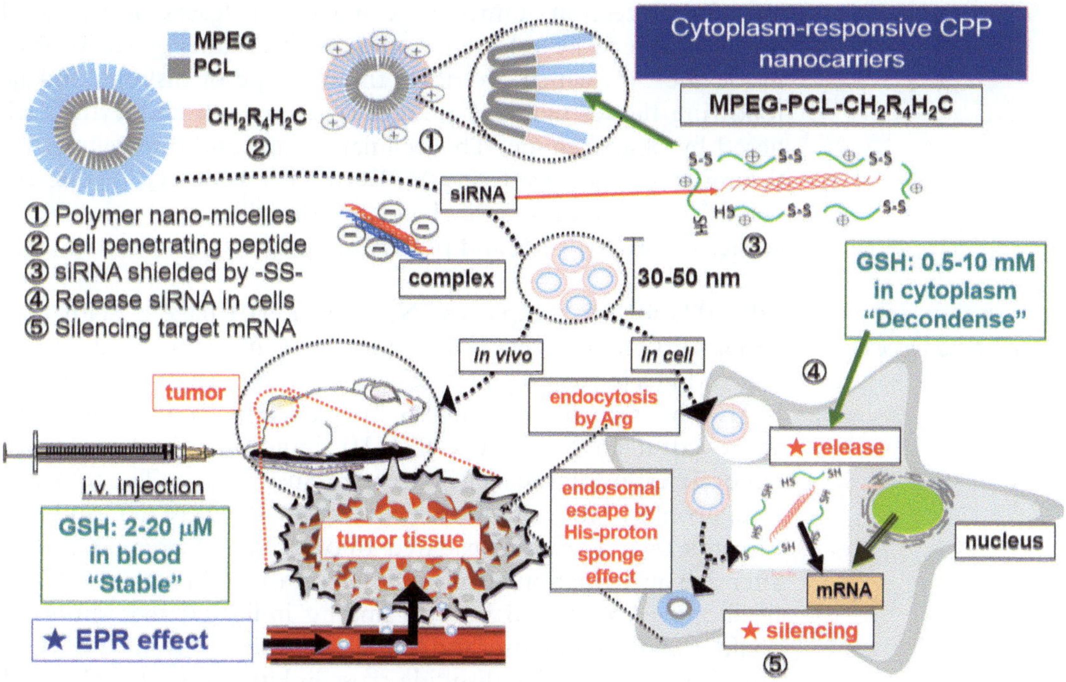

Fig. 7 Endocytosis and intracellular trafficking of cytoplasm-responsive CPP nanocarriers and MPEG-PCL-$CH_2R_4H_2C$ (OK-103)/siRNA complexes in cells (schematic) [25]

between intracellular and extracellular environments can be exploited for triggering intracellular delivery of various bioactive molecules [55]. Also of particular interest is that tumor tissues are highly reducing and hypoxic compared with normal tissues, with at least fourfold higher concentrations of GSH in tumor tissues than normal tissues [56]. The disulfide-linked complexes of nucleotides with cationic nanocarriers are very stable in blood, but complexes are easily cleaved and can release the nucleotides inside the cells efficiently.

3.2 Local Delivery of Genes

To develop a new gene carrier with higher efficacy of cellular uptake and greater intracellular release of nucleotides, we synthesized a new cytoplasm-responsive carrier peptide, stearoyl (STR)-$CH_2R_4H_2C$ (OK-102). Four Arg (R) residues and the STR moiety can induce endocytosis of the nucleotide complexes, and 4 His (H) residues and STR can promote early endosomal escape by the "proton sponge effect" and membrane fusion. Moreover, this carrier peptide can form rigid complexes with nucleotides not only through ionic interactions of negatively charged nucleotides with positively charged Arg moieties but also through trapping inside a CPP network of intermolecular and intramolecular disulfide cross-linkages between two Cys (C) residues in non-reducing environments (e.g., extracellular space and blood), which results in effective protection of nucleotides against nucleases. Subsequently, nucleotides can be released readily in the reducing environment inside the cell, which promotes the cleavage of disulfide linkages following higher uptake by target cells through endocytosis triggered by oligoarginine. This cellular uptake and intracellular trafficking also occurred in MPEG-PCL-$CH_2R_4H_2C$ (OK-103) (Fig. 7). Furthermore, we elucidated the efficacy of OK-102 as a carrier for siRNA [47] and pDNA [48].

3.2.1 Pharmacological Effects of Nanocomplexes

OK-102/siRNA complexes (N/P ratio, 10) have a diameter of about 100 nm and zeta potential of 18.2 mV, which indicate that Arg and His in the polymer appear on the surface of the complexes [47]. The shielding of 85–95 % siRNAs with this carrier was approved at an N/P ratio of 1–10, indicating rigid trapping in nanocarriers using the SYBR Green exclusion assay. The remaining thiol groups in the complexes (N/P ratio, 10) were determined by Elman's test. The non-oxidated thiol groups decreased to 60 % after 2-h air oxidation at room temperature and reached a *plateau* of about 40 % after 8 h. This finding indicated that the carrier could rapidly condense and physically shield siRNA via charge interaction and netlike disulfide cross-linking of double Cys in the peptide carrier.

The sequence-specific silencing effects by these carrier complexes of anti-VEGF siRNA (siVEGF) were evaluated by VEGF secretion in S-180 sarcoma cells using an enzyme-linked immunosorbent assay (ELISA) [47]. Increasing the N/P ratio of OK-102/siVEGF enhanced suppression of VEGF secretion. This complex exhibited distinctly greater inhibition on VEGF secretion than did siVEGF/STR-$GH_2R_4H_2G$ (no disulfide-binding carrier) and comparable inhibition with siVEGF/$CH_2R_4H_2C$ (no STR carrier) or LipoTrust (commercial cationic liposome vector) complexes in this in vitro study (Fig. 8). Naked siVEGF and non-silencing mock siRNA (siCont)/OK-102 did not show gene inhibition comparable with siVEGF/OK-102, suggesting that siVEGF can suppress VEGF expression in cancer cells in a highly sequence-specific manner. These pharmacological activities coincided with cellular uptake of siVEGF [47]. OK-102 complexes at any N/P ratio had higher cellular viability in the WST-8 assays in comparison to untreated cells. These results indicate that OK-102 may serve as a highly efficient and safe carrier of siRNA for local injection and mucosal application.

OK-102/siVEGF complexes were evaluated for in vivo therapeutic activity by determination of efficacy after intratumoral injection in mice subcutaneously inoculated with S-180 sarcoma cells [47]. Increased suppression of tumor growth by OK-102/siVEGF was achieved in comparison to complexation with a commercial vector. Naked siVEGF did not show suppression of tumor growth in this mouse model (Fig. 9).

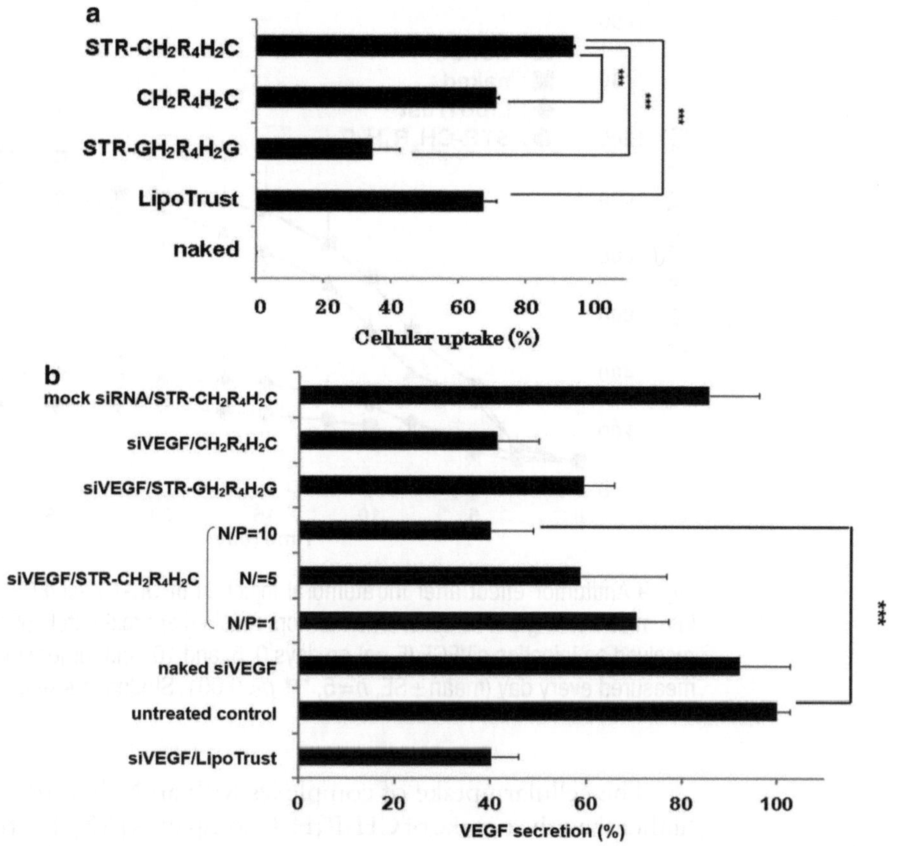

Fig. 8 Cellular uptake of siRNA and silencing effects by STR-$CH_2R_4H_2C$ (OK-102)/siVEGF in S-180 cells. (**a**) FAM-siRNA (1 μg) complexes with $CH_2R_4H_2C$-based carriers (N/P ratio, 10) were transfected into S-180 cells. After 4-h incubation, cellular uptake of FAM-siRNA was determined by flow cytometry. (**b**) siVEGF (1 μg) complexes with OK-102 (N/P ratio, 10) were transfected into S-180 cells for 12 h. After 48-h incubation, VEGF secretion in the culture medium was determined by ELISA (mean ± SD, $n = 3$, *** $p < 0.001$, Student's *t*-test)

3.3 Nanocarriers for Systemic Injection

To obtain nucleotide delivery systems with high stability in blood and high transfection efficiency to the target organ, a systemic delivery system for siRNAs using polymer micelles comprising amphiphilic block copolymers of MPEG and poly(ε-caprolactone), MPEG-PCL, conjugated with the Tat analog [51] and an artificial CPP, $CH_2R_4H_2C$ (OK-103) [52], was investigated.

The physical and chemical characterization of OK-103/siRNA complexes was evaluated [52]. OK-103/siVEGF complexes could be condensed effectively at N/P ratios >5, and the carrier had considerably higher compaction to physically shield siRNAs (Fig. 10a). Polymer-CPP carrier/siVEGF complexes at high N/P ratios of 5–20 were approximately 30–70 nm in diameter, and their zeta potential was positive (Fig. 10b). Formation of a complex of this polymer micelle with an artificial CPP (N/P ratio, 20) increased its RNAse resistance (Fig. 10c).

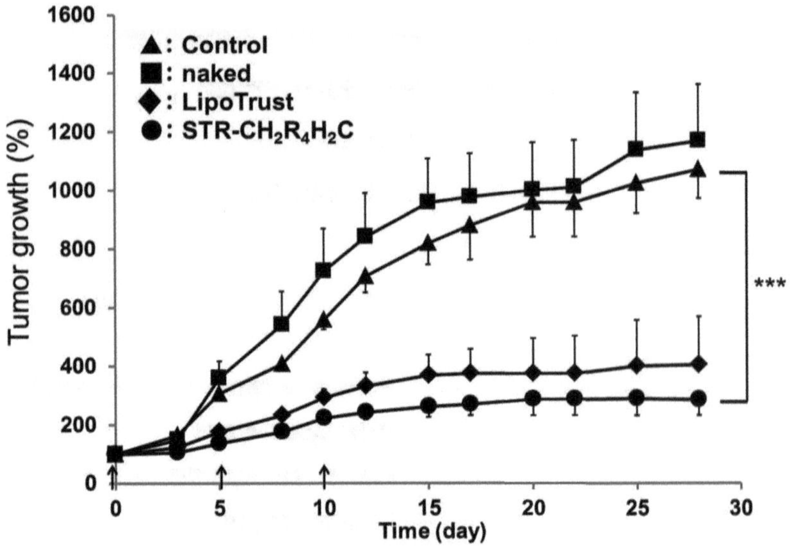

Fig. 9 Antitumor effect after intratumoral injection of OK-102/siVEGF complexes into mice bearing S-180 cells. When tumors reached approximately 50 mm^3, mice received an injection siVEGF (5 μg) on days 0, 5, and 10, and tumor volumes were measured every day (mean ± SE, $n = 5$, *** $p < 0.001$, Student's *t*-test)

The cellular uptake of complexes with an N/P ratio of 20 was higher than the uptake of $CH_2R_4H_2C$ complexes [52]. Furthermore, the cellular uptake of $CH_2R_4H_2C$ complexes decreased significantly in the presence of serum, while cellular uptake of OK-103 complexes remained unaffected. These results suggest that the PEG chain provides resistance against interactions with serum proteins and enzymatic attack in the blood. We hypothesized that our micelles form a "V" shape that exposes $CH_2R_4H_2C$ and the PEG chain on the surface of the micelle, which allows each moiety to exert its respective function (Fig. 7) [25].

PEI has strong ionic interaction with nucleotides, so PEI is taken into cells effectively. However, the release and transfection of the nucleotide is insufficient because of very strong ionic interactions, which also produces higher cytotoxicity. siRNAs in our carrier complexes could be released easily from the rigid complex after cleavage of disulfide linkages in the reductive environment of the cytoplasm.

Although tumor growth in mice treated with naked siVEGF and siCont (nonsense sequence control oligonucleotide) was not affected as well as untreated control mice, the tumor growth in tumor-bearing mice injected intravenously with the OK-103/siVEGF complex was suppressed significantly (Fig. 11) [52]. The ELISA assay revealed that VEGF secretion in tumor tissue after intravenous injection of the complex was suppressed significantly compared with that in mice treated with naked siVEGF and in untreated controls.

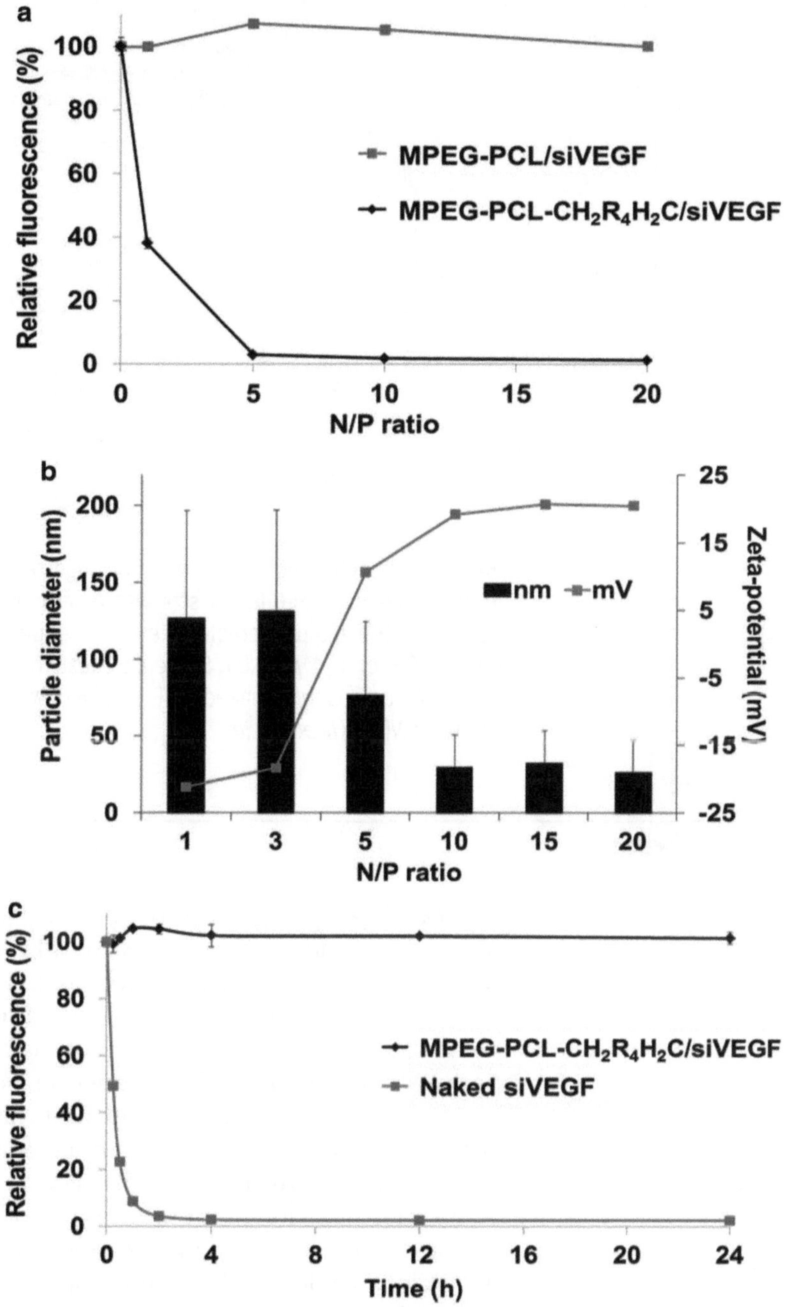

Fig. 10 Condensation by disulfide bonding and particle size/charge of siVEGF complexes with OK-103 and RNAse resistance of siVEGF. (**a**) Complexes were prepared at several N/P ratios by incubation at room temperature for 30 min. Fluorescence was measured using a microplate reader after labeling with SYBR Green. (**b**) Particle diameter (bar) and zeta potential (point) were measured using a dynamic light scattering and particle-sizing system, respectively. (**c**) RNAse A (RNAse A/siVEGF, 10 ng/μg) was added to naked siVEGF and the OK-103/siVEGF complex (N/P ratio, 20) solution and kept at room temperature until determination of intact siVEGF (mean ± SD, $n = 3$)

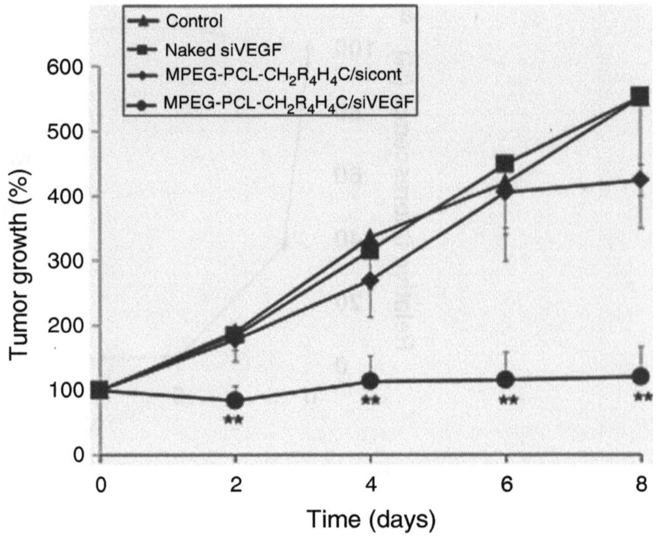

Fig. 11 Antitumor effect after intravenous injections of OK-103/siVEGF complexes in tumor-bearing mice. Tumor size was determined after intravenous injection of OK-103/siVEGF (25 μg) complexes every other day into S-180 tumor-bearing mice (mean ± SE, $n=5$, $^{**}p<0.01$: Student's *t*-test versus untreated control). Untreated control (*filled triangle*), naked siVEGF (*filled square*), OK-103/siCont (*diamond*), OK-103/siVEGF (*filled circle*)

4 Conclusion

Lupron Depot preparations (leuprorelin sustained-release injectable mcps with biodegradable PLGA and PLA) were found to exert persistent suppression of steroidogenesis and hormone-dependent diseases (e.g., prostate tumors, breast tumors, endometriosis, and precocious puberty) for 1 and 3 months by single injection, respectively. Mcps can encapsulate numerous peptide nanocores inside a polymer matrix. They have a rigid alkyl chain as a "diffusion barrier" and can release peptides as insulin nanoparticles inside small secretory granules of pancreatic β-cells. Thus, peptides can be released at a steady rate for a long time at the injection site. In this investigation, the novel microencapsulation method of in-water drying through the use of a stable W/O/W emulsion for water-soluble peptides was devised by our research team, resulting in the launch of a commercial product in the USA. These depot formulations have undoubtedly improved the quality of life and medication compliance of patients (90 % for those with prostate cancer) and have enhanced the medical usefulness of leuprorelin acetate dramatically. However, to achieve a more rational approach for most therapeutic peptides and proteins, DDSs providing more complex control of release (e.g., stimulus-mediated or biosensor-controlled) will be necessary. For example, we could treat diseases more precisely by taking into account circadian rhythms or disease symptoms using intelligent materials responsive to external stimuli.

Two functional CPPs, Tat analog and the artificial CPP, $CH_2R_4H_2C$, were conjugated with STR for local administration and MPEG-PCL for systemic injection. STR-$CH_2R_4H_2C$ (OK-102) promoted the delivery of siRNAs for treating rat tumors by direct intratumoral injection. Moreover, a novel diblock copolymer conjugated with a functional CPP, MPEG-PCL-$CH_2R_4H_2C$ (OK-103), safely promoted the delivery of siRNAs into tumor cells after intravenous injection in an in vivo study. OK-103/siRNA nanomicelles are very stable in blood of oxidative conditions after intravenous injection, because of complete physical shielding by 2 Cys in the CPP peptide network. These nanomicelles are delivered efficiently into tumor tissue by stabilizing the siRNA against nucleases, avoiding uptake by the reticuloendothelial system, and localizing by the enhanced permeability and retention effect (EPR effect). Therefore, these CPP carrier/siRNA complexes increase uptake by tumor cells (via Arg clusters on the surface of polymer micelles that promote endocytosis), ensure rapid escape from early endosomes (proton sponge effect by His residues), and achieve efficient release by decompaction of CPP nanocarrier complexes in the cytoplasm (cleavage of disulfide linkages by the reducing cytosol environment: "cytoplasm-responsive nanocarriers") and may efficiently exert persistent silencing effect and strong therapeutic effects.

Acknowledgments

In developing the Lupron Depot injection, I acknowledge and thank Mr. Masaki Yamamoto, Ms. Yayoi Doken, Dr. Toshiro Heya, Mr. Kenzo Ishizuka, Dr. Takatsuka Yashiki, Dr. Hiroyuki Mima, and many other researchers at Takeda Pharmaceutical Co., Ltd for excellent collaborations. In investigation of cytoplasm-responsive nanocarriers, I sincerely thank Dr. Tsunehiko Fukuda (Nagahama Institute of Bio-Science and Technology) for peptide synthesis and Mr. Takaya Ogawa, Dr. Ko Tanaka, Dr. Takanori Kanazawa, and Dr. Yuuki Takashima (School of Pharmacy, Tokyo University of Pharmacy and Life Sciences) for their excellent collaborations.

References

1. http://www.uniqure.com/
2. http://www.osiris.com/
3. Henriksen K, Neutzsky-Wulff AV, Bonewald LF, Karsdal MA (2009) Local communication on and within bone controls bone remodeling. Bone 44:1026–1033
4. Eismann EA, Lush E, Sephton SE (2010) Circadian effects in cancer-relevant psychoneuroendocrine and immune pathways. Psychoneuroendocrinology 35:963–976
5. Norman AW, Henry HL (2015) Calcium-regulating hormones: vitamin D, parathyroid hormone, calcitonin, and fibroblast growth

factor 23. In: Hormones, 3rd edn, Academic Press, Waltham, pp 189–221
6. Park H-K, Ahima RS (2015) Physiology of leptin: energy homeostasis, neuroendocrine function and metabolism. Metab Clin Exp 64:24–34
7. Commins SP, Borish L, Steinke JW (2010) Immunologic messenger molecules: cytokines, interferons, and chemokines. J Allergy Clin Immunol 125:S53–S72
8. Brotman RM, Ravel J, Bavoil PM, Gravitt PE, Ghanem KG (2014) Microbiome, sex hormones, and immune responses in the reproductive tract: challenges for vaccine development against sexually transmitted infections. Vaccine 32:1543–1552
9. Junqueira LC, Carneiro J (1983) Basic histology, 4th edn. Maruzen Asia, Singapore, pp 436–439
10. Okada H (1997) One- and three-month release injectable microspheres of the LH-RH superagonist leuprorelin acetate. Ad Drug Del Rev 28:43–70
11. Okada H, Ogawa Y, Yashiki T (1987) Prolonged release microcapsule and its production. US Patent 4652441 (Jpn Patent Appl 1983:207760)
12. Okada H, Heya T, Ogawa Y, Shimamoto T (1988) One-month release injectable microcapsules of a luteinizing hormone-releasing hormone agonist (leuprolide acetate) for treating experimental endometriosis in rats. J Pharmacol Exp Ther 244:744–750
13. Okada H, Heya T, Igari Y, Ogawa Y, Toguchi H, Shimamoto T (1989) One-month release injectable microspheres of leuprolide acetate inhibit steroidogenesis and genital organ growth in rats. Int J Pharm 54:231–239
14. Ogawa Y, Okada H, Heya T, Shimamoto T (1989) Controlled release of LH-RH agonist, leuprolide acetate, from microcapsules: serum drug level profiles and pharmacological effects in animals. J Pharm Pharmacol 41:439–444
15. Okada H, Heya T, Ogawa Y, Toguchi H, Shimamoto T (1991) Sustained pharmacological activities in rats following single and repeated administration of once-a-month injectable microspheres of leuprolide acetate. Pharm Res 8:584–587
16. Okada H, Inoue Y, Heya T, Ueno H, Ogawa H, Toguchi H (1991) Pharmacokinetics of once-a-month injectable microspheres of leuprolide acetate. Pharm Res 8:787–791
17. Okada H, Inoue Y, Ogawa Y (1996) Prolonged release microcapsules. US Patent: 5480656 (Jpn Patent App 1990:33133)
18. Okada H, Doken Y, Ogawa Y, Toguchi H (1994) Preparation of three-month depot injectable microspheres of leuprorelin acetate using biodegradable polymers. Pharm Res 11:1143–1147
19. Okada H, Doken Y, Ogawa Y, Toguchi H (1994) Sustained suppression of the pituitary-gonadal axis by leuprorelin three-month depot microspheres in rats and dogs. Pharm Res 11:1199–1203
20. Okada H, Doken Y, Ogawa Y (1996) Persistent suppression of the pituitary-gonadal system in female rats by three-month depot injectable microspheres of leuprorelin acetate. J Pharm Sci 85:1044–1048
21. Murata N, Takashima Y, Toyoshima K, Yamamoto M, Okada H (2008) Anti-tumor effects of anti-VEGF siRNA encapsulated with PLGA microspheres in mice. J Cont Rel 126:246–254
22. Yokoi Y, Takashima Y, Kanazawa T, Morisaki K, Osawa E, Okada H (2010) Therapeutic effects in arteriosclerosis obliterans (ASO) by sustained release microspheres of angiogenesis inducing siRNA. The 25th annual meeting of Academy of Pharmaceutical Science and Technology, Japan, Tokushima
23. Okada H (2011) Drug discovery by formulation design and innovative drug delivery systems (DDS). Yakugaku Zasshi 131:1271–1287, Japanese
24. Burnett JC, Rossi JJ (2012) RNA-based therapeutics-current progress and future prospects. Chem Biol 27:60–71
25. Okada H, Ogawa T, Tanaka K, Kanazawa T, Takashima Y (2014) Cytoplasm-responsive delivery systems for siRNA using cell-penetrating peptide nanomicelles. J Drug Del Sci Tech 24:3–11
26. Christensen LV, Chang C-W, Kim WJ, Kim SW (2006) Reducible poly(amido ethylenimine)s designed for triggered intracellular gene delivery. Bioconjug Chem 17:1233–1240
27. Ou M, Wang X-L, Xu R, Chang C-W, Bull DA, Kim SW (2008) Novel biodegradable poly(disulfide amine)s for gene delivery with high efficiency and low cytotoxicity. Bioconjug Chem 19:626–633
28. Kim SH, Jeong JH, Ou M, Yockman JW, Kim SW, Bull DA (2008) Cardiomyocyte-targeted siRNA delivery by prostaglandin E2-Fas siRNA polyplexes formulated with reducible poly(amido amine) for preventing cardiomyocyte apoptosis. Biomaterials 29:4439–4446
29. Ou M, Xu R, Kim SH, Bull DA, Kim SW (2009) A family of bioreducible poly(disulfide

amine)s for gene delivery. Biomaterials 30:5804–5814

30. Kim T-I, Ou M, Lee M, Kim SW (2009) Arginine-grafted bioreducible poly(disulfide amine) for gene delivery systems. Biomaterials 30:658–664
31. Kim SH, Jeong JH, Kim TI, Kim SW, Bull DA (2009) VEGF siRNA delivery system using arginine-grafted bioreducible poly(disulfide amine). Mol Pharm 6:718–726
32. Ou M, Kim T-I, Yockman JW, Borden BA, Bull DA, Kim SW (2010) Polymer transfected primary myoblasts mediated efficient gene expression and angiogenic proliferation. J Control Release 142:61–69
33. Kim T-I, Lee M, Kim SW (2010) A guanidinylated bioreducible polymer with high nuclear localization ability for gene delivery systems. Biomaterials 31:1798–1804
34. Nam HY, McGinn A, Kim P-H, Kim SW, Bull DA (2010) Primary cardiomyocyte targeted bioreducible polymer for efficient gene delivery to the myocardium. Biomaterials 31:8081–8087
35. Nam HY, Kim J, Kim S, Yockman JW, Kim SW, Bull DA (2011) Cell penetrating peptide conjugated bioreducible polymer for siRNA delivery. Biomaterials 32:5213–5222
36. Kim T-I, Rothmund T, Kissel T, Kim SW (2011) Bioreducible polymers with cell penetrating and endosome buffering functionality for gene delivery systems. J Control Release 152:110–119
37. Beloor J, Choi CS, Nam HY, Park M, Kim SH, Jackson A, Lee KY, Kim SW, Kumar P, Lee S-K (2012) Arginine-engrafted biodegradable polymer for the systemic delivery of therapeutic siRNA. Biomaterials 33:1640–1650
38. Ryu JK, Choi MJ, Kim TI, Jin HR, Kwon KD, Batbold D, Song KM, Kwon MH, Yin GN, Lee M, Kim SW, Suh JK (2013) A guanidinylated bioreducible polymer as a novel gene carrier to the corpus cavernosum of mice with high-cholesterol diet-induced erectile dysfunction. Andrology 1:216–222
39. Trubetskoy VS, Budker VG, Hanson LJ, Slattum PM, Wolff JA, Hagstrom JE (1998) Self-assembly of DNA-polymer complexes using template polymerization. Nucleic Acids Res 26:4178–4185
40. Stevenson M, Ramos-Perez V, Singh S, Soliman M, Preece JA, Briggs SS, Read ML, Seymour LW (2008) Delivery of siRNA mediated by histidine-containing reducible polycations. J Control Release 130:46–56
41. Mok H, Park TG (2008) Self-crosslinked and reducible fusogenic peptides for intracellular delivery of siRNA. Biopolymers 89:881–888
42. Hyun H, Won Y-W, Kim K-M, Lee J, Lee M, Kim Y-H (2010) Therapeutic effects of a reducible poly(oligo-D-arginine) carrier with the heme oxygenase-1 gene in the treatment of hypoxic-ischemic brain injury. Biomaterials 31:9128–9134
43. Won Y-W, Kim HA, Lee M, Kim Y-H (2010) Reducible poly(oligo-D-arginine) for enhanced gene expression in mouse lung by intratracheal injection. Mol Ther 18:734–742
44. Won Y-W, Kim K-M, An SS, Lee M, Ha Y, Kim Y-H (2011) Suicide gene therapy using reducible poly(oligo-D-arginine) for the treatment of spinal cord tumors. Biomaterials 32:9766–9775
45. Won Y-W, Yoon S-M, Lee K-M, Kim Y-H (2011) Poly(oligo-D-arginine) with internal disulfide linkages as a cytoplasm-sensitive carrier for siRNA delivery. Mol Ther 19:372–380
46. Kiselev A, Egorova A, Laukkanen A, Baranov V, Urtti A (2013) Characterization of reducible peptide oligomers as carriers for gene delivery. Int J Pharm 441:736–747
47. Tanaka K, Kanazawa T, Ogawa T, Takashima Y, Fukuda T, Okada H (2010) Disulfide crosslinked stearoyl carrier peptides containing arginine and histidine enhance siRNA uptake and gene silencing. Int J Pharm 398:219–224
48. Tanaka K, Kanazawa T, Ogawa T, Suda Y, Takashima Y, Fukuda T, Okada H (2011) A novel, bio-reducible gene vector containing arginine and histidine enhances gene transfection and expression of plasmid DNA. Chem Pharm Bull 59:202–207
49. Kanazawa T, Tamura T, Yamazaki M, Takashima Y, Okada H (2013) Needle-free intravaginal DNA vaccination using a stearoyl oligopeptide carrier promotes local gene expression and immune responses. Int J Pharm 447:70–74
50. Tanaka K, Kanazawa T, Shibata Y, Suda Y, Fukuda T, Takashima Y, Okada H (2010) Development of cell-penetrating peptide-modified MPEG-PCL diblock copolymeric nanoparticles for systemic gene delivery. Int J Pharm 396:229–238
51. Kanazawa T, Sugawara K, Tanaka K, Horiuchi S, Takashima Y, Okada H (2012) Suppression of tumor growth by systemic delivery of anti-VEGF siRNA with cell-penetrating peptide-modified MPEG-PCL nanomicelles. Eur J Pharm Biopharm 81:470–477
52. Tanaka K, Kanazawa T, Horiuchi S, Ando T, Sugawara K, Takashima Y, Seta Y, Okada H (2013) Cytoplasm-responsive nanocarriers conjugated with a functional cell-penetrating peptide for systemic siRNA delivery. Int J Pharm 455:40–47

53. Ichikawa T, Akimoto S, Shimazaki J (1988) Effect of leuprolide on growth of rat prostatic tumor (R 3327) and weight of male accessory sex organs. Endocr J 35:181–187
54. Wu G, Fang Y-Z, Yang S, Lupton JR, Turnere ND (2004) Glutathione metabolism and its implications for health. J Nutr 134:489–492
55. Saito G, Swanson JA, Lee KD (2003) Drug delivery strategy utilizing conjugation via reversible disulfide linkages: role and site of cellular reducing activities. Adv Drug Deliv Rev 55:199–214
56. Kuppusamy P, Li H, Ilangovan G, Cardounel AJ, Zweier JL, Yamada K, Krishna MC, Mitchell JB (2002) Noninvasive imaging of tumor redox status and its modification by tissue glutathione levels. Cancer Res 62: 307–312

Chapter 17

Nanoparticulate Drug Delivery Systems to Overcome the Blood–Brain Barrier

Tatsuaki Tagami, Moeko Taki, and Tetsuya Ozeki

Abstract

Nanomedicine, the term used to describe the combination of nanotechnology (or nanoparticles) with medicine, is now being used in the medical field worldwide. Researchers in the field of nanomedicine have been developing drug delivery strategies to overcome the blood–brain barrier (BBB) and have been investigating methods for penetrating the BBB for decades. However, effective nanoparticle-based formulations that successfully penetrate the BBB and reach the target site (e.g., brain cancer) in the brain have not yet been developed. In contrast, several drug-loaded nanoparticle formulations delivered via the systemic route have been approved by the FDA to treat various types of cancers. This review first discusses FDA-approved nanomedicines, including liposomal formulations of Doxil® and the albumin-based drug Abraxane®. Their characteristics are discussed, as are the challenging issues in the development of nanomedicine. Subsequently, recent progress toward nanoparticle-based formulations that have succeeded in delivering drugs to the brain is reviewed. The approaches used to overcome the BBB, including receptor-mediated transcytosis and other attractive strategies, are discussed. This information can be useful in understanding nanoparticle-based drug delivery to brain tissue and can provide hints for next-generation nanoparticle-based drug delivery systems and the future of personalized therapy.

Key words Nanoparticle-based drug delivery, Blood–brain barrier, Receptor-mediated transcytosis, Nanomedicine

1 Introduction

The blood–brain barrier (BBB) is the most important mechanism developed during the course of evolution to protect the central nervous system from invasion by foreign material. The tightly assembled endothelial cells comprising the BBB can exclude most of the substances present in the circulation, including useful substances such as drugs. Therefore, a variety of methods have been tested over the decades to transport drugs into the brain.

Nanoparticle-based drug delivery systems have been developed for treating systemic diseases. An overview of nanoparticulate drug delivery systems designed to overcome the BBB is shown in Fig. 1. Various drug nanocarriers have been developed and

Zheng-Rong Lu and Shinji Sakuma (eds.), *Nanomaterials in Pharmacology*, Methods in Pharmacology and Toxicology,
DOI 10.1007/978-1-4939-3121-7_17,

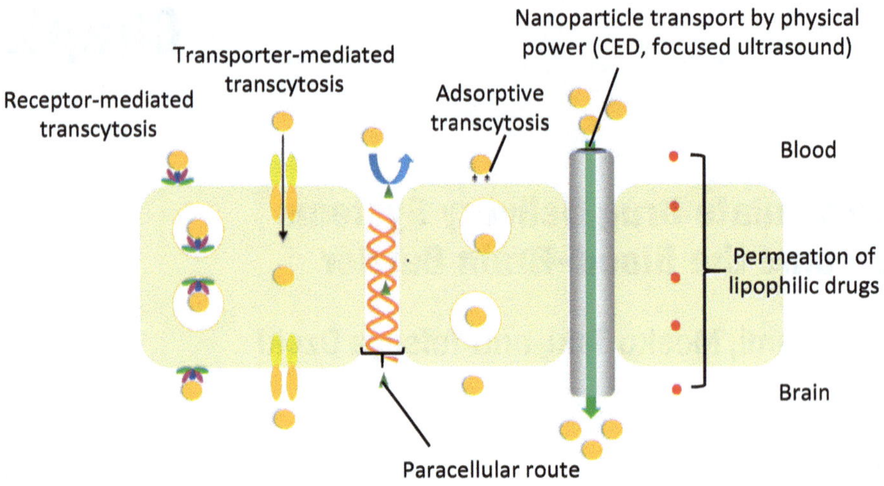

Fig. 1 Overview of nanoparticulate drug delivery systems to overcome the brain–blood barrier

investigated for brain-specific drug delivery [1, 2]. Nanoparticles can deliver drugs at high concentrations into the targeted tissues with less non-specific drug distribution to other organs compared to other carrier systems. Controlled drug release from these particles is also feasible. However, nanoparticles are large compared to a typical drug molecule, which hinders their transport across the BBB. One promising strategy for overcoming this drawback is to use the endothelial receptors and transporters, which transport essential substances such as nutrients through the BBB.

In this review, we first look at the characteristics of nanoparticle-based drug delivery nanomedicines approved by the FDA. Next, we discuss strategies for delivering nanoparticles to brain tissue. Several formulations for systemic administration have been developed and one or more could be adapted to deliver drugs to the brain. Several methods for delivering nanoparticle-based drugs to the brain using receptors and transporters are reviewed (summarized in Table 1), and methods for preparing drug-loaded nanoparticles are briefly described on a case-by-case basis. Finally, several attractive approaches, in addition to the use of receptors and transporters, are described.

2 FDA-Approved Nanomedicines

2.1 A Liposomal Drug Formulation: DOXIL®

Liposomes are among the best characterized and established drug nanocarriers. Liposomes are composed of lipids that are nonimmunogenic. Both water-soluble and poorly water-soluble drugs can be encapsulated in liposomes, including large molecules such as proteins and nucleic acids. Doxil, which consists of PEGylated liposomes containing doxorubicin, is the first nanoparticle-based

Table 1
Recent progress of transporter- and receptor-mediated drug delivery

Target	Ligand	Carrier	Size	Drug	Condition/disease	Reference
Tf-R	Tf Tf-R Ab	Human serum albumin	154–183 nm	Loperamide	Pain	[23]
Insulin-R	Insulin Insulin-R Ab	Human serum albumin	148–190 nm	Loperamide	Pain	[24]
Tf-R	Tf-cell penetrating peptides	Liposome	72.3–88.3 nm	Doxorubicin	Brain tumor	[25]
Tf-R	Tf-R Ab	PEG–PEI	116 nm	Oligonucleotide (NF-kB decoy)	Neuroinflammatory disease	[26]
Tf-R	Tf-R Ab	Liposome and PEI	142.7 nm	Oligonucleotide (NF-kB decoy)	Neuroinflammatory disease	[27]
LRP	Angiopep-2	None	None	Peptide (Neurotensin)	Pain	[30]
LRP	Angiopep-2	PEG–PLA micelle	38.4 nm	DiI (marker)	None	[31]
LDLR	ApoB/LDLR binding protein	None (viral vector)	None	GFP (marker)	None	[32]
LDLR	ApoB/LDLR binding protein	None (viral vector)	None	Peptide (neprilysin)	Alzheimer's disease	[33]
None	None	None (viral vector)	None	Peptide (neprilysin)	Alzheimer's disease	[34]
LDLR	LDLR binding peptide	Liposome	72.05 nm	Doxorubicin	Brain tumor	[35]
Others	Lactoferrin	PEG–PLGA polymersome	120 nm	Peptide (S14G-humanin)	Alzheimer's disease	[37]
Others	Lactoferrin	PEG–PLGA polymersome	90–120 nm	Peptide (S14G-humanin)	Alzheimer's disease	[38]
Others	Lactoferrin	PEG–PLGA nanoparticle	90 nm	Peptide (urocortin)	Parkinson's disease	[39]
Others	Lactoferrin	Iron nanoparticle	48.9 nm	None	Imaging	[40]
Others	Glutathione	Liposome	95 nm	Doxorubicin	Brain tumor	[42]
Others	Glutathione	Liposome	97 nm	Doxorubicin	Brain tumor	[43]
Others	Glutathione	Liposome	96–119 nm	Methylprednisolone	Multiple sclerosis	[44]
None	None	Liposome	80 nm	Tempamine	Multiple sclerosis	[45]

drug approved by the FDA and is used to treat recurrent ovarian cancer and Kaposi sarcoma. Non-PEGylated liposomal formulations that have been approved by the FDA, such as Daunosome® and Marquibo®, have been summarized in another review [3]. Two major technologies have contributed to the development of Doxil: PEGylation and active drug loading [4]. PEGylation coats the liposome with polyethylene glycol (PEG), allowing water to be trapped and form a layer around the liposome. This allows the liposome to escape recognition and phagocytosis by the mononuclear phagocyte system (MPS). Furthermore, PEGylation alters the form of the liposome and can help retain the drug in the liposome. Because they escape MPS, PEGylated liposomes can have a longer blood circulation time, allowing them to accumulate in solid tumor tissue. This is called the enhanced permeability and retention (EPR) effect [5]. New tumor blood vessels are leaky compared with normal, rigid blood vessels, and macromolecules can enter the tumor tissue by extravasation. The EPR effect is dependent upon the size of the macromolecule. Liposomes approximately 100 nm in diameter can accumulate in solid tumors.

The second major technology used to manufacture liposomal drug formulations is the active drug-loading method, which is also called the remote loading method. This method is used with pH-dependent basic drugs and acidic drugs. Due to the pH gradient between the inside and the outside of the liposome, a nonionic drug can migrate from the exterior membrane of the liposome to the interior membrane of the liposome and there assumes an ionic form. The drug interacts with salts in the liposome interior and sometimes precipitates. This drug-loading process is an equilibration reaction and the drugs are actively loaded into the liposome, resulting in almost 100 % of the drug being loaded into the liposome. This method is cost effective but is suitable only for pH-dependent drugs and its application is therefore limited. The efficacy of drug loading is dependent on the solubility, pKa, molecular weight, and other characteristics of both the liposomes and especially the drug. Specifically, the drug-loading efficiency is dependent on the physicochemical properties of the drug; a quantitative structural property relationship model to predict the efficacy has been proposed [6]. Methods using other gradients, such as polyphosphate [7], sucroseoctasulfate [8], and a metal ion gradient [9], are being developed.

The development of liposomes using these major technologies has allowed the passive targeting of PEGylated liposomes into tumor tissue. PEGylated liposomes can dramatically reduce the side effects of anticancer drugs. Cardiotoxicity, which is an irreversible effect of doxorubicin, has been greatly reduced with Doxil. However, the maximum tolerated dosage of Doxil is similar to that of the free formulation of doxorubicin. The doxorubicin concentration in the skin is increased by the administration of Doxil and incidents of hand–foot syndrome have been reported. Additionally, the low bioavailability of Doxil in tumor tissue is a challenging issue: the drug is not efficiently released from the liposomes after they reach the tumor tissue. Doxil as a treatment for glioblastoma is being investigated in clinical trials [10–12].

Strategies to move beyond Doxil and improve the bioavailability of liposome-entrapped drugs in tumor tissue are under development. The major strategy is active targeting and triggered release. Active targeting is a strategy that uses therapeutic molecules that home in on tumor cells and/or other components of the tumor tissue, such as blood vessels [13, 14]. Antibodies that recognize specific tumor tissue (antibody, Fab fragment, and bi-specific antibody) and ligands are commonly conjugated to liposomes at the end of the PEG–lipid molecule. Although this strategy is straightforward and novel liposome formulations are being developed, effective therapeutic results have not been demonstrated in clinical studies, although many studies have been conducted in animal models. Triggered release is a strategy to deliver the therapeutic drug at the target site. Physical power (heating, ultrasound, and light), endogenous reaction (pH and enzymatic reaction), or a combination of these methods are used to release the drug from the liposomes. Thermosensitive liposomes are among the best characterized of the triggered release liposomes and are used under conditions of mild hyperthermia [15, 16]. ThermoDOX, currently undergoing clinical trials, is used to treat liver cancer.

2.2 An Albumin/Drug Formulation: Abraxane®

Abraxane, comprising paclitaxel/albumin nanoparticles, is an FDA-approved nanomedicine and is used to treat metastatic breast cancer and non-small-cell lung cancer. Abraxane addresses several of the problems associated with paclitaxel [17]. Paclitaxel is a poorly water-soluble drug and an organic solvent is necessary to dissolve the drug. Taxol, which is a paclitaxel formulation dissolved in Cremophor and ethanol, can induce hypersensitivity; thus, the patient must be pretreated with steroids and antihistamine drugs. Abraxane does not contain alcohol, so no pretreatment is necessary. The infusion time of paclitaxel is a few hours, whereas that of Abraxane is 30 min. Other paclitaxel-loaded nanoparticles aside from Abraxane have been extensively investigated and several formulations are in clinical trials (please see review [18]).

The Abraxane nanoparticle is approximately 130 nm in diameter. After administration, Abraxane disintegrates into small paclitaxel/albumin complexes. Some of the Abraxane circulates in the blood and reaches the tumor tissues; subsequently, the albumin-conjugated Abraxane permeates through the endothelial cells by gp60 receptor-mediated transcytosis [19]. Transcytosis is related to caveolae [20] and results in increased binding and permeation through endothelial cells. Increased paclitaxel concentrations and therapeutic accumulation in tumors have been reported following administration of Abraxane [21]. Few investigations of the efficacy of Abraxane to treat brain cancer have been conducted to date but several paclitaxel nanoparticulate formulations and drug formulations which utilize albumin binding (e.g., aldoxorubicin) are under development for treating brain diseases such as glioblastoma [22].

3 Transporter- and Ligand-Mediated Nanoparticle Delivery to Brain Tissue

As described in the Introduction, the use of transporter- and receptor-mediated nanoparticle delivery is one of the most promising strategies to overcome the BBB. There are many different transporters and receptors in endothelial cells for transporting essential substances to brain tissue. Transferrin receptor, insulin receptor, low-density lipoprotein (LDL) receptor (LDLR), and LDL receptor-related protein (LRP) all hold promise and have been investigated. In this review, other targets, such as lactoferrin and glutathione, are described. Please see Table 1 for a summary of recent articles introduced in this review.

3.1 Transferrin Receptor

Actively targeting transferrin receptor is one of the most studied approaches and is an attractive option for guiding drug-loaded nanoparticles into brain tissue. Transferrin or anti-transferrin receptor antibodies have been conjugated with drug carriers and characterized. Kreuter's group developed nanoparticles that are composed of human serum albumin (HSA)/transferrin or HSA/transferrin receptor antibodies (OX26) [23]. The HSA/transferrin and HSA/OX26 conjugates were made using NHS–PEG–maleimide, a heterobifunctional crosslinker. Loperamide was included in HAS/conjugate nanoparticles. Kreuter's group focused on the synthetic strategy for generating the nanoparticles and did not investigate the biodistribution of the nanoparticles. The tail-flick test, used to evaluate the analgesic effect of loperamide, revealed that HSA/transferrin and HSA/OX26 nanoparticles induce an analgesic effect. The same group developed insulin/HSA and anti-insulin receptor antibody/HSA nanoparticles loaded with loperamide and evaluated the efficacy of the nanoparticles, again using the tail-flick test [24].

Sharma et al. developed Tf-cell penetrating peptide liposomes with a dual function [25]. In an in vitro study of endothelial permeability, Tf-Penetratin liposomes exhibited better permeation properties (14.9 %, after 8 h) than single ligand liposomes. This liposome formulation accumulated in the brain tissue (3.67 % per gram of tissue) in vivo, although accumulation in other organs was also detected.

Bickel's group prepared biotin–PEG–polyethylenimine (PEI) that was used as a carrier of NF-kB decoy, an anti-inflammatory oligonucleotide (ODN) [26]. This construct was first used to investigate adsorption-mediated endocytosis, and then they synthesized a conjugate of 8D3 antibody (anti-mouse Tf receptor antibody) and PEG–PEI for receptor-mediated endocytosis. Neither complex exhibited cytotoxicity in vitro and exhibited an anti-inflammatory effect by reducing the mRNA level of VCAM-1, ICAM-1, and other genes targeting endothelial cells. Bickel's group also used liposomes to encapsulate ODN/PEI complexes [27] both to protect ODN from degradation by nucleases and to aid its systemic delivery. They conjugated the 8D3 antibody to the end of a PEG–lipid using the streptavidin–biotin reaction and then prepared immunoliposomes. The immunoliposomes produced a remarkable nearly tenfold accumulation of radiolabeled ODN in the brain tissue of mice.

3.2 LRP and LDLR

LRP is a multiligand receptor; many kinds of proteins can interact with LRP, such as apolipoprotein E, alpha2 macroglobulin, tissue plasminogen activator, and plasminogen activator inhibitor-1 [28]. Angiopep-2 peptide has received considerable attention recently. Angiopep-2 is a novel brain ligand that can enter brain tissue via LRP-1-mediated transcytosis [29]. Angiopep-2 was conjugated with neurotensin, which has an antalgic effect. This peptide conjugate (10 mg peptide/kg and 20 mg peptide/kg, via intravenous injection) exhibited antalgic effects in the hot-plate and tail-flick assays, which are in vivo acute pain models in mice [30]. Lu et al. developed angiopep-2-conjugated PEG–PLA micelles [31] and investigated their biodistribution using radioisotope-labeled versions of the micelles. These studies revealed that angiopep-2-conjugated micellar formulations accumulated remarkably in brain tissue compared with the control PEG–PLA micelles.

LDL contains several apolipoproteins that can be recognized by the LDLR, which is expressed on neuronal and glial cells. Spencer et al. prepared a lentiviral vector that can be used to express the ApoB/LDLR binding domain conjugate. The conjugate acts as a ligand for LDLR and a fluorescent marker protein, GFP [32]. The lentiviral vector was intraperitoneally injected into mice. The expressed protein was primarily distributed in the liver and other tissues. Their report discussed that the liver acts as a depot for the expressed protein and that the protein can be sustainably released into the brain tissue. This group applied the same strategy to prepare a fusion protein of the ApoB/LDLR binding domain and neprilysin, a metalo-peptidase targeting amyloid beta peptide [33]. Peritoneal injection of this vector into amyloid protein precursor peptide (APP) transgenic mice, a model of Alzheimer's disease, resulted in a reduction in the amount of amyloid beta in the brain, but the vector did not reduce the synaptic protein level to that of non-transgenic (healthy) mice. In contrast, another group prepared an adeno-associated virus vector that can express neprilysin alone. This vector exhibited a therapeutic effect in APP transgenic mice [34].

A peptide containing the LDLR-binding site derived from ApoB-100 was incorporated into doxorubicin-loaded liposomes, and its ability to cross the BBB was investigated in vitro using the hCMEC/D3 coculture cell model in transwell plates [35]. The use of simvastatin enhanced drug permeability. The authors demonstrated that statins induce NO via the Rho A/Rho A kinase pathway and that the NO can enhance permeation of the drug through the BBB. The reduction in cholesterol induced by the statin may enhance drug permeability in vivo via the paracellular route.

3.3 Lactoferrin

Lactoferrin is a cationic iron-binding glycoprotein belonging to the transferrin family. It exhibits strong binding with LRP and conducts receptor-mediated transcytosis through the BBB [36]. Pang's group created a rat model for impaired learning and memory by microinjecting amyloid β into the hippocampus and then studied the effects of a neuroprotective peptide as a therapeutic compound [37]. Humanin is a 24-amino-acid peptide. The S14G variant exhibits 1000-fold higher efficacy than humanin in blocking Alzheimer's disease-related apoptosis and was used in the study. S14G-humanin was loaded into PEG–PLGA polymersomes. Polymersomes are prepared using asymmetric diblock polymers that self-assemble to form supermolecules in aqueous solution. Polymersomes are less permeable than liposomes and are amenable to active drug loading, described in the above section on liposomes. They conducted pH-gradient active loading of S14G-humanin into the polymersomes. S14G-humanin peptide is larger than conventional basic drugs typically loaded into liposomes, so they used 1,4-dioxane to improve the permeability of the polymersomes toward S14G-humanin. S14G-humanin was loaded for 30 min at 37 °C but the encapsulation efficiency was low (21.78 %), suggesting that S14-humanin cannot enter polymersomes efficiently and that the peptide may stay in the outer layer of the polymersome. The S14G-humanin peptide-loaded lactoferrin polymersome (HNG-Lf-POS) exhibited increased cellular uptake into brain capillary endothelial cells, providing an increased concentration of lactoferrin. The accumulation of Lf-POS (using coumarin as a marker) was comparable with that of other ligand (Tf)-conjugated polymersomes. Pang's group previously determined that 101 molecules of Lf per polymersome particle are optimal for brain delivery [38], and this was confirmed in their cellular uptake study. This group previously used another peptide (urocortin) against another disease (Parkinson's disease) using similar Lf-conjugated PEG–PLGA nanoparticles [39] and showed a therapeutic effect. The biodistribution and pharmacokinetics parameters of Lf-conjugated PEG–PLGA nanoparticles were different from those of unconjugated PEG–PLGA nanoparticles. Lf nanoparticles significantly accumulated in the brain, heart, and spleen tissues. Another group used Lf-conjugated (and PEG-conjugated) iron nanoparticles for monitoring the delivery of nanoparticles into the brain tissue [40]. The nanoparticles were approximately 50 nm in diameter, and on average 14.4 molecules of Lf were conjugated onto each nanoparticle. The nanoparticles accumulated in the brain tissue (thalamus, brain stem, and frontal cortex) as demonstrated by a decrease in T2 values during MRI monitoring.

3.4 Glutathione

Glutathione is a tripeptide comprising glutamic acid, cysteine, and glycine. The main function of glutathione is as an antioxidant. Glutathione can bind various compounds, including transmitter compounds and toxic substances, and is involved in moving compounds out of cells. Kannan et al. reported that glutathione can be transported through cerebrovascular endothelial cells [41].

Glutathione-conjugated PEGylated liposome formulations were developed to deliver compounds into the brain tissue. A thioether bond is formed between maleimide groups conjugated with PEG–lipids and the thiol group of glutathione. The resulting glutathione–PEG–lipid micelle is then mixed with a liposome suspension and penetrates the liposomal membrane upon heating; this is called the post-insertion method. Glutathione PEGylated liposomes containing doxorubicin showed a plasma elimination profile and biodistribution very similar to that of PEGylated liposomes [42], but the doxorubicin concentration in the brain tissue 96 h after glutathione PEGylated liposome injection was higher than that after PEGylated liposome delivery. As a result, the glutathione PEGylated liposome significantly inhibited tumor growth in experimental mouse brain tumor models and prolonged the survival of the mice compared with conventional PEGylated liposomes. In another study, Birngruber et al. reported a method to determine the doxorubicin concentration in the extracellular fluid of the brain using cerebral open flow microperfusion (cOFM) in rats [43]. OFM allows more ready determination of the concentration of a compound, regardless of its lipophilicity or molecular weight, than the microdialysis method. Sodium fluorescein was used to show that the BBB was intact after implantation of the cOFM probe. Brain–plasma ratios of AUC after the administration of glutathione PEGylated liposomes were significantly higher (4.8-fold) than those after the administration of PEGylated liposomes. In their previous report, methylprednisolone-loaded glutathione PEGylated liposomes were prepared for the treatment of experimental autoimmune encephalomyelitis (EAE), a model of multiple sclerosis, in rat [44]. Methylprednisolone hemisuccinate, a prodrug of methylprednisolone, was actively loaded using a calcium acetate gradient between the exterior and interior of the liposomal bilayer membrane. The glutathione PEGylated liposomes containing methylprednisolone exhibited an improved therapeutic effect compared to free methylprednisolone, using the EAE clinical scores as an index of the therapeutic effect. Other groups reported that non-ligand liposome formulations (PEGylated liposomes) containing tempamine, which has anti-oxidative and antiapoptotic effects, could treat EAE model mice after intravenous injection [45]. They showed that the amount of PEGylated liposome accumulated in EAE mice was higher than that in healthy mice.

3.5 Adsorptive Transcytosis by Cationic Substances

Capillary endothelial cells have a region enriched in clathrin-coated pits and vesicles that is negatively charged. Thus, positively charged compounds combined with drugs can be used to bind the negatively charged luminal surface of endothelial cells for drug delivery. A review reported the possibility [46] that the adsorbed cationic compounds may be taken up into endothelial cells by caveolae-mediated transcytosis, and/or the compounds may be endocytosed by clathrin-coated pits. Then, the uncoated vesicles may fuse with transcytotic endosomes, and the compound may move to the opposite abluminal membrane. Cationic compounds, including cationic albumin and cell penetrating peptides, have already been investigated. Brain-targeted peptides are summarized in another review [47]. For example, TAT peptide, which is derived from HIV virus, was conjugated with Bcl-xL, which has antiapoptotic effects [48]. The Bcl-xL-TAT fusion protein inhibited the apoptosis of primary cultured cortical neurons in vitro and protected against focal ischemic infarction in mice.

4 Other Strategies, Miscellaneous

4.1 Convection-Enhanced Delivery

Convection-enhanced delivery (CED), a method of local injection into the brain tissue, is accepted in clinical settings of neurooncology and neurodegenerative disease. This method can bypass the BBB with minimal mechanical stress and a wide drug distribution within the brain can be obtained. The combination of CED and nanoparticles has been reported by many groups. Bankiewicz's group conducted a series of investigations using liposomes with CED and reviewed their studies [49]. PEGylated liposome formulations can be distributed in the brain tissue by CED. In contrast, free doxorubicin solution was localized around the injected site. The co-encapsulation of MRI contrast agent can report on drug distribution and can monitor drug administration using CED. Remarkably, the free drug disappeared within hours, whereas liposomal formulations delivered using CED remained in the brain tissue for 12 days (small dose) or 50 days (high dose), resulting in prolonged survival. Therefore, the combination of CED and nanoparticles may be a practical method to deliver nanoparticles.

Kenny et al. prepared multifunctional nanoparticles for CED [50]. They used LPD nanoparticles which can encapsulate pDNA. Thus, LPD has been used in potential gene therapy approaches. Peptides that target neurotensin- and gadolinium-conjugated lipids for MRI monitoring have also been encapsulated in LPDs. They compared anionic and cationic LPDs and found that anionic LPDs can distribute widely in the rat brain with a transfection efficacy similar to that of cationic LPDs.

4.2 Nanoparticle Delivery in Pathogenic Condition

The BBB is intact under normal conditions, but may collapse under pathogenic conditions. In these circumstances, conventional PEGylated liposomes and ligand- and site specific antibody-spiked liposomes can be useful. Oku's group used an asialo-erythropoietin (AEPO)-conjugated PEGylated formulation for targeted delivery to cerebral ischemia–reperfusion model rats [51]. AEPO can bind with erythropoietin receptors on neuronal cells. AEPO-conjugated PEGylated liposomes were prepared by conjugating DSPE-PEG-NHS with AEPO. Approximately 100 nm diameter PEGylated liposomes accumulated significantly in the cerebral ischemia–reperfusion region. The same group used conventional PEGylated liposomes containing FK506, an immunosuppressive drug [52]. PEGylated liposomes containing FK506 exhibited neuroprotective effects in rats with transient middle cerebral artery occlusion.

Tomizawa et al. developed an immunoliposome formulation that targeted anti-EGFR antibody to glioma membranes [53]. Anti-EGFR antibody was conjugated with the adaptor ZZ (IgG Fc-binding motif). Since ZZ chelates nickel, ZZ was conjugated with nickel lipid (DOTG-NTA-Ni). This liposome was PEGylated by the incorporation of PEGylated lipid and sodium borocaptate for boron neutron capture therapy. The liposomal formulation exhibited remarkable ^{10}B uptake in glioma cells in vitro and ^{10}B accumulation in a brain tumor model in mice. In contrast, the liposomal formulation did not accumulate in the normal brain, i.e., the brain tissue in healthy mice. They further improved the immunoliposomal formulation in a subsequent study [54]. The antibody was conjugated with ZZ adaptor-luciferase protein and the protein was then thiolated and conjugated with maleimide–PEG lipid. The accumulation of the immunoliposomal formulation in tumor tissue could be monitored by bioluminescence imaging.

4.3 Image-Guided Drug Delivery Using MRI with Focused Ultrasound

Transient BBB disruption by the combination of microbubbles and focused ultrasound has been investigated. Ultrasound can compromise the integrity of the BBB and enhance the EPR effect described in Sect. 2.1. The compromised integrity of the BBB is reversible (within a few hours), making this a relatively safe method. Liu et al. combined magnetic nanoparticles with focused ultrasound for effective MRI monitoring [55]. This novel therapy combined with image-guided drug delivery, along with the physical device used to deliver the drug, is called "theranostics." Numerous theranostics studies have recently been conducted (please see reviews [56–58]).

4.4 The Use of Cells to Deliver Drugs into the Brain

An interesting strategy to deliver drugs into the brain tissue uses cells (monocytes and neutrophils) as drug transporters [59]. Non-PEGylated liposomes were administered to rats. Most of the drug-loaded liposomes were trapped in the mononuclear phagocyte system, but the drug concentration in the brain was twofold higher than that after the administration of free drug. Depletion of the drug in the mononuclear phagocyte system did not lead to the accumulation of fluorescent liposomes in the brain tissue. Therefore, these results indirectly suggested that monocytes, which induce phagocytosis, act as transporters across the BBB and into brain tissue. Although the bioavailability of the drug in the brain tissue was unclear from the results of the study and more delivery efficacy is necessary to achieve a therapeutic effect, this strategy may hold promise for transporting drugs across the BBB.

5 Conclusion

Many kinds of drug-loaded nanoparticle formulations targeting the BBB described in this review exhibited a therapeutic effect, with increased accumulation of drugs in the brains of animal models. The therapeutic efficacy and drug delivery efficiency are dependent on multiple factors, including carrier design, drug properties, and the pathogenic condition. Further studies, including investigations assessing the safety with respect to other tissues and the transport mechanism, will be necessary. The technologies used to develop nanomedicines and imaging technologies will be useful for the development of future brain-targeted nanomedicines as personalized therapies.

References

1. Alyautdin R, Khalin I, Nafeeza MI, Haron MH, Kuznetsov D (2014) Nanoscale drug delivery systems and the blood-brain barrier. Int J Nanomedicine 9:795–811. doi:10.2147/IJN.S52236
2. Yang H (2010) Nanoparticle-mediated brain-specific drug delivery, imaging, and diagnosis. Pharm Res 27(9):1759–1771. doi:10.1007/s11095-010-0141-7
3. Dawidczyk CM, Kim C, Park JH, Russell LM, Lee KH, Pomper MG, Searson PC (2014) State-of-the-art in design rules for drug delivery platforms: lessons learned from FDA-approved nanomedicines. J Control Release 187C:133–144. doi:10.1016/j.jconrel.2014.05.036
4. Barenholz Y (2012) Doxil(R)-the first FDA-approved nano-drug: lessons learned. J Control Release 160(2):117–134. doi:10.1016/j.jconrel.2012.03.020
5. Fang J, Nakamura H, Maeda H (2011) The EPR effect: unique features of tumor blood vessels for drug delivery, factors involved, and limitations and augmentation of the effect. Adv Drug Deliv Rev 63(3):136–151. doi:10.1016/j.addr.2010.04.009

6. Cern A, Golbraikh A, Sedykh A, Tropsha A, Barenholz Y, Goldblum A (2012) Quantitative structure-property relationship modeling of remote liposome loading of drugs. J Control Release 160(2):147–157. doi:10.1016/j.jconrel.2011.11.029
7. Drummond DC, Noble CO, Guo Z, Hayes ME, Connolly-Ingram C, Gabriel BS, Hann B, Liu B, Park JW, Hong K, Benz CC, Marks JD, Kirpotin DB (2010) Development of a highly stable and targetable nanoliposomal formulation of topotecan. J Control Release 141(1): 13–21. doi:10.1016/j.jconrel.2009.08.006
8. Noble CO, Guo Z, Hayes ME, Marks JD, Park JW, Benz CC, Kirpotin DB, Drummond DC (2009) Characterization of highly stable liposomal and immunoliposomal formulations of vincristine and vinblastine. Cancer Chemother Pharmacol 64(4):741–751. doi:10.1007/s00280-008-0923-3
9. Kheirolomoom A, Mahakian LM, Lai CY, Lindfors HA, Seo JW, Paoli EE, Watson KD, Haynam EM, Ingham ES, Xing L, Cheng RH, Borowsky AD, Cardiff RD, Ferrara KW (2010) Copper-doxorubicin as a nanoparticle cargo retains efficacy with minimal toxicity. Mol Pharm 7(6):1948–1958. doi:10.1021/mp100245u
10. Ananda S, Nowak AK, Cher L, Dowling A, Brown C, Simes J, Rosenthal MA, Cooperative Trials Group for Neuro-Oncology (COGNO) (2011) Phase 2 trial of temozolomide and pegylated liposomal doxorubicin in the treatment of patients with glioblastoma multiforme following concurrent radiotherapy and chemotherapy. J Clin Neurosci 18(11):1444–1448. doi:10.1016/j.jocn.2011.02.026
11. Beier CP, Schmid C, Gorlia T, Kleinletzenberger C, Beier D, Grauer O, Steinbrecher A, Hirschmann B, Brawanski A, Dietmaier C, Jauch-Worley T, Kölbl O, Pietsch T, Proescholdt M, Rümmele P, Muigg A, Stockhammer G, Hegi M, Bogdahn U, Hau P (2009) RNOP-09: pegylated liposomal doxorubicine and prolonged temozolomide in addition to radiotherapy in newly diagnosed glioblastoma – a phase II study. BMC Cancer 9:308. doi:10.1186/1471-2407-9-308
12. Chua SL, Rosenthal MA, Wong SS, Ashley DM, Woods AM, Dowling A, Cher LM (2004) Phase 2 study of temozolomide and Caelyx in patients with recurrent glioblastoma multiforme. Neuro Oncol 6(1):38–43
13. Gabizon AA, Shmeeda H, Zalipsky S (2006) Pros and cons of the liposome platform in cancer drug targeting. J Liposome Res 16(3):175–183. doi:10.1080/08982100600848769
14. Maruyama K (2011) Intracellular targeting delivery of liposomal drugs to solid tumors based on EPR effects. Adv Drug Deliv Rev 63(3): 161–169. doi:10.1016/j.addr.2010.09.003
15. Ta T, Porter TM (2013) Thermosensitive liposomes for localized delivery and triggered release of chemotherapy. J Control Release 169(1-2):112–125. doi:10.1016/j.jconrel.2013.03.036
16. Koning GA, Eggermont AM, Lindner LH, ten Hagen TL (2010) Hyperthermia and thermosensitive liposomes for improved delivery of chemotherapeutic drugs to solid tumors. Pharm Res 27(8):1750–1754. doi:10.1007/s11095-010-0154-2
17. Gupta N, Hatoum H, Dy GK (2014) First line treatment of advanced non-small-cell lung cancer - specific focus on albumin bound paclitaxel. Int J Nanomedicine 9:209–221. doi:10.2147/IJN.S41770
18. Ma P, Mumper RJ (2013) Paclitaxel nanodelivery systems: a comprehensive review. J Nanomed Nanotechnol 4(2):1000164. doi:10.4172/2157-7439.1000164
19. John TA, Vogel SM, Tiruppathi C, Malik AB, Minshall RD (2003) Quantitative analysis of albumin uptake and transport in the rat microvessel endothelial monolayer. Am J Physiol Lung Cell Mol Physiol 284(1):L187–L196. doi:10.1152/ajplung.00152.2002
20. Schubert W, Frank PG, Razani B, Park DS, Chow CW, Lisanti MP (2001) Caveolae-deficient endothelial cells show defects in the uptake and transport of albumin in vivo. J Biol Chem 276(52):48619–48622. doi:10.1074/jbc.C100613200
21. Desai N, Trieu V, Yao Z, Louie L, Ci S, Yang A, Tao C, De T, Beals B, Dykes D, Noker P, Yao R, Labao E, Hawkins M, Soon-Shiong P (2006) Increased antitumor activity, intratumor paclitaxel concentrations, and endothelial cell transport of cremophor-free, albumin-bound paclitaxel, ABI-007, compared with cremophor-based paclitaxel. Clin Cancer Res 12(4):1317–1324. doi:10.1158/1078-0432.CCR-05-1634
22. Marrero L, Wyczechowska D, Musto AE, Wilk A, Vashistha H, Zapata A, Walker C, Velasco-Gonzalez C, Parsons C, Wieland S, Levitt D, Reiss K, Prakash O (2014) Therapeutic efficacy of aldoxorubicin in an intracranial xenograft mouse model of human glioblastoma. Neoplasia 16(10):874–882. doi:10.1016/j.neo.2014.08.015
23. Ulbrich K, Hekmatara T, Herbert E, Kreuter J (2009) Transferrin- and transferrin-receptor-antibody-modified nanoparticles enable drug

delivery across the blood-brain barrier (BBB). Eur J Pharm Biopharm 71(2):251–256. doi:10.1016/j.ejpb.2008.08.021

24. Ulbrich K, Knobloch T, Kreuter J (2011) Targeting the insulin receptor: nanoparticles for drug delivery across the blood-brain barrier (BBB). J Drug Target 19(2):125–132. doi:10.3109/10611861003734001
25. Sharma G, Modgil A, Zhong T, Sun C, Singh J (2014) Influence of short-chain cell-penetrating peptides on transport of Doxorubicin encapsulating receptor-targeted liposomes across brain endothelial barrier. Pharm Res 31(5):1194–1209. doi:10.1007/s11095-013-1242-x
26. Bhattacharya R, Osburg B, Fischer D, Bickel U (2008) Targeted delivery of complexes of biotin-PEG-polyethylenimine and NF-kappaB decoys to brain-derived endothelial cells in vitro. Pharm Res 25(3):605–615. doi:10.1007/s11095-007-9389-y
27. Ko YT, Bhattacharya R, Bickel U (2009) Liposome encapsulated polyethylenimine/ODN polyplexes for brain targeting. J Control Release 133(3):230–237. doi:10.1016/j.jconrel.2008.10.013
28. Gabathuler R (2010) Approaches to transport therapeutic drugs across the blood-brain barrier to treat brain diseases. Neurobiol Dis 37(1):48–57.doi:10.1016/j.nbd.2009.07.028
29. Demeule M, Regina A, Che C, Poirier J, Nguyen T, Gabathuler R, Castaigne JP, Beliveau R (2008) Identification and design of peptides as a new drug delivery system for the brain. J Pharmacol Exp Ther 324(3):1064–1072. doi:10.1124/jpet.107.131318
30. Demeule M, Beaudet N, Regina A, Besserer-Offroy E, Murza A, Tetreault P, Belleville K, Che C, Larocque A, Thiot C, Beliveau R, Longpre JM, Marsault E, Leduc R, Lachowicz JE, Gonias SL, Castaigne JP, Sarret P (2014) Conjugation of a brain-penetrant peptide with neurotensin provides antinociceptive properties. J Clin Invest 124(3):1199–1213. doi:10.1172/JCI70647
31. Shen J, Zhan C, Xie C, Meng Q, Gu B, Li C, Zhang Y, Lu W (2011) Poly(ethylene glycol)-block-poly(d, l-lactide acid) micelles anchored with angiopep-2 for brain-targeting delivery. J Drug Target 19(3):197–203. doi:10.3109/1061186X.2010.483517
32. Spencer BJ, Verma IM (2007) Targeted delivery of proteins across the blood-brain barrier. Proc Natl Acad Sci U S A 104(18):7594–7599. doi:10.1073/pnas.0702170104
33. Spencer B, Marr RA, Gindi R, Potkar R, Michael S, Adame A, Rockenstein E, Verma IM, Masliah E (2011) Peripheral delivery of a CNS targeted, metalo-protease reduces abeta toxicity in a mouse model of Alzheimer's disease. PLoS One 6(1), e16575. doi:10.1371/journal.pone.0016575
34. Iwata N, Sekiguchi M, Hattori Y, Takahashi A, Asai M, Ji B, Higuchi M, Staufenbiel M, Muramatsu S, Saido TC (2013) Global brain delivery of neprilysin gene by intravascular administration of AAV vector in mice. Sci Rep 3:1472. doi:10.1038/srep01472
35. Pinzon-Daza M, Garzon R, Couraud P, Romero I, Weksler B, Ghigo D, Bosia A, Riganti C (2012) The association of statins plus LDL receptor-targeted liposome-encapsulated doxorubicin increases in vitro drug delivery across blood-brain barrier cells. Br J Pharmacol 167(7):1431–1447. doi:10.1111/j.1476-5381.2012.02103.x
36. Fillebeen C, Descamps L, Dehouck MP, Fenart L, Benaissa M, Spik G, Cecchelli R, Pierce A (1999) Receptor-mediated transcytosis of lactoferrin through the blood-brain barrier. J Biol Chem 274(11):7011–7017
37. Yu Y, Jiang X, Gong S, Feng L, Zhong Y, Pang Z (2014) The proton permeability of self-assembled polymersomes and their neuroprotection by enhancing a neuroprotective peptide across the blood-brain barrier after modification with lactoferrin. Nanoscale 6(6):3250–3258. doi:10.1039/c3nr05196j
38. Yu Y, Pang Z, Lu W, Yin Q, Gao H, Jiang X (2012) Self-assembled polymersomes conjugated with lactoferrin as novel drug carrier for brain delivery. Pharm Res 29(1):83–96. doi:10.1007/s11095-011-0513-7
39. Hu K, Shi Y, Jiang W, Han J, Huang S, Jiang X (2011) Lactoferrin conjugated PEG-PLGA nanoparticles for brain delivery: Preparation, characterization and efficacy in Parkinson's disease. Int J Pharm 415(1-2): 273–283. doi:10.1016/j.ijpharm
40. Qiao R, Jia Q, Huwel S, Xia R, Liu T, Gao F, Galla HJ, Gao M (2012) Receptor-mediated delivery of magnetic nanoparticles across the blood-brain barrier. ACS Nano 6(4):3304–3310. doi:10.1021/nn300240p
41. Kannan R, Chakrabarti R, Tang D, Kim KJ, Kaplowitz N (2000) GSH transport in human cerebrovascular endothelial cells and human astrocytes: evidence for luminal localization of Na+-dependent GSH transport in HCEC. Brain Res 852(2):374–382
42. Gaillard PJ, Appeldoorn CC, Dorland R, van Kregten J, Manca F, Vugts DJ, Windhorst B, van Dongen GA, de Vries HE, Maussang D, van Tellingen O (2014) Pharmacokinetics, brain delivery, and efficacy in brain tumor-bearing mice of glutathione pegylated liposomal

doxorubicin (2B3-101). PLoS One 9(1), e82331. doi:10.1371/journal.pone.0082331

43. Birngruber T, Raml R, Gladdines W, Gatschelhofer C, Gander E, Ghosh A, Kroath T, Gaillard PJ, Pieber TR, Sinner F (2014) Enhanced doxorubicin delivery to the brain administered through glutathione PEGylated liposomal doxorubicin (2B3-101) as compared with generic Caelyx,((R))/Doxil((R)) – a cerebral open flow microperfusion pilot study. J Pharm Sci 103(7):1945–1948. doi:10.1002/jps.23994
44. Gaillard PJ, Appeldoorn CC, Rip J, Dorland R, van der Pol SM, Kooij G, de Vries HE, Reijerkerk A (2012) Enhanced brain delivery of liposomal methylprednisolone improved therapeutic efficacy in a model of neuroinflammation. J Control Release 164(3):364–369. doi:10.1016/j.jconrel.2012.06.022
45. Kizelsztein P, Ovadia H, Garbuzenko O, Sigal A, Barenholz Y (2009) Pegylated nanoliposomes remote-loaded with the antioxidant tempamine ameliorate experimental autoimmune encephalomyelitis. J Neuroimmunol 213(1-2):20–25. doi:10.1016/j.jneuroim.2009.05.019
46. Herve F, Ghinea N, Scherrmann JM (2008) CNS delivery via adsorptive transcytosis. AAPS J 10(3):455–472. doi:10.1208/s12248-008-9055-2
47. Lalatsa A, Schatzlein AG, Uchegbu IF (2014) Strategies to deliver peptide drugs to the brain. Mol Pharm 11(4):1081–1093. doi:10.1021/mp400680d
48. Cao G, Pei W, Ge H, Liang Q, Luo Y, Sharp FR, Lu A, Ran R, Graham SH, Chen J (2002) In vivo delivery of a Bcl-xL fusion protein containing the TAT protein transduction domain protects against ischemic brain injury and neuronal apoptosis. J Neurosci 22(13):5423–5431, doi: 20026550
49. Krauze MT, Forsayeth J, Park JW, Bankiewicz KS (2006) Real-time imaging and quantification of brain delivery of liposomes. Pharm Res 23(11):2493–2504. doi:10.1007/s11095-006-9103-5
50. Kenny GD, Bienemann AS, Tagalakis AD, Pugh JA, Welser K, Campbell F, Tabor AB, Hailes HC, Gill SS, Lythgoe MF, McLeod CW, White EA, Hart SL (2013) Multifunctional receptor-targeted nanocomplexes for the delivery of therapeutic nucleic acids to the brain. Biomaterials 34(36):9190–9200. doi:10.1016/j.biomaterials.2013.07.081
51. Ishii T, Asai T, Oyama D, Fukuta T, Yasuda N, Shimizu K, Minamino T, Oku N (2012) Amelioration of cerebral ischemia-reperfusion injury based on liposomal drug delivery system with asialo-erythropoietin. J Control Release 160(1):81–87. doi:10.1016/j.jconrel.2012.02.004
52. Ishii T, Asai T, Oyama D, Agato Y, Yasuda N, Fukuta T, Shimizu K, Minamino T, Oku N (2013) Treatment of cerebral ischemia-reperfusion injury with PEGylated liposomes encapsulating FK506. FASEB J 27(4):1362–1370. doi:10.1096/fj.12-221325
53. Feng B, Tomizawa K, Michiue H, Miyatake S, Han XJ, Fujimura A, Seno M, Kirihata M, Matsui H (2009) Delivery of sodium borocaptate to glioma cells using immunoliposome conjugated with anti-EGFR antibodies by ZZ-His. Biomaterials 30(9):1746–1755. doi:10.1016/j.biomaterials.2008.12.010
54. Feng B, Tomizawa K, Michiue H, Han XJ, Miyatake S, Matsui H (2010) Development of a bifunctional immunoliposome system for combined drug delivery and imaging in vivo. Biomaterials 31(14):4139–4145. doi:10.1016/j.biomaterials.2010.01.086
55. Liu HL, Hua MY, Yang HW, Huang CY, Chu PC, Wu JS, Tseng IC, Wang JJ, Yen TC, Chen PY, Wei KC (2010) Magnetic resonance monitoring of focused ultrasound/magnetic nanoparticle targeting delivery of therapeutic agents to the brain. Proc Natl Acad Sci U S A 107(34):15205–15210. doi:10.1073/pnas.1003388107
56. Kievit FM, Zhang M (2011) Cancer nanotheranostics: improving imaging and therapy by targeted delivery across biological barriers. Adv Mater 23(36):H217–H247. doi:10.1002/adma.201102313
57. Bhojani MS, Van Dort M, Rehemtulla A, Ross BD (2010) Targeted imaging and therapy of brain cancer using theranostic nanoparticles. Mol Pharm 7(6):1921–1929. doi:10.1021/mp100298r
58. Lammers T, Kiessling F, Hennink WE, Storm G (2010) Nanotheranostics and image-guided drug delivery: current concepts and future directions. Mol Pharm 7(6):1899–1912. doi:10.1021/mp100228v
59. Afergan E, Epstein H, Dahan R, Koroukhov N, Rohekar K, Danenberg HD, Golomb G (2008) Delivery of serotonin to the brain by monocytes following phagocytosis of liposomes. J Control Release 132(2):84–90. doi:10.1016/j.jconrel.2008.08.017

Chapter 18

Transcutaneous Immunization Using Nano-sized Drug Carriers

Momoko Kitaoka and Masahiro Goto

Abstract

Growing knowledge about the immune system in the skin and recent advances in the preparation of nano-sized particles have encouraged research into the induction of an adaptive immune response via the transcutaneous route. Because the skin is abundant in dendritic cell subsets, vaccine administration through the transcutaneous route has promise for simple and efficient immunization and immunotherapy methods, which would provide a welcome alternative to the conventional injection technique. Strategies using a nanoparticle-based protein delivery into the skin depend on the types of nanoparticles, such as soft vesicular nanoparticles, hard inorganic and polymer nanoparticles, and surfactant-coated solid-in-oil nanoparticles. Here, we discuss the skin structure and the immune system in the skin, as well as the types of nanoparticles, routes of administration, and effects of adjuvants. In addition, a detailed description of the preparation and characteristics of solid-in-oil nanoparticles is provided for the future development of an efficient transcutaneous immunization system.

Key words Transcutaneous immunization, Transdermal drug delivery, Solid-in-oil nanodispersion, Vaccine

1 Introduction

1.1 Skin Structure and Functions

The skin consists of three main layers, namely, the epidermis, dermis, and subcutaneous tissue. The epidermis is the outermost layer, and the human epidermis is 50–200 μm in thickness varying throughout the body [1, 2]. The epidermis is further comprised of five strata (Fig. 1), from outer to inner: stratum corneum (SC), stratum lucidum, stratum granulosum, stratum spinosum, and stratum basale [3]. The SC is a hydrophobic layer (15 μm thick in human) in which 10–20 layers of flattened corneocytes [4, 5] are embedded in lipid lamellae composed of phospholipids, cholesterols, triglycerides, and other lipid elements [6]. The corneocytes contain more keratin than other cells, and the SC layer functions as a primary barrier to the invasion of pathogens and foreign chemicals, or to water loss by evaporation. The moisture content of the SC is

Zheng-Rong Lu and Shinji Sakuma (eds.), *Nanomaterials in Pharmacology*, Methods in Pharmacology and Toxicology, DOI 10.1007/978-1-4939-3121-7_18,

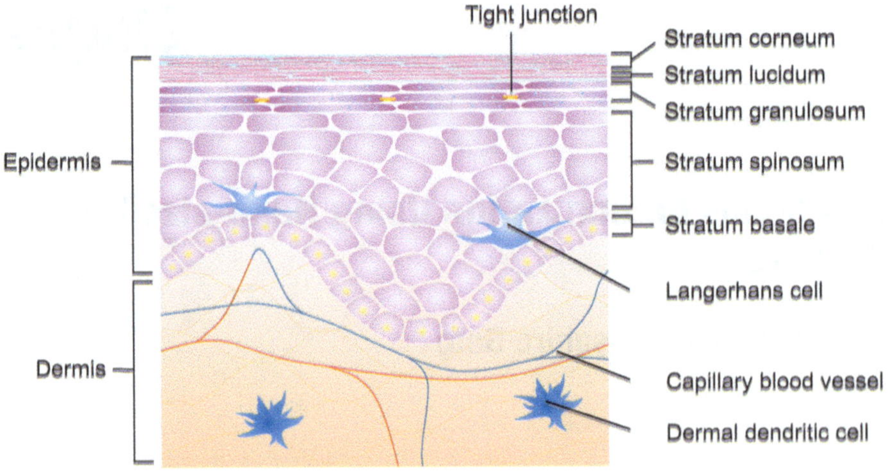

Fig. 1 Illustration of the epidermis and dermis

10–25 %; however, it gradually increases from the outer to inner layers and becomes 70 % at the bottom of the epidermis and at the dermis [7, 8]. In the stratum granulosum, cells are rigidly bound with membrane proteins, which form tight junctions and limit the infiltration of microorganisms and endotoxins [9, 10]. Tight junctions act as the second physical barrier in the skin. Beneath the SC, keratinocytes, melanocytes, Langerhans cells (LCs), and Merkel cells exist in the epidermis [3]. The dermis is the layer between the epidermis and subcutaneous tissues. In humans, the dermis is approximately 2 mm thick and is composed of collagen and elastin fibers, capillary blood vessels, lymph vessels, and nerves. Dermal dendritic cells (dDCs), mast cells, and fibroblasts are located in the dermis. A transdermal delivery system aims to deliver drug compounds to the blood vessels in the dermis from which they could enter systemic circulation.

The term “transcutaneous delivery” denotes the delivery of drug compounds beneath the SC, specifically to the epidermis, whereas “transdermal delivery” indicates the delivery of a drug through the skin for systemic distribution [11–13]. The routes of transdermal drug delivery are classified into three main types: (1) through the sweat glands and hair follicles associated with sebaceous glands for large molecules, such as proteins, and across the SC layer by (2) intercellular or (3) transcellular routes for smaller compounds (Fig. 2). Most molecules permeate through the intercellular spaces, which are filled with multiple lipid bilayers, and thus hydrophobic substances dissolved or dispersed in oil vehicles are prone to permeate more easily into the skin [14]. Hydrophilic molecules of low molecular weights are capable of permeating the skin; however, the degree of permeability drops an order of magnitude when the molecular weight is over 500 Da [14, 15].

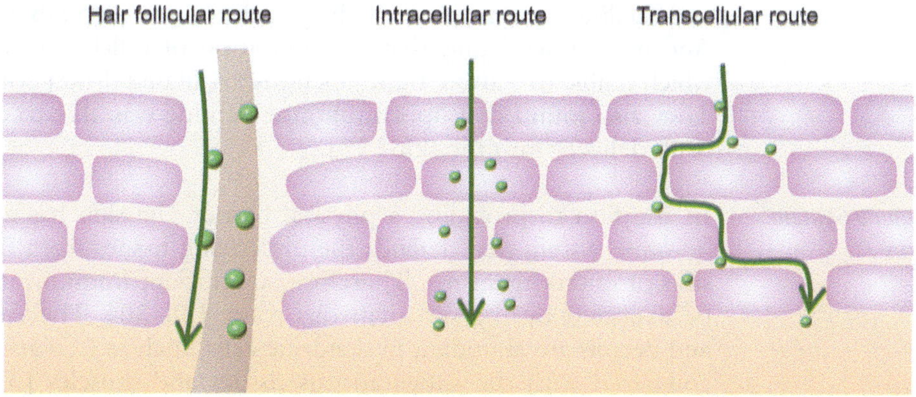

Fig. 2 Representative routes of transdermal drug delivery

1.2 Skin Permeation Enhancers

The skin permeation enhancers ideally are nonirritating and do not cause allergic reactions. However, because the outermost layer in the skin is composed of a lipid bilayer, most skin permeation enhancers act to disorder the lipid bilayer and increase the lipid fluidity. To date, several compounds are known as skin permeation enhancers, such as water, alcohols, lipids, and surfactants [16]. Short-chain alcohols, such as ethanol and isopropanol, are often employed as transcutaneous drug delivery enhancers [17–20]. Ethanol disorders the lipid matrix and increases the fluidity of lipids in the SC layer. However, short-chain alcohols are volatile, and their effect as skin permeation enhancers is limited to a short period following administration to the skin. Long-chain alcohols also enhance the permeation of drugs into the skin. Previous research found that alcohol with a carbon length of 10 showed the highest permeation-enhancing ability [21]. Moreover, those compounds containing one or two unsaturated bonds showed higher skin permeation effects [22]. Oleic acid was also demonstrated to enhance the skin permeability of drugs [23]. Oleic acid in *cis* form is considered to disorder the lipid bilayer in the SC, presumably because this form of oleic acid is capable of being packed rather than distributed in the skin lipids [24, 25]. Anionic and cationic surfactants have the ability to accelerate permeation of drugs; however, many of them cause skin irritation and damage. Nonionic surfactants are less irritating and enhance skin permeability of drug molecules by disrupting skin lipids. Water molecules are known to hydrate the skin, which enhances the permeability of hydrophilic drug compounds. Therefore, occlusive patches are used to exploit this feature of water molecules.

Recently, peptides composed of cationic or amphipathic amino acids were used as skin penetration enhancers. These peptides are called cell-penetrating peptides (CPP) or protein transduction domains and are able to penetrate the cell membrane [26]. Some CPP, such as oligoarginine, interact with tight junction proteins and facilitate permeation of drug compounds through the skin. Another report found that the inhibition of toll-like receptor 2, which is able to activate tight junctions, facilitated drug permeation. They also found that lipolanthionine peptide was able to enhance drug delivery into the skin [27].

1.3 Immune System in the Skin

In addition to providing a physical barrier, the skin has a unique immune system that defends the underlying tissues from the invasion of microorganisms. Therefore, an efficient immunization can be expected by the subcutaneous route [28–30]. The epidermis and dermis are abundant in dendritic cells, such as LCs and dDCs, compared with the subcutaneous tissues and muscles [31]. LCs reside at the bottom of the stratum spinosum and form a network with the dendrites in keratinocytes. An LC is demonstrated to migrate to the skin-draining lymph node when it captures an extraneous antigen compound and then stimulate naïve T cells [32, 33]. However, recent reports revealed that the migration of LCs is slow compared with that of dDCs [34]. The dDCs are also assumed to capture extraneous compounds and migrate to skin-draining lymph nodes at the initiation of antigen-specific immune responses [35]. There are multiple dDC subsets; however, their exact contributions in the skin's immune system are still unclear. Some dDC subsets are reported to promote a T helper type 1 (Th1-type) immune response, while the others promote a T helper type 2 (Th2-type) immune response [36]. Because attaining a long-lasting immunization is possible through the skin's adaptive immune response, studies investigating transcutaneous vaccine delivery are currently focused on the enhancement of antigen uptake by DCs using adjuvants, as well as on overcoming the physical skin barrier.

1.4 Particle Sizes and Immune Responses

Ex vivo studies have indicated that the particle size of drug carriers influences the type of immune responses [37, 38]. In one report, antigens were conjugated with carboxyl-modified polystyrene beads and applied to splenocytes. They found that nanoparticles of 40–50 nm induced interferon (IFN)-γ cytokines from $CD8^+$ T cells, whereas those of 90–120 nm stimulated $CD4^+$ T cells to induce interleukin (IL)-4 [39, 40]. In another report using macrophage cell lines, nanoparticles (200–600 nm) were taken up by macrophages; however, larger particles (2–8 μm) were more likely to be attached to the surface of macrophages [41]. In addition, an increased induction of IFN-γ was observed when antigen-bound nanoparticles of 200 nm were administered to mice, and antigen-bound microparticles induced a higher level of IL-4 cytokine. In an in vivo experiment where polystyrene particles labeled with fluorescent dyes were administered to mice by injection, large particles of 500–2000 nm were only found in dendritic cells at the site where the particles were administered; however, small nanoparticles (20–200 nm) were also found in dendritic cells in the lymph nodes and in macrophages, indicating that small particles may drain to lymph nodes [42]. These results indicate that small nanoparticles whose sizes correspond to those of viruses (<200 nm) are preferentially taken up by dendritic cells via endocytosis and induce a Th1-type immune response, while larger particles, such as microparticles (whose sizes correspond to that of bacteria), are prone to uptake by macrophages and elicit a Th2-type immune response. Consequently, their size allows nanoparticles to be used as adjuvants [43].

1.5 Advantages and Disadvantages of Transdermal Drug Delivery

Transdermal drug delivery has advantages over the conventional subcutaneous delivery using needles and syringes. It can reduce the pain inherent in the injection method and the poor patient compliance caused by that pain, as well as reduce the risks of needlestick-related injuries and transmission of blood-borne infectious diseases [13, 44]. Transcutaneous administrations using simple systems, such as patches or ointments, are advantageous because they do not require medically trained personnel, and self-administration of medicines/vaccines would be possible. The use of the patch would also decrease the amount of sharp waste produced by injections. In addition, the transdermal route of delivery avoids the first-pass effect on the liver, which also occurs during oral drug delivery. Compared with the injection method, the delivery of drug compounds is relatively slow in the transdermal route. However, the long-lasting administration could be useful in cases where the drug level in blood needs to be controlled. Slow drug delivery is also favorable when administering vaccines that have the potential to cause serious side effects, such as anaphylaxis. To deliver medically active compounds to the systemic circulation, these compounds must diffuse in the dermis and then penetrate capillary blood vessels. Because of the protective functions of the skin, however, the amount of drugs that could be approved for practical use is limited to small molecules, e.g., scopolamine, fentanyl, nicotine, and hormones. To help overcome this issue, transdermal drug deliveries administered by physical permeation-enhancing equipment were invented, such as electroporation and iontophoresis methods, ultrasonication methods, jet-injection methods, and microneedle methods [45]. In contrast, transcutaneous immunizations will be possible when vaccines can be permeated through the epidermis, and recent research has aimed to develop efficient transcutaneous immunization methods.

2 Transdermal Drug Delivery Using Nano-sized Carriers

Transdermal drug delivery methods are categorized into two main types: the physically facilitated techniques and the techniques using chemical permeation enhancers. The physical techniques use microneedles, electroporations, ultrasound, and jet injections and can efficiently deliver drugs to the dermis and epidermis. However, some devices may induce pain when delivering active compounds to the dermis, where nerve terminals lay, and the simplicity and convenience of transdermal administration might be lost when using electrical equipment. Chemical techniques, such as lipid-, surfactant-, and polymer-based nanoparticles, inorganic compounds, hydrogel patches, and microemulsions, are expected to allow a simple and noninvasive transcutaneous drug delivery. Permeation of inorganic nanoparticles through the skin has been tested; however, particles larger than 20 nm did not penetrate the skin because they were unable to pass through pores smaller than 10 nm between corneocytes in the SC layer [46–49]. The particles accumulated in hair follicles, and the follicular canals acted as reservoirs. In contrast, some soft nanoparticles are thought to penetrate into the epidermis.

2.1 Liposomes

Liposomes are composed of a phospholipid bilayer which resembles the cell membrane and are capable of entrapping both hydrophilic and hydrophobic molecules [50–52]. Several derivations of liposomes containing some additional compounds, such as surfactants, alcohols, and amphiphiles, have been developed to enhance the permeation of active compounds into the skin [53–55]. Transfersomes, which are elastic liposomes composed of phospholipid and sodium cholate, accelerated the transdermal delivery of insulin in mouse models and in clinical trials [56–60]. The ultradeformable transfersome vesicles can squeeze into the nano-sized pores between the cells in the skin and pass through the skin barrier without changing the vesicle size [61]. The surfactants and/or short-chain alcohols (edge-active molecules) composing the bilayers of vesicles localize in the vesicles and shape smaller spherical aggregates, thus enabling stable permeation through a narrow intercellular pore.

Other liposome derivatives likely permeate into the skin by a similar mechanism. Exemplified are ethosomes which are composed of lipids and ethanol. Transcutaneous immunization using ethosomes containing hepatitis B virus induced comparable levels of IgG and higher levels of IgA compared to those induced by the injection method [62, 63]. Other liposome derivatives are cationic liposomes which were investigated for the transcutaneous delivery of DNA vaccines. A cationic liposome composed of lipids and octadecylamine induced production of IFN-γ, a Th1-type cytokine [64]. Conversely, a cationic liposome composed of lipids and 1,2-dioleoyl-3-trimethylammonium-propane induced IgG1 and IgE, indicating that a Th2-type immune response was induced. These findings suggest the possibility of manipulating the Th1/Th2 balance of the immune response [65]. Vesosome, in which a cationic liposome is encapsulated in the lipid bilayer, successfully demonstrated transcutaneous immunization using tetanus toxoid (molecular weight, 150 kDa) [66]. SECosomes, surfactant-ethanol-cholesterol-osomes, are flexible nanosomes that have shown high transfection efficiencies with siRNA [67].

2.2 Niosome

Niosomes are composed of nonionic surfactants and cholesterols and may contain charge-inducing agents [68–71]. The vesicles can be stored stably and prepared at low costs. Niosomes have similar physical characteristics to liposomes and are capable of delivering hydrophilic and hydrophobic compounds. Niosomes prepared with Span 85 and cholesterol and contained a tetanus toxoid were able to induce rat serum IgG. Even higher levels of rat serum IgG were elicited by BSA-loaded niosomes prepared with Span 60 or Span 85 combined with cholesterol and stearylamine, which were coated with O-palmitoyl mannan to efficiently target them to Langerhans cells [72]. The Th2-predominant immune balance did not change regardless of the administration method, either intramuscular injection or topical administration. Like liposomes, niosomes can be used to deliver DNA vaccines. Transcutaneous administration of DNA encoding hepatitis surface antigen (HBsAg) loaded in niosomes induced high levels of HBsAg-specific antibody, IL-2, and IFN-γ, which were comparable to those induced by the same DNA vaccine administered in liposome carriers [73].

2.3 Polymer Nanoparticles

Polylactic acid (PLA) and poly(lactide-co-glycolic acid) (PLGA) nanoparticles are the most common and well-investigated nanoparticle carriers for transcutaneous vaccines [74–76]. The polymers are biodegradable and biocompatible, and their constituents, lactic acid and glycolic acid, are excreted from the body after degradation of the polymer [77]. In one study, PLA nanoparticles (approximately 150 nm in size) loaded with ovalbumin (OVA) or with fluorescence-labeled albumin were prepared and transcutaneously administered to mice [78]. As a result, permeation of PLA nanoparticles via hair follicles was observed in fluorescence microscopy images. Although induction of anti-OVA IgG titer by the transfollicular administration of PLA nanoparticles was limited, the nanoparticles induced high levels of IFN-γ and IL-2 in the presence of cholera toxin, indicating that the PLA nanoparticle could act as an adjuvant to elicit a Th1-type immune response.

Another study revealed that the follicular uptake of OVA was increased more than twofold by encapsulation of the antigen in chitosan-coated PLGA nanoparticles, and that induction of the immune response was possible [79]. Chitosan is a biopolymer of cationic polysaccharides consisting of glucosamine monomers that is applied as a carrier for transcutaneous drug delivery [80, 81]. Chitosan derivatives interact with keratin in the SC and increase the SC water content [82]. Moreover, chitosan-tripolyphosphate complex was recently applied to nanoparticle-based transcutaneous immunization to enhance the permeation of nanoparticles by interacting with negatively charged cell membranes and increasing drug entrapment inside the nanoparticles [83]. OVA-loaded chitosan nanoparticles administered to intact the skin induced a high level of OVA-specific IgG, comparable to that induced by injected OVA [84]. The antigen uptake by antigen-presenting cells was increased by using nanoparticles, and the chitosan nanoparticles containing melanocyte-associated antigen, gp100, suppressed tumor growth, indicating that these particles have a potential for an antitumor immunotherapy use [85]. As particle modifiers, other natural polymers, such as guar gum [86], hyaluronic acid [87, 88], and their derivatives, can be employed.

2.4 Metal Nanoparticles

It is known that small (<10 nm) metal nanoparticles are capable of permeating the skin. Huang et al. investigated the effect of gold nanoparticles (Au-NPs) having a mean particle size of 5 nm on transcutaneous immunization [89]. They found that coadministration of Au-NPs enhanced both the permeation of OVA throughout the skin and the induction of anti-OVA IgG.

2.5 Viruslike Particles

Viruslike particles are composed of virus-derived capsid protein without DNA/RNA and, hence, do not have the ability to replicate. They can provide an adjuvant effect and carry specific antigens when fused by genetic engineering [90, 91]. In one study, when approximately 40 nm of viruslike particles derived from *rabbit hemorrhagic disease virus* (VP60) were transcutaneously administered to mice in conjunction with CpG oligodeoxynucleotide and cholera toxin, they induced antigen-specific antibody and cytokine responses [92].

2.6 Other Chemical Approaches

Patches are also used for the topical application of vaccines. Occlusive patches prevent evaporation of water from the vehicle and hydrate the skin. It is theorized that a high-concentration antigen layer emerges between the vehicle and the skin as a result of the formation of an antigen concentration gradient in the vehicle, leading to an accelerated permeation of antigens when the patch system is applied. The simple application of hydrogel patches was demonstrated to induce effective immune responses to OVA [93, 94].

3 Solid-in-Oil Nanodispersions

Solid-in-oil (S/O) nanodispersions are nano-sized particles composed of hydrophobic surfactant and hydrophilic medically active macromolecules (i.e., proteins) that are dispersed in oil vehicles [95]. The first report of an S/O nanodispersion system employed a nonirritating organic solvent, soybean oil, as a vehicle [96].

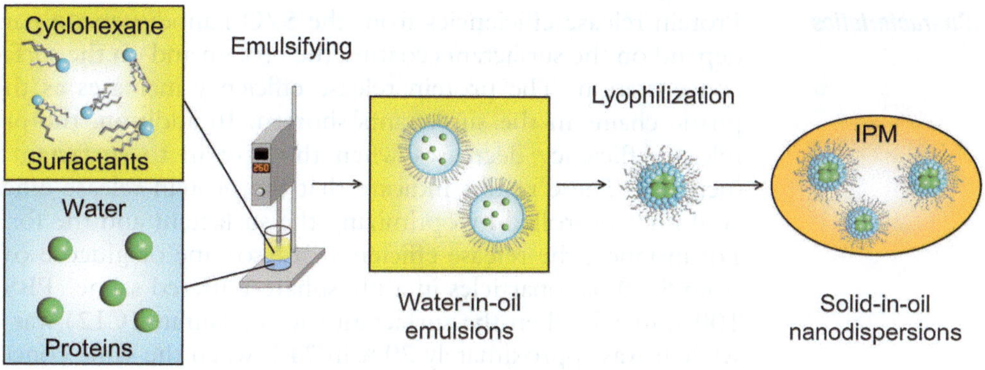

Fig. 3 Schematic representation of solid-in-oil nanodispersion preparation

In that report, insulin was dispersed in an oil vehicle and orally administered to rat models of diabetes to reduce serum glucose levels. Application of an S/O nanodispersion system to transdermal drug delivery was first performed by Piao et al. [97]. They successfully delivered a small hydrophilic compound, diclofenac sodium, to the Yucatan micropig skin. Thereafter, S/O nanodispersion systems were applied to transcutaneous administration of vitamin C [98], insulin [99], and OVA [100].

3.1 Preparation

The preparation of S/O nanodispersions occurs as follows: An aqueous solution of proteins and a cyclohexane solution of surfactants are mixed using a Polytron homogenizer to allow the formation of a white-colored water-in-oil emulsion (Fig. 3). The emulsion is quickly frozen in liquid nitrogen and then lyophilized for 12 h. After the water and cyclohexane are sublimed, a solid-state protein surrounded by surfactants can be obtained. Then, the surfactant-protein complex is dispersed in skin-permeable oil vehicles, such as isopropyl myristate (IPM), to yield a "solid-in-oil" nanodispersion. Proteins are encapsulated in the S/O nanoparticles without loss, and the particles are dispersed homogeneously in an oil vehicle by selecting the optimal surfactant concentration and protein to surfactant ratio.

Dynamic light scattering analysis indicated that the size of typical S/O nanodispersions in IPM is 100–400 nm. IPM is a safe and easy-to-treat aliphatic ester that is thought to interact with the intracellular matrix and enhance diffusivity of both the medical compound and the solvent itself [101, 102]. To our knowledge, IPM is the most suitable transcutaneous drug administration vehicle for the S/O nanodispersion system. Cholesterol can be used as a surfactant surrounding proteins; however, sucrose erucate and sucrose laurate (ER-290 and L-195, both from Mitsubishi-Kagaku Foods, Tokyo, Japan) form the most stable S/O nanodispersions. The S/O nanodispersions with optimized formula were stable for more than 3 months [99].

3.2 Characteristics

Protein release efficiencies from the S/O nanodispersion particles depend on the surfactants coating the protein and on the surfactant concentration. The protein release efficiency increases as the aliphatic chains in the surfactants shorten. In addition, the protein release efficiency decreases when the protein to surfactant ratio increases. These results indicate that the protein release efficiency could be controlled by optimizing the surfactant and the formula. For instance, the release efficiency of lysozyme or glucose oxidase from S/O nanoparticles in a phosphate-buffered saline (PBS) was 100 % in 3 h when the surfactant sucrose laurate (C12) was used, while it was approximately 30 % in 24 h when the same concentration of sucrose erucate (C22) was applied [103]. Furthermore, over 90 % of enzymatic activity remained in the S/O nanoparticles composed of sucrose laurate after 24 h. A similar observation was reported when horseradish peroxidase was encapsulated in S/O nanodispersions prepared with sucrose laurate [104]. The S/O nanodispersion system exhibits behaviors similar to water-in-oil emulsions and microemulsions; however, S/O nanodispersions are stable after longtime storage, presumably because of their smaller particle sizes. Additionally, protein drugs can be dispersed in an oil phase at a very high concentration of up to 5 mg/mL. Lastly, smaller amounts of surfactants are enough for the preparation of S/O nanoparticles as compared with those needed for emulsions.

Histological observations indicate that S/O nanodispersions administered using patches mainly accumulate in the SC layer. Since the whole SC layer serves as a reservoir for the S/O nanodispersions, drug compounds might continue to be released even after removal of the patch [99]. Fluorescence microscopy investigations suggested that the hydrophobic surfactants surrounding proteins are removed and accumulate in the SC layer and that only the proteins further permeate through the hydrophilic epidermis and dermis (Fig. 4). This idea could also explain the fact that IPM mainly accelerates the permeation of drugs through the SC layer and that IPM had little effect as a skin permeation enhancer when the SC layer was removed by tape stripping [101]. Additionally, in an in vitro experiment, insulin, a smaller protein (molecular weight, 6 kDa), permeated more efficiently than horseradish peroxidase (HRP), a larger protein (molecular weight, 40 kDa). Therefore, it is conceivable that IPM assists the permeation of S/O nanodispersions through the SC layer, and the hydrophilicity and size of proteins affect the permeability of proteins into the deeper layers of the skin. Another investigation using confocal laser scanning microscopy revealed that the surfactants and proteins permeated the SC layer via intracellular matrix [105].

3.3 Delivery of Protein Drugs and Vaccines

According to an in vitro examination using fluorescein isothiocyanate (FITC)-labeled insulin, the protein slowly permeated the epidermis and dermis in the porcine skin within 48 h, while an aqueous

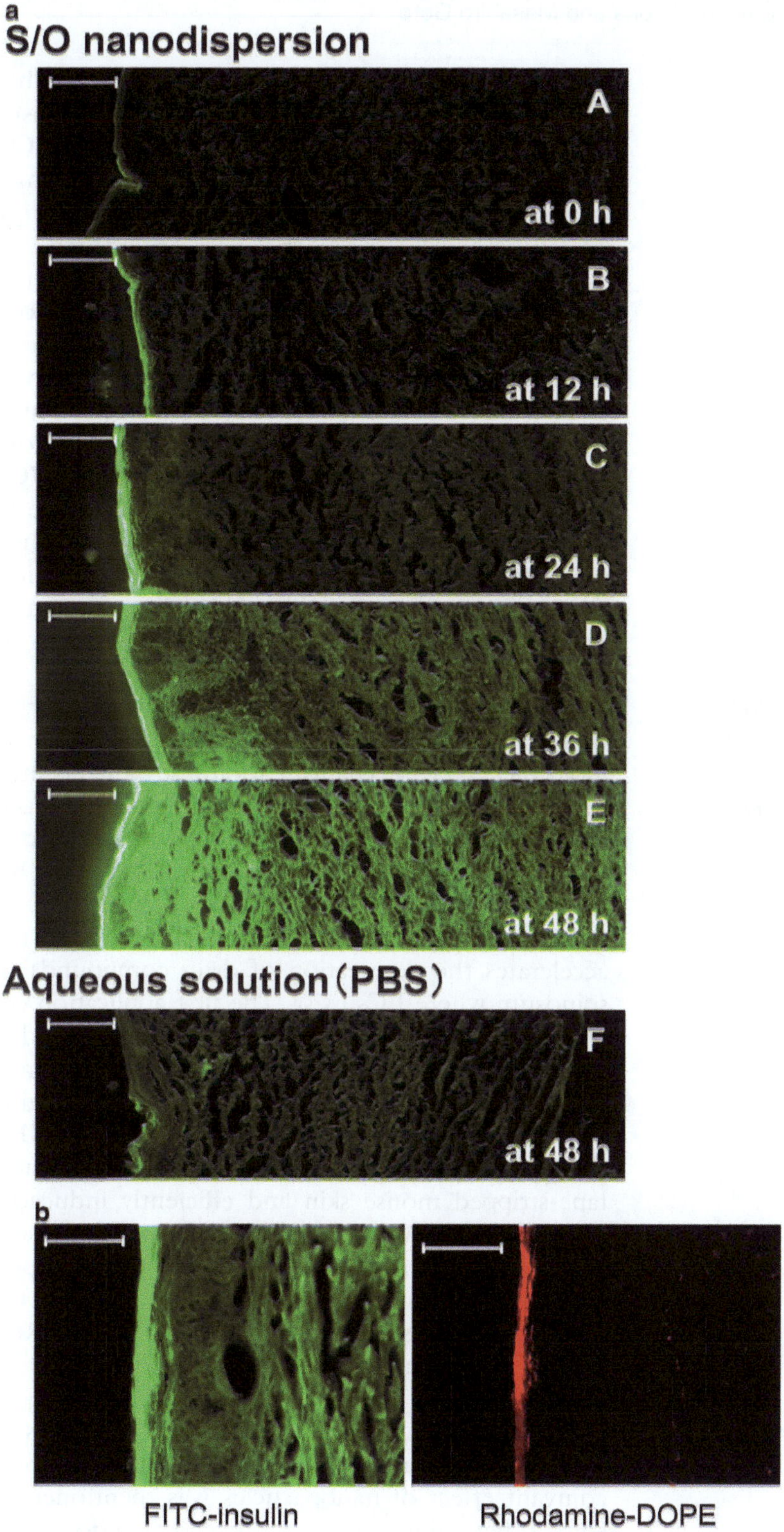

Fig. 4 Fluorescence microscopy images of the Yucatan micropig skin sections treated with solid-in-oil (S/O) nanodispersions composed of fluorescein isothiocyanate-labeled insulin (FITC-insulin) and Rhodamine-labeled 1,2-dioleoyl-sn-glycero-3-phosphoethanolamine (Rhodamine-DOPE) (**a**), the S/O nanodispersions containing FITC-insulin (**b**), and schematic illustration of transcutaneous protein delivery using S/O nanodispersion (**c**). Scale bars show 200 μm

solution of FITC-insulin did not permeate much and only did so in the SC layer (Fig. 4b). The permeation of insulin through the skin was accelerated sevenfold by using the S/O nanodispersion system. HRP administered to the epidermis using the S/O nanodispersion system displayed enzymatic activity, suggesting that the proteins are protected from denaturation [99].

The S/O nanodispersion system has also been applied to transcutaneous immunization [100, 105]. This method induced serum anti-OVA IgG efficiently in guinea pig, rabbit, and mouse models. A higher level of antibody was induced when a lower concentration of surfactant was used, indicating that the protein release efficiency from the nanoparticle affected the efficiency of immunization. However, the antibody level induced with the S/O nanodispersion system was still lower than that induced by the same amount of OVA administered via subcutaneous injection when a transcutaneous permeation enhancer was not applied. Additionally, the induction of antigen-specific antibody by the transcutaneous system was slower than the induction by the injection method.

3.4 Application of Skin Penetration Enhancers and Adjuvants

As mentioned above, it is known that particular peptides act as a skin penetration enhancers when they are administered with drug molecules. The mechanism for these skin penetration-enhancing peptides is still unclear; however, the condensation of the proteins in keratinocytes [106], induction of macropinocytosis [107], and denaturation of the tight junction proteins [108] have all been suggested. Because the tight junction proteins are located between epithelial cells in the stratum granulosum [109, 110], their denaturation accelerates the permeation of drug compounds through stratum spinosum where LCs exist. The first application of a skin penetration-enhancing peptide was reported by Rothbard et al. in which an enhancement of skin permeability of cyclosporin A was observed when it was chemically conjugated with oligoarginine (R7) [106]. In another report, an OVA peptide epitope (SIINFEKL) fused with the antennapedia homeodomain peptide was administered to a tape-stripped mouse skin and efficiently induced antigen-specific antibody [111]. When a series of lengths of oligoarginines (R3, R6, and R9) were co-encapsulated in S/O nanodispersions, R6 most efficiently enhanced the permeation of insulin [100]. Additionally, the S/O nanodispersion containing OVA and R6 induced a high level of OVA-specific IgG, as does subcutaneous injection of OVA (Fig. 5).

Transcutaneous administration of antigens in combination with adjuvants also facilitates the immunization efficiency. The adjuvant effect of nanoparticles was mentioned above; however, some other adjuvants, such as bacterial endotoxins and ligands for pattern recognition receptors (PRRs), are known to be effective in transcutaneous immunization. Bacterial endotoxins, such as cholera toxin [113] and heat-labile enterotoxins from *Escherichia coli* [114],

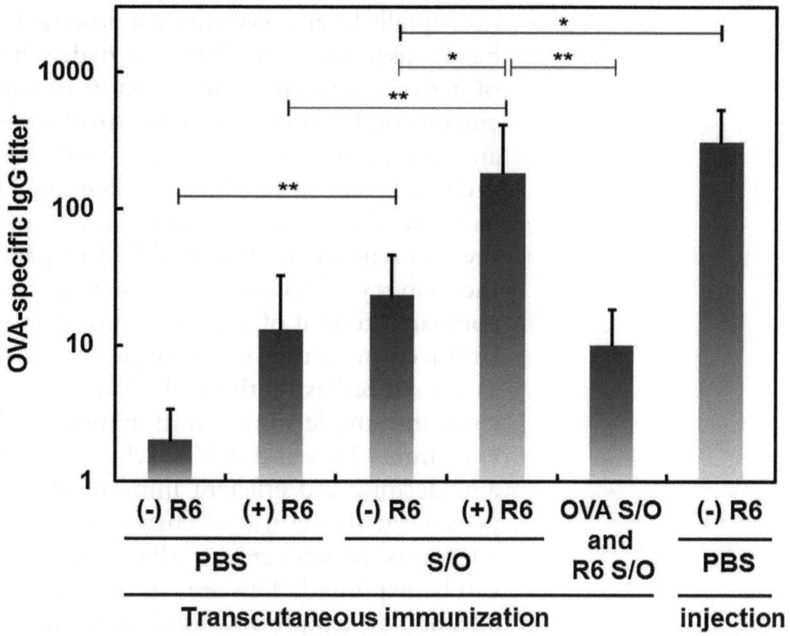

Fig. 5 Serum IgG response to ovalbumin (OVA) in ddY mice [112]. OVA with (+) or without (–) hexa-arginine (R6) was transcutaneously administered (in PBS solutions or S/O nanodispersions) three times at 1 week intervals. Data represent the mean ± SD of results from 5 mice. *$p < 0.05$ and **$p < 0.01$

interact with dendritic cells and gangliosides, which are located on cells in the skin and mucosa [115]. The bacterial endotoxins enhance antigen capture by LCs and induce strong immune responses [116–118]. Toll-like receptors (TLRs) are members of a family of PRRs found only in mammalian cells that recognize pathogen-associated molecular patterns (PAMPs) to regulate signal transduction pathways involved in the immune response [119, 120]. Unmethylated CpG DNA motifs in bacteria known as CpG oligodeoxynucleotides (ODNs) are ligands of TLR9 [121]. CpG ODNs strongly induce a Th1-biased immune response and enhance the body's immune response against antigens administered by several routes, including intramuscular, oral, nasal, and transcutaneous routes [122–124]. In our preliminary investigation, CpG ODN co-encapsulated with OVA in S/O nanodispersions enhanced an induction of OVA-specific IgG in mouse, indicating that CpG ODN is an effective adjuvant.

4 Future Prospects

Transdermal drug/vaccine delivery aims to provide a simple, noninvasive, and nonirritating delivery method for medically active compounds. Because the skin consists of hydrophobic and hydrophilic layers, conventional drug design for transdermal delivery has focused on controlling the hydrophobicity and hydrophilicity of active compounds, in addition to the application of chemical enhancers. Furthermore, only small molecules permeate the skin, and the transcutaneous delivery of hydrophilic macromolecules, such as proteins, has been challenging. Recent technology using nano-sized drug carriers posed a way to deliver proteins through the transcutaneous hair follicle and paracellular routes; however, the delivery of proteins by these methods is slow and less efficient compared to that of the conventional subcutaneous or intramuscular injection methods. A synergistic use of physical enhancers, such as microneedles or thermal ablation, has promise as a more efficient and simple administration method. In contrast, vaccine delivery targets LCs and dDCs, which are abundant in the epidermis and dermis, and efficient immunization with a low dose may be possible with the use of chemical skin permeation enhancers and adjuvants. Moreover, the adjuvanticity of nanoparticles themselves can be exploited. This area of research is still in an early stage, and advances in simple and efficient immunization techniques will be facilitated with the elucidation of signal transduction during the immune response in the skin.

Glossary

Au-NPs	Gold nanoparticles
CPP	Cell-penetrating peptides
dDC	Dermal dendritic cell
FITC	Fluorescein isothiocyanate
HBsAg	Hepatitis B surface antigen
HRP	Horseradish peroxidase
IFN	Interferon
IL	Interleukin
IPM	Isopropyl myristate
LC	Langerhans cell
ODN	Oligodeoxynucleotide
OVA	Ovalbumin
PBS	Phosphate-buffered saline
PLA	Polylactic acid
PLGA	Poly(lactide-co-glycolic acid)
PRR	Pattern recognition receptor
PAMP	Pathogen-associated molecular pattern
SC	Stratum corneum
S/O	Solid-in-oil
Th1-type	T helper type 1
Th2-type	T helper type 2
TLR	Toll-like receptor

References

1. Sandby-Møller J, Poulsen T, Wulf HC (2003) Epidermal thickness at different body sites: relationship to age, gender, pigmentation, blood content, skin type and smoking habits. Acta Derm Venereol 83:410–413
2. Yudovsky D, Pilon L (2010) Rapid and accurate estimation of blood saturation, melanin content, and epidermis thickness from spectral diffuse reflectance. Appl Opt 49:1707–1719
3. Watt FM (1989) Terminal differentiation of epidermal keratinocytes. Curr Opin Cell Biol 1:1107–1115
4. Madison KC (2003) Barrier function of the skin: "la raison d'être" of the epidermis. J Invest Dermatol 121:231–241
5. Bouwstra JA, Honeywell-Nguyen PL, Gooris GS et al (2003) Structure of the skin barrier and its modulation by vesicular formulations. Prog Lipid Res 42:1–36
6. Ho NFH, Barsuhn CL, Burton PS et al (1992) (D) Routes of delivery: case studies: (3) mechanistic insights to buccal delivery of proteinaceous substances. Adv Drug Deliv Rev 8:97–236
7. Cevc G, Blume G (1992) Lipid vesicles penetrate into intact skin owing to the transdermal osmotic gradients and hydration force. Biochim Biophys Acta 1104:226–232
8. Caspers PJ, Lucassen GW, Carter EA et al (2001) In vivo confocal Raman microspectroscopy of the skin: noninvasive determination of molecular concentration profiles. J Invest Dermatol 116:434–442
9. Denker BM, Nigam SK (1998) Molecular structure and assembly of the tight junction. Am J Physiol 274:F1–F9
10. Farquhar MG, Palade GE (1963) Junctional complexes in various epithelia. J Cell Biol 17:375–412
11. Barry BW (2001) Novel mechanisms and devices to enable successful transdermal drug delivery. Eur J Pharm Sci 14:101–114
12. Thomas BJ, Finnin BC (2004) The transdermal revolution. Drug Discov Today 9: 697–703
13. Prausnitz MR, Langer R (2008) Transdermal drug delivery. Nat Biotechnol 26: 1261–1268
14. Mitragotri S (2003) Modeling skin permeability to hydrophilic and hydrophobic solutes based on four permeation pathways. J Control Release 86:69–92
15. Bos JD, Meinardi MM (2000) The 500 Dalton rule for the skin penetration of chemical compounds and drugs. Exp Dermatol 9:165
16. Lane ME (2013) Skin penetration enhancers. Int J Pharm 447:12–21
17. Kurihara-Bergstrom T, Knutson K, DeNoble LJ et al (1990) Percutaneous absorption enhancement of an ionic molecule by ethanol-water systems in human skin. Pharm Res 7:762–766
18. Liu P, Cettina M, Wong J (2009) Effects of isopropanol-isopropyl myristate binary enhancers on in vitro transport of estradiol in human epidermis: a mechanistic evaluation. J Pharm Sci 98:565–572
19. Bommanam D, Potts RO, Guy RH (1991) Examination of the effect of ethanol on human stratum corneum in vivo using infrared spectroscopy. J control Release 16:299–304
20. Goates CY, Knutson K (1994) Enhanced permeation of polar compounds through human epidermis. I. Permeability and membrane structural changes in the presence of short chain alcohols. Biochim Biophys Acta 1195:169–179
21. Dias M, Naik A, Guy RH et al (2008) In vivo infrared spectroscopy studies of alkanol effects on human skin. Eur J Pharm Biopharm 69:1171–1175
22. Andega S, Kanikkannan N, Singh M (2001) Comparison of the effect of fatty alcohols on the permeation of melatonin between porcine and human skin. J Control Release 77:17–25
23. Mak VH, Potts RO, Guy RH (1990) Percutaneous penetration enhancement in vivo measured by attenuated total reflectance infrared spectroscopy. Pharm Res 7:835–841
24. Naik A, Pechtold LARM, Potts RO et al (1995) J Controll Release 37:299–306
25. Ongpipattanakul B, Burnette RR, Potts RO et al (1991) Evidence that oleic acid exists in a separate phase within stratum corneum lipids. Pharm Res 8:350–354
26. Desai P, Patlolla RR, Singh M (2010) Interaction of nanoparticles and cell-penetrating peptides with skin for transdermal drug delivery. Mol Membr Biol 27:247–259
27. Chen B, Liu DL, Pan WY et al (2014) Use of lipolanthionine peptide, a toll-like receptor 2 inhibitor, enhances transdermal delivery efficiency. Mol Med Rep 10:593–598
28. Glenn GM, Rao M, Matyas GR et al (1998) Skin immunization made possible by cholera toxin. Nature 391:851
29. Weiss R, Scheiblhofer S, Machado Y et al (2013) New approaches to transcutaneous immunotherapy: targeting dendritic cells with novel allergen conjugates. Curr Opin Allergy Clin Immunol 13:669–676

30. Bal SM, Ding Z, van Riet E et al (2010) Advances in transcutaneous vaccine delivery: do all ways lead to Rome? J Control Release 148:266–282
31. Kissenpfennig A, Henri S, Dubois B (2005) Dynamics and function of Langerhans cells in vivo: dermal dendritic cells colonize lymph node areas distinct from slower migrating Langerhans cells. Immunity 22:643–654
32. Silberberg I, Baer RL, Rosenthal SA (1976) The role of Langerhans cells in allergic contact hypersensitivity. A review of findings in man and guinea pigs. J Invest Dermatol 66: 210–217
33. Yu RC, Abrams DC, Alaibac M et al (1994) Morphological and quantitative analyses of normal epidermal Langerhans cells using confocal scanning laser microscopy. Br J Dermatol 131:843–848
34. Sen D, Forrest L, Kepler TB et al (2010) Selective and site-specific mobilization of dermal dendritic cells and Langerhans cells by Th1- and Th2-polarizing adjuvants. Proc Natl Acad Sci 107:8334–8339
35. Kissenpfennig A, Malissen B (2006) Langerhans cells – revisiting the paradigm using genetically engineered mice. Trends Immunol 27:132–139
36. Murakami R, Denda-Nagai K, Hashimoto S et al (2013) A unique dermal dendritic cell subset that skews the immune response toward Th2. PLoS One 8:e73270
37. Hansen S, Lehr CM (2012) Nanoparticles for transcutaneous vaccination. Microb Biotechnol 5:156–167
38. Xiang SD, Scholzen A, Minigo G et al (2006) Pathogen recognition and development of particulate vaccines: does size matter? Methods 40:1–9
39. Fifis T, Gamvrellis A, Crimeen-Irwin B et al (2004) Size-dependent immunogenicity: therapeutic and protective properties of nanovaccines against tumors. J Immunol 173: 3148–3154
40. Mottram PL, Leong D, Crimeen-Irwin B et al (2007) Type 1 and 2 immunity following vaccination is influenced by nanoparticle size: formulation of a model vaccine for respiratory syncytial virus. Mol Pharm 4:73–84
41. Kanchan V, Panda AK (2007) Interactions of antigen-loaded polylactide particles with macrophages and their correlation with the immune response. Biomaterials 28:5344–5357
42. Manolova V, Flace A, Bauer M et al (2008) Nanoparticles target distinct dendritic cell populations according to their size. Eur J Immunol 38:1404–1413
43. Wibowo N, Chuan YP, Seth A et al (2014) Co-administration of non-carrier nanoparticles boosts antigen immune response without requiring protein conjugation. Vaccine 32: 3664–3669
44. Mitragotri S (2005) Immunization without needles. Nat Rev 5:905–916
45. Matsuo K, Hirobe S, Okada N et al (2013) Frontiers of transcutaneous vaccination systems: novel technologies and devices for vaccine delivery. Vaccine 31:2403–2415
46. Baroli B, Ennas MG, Loffredo F et al (2007) Penetration of metallic nanoparticles in human full-thickness skin. J Invest Dermatol 127:1701–1712
47. Prow TW, Grice JE, Lin LL et al (2011) Nanoparticles and microparticles for skin drug delivery. Adv Drug Deliv Rev 63: 470–491
48. Labouta HI, Schneider M (2013) Interaction of inorganic nanoparticles with the skin barrier: current status and critical review. Nanomedicine 9:39–54
49. Papakostas D, Rancan F, Sterry W et al (2011) Nanoparticles in dermatology. Arch Dermatol Res 303:533–550
50. de Leeuw J, de Vijlder HC, Bjerring P et al (2009) Liposomes in dermatology today. J Eur Acad Dermatol Venereol 23:505–516
51. Duangjit S, Pamornpathomkul B, Opanasopit P et al (2014) Role of the charge, carbon chain length, and content of surfactant on the skin penetration of meloxicam-loaded liposomes. Int J Nanomedicine 29:2005–2017
52. Rattanapak T, Young K, Rades T et al (2012) Comparative study of liposomes, transfersomes, ethosomes and cubosomes for transcutaneous immunisation: characterisation and in vitro skin penetration. J Pharm Pharmacol 64:1560–1569
53. Ghanbarzadeh S, Arami S (2013) Enhanced transdermal delivery of diclofenac sodium via conventional liposomes, ethosomes, and transfersomes. Biomed Res Int 2013:616810
54. Li N, Peng LH, Chen X et al (2011) Effective transcutaneous immunization by antigen-loaded flexible liposome in vivo. Int J Nanomedicine 6:3241–3250
55. Romero EL, Morilla MJ (2013) Highly deformable and highly fluid vesicles as potential drug delivery systems: theoretical and practical considerations. Int J Nanomedicine 8:3171–3186
56. Cevc G, Gebauer D, Stieber J et al (1998) Ultraflexible vesicles, transfersomes, have an extremely low pore penetration resistance and transport therapeutic amounts of insulin

across the intact mammalian skin. Biochim Biophys Acta 1368:201–215
57. Cevc G, Richardsen H (1999) Lipid vesicles and membrane fusion. Adv Drug Deliv Rev 38:207–232
58. Gupta PN, Mishra V, Rawat A et al (2005) Non-invasive vaccine delivery in transfersomes, niosomes and liposomes: a comparative study. Int J Pharm 293:73–82
59. Mahor S, Rawat A, Dubey PK et al (2007) Cationic transfersomes based topical genetic vaccine against hepatitis B. Int J Pharm 340:13–19
60. Cevc G, Vierl U (2010) Nanotechnology and the transdermal route: a state of the art review and critical appraisal. J Control Release 141:277–299
61. Kumar A, Pathak K, Bali V (2012) Ultra-adaptable nanovesicular systems: a carrier for systemic delivery of therapeutic agents. Drug Discov Today 17:1233–1241
62. Mishra D, Dubey V, Asthana A et al (2006) Elastic liposomes mediated transcutaneous immunization against Hepatitis B. Vaccine 24:4847–4855
63. Mishra D, Mishra PK, Dubey V et al (2008) Systemic and mucosal immune response induced by transcutaneous immunization using Hepatitis B surface antigen-loaded modified liposomes. Eur J Pharm Sci 33: 424–433
64. Wang J, Hu JH, Li FQ et al (2007) Strong cellular and humoral immune responses induced by transcutaneous immunization with HBsAg DNA-cationic deformable liposome complex. Exp Dermatol 16:724–729
65. Cheng JY, Huang HN, Tseng WC et al (2009) Transcutaneous immunization by lipoplex-patch based DNA vaccines is effective vaccination against Japanese encephalitis virus infection. J Control Release 135:242–249
66. Mishra V, Mahor S, Rawat A et al (2006) Development of novel fusogenic vesosomes for transcutaneous immunization. Vaccine 24:5559–5570
67. Bracke S, Carretero M, Guerrero-Aspizua S et al (2014) Targeted silencing of DEFB4 in a bioengineered skin-humanized mouse model for psoriasis: development of siRNA SECosome-based novel therapies. Exp Dermatol 23:199–201
68. Moghassemi S, Hadjizadeh A (2014) Nano-niosomes as nanoscale drug delivery systems: an illustrated review. J Control Release 185C:22–36
69. El-Laithy HM, Shoukry O, Mahran LG (2011) Novel sugar esters proniosomes for transdermal delivery of vinpocetine: preclinical and clinical studies. Eur J Pharm Biopharm 77:43–55
70. Junyaprasert VB, Singhsa P, Suksiriworapong J et al (2012) Physicochemical properties and skin permeation of Span 60/Tween 60 niosomes of ellagic acid. Int J Pharm 423: 303–311
71. El-Ridy MS, Badawi AA, Safar MM et al (2012) Niosomes as a novel pharmaceutical formulation encapsulating the hepatoprotective drug silymarin. Int J Pharm Pharm Sci 4:549–559
72. Jain S, Vyas SP (2005) Mannosylated niosomes as carrier adjuvant system for topical immunization. J Pharm Pharmacol 57: 1177–1184
73. Vyas SP, Singh RP, Jain S et al (2005) Non-ionic surfactant based vesicles (niosomes) for non-invasive topical genetic immunization against hepatitis B. Int J Pharm 296:80–86
74. Panyam J, Labhasetwar V (2003) Biodegradable nanoparticles for drug and gene delivery to cells and tissue. Adv Drug Deliv Rev 55:329–347
75. Combadière B, Mahé B (2008) Particle-based vaccines for transcutaneous vaccination. Comp Immunol Microbiol Infect Dis 31: 293–315
76. Kumar A, Wonganan P, Sandoval MA et al (2012) Microneedle-mediated transcutaneous immunization with plasmid DNA coated on cationic PLGA nanoparticles. J Control Release 163:230–239
77. Sahdev P, Ochyl LJ, Moon JJ (2014) Biomaterials for nanoparticle vaccine delivery systems. Pharm Res. doi:10.1007/s110950141419-y
78. Mattheolabakis G, Lagoumintzis G, Panagi Z et al (2010) Transcutaneous delivery of a nano-encapsulated antigen: induction of immune responses. Int J Pharm 385:187–193
79. Mittal A, Raber AS, Schaefer UF et al (2013) Non-invasive delivery of nanoparticles to hair follicles: a perspective for transcutaneous immunization. Vaccine 31:3442–3451
80. Zhou X, Liu D, Liu H et al (2010) Effect of low molecular weight chitosans on drug permeation through mouse skin: 1. Transdermal delivery of baicalin. J Pharm Sci 99:2991–2998
81. Li N, Peng LH, Chen X et al (2011) Transcutaneous vaccines: novel advances in technology and delivery for overcoming the barriers. Vaccine 29:6179–6190
82. He W, Guo X, Xiao L et al (2009) Study on the mechanisms of chitosan and its derivatives

used as transdermal penetration enhancers. Int J Pharm 382:234–243
83. Hasanovic A, Zehl M, Reznicek G et al (2009) Chitosan-tripolyphosphate nanoparticles as a possible skin drug delivery system for aciclovir with enhanced stability. J Pharm Pharmacol 61:1609–1616
84. Slütter B, Plapied L, Fievez V et al (2009) Mechanistic study of the adjuvant effect of biodegradable nanoparticles in mucosal vaccination. J Control Release 138:113–121
85. Li N, Peng LH, Chen X et al (2014) Antigen-loaded nanocarriers enhance the migration of stimulated Langerhans cells to draining lymph nodes and induce effective transcutaneous immunization. Nanomedicine 10:215–223
86. Prabaharan M (2011) Prospective of guar gum and its derivatives as controlled drug delivery systems. Int J Biol Macromol 49:117–124
87. Mummert ME (2005) Immunologic roles of hyaluronan. Immunol Res 31:189–206
88. Singh M, Briones M, O'Hagan DT (2001) A novel bioadhesive intranasal delivery system for inactivated influenza vaccines. J Control Release 70:267–276
89. Huang Y, Yu F, Park YS et al (2010) Co-administration of protein drugs with gold nanoparticles to enable percutaneous delivery. Biomaterials 31:9086–9091
90. Kürsteiner O, Moser C, Lazar H et al (2006) Inflexal® V – the influenza vaccine with the lowest ovalbumin content. Vaccine 24: 6632–6635
91. Vacher G, Kaeser MD, Moser C et al (2013) Recent advances in mucosal immunization using virus-like particles. Mol Pharm 10: 1596–1609
92. Young SL, Wilson M, Wilson S et al (2006) Transcutaneous vaccination with virus-like particles. Vaccine 24:5406–5412
93. Matsuo K, Ishii Y, Quan YS et al (2011) Compositional optimization and safety assessment of a hydrogel patch as a transcutaneous immunization device. Biol Pharm Bull 34:1835–1840
94. Matsuo K, Ishii Y, Kawai Y et al (2013) Analysis of transcutaneous antigenic protein delivery by a hydrogel patch formulation. J Pharm Sci 102:1936–1947
95. Tahara Y, Kamiya N, Goto M (2012) Solid-in-oil dispersion: a novel core technology for drug delivery systems. Int J Pharm 438: 249–257
96. Toorisaka E, Ono H, Arimori K et al (2003) Hypoglycemic effect of surfactant-coated insulin solubilized in a novel solid-in-oil-in-water (S/O/W) emulsion. Int J Pharm 252: 271–274
97. Piao H, Kamiya N, Hirata A et al (2007) A novel solid-in-oil nanosuspension for transdermal delivery of diclofenac sodium. Pharm Res 25:896–901
98. Piao H, Kamiya N, Cui F et al (2011) Preparation of a solid-in-oil nanosuspension containing L-ascorbic acid as a novel long-term stable topical formulation. Int J Pharm 420:156–160
99. Tahara Y, Honda S, Kamiya N et al (2008) A solid-in-oil nanodispersion for transcutaneous protein delivery. J Control Release 131: 14–18
100. Tahara Y, Namatsu K, Kamiya N et al (2010) Transcutaneous immunization by a solid-in-oil nanodispersion. Chem Commun 46:9200–9202
101. Sato K, Sugibayashi K, Morimoto Y (1988) Effect and mode of action of aliphatic esters on the in vitro skin permeation of nicorandil. Int J Pharm 43:31–40
102. Santos P, Watkinson AC, Hadgraft J et al (2012) Influence of penetration enhancer on drug permeation from volatile formulations. Int J Pharm 439:260–268
103. Yoshiura H, Hashida M, Kamiya N et al (2007) Factors affecting protein release behavior from surfactant-protein complexes under physiological conditions. Int J Pharm 338:174–179
104. Yoshiura H, Tahara Y, Hashida M et al (2008) Design and in vivo evaluation of solid-in-oil suspension for oral delivery of human growth hormone. Biochem Eng J 41:106–110
105. Kitaoka M, Imamura K, Hirakawa Y et al (2014) Sucrose laurate-enhanced transcutaneous immunization with a solid-in-oil nanodispersion. Med Chem Commun 5:20–24
106. Rothbard JB, Garlington S, Lin Q et al (2000) Conjugation of arginine oligomers to cyclosporin A facilitates topical delivery and inhibition of inflammation. Nat Med 6:1253–1257
107. Nakase I, Takeuchi T, Tanaka G et al (2008) Methodological and cellular aspects that govern the internalization mechanisms of arginine-rich cell-penetrating peptides. Adv Drug Deliv Rev 60:598–607
108. Lopes LB, Furnish E, Komalavilas P et al (2008) Enhanced skin penetration of P20 phosphopeptide using protein transduction domains. Eur J Pharm Biopharm 68: 441–445
109. Langbein L, Grund C, Kuhn C et al (2002) Tight junctions and compositionally related junctional structures in mammalian stratified epithelia and cell cultures derived therefrom. Eur J Cell Biol 81:419–435

110. Brandner JM, Kief S, Grund C et al (2002) Organization and formation of the tight junction system in human epidermis and cultured keratinocytes. Eur J Cell Biol 81: 253–263
111. Schutze-Redelmeier MP, Kong S, Bally MB et al (2004) Antennapedia transduction sequence promotes anti tumour immunity to epicutaneously administered CTL epitopes. Vaccine 22:1985–1991
112. Kitaoka M, Imamura K, Hirakawa Y et al (2013) Needle-free immunization using a solid-in-oil nanodispersion enhanced by a skin-permeable oligoarginine peptide. Int J Pharm 458:334–339
113. Anjuère F, George-Chandy A, Audant F et al (2003) Transcutaneous immunization with cholera toxin B subunit adjuvant suppresses IgE antibody responses via selective induction of Th1 immune responses. J Immunol 170:1586–1592
114. Pitcovski J, Bazak Z, Wasserman E et al (2006) Heat labile enterotoxin of E. coli: a potential adjuvant for transcutaneous cancer immunotherapy. Vaccine 24:636–643
115. Connell TD (2007) Cholera toxin, LT-I, LT-IIa and LT-IIb: the critical role of ganglioside binding in immunomodulation by type I and type II heat-labile enterotoxins. Expert Rev Vaccines 6:821–834
116. Glenn GM, Flyer DC, Ellingsworth LR et al (2007) Transcutaneous immunization with heat-labile enterotoxin: development of a needle-free vaccine patch. Expert Rev Vaccines 6:809–819
117. Mkrtichyan M, Ghochikyan A, Movsesyan N et al (2008) Immunostimulant adjuvant patch enhances humoral and cellular immune responses to DNA immunization. DNA Cell Biol 27:19–24
118. Guebre-Xabier M, Hammond SA, Ellingsworth LR et al (2004) Immunostimulant patch enhances immune responses to influenza virus vaccine in aged mice. J Virol 78:7610–7618
119. Akira S, Uematsu S, Takeuchi O (2006) Pathogen recognition and innate immunity. Cell 124:783–801
120. Aguilar JC, Rodríguez EG (2007) Vaccine adjuvants revisited. Vaccine 25:3752–3762
121. Hemmi H, Takeuchi O, Kawai T et al (2000) A toll-like receptor recognizes bacterial DNA. Nature 408:740–745
122. Klinman DM (2004) Immunotherapeutic uses of CpG oligodeoxynucleotides. Nat Rev Immunol 4:249–258
123. Ilyinskii PO, Roy CJ, O'Neil CP et al (2014) Adjuvant-carrying synthetic vaccine particles augment the immune response to encapsulated antigen and exhibit strong local immune activation without inducing systemic cytokine release. Vaccine 32:2882–2895
124. Slütter B, Bal SM, Ding Z et al (2011) Adjuvant effect of cationic liposomes and CpG depends on administration route. J Control Release 154:123–130

Chapter 19

Nanomaterials for Treating Ocular Diseases

Guanping Yu, Amita Vaidya, Da Sun, and Zheng-Rong Lu

Abstract

Over 5 % of the world population is visually impaired. Despite extensive advances in ocular drug R&D, intraocular drug delivery remains a daunting challenge, by virtue of the unique anatomy and physiology of the eye. In recent years, the development of nanomaterial-based drug delivery systems has opened up new avenues for treating ocular diseases. This chapter provides a summary of the ocular barriers that restrict drug delivery, some of the recent nanomaterial-based drug delivery studies, their advantages and toxicity, and future implications of using nanoparticle-based drug delivery for ocular therapy.

Key words Nanomaterials, Eye disease, Ocular drug delivery, Safety

1 Introduction

As of 2010, visual impairment is estimated to have affected over 285 million people worldwide [1]. Among these, 86 % experienced partial vision loss, while 14 % exhibited ocular blindness. In 2013 alone, the direct and indirect costs of ocular disorder management in the United States amounted to about $139 billion [2], indicating that the rising healthcare expenses and the chronic nature of most ocular problems are a major source of economic burden. The unique anatomy and physiology of the eye present a major challenge to drug delivery for treating diseases associated with the anterior and posterior segments of the eye [3, 4]. While naturally occurring static and dynamic barriers, such as the cornea, blood–retinal barrier, lacrimal system, intraocular convection, episcleral pressure, blood flow, and efflux pumps, function to protect the eyes from foreign pathogens, circulating antigens, and inflammatory mediators, they also limit the bioavailability of locally and systemically administered drugs [5, 6].

Diseases of the anterior segments of the eye are commonly treated by topical drug application. Although this route of administration may exhibit high patient compliance, drug penetration to the intraocular tissue is limited, with less than 5 % bioavailability

Zheng-Rong Lu and Shinji Sakuma (eds.), *Nanomaterials in Pharmacology*, Methods in Pharmacology and Toxicology, DOI 10.1007/978-1-4939-3121-7_19, © Springer Science+Business Media New York 2016

[4]. Since the posterior segments of the eye are refractory to oral drugs, higher doses are necessary to achieve therapeutic drug concentrations, leading to concerns of toxicity and adverse side effects [7]. Intraocular drug delivery can be accomplished by intravitreal injections and implants, but he invasiveness and increased likelihood of infections and injury caused by these routes leads to reduced patient compliance [7, 8]. To circumvent these problems, it is essential to develop an optimal drug delivery system that will enable controlled and sustained release, superior targeting, and prolonged retention of the drug in ocular tissues, so as to improve therapeutic efficiency, reduce the frequency of dosing, minimize side effects, and improve patient compliance [9].

In recent years, the development of novel and ingenious nanomaterial-based drug delivery systems has opened up new avenues to facilitate efficient drug delivery and gene therapy for ocular diseases [10]. By virtue of their small size and high surface-area-to-volume ratio, nanomaterials are likely to exhibit higher diffusivity across ocular membranes, increased interaction with the outer mucous membrane of the corneal surface, and prolonged retention of the encapsulated drug. Multiple studies have demonstrated significant improvement in the corneal permeability of topically administered drugs using nanomaterials [11–14]. In addition to drug delivery to the anterior segments of the eye, nanomaterials are also being used for noninvasive delivery and targeting of therapeutic agents to the posterior segments such as the retina, retinal pigment epithelium (RPE), and choroid [8, 15–17].

This chapter provides a brief summary of the primary routes of ocular drug administration and the various ocular barriers that limit the efficiency of drug absorption, followed by a discussion of some of the most recent findings in the utilization of nanomaterials for enhancing ocular drug delivery to cure ocular disease. The benefits and risks involved in the use of nanomaterials in ocular medicine are also outlined.

2 Administration Modes and Barriers in Ocular Drug Delivery

2.1 Eye Structure and Related Disease

Known as the "window to the brain," the eye is a unique photosensory organ, which is responsible for 38 % of the neuronal input to the brain [18]. Because of their complex and fragile nature, damage to the various ocular structures can result in physical disruption, malfunction, partial or complete loss of vision (Fig. 1), culminating in ocular diseases such as cataract, glaucoma, uveitis, keratitis, age-related macular degeneration (AMD), dry eye, diabetic retinopathy, and retinal degeneration [19].

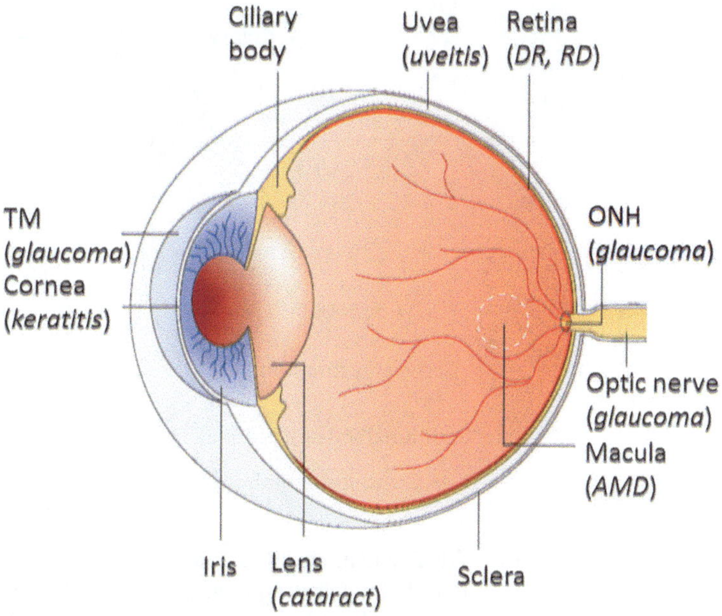

Fig. 1 Ocular tissues and the associated ocular diseases. The anatomical components of the eye and their associated ocular diseases (in parentheses) are depicted. *AMD* age-related macular degeneration, *DR* diabetic retinopathy, *ONH* optic nerve head, *RD* retinal degeneration, *TM* trabecular meshwork (Reproduced by permission from Clark, A. F, and Yorio, T. (2003). *Nat Rev Drug Discov.* 2, 448–459. Reference [19]. Copyright 2003 by Macmillan Publishers)

2.2 Barriers in Ocular Drug Delivery

Ocular drugs are typically administered by topical application or oral delivery. However, these drugs exhibit poor penetration and limited access to their ocular targets, due to the action of numerous static and dynamic ocular barriers that safeguard the eye from foreign particles and injury [3] (Fig. 2). The absorption of eyedrop formulations is impeded by barriers formed by the cornea, conjunctival epithelium, and lacrimal system [20]. Systemically circulating drugs must traverse through the blood–aqueous barrier to access the anterior chamber and through the blood–retinal barrier formed by the RPE and the tight retinal capillary walls to access the neural retina [8]. To circumvent these problems, invasive intravitreal and periocular injections are performed to enhance drug absorption, but they can in turn increase the risk of ocular complications [7]. Thus, during drug design, it is crucial to consider the mode of administration of the ocular drug therapy to ensure safety and patient compliance. The advantages and disadvantages of the current and potential drug delivery systems used to treat ocular diseases are enlisted in Table 1. The development of an efficient drug delivery system that can enhance ocular targeting, bioavailability, and tissue retention and activity, while minimizing the risk of toxicity and adverse side effects, remains a daunting challenge.

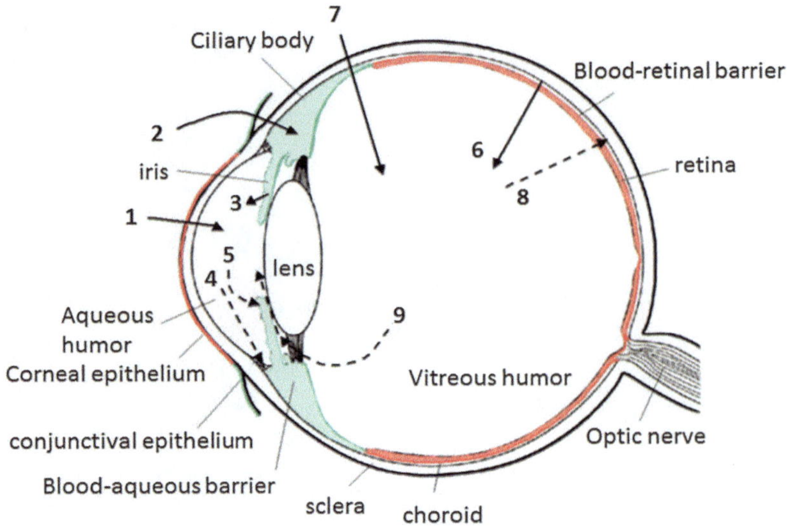

Fig. 2 Schematic presentation of the routes of ocular drug delivery. The numbers refer to the following processes: (1) trans-corneal permeation from the lacrimal fluid into the anterior chamber, (2) non-corneal drug permeation across the conjunctiva and sclera into the anterior uvea, (3) drug distribution from the blood stream via blood–aqueous barrier into the anterior chamber, (4) elimination of a drug from the anterior chamber by aqueous humor turnover to the trabecular meshwork and Schlemm's canal, (5) drug elimination from the aqueous humor into the systemic uveoscleral circulation, (6) drug distribution from the blood into the posterior eye across the blood-retinal barrier, (7) intravitreal drug administration, (8) drug elimination from the vitreous via posterior route across the blood-retinal barrier, and (9) drug elimination from the vitreous via anterior route to the posterior chamber (Reproduced by permission from Urtti, A. (2006). *Adv Drug Deliv Rev*. 58, 1131–1135. Reference [3]. Copyright 2006 by Elsevier)

3 Nanomaterials

Nanomaterial-based therapeutics, sized between 1 and 1000 nm, have demonstrated improved drug solubility and therapeutic index, longer half-life, lower immunogenicity, and targeted drug delivery, and have consequently been used to treat cancer, pain, and infectious diseases [24–28]. The discovery of liposomes in 1966 [29] and polymer–drug conjugates in 1976 [30] laid the foundation for the use of first generation of nanoparticles in medicinal therapeutic applications, further paving the way for major advances in polymer chemistry and the marketing of new and improved generations of drug formulations [25, 31–35]. In 1989, the FDA approved Zoladex, the first polymer–drug formulation, comprising an implantable depot for the controlled release of gonadotropin-releasing hormone (GnRH) agonist, to treat certain breast and prostate cancers [36]. This was followed by the approval

Table 1
Advantages and disadvantages of the current and potential drug delivery systems to treat ocular diseases

	Advantages	Disadvantages
Drops	– Easy application – Least invasive – Good patient acceptance	– Poor ocular bioavailability, less than 5 % [21] – Short duration of action – Ineffective in treatment of diseases of the posterior segments of the eye – High concentrations or frequent instillations may lead to ocular and systemic toxicity – Sometimes low patient compliance
Systemic administration	– More effective in treatment of diseases of the posterior segment of the eye than drops	– Most of the administered drugs cannot bypass the blood–ocular barrier – Side effects: systemic toxicity
Intravitreal, periocular, and subconjunctival injections [22]	– Improved drug absorption over systemically and topically delivered agents – Safer drug delivery to the posterior segment of the eye than systemic administration (no systemic toxicity) – Drug delivery to the target sites of the eye	– Injections display first-order kinetics (this rapid rise may cause difficulties with toxicity, and drug efficacy can diminish as the drug concentration falls below the targeted range) – Injections have short half-life (few hours) and need to be administered repeatedly – Side effects: repeated injections can cause pain, discomfort, increased IOP, intraocular bleeding, increased chances of infection, and possible retinal detachment; the major complication for intravitreal injection is endophthalmitis – Poor patient acceptance
Implants [23]	– An alternative to repeated injections because they increase half-life of the drug and may help to minimize peak plasma level; they may also improve patient acceptance and compliance – Stabilization of the drug – The non-biodegradable implants exhibit a more controlled delivery profile and longer periods of drug release than biodegradable ones – The biodegradable implants do not need to be removed	– Side effects: insertion of these devices is invasive and is associated with ocular complications (retinal detachment and intravitreal hemorrhage for intravitreal implant) – The non-biodegradable devices have to be surgically retrieved once the drug is depleted (risk of ocular complications) – The biodegradable implants have a final uncontrollable "burst" in their drug release profile

(continued)

Table 1
(continued)

	Advantages	Disadvantages
Microparticles, nanoparticles, and liposomes	– Stabilization of the drug – Increased half-life of drugs (the frequency of injections diminishes) – Decrease in peak concentration resulting in decreased toxicity (micro- and nanoparticles minimize "burst" in their drug delivery profile because the dose volume is limited) – Localized delivery of drugs (RPE cells) – Improved patient compliance and convenience	– Side effects: risks associated with injections and vitreous clouding
Cell encapsulation	– Long-lasting and continuous expression of the given protein (avoids repeated injections) without genetic alteration of the host tissues – Direct delivery to the target site (limiting toxicity) – Easy retrieval of the implant when desired (making the treatment reversible) – Improved patient compliance	– Side effects: invasive method involving complications related to surgical insertion and removal – Patient acceptance to be seen
Iontophoresis	– Noninvasive method and easy to use – May be combined with other drug delivery systems – Ability to modulate dosage (low risk of toxicity) – Good drug penetration to anterior and posterior segment of the eye – Good acceptance by patients – A broad applicability to deliver a broad range of drugs or genes to treat several ophthalmic diseases in the posterior segment of the eye	– No sustained half-life: requires repeated administrations – Side effects: mild pain in some cases, but no risk of infections or ulcerations – Risk of low patient compliance because frequent administrations may be needed

Adapted from Ref. [8] (Reproduced by permission from Del Amo, E.M. and Urtti, A. (2008). *Drug Discov Today* 13, 135–143. Copyright 2008 by Elsevier) and marketing of a myriad of nanomedicines including polyethylene glycol (PEG)-protein conjugates and PEGylated liposomes [15, 37, 38]. By virtue of their optimal properties such as enhanced drug efficacy through improved drug encapsulation, sustained or triggered drug release, and preferential targeting to disease sites, various nanomedicines, including polymeric nanoparticles, dendrimers, hydrogels, micelles, and nanoconjugates, which were originally developed for cancer treatment, have been expanded for drug delivery in ophthalmology [9, 39–43]. For example, pegaptanib (Macugen) [36], an anti-VEGF aptamer conjugated with branched PEG, has been clinically approved for treating wet AMD [25]. Recent decades have seen a tremendous increase in the number of patents on nanotechnology-based applications for controlled and targeted ocular drug delivery, as reviewed by Gupta [44] and Pignatello [45].

3.1 Nanoparticles for Ocular Drug Delivery

The past three decades have witnessed significant progress in the development of advanced ocular drug delivery systems. A comprehensive review of the design and development of nanoparticles for ocular drug delivery is provided by Liu et al. [9]. Here, we provide a summary of nanomaterial-based drug research conducted in the last 2 years.

Recently, our group achieved prolonged prevention of bright light-induced retinal degeneration by subcutaneous administration of polylactic acid (PLA) nanoparticles containing retinylamine in *Abca4*$^{-/-}$*Rdh8*$^{-/-}$ mice, which are models for Stargardt disease (STGD) and AMD (Fig. 3) [46]. Retinylamine facilitates the

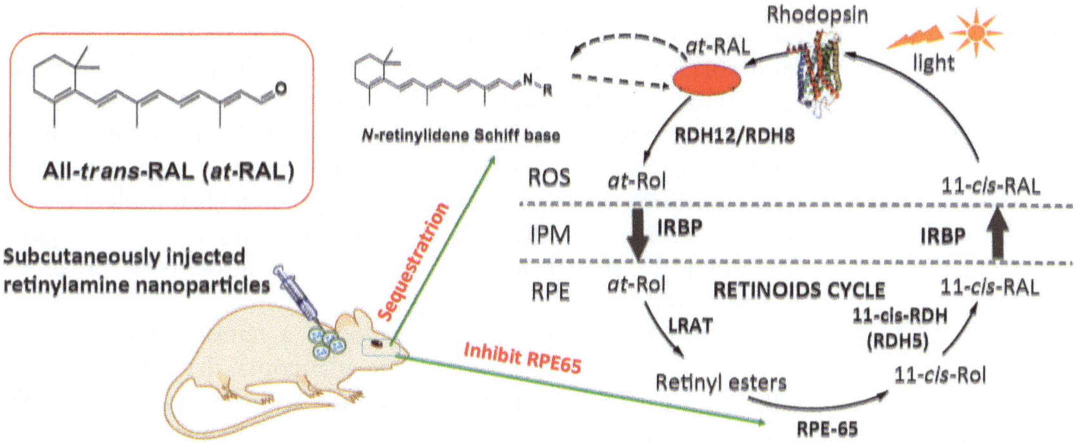

Fig. 3 Retinylamine-loaded PLA nanoparticles provide prolonged protection against light-induced retinal degeneration in *Abca4*$^{-/-}$*Rdh8*$^{-/-}$ mice. After subcutaneous administration of the biodegradable nanoparticles, retinylamine is gradually released in the body, and a sufficient amount of the drug is available in the eye to sequester all-*trans*-retinal (*at*RAL) for a prolonged period to effectively protect against light-induced retinal degeneration (Reprinted from Ref. [46], Puntel et al. (2015). *Biomaterials,* 44, 103–110. Copyright (2015) with permission from Elsevier)

clearance of all-*trans*-retinal (*at*RAL) and its toxic condensation byproducts (formed due to the absence of the mutated gene products), which are known to cause irreversible loss of photoreceptor cells, culminating in various retinal degenerative diseases, including STGD and AMD [47]. To circumvent the ocular barriers, the retinylamine-containing nanoparticles were administered via subcutaneous injections into the neck pad of the DKO mice. Being a retinoid derivative, retinylamine is transported across the blood–retinal barrier via the vitamin A transport machinery. Formulated using the single emulsion technique, the drug-loaded PLA nanoparticles are about 730 ± 310 nm in diameter, with a loading capacity of 6.9 ± 0.3 % (w/w), and were found to display an initial burst of drug release within the first 24 h, followed by zero-order release kinetics in PBS at 37°C for as long as 4 weeks. On the other hand, under in vivo conditions, the PLA nanoparticles facilitated sustained supply of the drug for about 7 days, even at low drug dosage, resulting in visible protection of the structure and functions of rod and cone photoreceptor cells, and preserved thickness of the retinal outer nuclear layer (ONL) in the treated DKO mice. It is possible that this inconsistency arises due to the in vivo degradation of the nanoparticles by phagosomes or clearance by the immune system, which can be circumvented by modifications, such as copolymerization of PLA with PEG [48]. This study shows that the biocompatible PLA nanoparticles can be potentially used for drug delivery and prolonged prophylactic treatment of human retinal degenerative diseases.

Previous research by Giannaccini et al. demonstrated that the RPE layer can be specifically targeted for prolonged drug retention by intraocular injections of magnetic nanoparticles (MNPs) in *Xenopus* and zebrafish embryos, irrespective of the charge, size, and surface properties of the MNPs [49]. This study employed Feraheme MNPs, which are FDA-approved for the treatment of iron deficiency anemia in adult patients with chronic kidney disease and as contrast agents for molecular resonance imaging (MRI) [50]. Although MNPs are thought to possess ideal molecular carrier properties, e.g., their surface can be functionalized for targeted therapy [51], their role in human ocular drug delivery remains to be determined.

Tuomela and colleagues developed a nanocrystalline topical formulation of the poorly soluble glaucoma drug brinzolamide (BRA), a carbonic anhydrase inhibitor, and demonstrated significant reduction of intraocular pressure (IOP) in a rat ocular hypertension model [52]. Nanocrystal-based ocular drug delivery is advantageous in that the nanocrystals are carrier-free crystalline clusters of drug (10–1000 nm in size) and devoid of matrix material, facilitating high bioavailability, low irritation, enhanced dissolution velocity, and saturation solubility of drugs in the lacrimal fluid [53]. Nevertheless, it is important to note that increased dosage and longer incubation times of the BRA nanocrystals caused cell toxicity, warranting further pharmacokinetic and pharmacodynamic studies for their human ocular applications. Besides nanocrystal technology, cyclodextrins (CDs) function as suitable candidates for the delivery of lipophilic drugs by forming water-soluble drug–CD nano-complexes that facilitate drug delivery and permeation. Stefansson's group conducted a randomized, cross-over trial to evaluate IOP control by dorzolamide hydrochloride (marketed as Trusopt®) administered three times a day (TID) versus dorzolamide γ-cyclodextrin (D-γCD) nanoparticle eye drops administered once a day (QD) for glaucoma therapy [54]. The investigators demonstrated that compared to Trusopt TID, D-γCD QD treatment may lower IOP with a better safety profile, prompting the need for long-term experiments for safety and efficacy. It is important to note that the drug–CD ratio is critical for efficient delivery; too much CD decreases bioavailability, while too less CD may not form sufficient nanoparticle complexes [55].

Solinís et al. designed a vector system containing solid lipid nanoparticles (SLNs), protamine (P), and hyaluronic acid (HA), which exhibits remarkable cellular uptake by calveolar/lipid raft-mediated endocytosis. The three components form a stable positively charged complex, between 240 and 340 nm, and the combination of P and HA serves to significantly enhance the cell transfection efficiency, compared to SLNs alone [56]. Although the authors demonstrate efficient plasmid delivery and increased production of the protein retinoschisin in ARPE19 cells, comprehensive in vivo studies are required to determine if this vector system can treat human X-linked juvenile retinoschisis.

To circumvent the local toxicity caused by periocular carboplatin injections in retinoblastoma patients, Bellare and colleagues loaded the carboplatin on polymethylmethacrylate (PMMA) nanoparticles to improve stability, circulation time, and sustained delivery of the drug. Following single posterior subtenon injections, the patients exhibited increased trans-scleral transport of carboplatin in the retina, with no acute ocular and systemic toxicity [57]. Although PMMA nanoparticle therapy has never been investigated in retinoblastoma patients, the encouraging results suggest that pending long-term efficacy studies, this technology could be used for adjunctive treatment of advanced intraocular retinoblastoma in the clinic.

3.2 Dendrimers for Ocular Drug Delivery

Dendrimers (dendron = tree) are three-dimensional, well-organized nanoscopic macromolecules, with a central core that is surrounded by overlapping and branched repeating units containing the active sites. By virtue of their multivalency, versatility, and functionality, dendrimers have gained increasing attention in the field of targeted and multidrug delivery [41, 58].

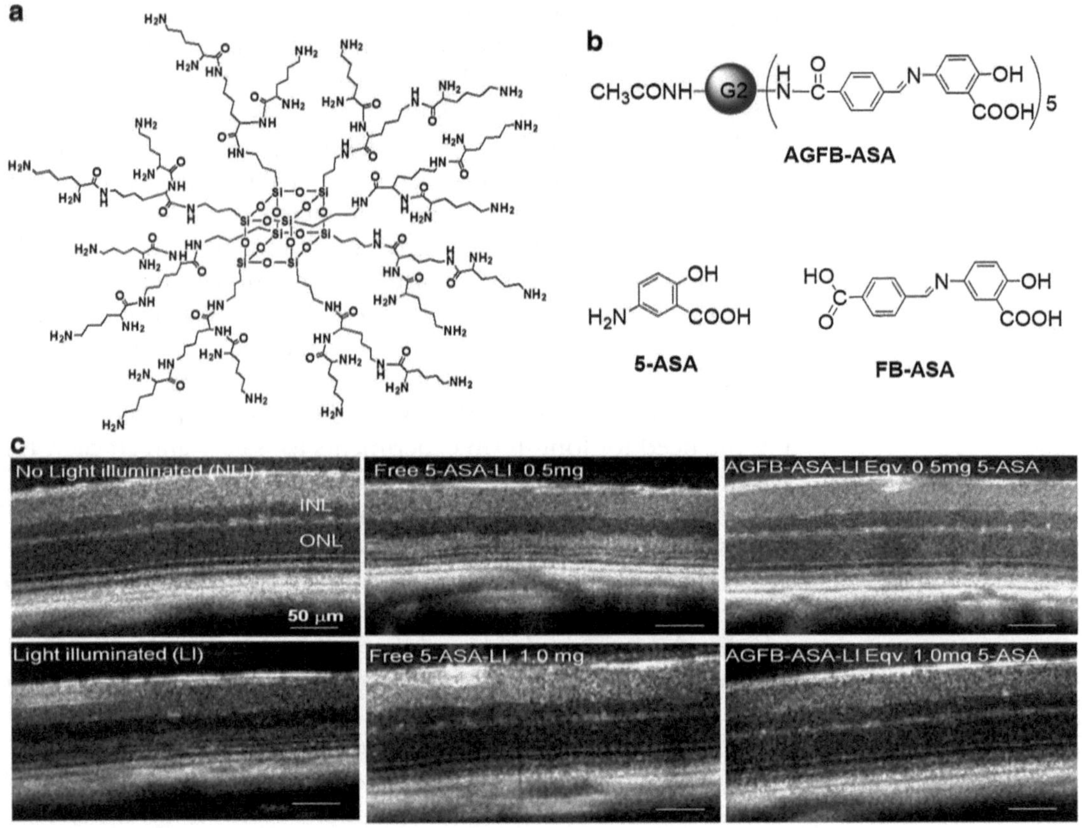

Fig. 4 The AGFB-ASA conjugate: structure and in vivo efficacy. (**a**) Structure of the nanoglobular dendrimer G_2 and (**b**) scheme of AGFB-ASA conjugate. (**c**) OCT images indicate representative morphology of *Abca4–/–Rdh8–/–* mouse retinas. Scale bar indicates 50 μm in the OCT image. AGFB-ASA-pretreated light-illuminated *Abca4–/–Rdh8–/–*mice exhibit increased preservation of the ONL thickness than free 5-ASA-pretreated light-illuminated mice, which failed to exhibit any protection against light-induced retinal degeneration at 0.5 mg 5-ASA per mouse (adapted with permission from Wu X. et al. (2013) *ACS Nano* 8, 153-161. Reference [15]. Copyright 2013 by American Chemical Society)

We synthesized a nanoglobular dendrimer of the drug 5-aminosalicylic acid (5-ASA), which is FDA-approved for treating retinal degeneration [15]. As a free drug, 5-ASA exhibits rapid pharmacokinetics and low bioavailability, necessitating the design of a suitable drug delivery system, in which 5-ASA was conjugated to a generation 2 (G2) lysine dendrimer with an octa(3-aminopropyl)silsesquioxane core, and sustained drug release via hydrolysis was facilitated by an acid-sensitive Schiff base spacer (Fig. 4a and b). Compared to 5-ASA alone, the nanoglobular 5-ASA conjugate (five 5-ASA molecules per nanoglobule) exhibited controlled release with reduced systemic clearance of the drug as well as prolonged protection against bright light-induced retinal degeneration in the *Abca4–/–Rdh8–/–* STGD mouse model (Fig. 4c). It is also evident that intraperitoneal administration of the drug conjugate permits sufficient drug delivery to the posterior segments of the eye, indicating that the nanoglobular dendrimer is a promising tool for noninvasive ocular delivery of drugs, gene therapy, and imaging agents [59, 60]. The presence of 32 surface amino acids on the nanoglobule, the modifiable spacer linkage, and other versatile properties can further enable the modification of this system for optimized drug load, solubility, rate of drug release, reduced cytotoxicity, and tissue-specific targeting.

In addition, poly(amidoamine) (PAMAM) dendrimers, which are polymers that can be synthesized to create precise molecular architectures, possess amino, hydroxyl, or carboxylic surface groups, to which drug molecules can be covalently attached. For example, PAMAM dendrimers conjugated to the inflammatory mediators, glucosamine and glucosamine 6-sulfate, have been demonstrated to prevent scar formation after glaucoma filtration surgery in rabbits [61]. Conjugation to PAMAM dendrimer increases the bioavailability of topically applied pilocarpine nitrate and tropicamide in albino rabbits [62] and enhances the solubility and antibacterial activity of quinolones [63]. A hybrid linear-dendritic-copolymer, poly(glycerol-co-succinic acid)-poly(ethylene glycol), synthesized from biodegradable components including succinic acid and glycerol, undergoes photopolymerization to form an interpenetrating network with the surrounding tissue to facilitate rapid sealing of corneal lacerations, compared to conventional sutures [64]. Phthalocyanine dendrimers complexed with plasmid DNA and cationic peptides have been designed to enable photosensitive enhancement of gene expression in rat conjunctival tissues [65]. Similarly, polycationic dendrimers complexed with lipoamino acids have been developed for the delivery of anti-VEGF oligonucleotides in human RPE51 cells [66]. Additional research for optimizing the physical properties, delivery routes, safety, and efficacy of these dendrimers may provide strategies for treating choroidal neovascularization (CNV). Phosphorous dendrimers have been demonstrated to deliver the antihypertensive drug carteolol across corneal barriers into the aqueous humor of albino rabbits [67]. Indeed, preclinical trials involving dendrimer-mediated ocular drug delivery are already under way and are reviewed in [68].

3.3 Nanoconjugates

Among the numerous delivery systems discussed so far, polymer-based carriers are powerful delivery tools and are being widely investigated for ocular drug delivery. *N*-(2-Hydroxypropyl)methacrylamide (HPMA) polymer–drug conjugates with oligopeptide spacers that can be cleaved by pancreatic and intestinal enzymes have been tested for the site-specific release of anticancer therapeutics [69, 70].

On similar lines, our group designed a PEG-retinylamine (Ret-NH_2) conjugate PEG-GFL-NH-Ret with a

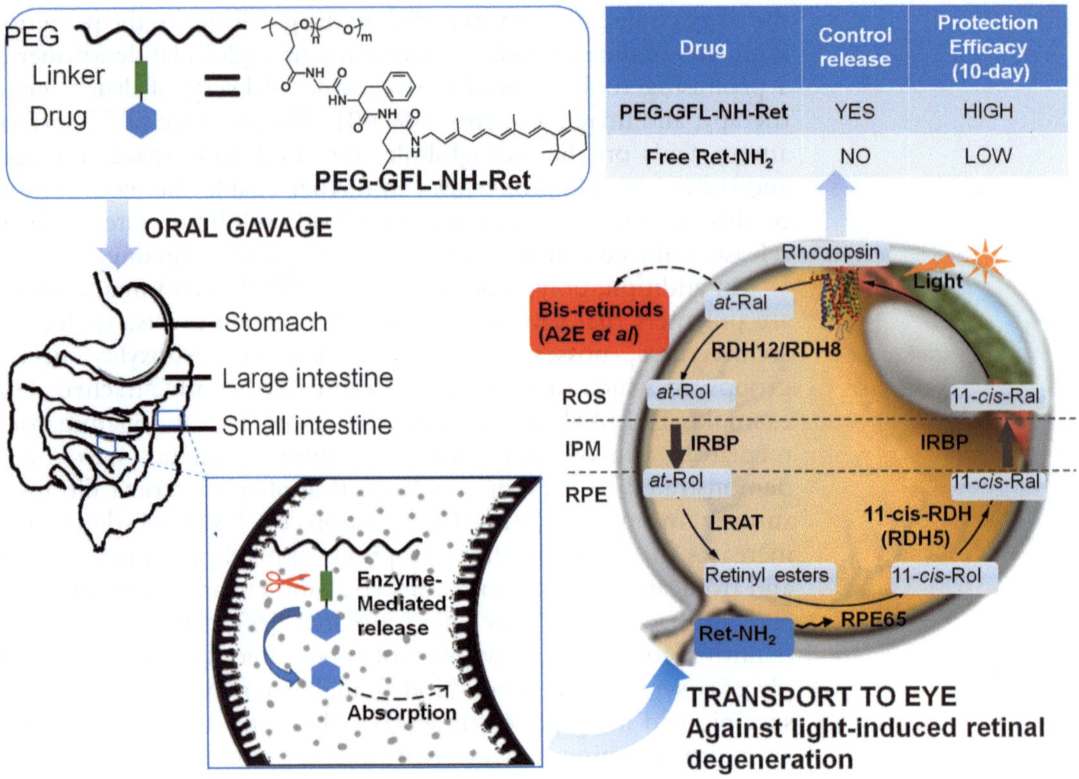

Fig. 5 An oral PEG-retinylamine conjugate for prolonged protection against light-induced retinal degeneration in *Abca4−/−Rdh8−/−* mice. After oral administration of PEG-GFL-NH-Ret conjugate, Ret-NH_2 is gradually released into the small intestine and colon to maintain a relatively stable effective drug concentration in the circulation and a sufficient amount of the drug in the eye for an extended period. Sustained drug release from the conjugate provides prolonged protection against light-induced retinal degeneration, with a possible reduction in the overall dose and dosing frequency (Reprinted with permission from Yu G. et al. (2014). *Biomacromolecules* 15, 4570–4578. Reference [71]. Copyright 2014 by American Chemical Society)

glycine-phenylalanine-leucine (GFL) spacer for controlled oral delivery of Ret-NH_2, for the treatment of retinal degenerative diseases, including STGD and AMD [71]. Cleavage of the GFL peptide spacer by digestive enzymes of the gastrointestinal tract facilitates sustained release of Ret-NH_2 from the biocompatible drug-polymer conjugate, thus increasing the residence time of therapeutically effective concentration of Ret-NH_2 in the eyes and circulation for up to 72 h. Compared to free Ret-NH_2, the conjugate also protected the STGD mouse model from retinal degeneration induced by bright light (Fig. 5). Thus, this conjugate-mediated drug delivery promises to be highly advantageous over free drug delivery to ocular tissues, by facilitating sustained drug release, reduction of drug dose, dosing frequency, and dose-related toxic side effects.

3.4 Hydrogel

Although topical application of eye drops is the most common route of administration of ocular drugs to the anterior segments, it leads to a significant reduction in the drug bioavailability to target tissues, due to lacrimal drainage, and other ocular barriers. Hydrogel formulations can be used to overcome such barriers, by increasing the viscosity and, consequently, the residence time of the drugs on the ocular surface. When topically applied, most of the antiglaucoma drug timolol is lost through systemic drainage, resulting in numerous adverse side effects. On the other hand, ophthalmic application of 0.1 % hydrogel formulation of timolol exhibits almost 100 % receptor occupancy and reduced loss to the aqueous humor in human patients [72]. The controlled and sustained release profile reduces the probability of having insufficient local drug concentration. It also reduces the risk of toxic side-effects caused by repetitive administration. Lou et al. developed a thermoresponsive ophthalmic in situ gel system for the delivery of curcumin loaded on to albumin nanoparticles (Cur-BSA-NPs-Gel) in albino rabbits. This gel formulation showed increased viscosity, prolonged release times, little ocular irritation, and enhanced ocular bioavailability of curcumin in vivo, indicating that it may serve as a possible approach for safe ocular curcumin delivery in patients with diabetic retinopathy [73]. In addition, hydrogel iontophoresis, in which hydrogel sponges loaded with charged nanoparticles are applied along with low electric current, is also an attractive noninvasive strategy for drug delivery to the anterior and posterior ocular tissues [74]. Trans-scleral iontophoresis using polyacrylic hydrogel sponges enhances the ocular delivery of drugs like dexamethasone, methotrexate, and methylprednisolone, compared to conventional injections [75, 76]. Preliminary safety and tolerance studies of iontophoresis with balanced salt solution demonstrate that a total charge of less than 60 mAmin is well tolerated by healthy human subjects [77], indicating that this technique could indeed be used for noninvasive ocular drug delivery in the clinic.

3.5 Preclinical Studies of Ocular Nanomedicine

Although numerous ocular nanomedicines and nanomaterial-based strategies progress to preclinical studies, for the characterization of their pharmacokinetic properties in the physiological environment, only a small percentage of the novel drugs actually make it to clinical trials [9]. Numerous eye-drop formulations that exploit the interactions between drug carriers and ocular milieu are currently available in the market [78]. In addition, contact lenses, intravitreal implants, cul-de-sac inserts, and punctal plugs are also being developed by various pharmaceutical companies [78]. Table 2 summarizes the progress of nanomaterial-based ocular drug delivery systems that are currently in the clinical stages.

Table 2
List of preclinical and clinical studies using nanomaterials in ocular drug delivery system

Nanomaterial	Drug	Formulation	Administration	Treatment	Clinical stage	Reference
Microspheres	Triamcinolone acetonide	PLGA (RETAAC)	Intravitreal injection	Diabetic macular edema	Launched	[79]
Micelles	Dexamethasone	NIPAAM-VP-MAA	Eye-drop	Inflammation	Preclinical	[80]
	Dexamethasone	Pluronic F127/chitosan	Eye-drop	Ocular hypertension	Preclinical	[81]
	Cyclosporin A	MPEG-hexPLA	Eye-drop	Dry eye, autoimmune uveitis	Preclinical	[82]
	Dexamethasone	PHEA-PEG	Eye-drop	Ocular hypertension	Preclinical	[83]
Hydrogels	Timolol		Topical	Ocular hypertension	Randomized human	[72]
			Trans-scleral iontophoresis		Randomized human	[77]
Liposomes	Flurbiprofen	Stearic acid + castor oil	Eye-drop	Inflammation	Preclinical	[84]
	Ciprofloxacin HCl	Chitosan-coated liposomes	Eye-drop	Conjunctivitis	Preclinical	[85]
	Fluconazole	Liposomes	Eye-drop	Fungal infection	Preclinical	[86]
	Ciprofloxacin HCl	Chitosan-coated liposomes	Eye-drop	Bacterial growth of *P. aeruginosa*	Preclinical	[87]
	Bevacizumab	Liposomes	Intravitreal injection	Ocular neovascular activity	Preclinical	[88]
	Verteporfin	Liposomes (Visudyne)	Intravitreal injection	Classic subfoveal choroidal neovascularization	Launched	[78]
Dendrimers	Pilocarpine nitrate and tropicamide	PAMAM	Eye-drop	Myosis and mydriasis	Preclinical	[62]
	Carteolol	Phosphorus-containing dendrimers	Eye-drop	Glaucoma	Preclinical	[67]
Cyclodextrins	Methazolamide	HPβCD and HPMC	Eye-drop	Ocular hypertension	Randomized human	[89]
	Latanoprost		Eye-drop	Open-angle glaucoma	Randomized human	[90]

Adapted from Ref. [9] (Reproduced by permission from Liu S. et al. (2012). *Macromol Biosci*. 12, 608–620. Copyright 2012 by John Wiley and Sons)

4 Nanoparticle Safety

In general, nanomedicines and nanomaterial-based formulations are subject to the same stringent rules and regulations as other conventional medications and treatments for use in humans and animals. Extensive research is essential to comprehensively understand the effects of nanomaterial-based drugs, in terms of their safety, toxicity, and efficacy, and for formulating appropriate guidelines and laws for regulating their use in human patients [35, 36, 91, 92]. Different types of nanomaterials are known to cause toxic side effects in several organ systems [93]. Nanoparticles can lead to enhanced oxidative stress, triggering the expression of transcription factors that may harm cells and tissues via oxidative stress generation, which may consequently lead to the activation of different transcription factors [93]. Generally, nanoparticles distributed through the lymphatic system in parallel with the blood vascular system are taken up by lymph nodes. The ocular mucosa contains lymphoid tissue that drains to different face and neck lymphatic ganglia [94]. Prow [95] provides a summary of the toxicity of about thirty kinds of nanoparticles and other nanocarriers tested for ocular applications in vitro and in vivo and highlighting the significance of conducting toxicity testing for cell morphology, cell viability, clinical signs evaluation, gross tissue examination, irritation test, histology and functional analyses, and inflammatory response for newly developed drug carriers. The development of a viable commercial nanomaterial-based delivery system poses significant challenges, such as biomaterial and drug compatibility, mass production and scalability, and long-term stability and reactability of the biomaterial and drug [96].

In summary, the currently marketed nanomaterial-based drugs have already ushered in the era of nanomedicine [35]. The application of nanotechnology will undoubtedly enable researchers to improve and develop novel ocular drug delivery systems, so as to achieve therapeutic efficacy, patient-compliance, and negligible side-effects in a cost-effective manner. Despite the publication of several prominent researches and studies, the design of efficient nanomaterial platforms for perfectly controlled drug delivery in human patients remains a daunting task. Safety is also an important issue for the nanomaterials; consequently, the development of appropriate and well-validated methods of characterization is imperative for assessing the biodistribution and toxicity profile of the biomaterial-encapsulated drug, biodegradability, and sustained release under physiological conditions [34].

References

1. Pascolini D, Mariotti SP (2012) Global estimates of visual impairment: 2010. Br J Ophthalmol 96(5):614–618. doi:10.1136/bjophthalmol-2011-300539
2. NORC at the University of Chicago (2013) Cost of vision problems: the economic burden of vision loss and eye disorders in the United States. Prepared for Prevent Blindness America, Chicago, IL. http://costofvision.preventblindness.org [database on the Internet]2013
3. Urtti A (2006) Challenges and obstacles of ocular pharmacokinetics and drug delivery. Adv Drug Deliv Rev 58(11):1131–1135. doi:10.1016/j.addr.2006.07.027
4. Short BG (2008) Safety evaluation of ocular drug delivery formulations: techniques and practical considerations. Toxicol Pathol 36(1):49–62. doi:10.1177/0192623307310955
5. Davis JL, Gilger BC, Robinson MR (2004) Novel approaches to ocular drug delivery. Curr Opin Mol Ther 6(2):195–205
6. Yasukawa T, Ogura Y, Kimura H, Sakurai E, Tabata Y (2006) Drug delivery from ocular implants. Expert Opin Drug Deliv 3(2):261–273. doi:10.1517/17425247.3.2.261
7. Gaudana R, Ananthula HK, Parenky A, Mitra AK (2010) Ocular drug delivery. AAPS J 12(3):348–360. doi:10.1208/s12248-010-9183-3
8. Del Amo EM, Urtti A (2008) Current and future ophthalmic drug delivery systems. A shift to the posterior segment. Drug Discov Today 13(3-4):135–143. doi:10.1016/j.drudis.2007.11.002
9. Liu S, Jones L, Gu FX (2012) Nanomaterials for ocular drug delivery. Macromol Biosci 12(5):608–620. doi:10.1002/mabi.201100419
10. Mudgil M, Gupta N, Nagpal M, Pawar P (2012) Nanotechnology: a new approach for ocular drug delivery system. Int J Pharm Pharm Sci 4(2):105–112
11. Nagarwal RC, Kant S, Singh PN, Maiti P, Pandit JK (2009) Polymeric nanoparticulate system: a potential approach for ocular drug delivery. J Control Release 136(1):2–13. doi:10.1016/j.jconrel.2008.12.018
12. Wadhwa S, Paliwal R, Paliwal SR, Vyas SP (2009) Nanocarriers in ocular drug delivery: an update review. Curr Pharm Des 15(23):2724–2750
13. Zarbin MA, Montemagno C, Leary JF, Ritch R (2010) Nanomedicine in ophthalmology: the new frontier. Am J Ophthalmol 150(2):144–162. doi:10.1016/j.ajo.2010.03.019, e2
14. Tong YC, Chang SF, Liu CY, Kao WW, Huang CH, Liaw J (2007) Eye drop delivery of nano-polymeric micelle formulated genes with cornea-specific promoters. J Gene Med 9(11):956–966. doi:10.1002/jgm.1093
15. Wu X, Yu G, Luo C, Maeda A, Zhang N, Sun D et al (2014) Synthesis and evaluation of a nanoglobular dendrimer 5-aminosalicylic Acid conjugate with a hydrolyzable schiff base spacer for treating retinal degeneration. ACS Nano 8(1):153–161. doi:10.1021/nn4054107
16. Thrimawithana TR, Young S, Bunt CR, Green C, Alany RG (2011) Drug delivery to the posterior segment of the eye. Drug Discov Today 16(5-6):270–277. doi:10.1016/j.drudis.2010.12.004
17. Kaur IP, Kakkar S (2014) Nanotherapy for posterior eye diseases. J Control Release 193:100–112. doi:10.1016/j.jconrel.2014.05.031
18. Alward WL (2003) Biomedicine. A new angle on ocular development. Science 299(5612):1527–1528. doi:10.1126/science.1082933
19. Clark AF, Yorio T (2003) Ophthalmic drug discovery. Nat Rev Drug Discov 2(6):448–459. doi:10.1038/nrd1106
20. Nagai N, Ito Y (2014) A new preparation method for ophthalmic drug nanoparticles. Pharm Anal Acta. 5(7):305. doi: 10.4172/2153-2435.1000305
21. Urtti A, Pipkin JD, Rork G, Sendo T, Finne U, Repta AJ (1990) Controlled drug delivery devices for experimental ocular studies with timolol 2. Ocular and systemic absorption in rabbits. Int J Pharm 61(3):241–249, doi: http://dx.doi.org/10.1016/0378-5173(90)90215-P
22. Maurice DM, Mishima S (1984) Ocular pharmacokinetics. In: Sears M (ed) Pharmacology of the eye. Handbook of experimental pharmacology. Springer, Berlin, pp 19–116
23. Bourges JL, Bloquel C, Thomas A, Froussart F, Bochot A, Azan F et al (2006) Intraocular implants for extended drug delivery: therapeutic applications. Adv Drug Deliv Rev 58(11):1182–1202. doi:10.1016/j.addr.2006.07.026
24. Davis ME, Chen Z, Shin DM (2008) Nanoparticle therapeutics: an emerging treatment modality for cancer. Nat Rev Drug Discov 7(9):771–782
25. Zhang L, Gu FX, Chan JM, Wang AZ, Langer RS, Farokhzad OC (2008) Nanoparticles in medicine: therapeutic applications and developments. Clin Pharmacol Ther 83(5):761–769. doi:10.1038/sj.clpt.6100400
26. Petros RA, DeSimone JM (2010) Strategies in the design of nanoparticles for therapeutic applications. Nat Rev Drug Discov 9(8):615–627. doi:10.1038/nrd2591

27. Park J, Fong PM, Lu J, Russell KS, Booth CJ, Saltzman WM et al (2009) PEGylated PLGA nanoparticles for the improved delivery of doxorubicin. Nanomedicine 5(4):410–418. doi:10.1016/j.nano.2009.02.002
28. Wang X, Li J, Wang Y, Cho KJ, Kim G, Gjyrezi A et al (2009) HFT-T, a targeting nanoparticle, enhances specific delivery of paclitaxel to folate receptor-positive tumors. ACS Nano 3(10):3165–3174. doi:10.1021/nn900649v
29. Bangham AD, Standish MM, Weissmann G (1965) The action of steroids and streptolysin S on the permeability of phospholipid structures to cations. J Mol Biol 13(1): 253–259
30. Kopf H, Joshi RK, Soliva M, Speiser P (1976) Study on micelle polymerization in the presence of low-molecular-weight drugs. 1. Production and isolation of nanoparticles, residual monomer determination, physical-chemical data. Pharm Ind 38:281–284
31. Adler-moore JP, Proffitt RT (1993) Development, characterization, efficacy and mode of action of Am Bisome, a unilamellar liposomal formulation of amphotericin B. J Liposome Res 3(3):429–450. doi:10.3109/08982109309150729
32. Haley B, Frenkel E (2008) Nanoparticles for drug delivery in cancer treatment. Urol Oncol 26(1):57–64. doi:10.1016/j.urolonc.2007.03.015
33. Miele E, Spinelli GP, Miele E, Tomao F, Tomao S (2009) Albumin-bound formulation of paclitaxel (Abraxane ABI-007) in the treatment of breast cancer. Int J Nanomedicine 4:99–105
34. Murday JS, Siegel RW, Stein J, Wright JF (2009) Translational nanomedicine: status assessment and opportunities. Nanomedicine 5(3):251–273. doi:10.1016/j.nano.2009.06.001
35. Vauthier C, Couvreur P, Fattal E (2012) Nanomaterials: applications in drug delivery. In: Brayner R, Fiévet F, Coradin T (eds) Nanomaterials: a danger or a promise?: A chemical and biological perspective. Springer, London, pp 131–151
36. FDA (2002) Guidance for industry, liposome drug products chemistry, manufacturing, and controls; human, pharmacokinetics and bioavailability; and labeling documentation. J:\!GUIDANC\2191dft.doc, 07/29/02. http://www.fda.gov/downloads/Drugs/GuidanceComplianceRegulatoryInformation/Guidances/ucm070570.pdf. Accessed 8 Aug 2014
37. Adair JH, Parette MP, Altinoglu EI, Kester M (2010) Nanoparticulate alternatives for drug delivery. ACS Nano 4(9):4967–4970. doi:10.1021/nn102324e
38. Peer D, Karp JM, Hong S, Farokhzad OC, Margalit R, Langer R (2007) Nanocarriers as an emerging platform for cancer therapy. Nat Nanotechnol 2(12):751–760
39. Zhang K, Zhang L, Weinreb RN (2012) Ophthalmic drug discovery: novel targets and mechanisms for retinal diseases and glaucoma. Nat Rev Drug Discov 11(7):541–559. doi:10.1038/nrd3745
40. Sultana Y, Maurya DP, Iqbal Z, Aqil M (2011) Nanotechnology in ocular delivery: current and future directions. Drugs Today (Barc) 47(6):441–455. doi:10.1358/dot.2011.47.6.1549023
41. Chaplot SP, Rupenthal ID (2014) Dendrimers for gene delivery – a potential approach for ocular therapy? J Pharm Pharmacol 66(4):542–556. doi:10.1111/jphp.12104
42. Vadlapudi AD, Mitra AK (2013) Nanomicelles: an emerging platform for drug delivery to the eye. Ther Deliv 4(1):1–3. doi:10.4155/tde.12.122
43. Sahoo SK, Dilnawaz F, Krishnakumar S (2008) Nanotechnology in ocular drug delivery. Drug Discov Today 13(3–4):144–151. doi:10.1016/j.drudis.2007.10.021
44. Gupta N, Goel S, Gupta H (2013) Patent review on nanotechnology in ocular drug delivery. Recent Pat Nanomed 3(1):37–46. doi:10.2174/18779123112029990004
45. Pignatello R, Puglisi G (2011) Nanotechnology in ophthalmic drug delivery: a survey of recent developments and patenting activity. Recent Pat Nanomed 1(1):42–54. doi:10.2174/1877912311101010042
46. Puntel A, Maeda A, Golczak M, Gao S-Q, Yu G, Palczewski K et al (2015) Prolonged prevention of retinal degeneration with retinylamine loaded nanoparticles. Biomaterials 44:103–110, doi: http://dx.doi.org/10.1016/j.biomaterials.2014.12.019
47. Palczewski K (2010) Retinoids for treatment of retinal diseases. Trends Pharmacol Sci 31(6):284–295. doi:10.1016/j.tips.2010.03.001
48. Xiao RZ, Zeng ZW, Zhou GL, Wang JJ, Li FZ, Wang AM (2010) Recent advances in PEG-PLA block copolymer nanoparticles. Int J Nanomedicine 5:1057–1065. doi:10.2147/IJN.S14912
49. Giannaccini M, Giannini M, Calatayud MP, Goya GF, Cuschieri A, Dente L et al (2014) Magnetic nanoparticles as intraocular drug delivery system to target retinal pigmented epithelium (RPE). Int J Mol Sci 15(1):1590–1605. doi:10.3390/ijms15011590

50. Bullivant JP, Zhao S, Willenberg BJ, Kozissnik B, Batich CD, Dobson J (2013) Materials characterization of Feraheme/ferumoxytol and preliminary evaluation of its potential for magnetic fluid hyperthermia. Int J Mol Sci 14(9): 17501–17510. doi:10.3390/ijms140917501
51. Misra RD (2008) Magnetic nanoparticle carrier for targeted drug delivery: perspective, outlook and design. Mater Sci Technol 24(9):1011–1019. doi:10.1179/174328408X341690
52. Tuomela A, Liu P, Puranen J, Ronkko S, Laaksonen T, Kalesnykas G et al (2014) Brinzolamide nanocrystal formulations for ophthalmic delivery: reduction of elevated intraocular pressure in vivo. Int J Pharm 467(1-2):34–41. doi:10.1016/j.ijpharm.2014.03.048
53. Nagarwal RC, Kumar R, Dhanawat M, Das N, Pandit JK (2011) Nanocrystal technology in the delivery of poorly soluble drugs: an overview. Curr Drug Deliv 8(4):398–406
54. Gudmundsdottir BS, Petursdottir D, Asgrimsdottir GM, Gottfredsdottir MS, Hardarson SH, Johannesson G et al (2014) γ-Cyclodextrin nanoparticle eye drops with dorzolamide: effect on intraocular pressure in man. J Ocul Pharmacol Ther 30(1):35–41. doi:10.1089/jop.2013.0060
55. Loftsson T, Brewster ME (2011) Pharmaceutical applications of cyclodextrins: effects on drug permeation through biological membranes. J Pharm Pharmacol 63(9):1119–1135. doi:10.1111/j.2042-7158.2011.01279.x
56. Apaolaza PS, Delgado D, del Pozo-Rodriguez A, Gascon AR, Solinis MA (2014) A novel gene therapy vector based on hyaluronic acid and solid lipid nanoparticles for ocular diseases. Int J Pharm 465(1-2):413–426. doi:10.1016/j.ijpharm.2014.02.038
57. Kalita D, Shome D, Jain VG, Chadha K, Bellare JR (2014) In vivo intraocular distribution and safety of periocular nanoparticle carboplatin for treatment of advanced retinoblastoma in humans. Am J Ophthalmol 157(5):1109–1115. doi:10.1016/j.ajo.2014.01.027
58. Madaan K, Kumar S, Poonia N, Lather V, Pandita D (2014) Dendrimers in drug delivery and targeting: drug-dendrimer interactions and toxicity issues. J Pharm Bioallied Sci 6(3):139–150. doi:10.4103/0975-7406.130965
59. Kaneshiro TL, Wang X, Lu ZR (2007) Synthesis, characterization, and gene delivery of poly-L-lysine octa(3-aminopropyl)silsesquioxane dendrimers: nanoglobular drug carriers with precisely defined molecular architectures. Mol Pharm 4(5):759–768. doi:10.1021/mp070036z
60. Kaneshiro TL, Jeong EK, Morrell G, Parker DL, Lu ZR (2008) Synthesis and evaluation of globular Gd-DOTA-monoamide conjugates with precisely controlled nanosizes for magnetic resonance angiography. Biomacromolecules 9(10):2742–2748. doi:10.1021/bm800486c
61. Shaunak S, Thomas S, Gianasi E, Godwin A, Jones E, Teo I et al (2004) Polyvalent dendrimer glucosamine conjugates prevent scar tissue formation. Nat Biotechnol 22(8):977–984. doi:10.1038/nbt995
62. Vandamme TF, Brobeck L (2005) Poly(amidoamine) dendrimers as ophthalmic vehicles for ocular delivery of pilocarpine nitrate and tropicamide. J Control Release 102(1):23–38. doi:10.1016/j.jconrel.2004.09.015
63. Cheng Y, Qu H, Ma M, Xu Z, Xu P, Fang Y et al (2007) Polyamidoamine (PAMAM) dendrimers as biocompatible carriers of quinolone antimicrobials: an in vitro study. Eur J Med Chem 42(7):1032–1038. doi:10.1016/j.ejmech.2006.12.035
64. Carnahan MA, Middleton C, Kim J, Kim T, Grinstaff MW (2002) Hybrid dendritic-linear polyester-ethers for in situ photopolymerization. J Am Chem Soc 124(19):5291–5293
65. Nishiyama N, Iriyama A, Jang WD, Miyata K, Itaka K, Inoue Y et al (2005) Light-induced gene transfer from packaged DNA enveloped in a dendrimeric photosensitizer. Nat Mater 4(12):934–941. doi:10.1038/nmat1524
66. Parekh HS, Marano RJ, Rakoczy EP, Blanchfield J, Toth I (2006) Synthesis of a library of polycationic lipid core dendrimers and their evaluation in the delivery of an oligonucleotide with hVEGF inhibition. Bioorg Med Chem 14(14):4775–4780. doi:10.1016/j.bmc.2006.03.029
67. Spataro G, Malecaze F, Turrin CO, Soler V, Duhayon C, Elena PP et al (2010) Designing dendrimers for ocular drug delivery. Eur J Med Chem 45(1):326–334. doi:10.1016/j.ejmech.2009.10.017
68. Xu Q, Kambhampati SP, Kannan RM (2013) Nanotechnology approaches for ocular drug delivery. Middle East Afr J Ophthalmol 20(1):26–37. doi:10.4103/0974-9233.106384
69. Kopečková P, Ikesue K, Kopeček J (1992) Cleavage of oligopeptide p-nitroanilides attached to N-(2-hydroxypropyl)methacrylamide copolymers by guinea pig intestinal enzymes. Macromol Chem Phys 193(10):2605–2619. doi:10.1002/macp.1992.021931010
70. Heizmann J, Langguth P, Biber A, Oschmann R, Merkle HP, Wolffram S (1996) Enzymatic cleavage of thymopoietin oligopeptides by

pancreatic and intestinal brush-border enzymes. Peptides 17(7):1083–1089

71. Yu G, Wu X, Ayat N, Maeda A, Gao SQ, Golczak M et al (2014) Multifunctional PEG retinylamine conjugate provides prolonged protection against retinal degeneration in mice. Biomacromolecules 15(12):4570–4578. doi:10.1021/bm501352s
72. Volotinen M, Maenpaa J, Kautiainen H, Tolonen A, Uusitalo J, Ropo A et al (2009) Ophthalmic timolol in a hydrogel vehicle leads to minor inter-individual variation in timolol concentration in aqueous humor. Eur J Pharm Sci 36(2-3):292–296. doi:10.1016/j.ejps.2008.10.004
73. Lou J, Hu W, Tian R, Zhang H, Jia Y, Zhang J et al (2014) Optimization and evaluation of a thermoresponsive ophthalmic in situ gel containing curcumin-loaded albumin nanoparticles. Int J Nanomedicine 9:2517–2525. doi:10.2147/ijn.s60270
74. Eljarrat-Binstock E, Orucov F, Aldouby Y, Frucht-Pery J, Domb AJ (2008) Charged nanoparticles delivery to the eye using hydrogel iontophoresis. J Control Release 126(2):156–161. doi:10.1016/j.jconrel.2007.11.016
75. Eljarrat-Binstock E, Orucov F, Frucht-Pery J, Pe'er J, Domb AJ (2008) Methylprednisolone delivery to the back of the eye using hydrogel iontophoresis. J Ocul Pharmacol Ther 24(3):344–350. doi:10.1089/jop.2007.0097
76. Eljarrat-Binstock E, Domb AJ (2006) Iontophoresis: a non-invasive ocular drug delivery. J Control Release 110(3):479–489. doi:10.1016/j.jconrel.2005.09.049
77. Parkinson TM, Ferguson E, Febbraro S, Bakhtyari A, King M, Mundasad M (2003) Tolerance of ocular iontophoresis in healthy volunteers. J Ocul Pharmacol Ther 19(2):145–151. doi:10.1089/108076803321637672
78. Kuno N, Fujii S (2011) Recent advances in ocular drug delivery systems. Polymers 3(1):193–221
79. Cardillo JA, Souza-Filho AA, Oliveira AG (2006) Intravitreal bioerudivel sustained-release triamcinolone microspheres system (RETAAC). Preliminary report of its potential usefulness for the treatment of diabetic macular edema. Arch Soc Esp Oftalmol 81(12):675–677
80. Rafie F, Javadzadeh Y, Javadzadeh AR, Ghavidel LA, Jafari B, Moogooee M et al (2010) In vivo evaluation of novel nanoparticles containing dexamethasone for ocular drug delivery on rabbit eye. Curr Eye Res 35(12):1081–1089. doi:10.3109/02713683.2010.508867
81. Pepić I, Hafner A, Lovrić J, Pirkić B, Filipović-Grčić J (2010) A nonionic surfactant/chitosan micelle system in an innovative eye drop formulation. J Pharm Sci 99(10):4317–4325. doi:10.1002/jps.22137
82. Di Tommaso C, Torriglia A, Furrer P, Behar-Cohen F, Gurny R, Moller M (2011) Ocular biocompatibility of novel Cyclosporin A formulations based on methoxy poly(ethylene glycol)-hexylsubstituted poly(lactide) micelle carriers. Int J Pharm 416(2):515–524. doi:10.1016/j.ijpharm.2011.01.004
83. Civiale C, Licciardi M, Cavallaro G, Giammona G, Mazzone MG (2009) Polyhydroxyethylaspartamide-based micelles for ocular drug delivery. Int J Pharm 378(1–2):177–186. doi:10.1016/j.ijpharm.2009.05.028
84. Gonzalez-Mira E, Egea MA, Garcia ML, Souto EB (2010) Design and ocular tolerance of flurbiprofen loaded ultrasound-engineered NLC. Colloids Surf B Biointerfaces 81(2):412–421, doi: http://dx.doi.org/10.1016/j.colsurfb.2010.07.029
85. Abdelbary G (2011) Ocular ciprofloxacin hydrochloride mucoadhesive chitosan-coated liposomes. Pharm Dev Technol 16(1):44–56. doi:10.3109/10837450903479988
86. Habib FS, Fouad EA, Abdel-Rhaman MS, Fathalla D (2010) Liposomes as an ocular delivery system of fluconazole: in-vitro studies. Acta Ophthalmol 88(8):901–904. doi:10.1111/j.1755-3768.2009.01584.x
87. Mehanna MM, Elmaradny HA, Samaha MW (2010) Mucoadhesive liposomes as ocular delivery system: physical, microbiological, and in vivo assessment. Drug Dev Ind Pharm 36(1):108–118. doi:10.3109/03639040903099751
88. Abrishami M, Zarei-Ghanavati S, Soroush D, Rouhbakhsh M, Jaafari MR, Malaekeh-Nikouei B (2009) Preparation, characterization, and in vivo evaluation of nanoliposomes-encapsulated bevacizumab (avastin) for intravitreal administration. Retina 29(5):699–703. doi:10.1097/IAE.0b013e3181a2f42a
89. Gudmundsdottir E, Stefansson E, Bjarnadottir G, Sigurjonsdottir JF, Gudmundsdottir G, Masson M et al (2000) Methazolamide 1 % in cyclodextrin solution lowers IOP in human ocular hypertension. Invest Ophthalmol Vis Sci 41(11):3552–3554
90. Gonzalez JR, Baiza-Duran L, Quintana-Hau J, Tornero-Montano R, Castaneda-Hernandez G, Ortiz M et al (2007) Comparison of the stability, efficacy, and adverse effect profile of the innovator 0.005 % latanoprost ophthalmic

solution and a novel cyclodextrin-containing formulation. J Clin Pharmacol 47(1):121–126. doi:10.1177/0091270006292626

91. Bawa R (2009) NanoBiotech 2008: exploring global advances in nanomedicine. Nanomedicine 5(1):5–7
92. Gaspar R (2007) Regulatory issues surrounding nanomedicines: setting the scene for the next generation of nanopharmaceuticals. Nanomedicine (Lond) 2(2):143–147. doi:10.2217/17435889.2.2.143
93. Medina C, Santos-Martinez MJ, Radomski A, Corrigan OI, Radomski MW (2007) Nanoparticles: pharmacological and toxicological significance. Br J Pharmacol 150(5): 552–558. doi:10.1038/sj.bjp.0707130
94. Diebold Y, Calonge M (2010) Applications of nanoparticles in ophthalmology. Prog Retin Eye Res 29(6):596–609. doi:10.1016/j.preteyeres.2010.08.002
95. Prow TW (2010) Toxicity of nanomaterials to the eye. Wiley interdisciplinary reviews. Nanomed Nanobiotechnol 2(4):317–333. doi:10.1002/wnan.65
96. Weiner AL, Gilger BC (2010) Advancements in ocular drug delivery. Vet Ophthalmol 13(6):395–406. doi:10.1111/j.1463-5224.2010.00835.x

Chapter 20

Nanomedicine for the Treatment of Musculoskeletal Diseases

Ke Ren, Xin Wei, Lingli Zhang, and Dong Wang

Abstract

The human adult skeletal system is comprised of 206 bones, along with a network of ligaments, tendons and cartilage. In addition to providing locomotion, the skeletal tissues serve as attachment sites for muscles and as protection for vital soft tissue organs. They harbor hematopoietic tissues (bone marrow) and act as a reservoir for calcium and phosphorus. Just as with any other organ systems, many pathological conditions are associated with musculoskeletal tissues, such as osteoporosis, arthritis, impaired fracture healing, and bone cancers, etc. These diseases affect many people, especially the geriatric population, resulting in pain, stiffness, loss of body function and even mortality. The health-related quality of life in patients with musculoskeletal diseases is significantly reduced, and the rising number of patients suffering from age-related musculoskeletal diseases can become a significant economic burden in an aging society.

To address this issue, many clinical interventions, ranging from new therapeutic treatments to novel surgical procedures, have been developed. Due to the inherent nature of the musculoskeletal system and its clinical relevance, extensive work has been done in the development of nanomaterials scaffolding and the local delivery of functional agents to improve bone repair/regeneration, osseointegration with orthopedic implants and prevention or treatment of postoperative infections. This is a rather crowded field with many high quality reviews being published (Tran and Webster. Wiley Interdiscip Rev Nanomed Nanobiotechnol 1(3): 336–351, 2009; Harvey et al. J Orthop Trauma 24(Suppl 1): S25–S30, 2010; Stylios et al. Injury 38(Suppl 1): S63–S74, 2007; Sato and Webster. Expert Rev Med Devices 1(1): 105–114, 2004; Webster and Ahn. Adv Biochem Eng Biotechnol 103: 275–308, 2007), which the readers are encouraged to explore. This chapter, however, will be mainly focused on several new directions in the field, especially on the use of nanomaterials as carriers to target therapeutic agents to the musculoskeletal lesions after systemic administration. In contrast to the local nanomaterial depot approach, of which the material design and drug release/activation are somewhat arbitrary, the systemically administered carriers would "seek out" its target and deliver the drugs according to the pathological conditions present.

Key words Musculoskeletal disease, Nanomedicine, Bone-targeting, ELVIS mechanism, Bone anabolic agent, Regenerative medicine, Inflammation, arthritis, Osteoporosis, Bone cancer

1 Basic Bone Biology

The composition of bone varies with age, gender, general health, anatomical location, and nutritional status. Generally, adult bone is composed of 50–70 % mineral, 20–40 % organic matrix, 5–10 %

Zheng-Rong Lu and Shinji Sakuma (eds.), *Nanomaterials in Pharmacology*, Methods in Pharmacology and Toxicology, DOI 10.1007/978-1-4939-3121-7_20,

water, and 1–5 % lipids [1]. The mineral content of the bone is mostly hydroxyapatites [HA, $Ca_{10}(PO_4)_6(OH)_2$], an insoluble salt of calcium and phosphate with small amounts of F^-, Cl^-, Na^+, K^+, Fe^{2+}, Zn^{2+}, Sr^{2+}, Mg^{2+}, citrate, and carbonate. The bone apatite is in the form of small needle-like crystals around 200 Å in their largest dimension [2]. About 90 % of the bone organic matrix is composed of type I collagen [3]. The collagen fibrils form a scaffold for a highly organized arrangement of uniaxially oriented bone apatite crystals. Bone minerals provide mechanical rigidity and load-bearing strength to bone, whereas the organic matrices are responsible for flexibility and elasticity.

Bone is a metabolically active organ that undergoes continuous remodeling throughout an individual's life. Bone remodeling helps to repair micro-damages in the bone matrix, prevents old bone accumulation and plays an important role in maintaining plasma mineral homeostasis. Remodeling involves continuous removal of discrete packets of old bone, replacement with newly synthesized matrix, and subsequent mineralization of the matrix to form new bone [4]. The remodeling cycle consists of five consecutive phases: activation (differentiation of preosteoclasts into mature osteoclasts); resorption (osteoclasts digest old bone); reversal (mononuclear cells appear on the surface of bone); formation (osteoblasts synthesize new bone matrix); and quiescence (osteoblasts become resting bone-lining cells on the newly formed bone surface) [5, 6]. During the bone remodeling process, the balance between the removal of mineralized tissue by osteoclasts and the formation of bone matrix through osteoblasts are of critical importance. Osteoclasts are the only cells that are known to be capable of resorbing bone. They are large, multinucleated cells derived from mononuclear precursor cells of the monocyte/macrophage lineage [7]. Resorbing osteoclasts secrete proton via H^+-ATP pump and chloride channels to decrease the pH within the bone resorption lacunae to as low as 4.5, which helps mobilize bone minerals [8]. In the meantime, they secrete cathepsin K, matrix metalloproteinase 9 and gelatinase to digest the organic matrix [9]. Osteoblasts are bone-forming cells derived from mesenchymal stem cells. They are responsible for the synthesis of new collagenous organic matrix and regulate mineralization by releasing small membrane-bound matrix vesicles that concentrate calcium and phosphate and enzymatically destroy mineralization inhibitors [10]. The bone remodeling through osteoclasts/osteoblasts and their regulation are shown in Fig. 1.

Many pathways regulate the bone remodeling cycle. The receptor activator of nuclear factor kappa B (NF-κB) ligand/receptor activator of NF-κB/osteoprotegerin (RANKL/RANK/OPG) pathway plays an essential role in the formation, activation,

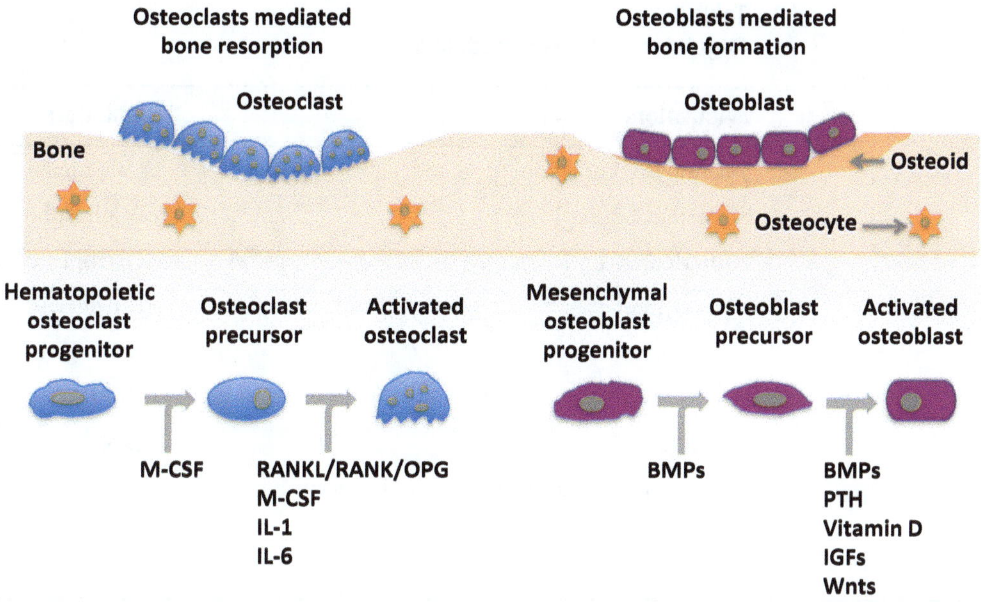

Fig. 1 During the bone remodeling process, the balance between the removal of mineralized bone by osteoclasts and the formation of bone matrix through osteoblasts are of critical importance. Hormones, cytokines, and growth factors that control cell proliferation and differentiation of osteoclasts and osteoblasts are shown below the *arrows*. *M-CSF* macrophage colony-stimulating factor, *RANK* receptor activator of NF-κB ligand, *RANKL* RANK ligand, *OPG* osteoprotegerin, *IL-1* interleukin-1, *IL-6* interleukin-6, *BMPs* bone morphogenetic proteins, *PTH* parathyroid hormone, *IGFs* insulin-like growth factors, *Wnts* wingless-type, mouse mammary tumor virus integration site

and function of osteoclasts [11]. When RANKL, expressed by osteoblasts, and stromal stem cells bind to RANK on the surface of osteoclasts and their precursors, the recruitment and activation of osteoclasts are stimulated. On the other hand, OPG, produced by osteoblasts and osteogenic stromal stem cells, acts as a decoy receptor to prevent RANKL from interacting with RANK. It protects the skeleton from excessive bone resorption [12, 13]. Thus, the RANKL/OPG ratio is an important determinant of bone mass and skeletal integrity in normal and disease states. Besides the RANKL/RANK/OPG system, a number of endocrine, immune, and cytokine mediators also influence or regulate bone remodeling. The major systemic regulators include calcitriol, parathyroid hormone (PTH), and hormones such as glucocorticoids (GC), growth hormones, sex hormones and thyroid hormones. Other factors such as prostaglandins, insulin-like growth factors, tumor growth factor-beta (TGF-beta), colony stimulating factor (CSF) and bone morphogenetic proteins (BMPs) are also involved [5]. Some of these regulators for bone remodeling are summarized in Table 1.

Table 1
Regulators of bone remodeling

Activators	Inhibitors
Parathyroid hormone[a]	Calcitonin
Prostaglandins	Bisphosphonates
Interleukin-1	Osteoprotegerin
Interleukin-1	Estrogens
Thyroxine	Androgens
1, 25 $(OH)_2$ Vitamin D	IL-18
RANK ligand	IFN-γ

[a]Parathyroid hormone's effect is dose dependent

2 Current Treatments and Proposed Novel Strategies for Improvement

2.1 Current Treatments

To maintain bone hemostasis, two classes of drugs have been developed. Bisphosphonates (BPs), cathepsin K inhibitiors, RANKL antibodies, calcitonin, estrogen, and estrogen agonists are commonly used as antiresorptive agents [14]. They inhibit osteoclast-mediated bone resorption and slow bone loss through multiple mechanisms, such as decreasing osteoclast activity and inducing osteoclast apoptosis [15]. Anabolic drugs, such as parathyroid hormone (PTH) analogs and sclerostin antibodies, are another type of medication, which stimulate bone formation by regulating osteoblast functions [16–18]. Other drugs have also been developed for particular musculoskeletal disorders such as rheumatoid arthritis and osteomyelitis [19–21].

Of these pharmacologically active drugs developed for musculoskeletal diseases, rarely do any of the drugs demonstrate tissue specificity to the bone, with the exception of bisphosphonates. When surgical procedure is part of the treatment protocol, a nanomaterial-based drug depot may be implanted to provide the needed local drug concentration [3, 22–25]. When used to treat systemic conditions or when there is no opportunity for implantation of a local drug depot, high systemic dose is often required to reach the drug's pharmacological activity at the peripheral skeletal site. The distribution of drugs to other normal organs and tissues, however, carries a considerable risk of adverse effects, which can be severe or even life threatening [26]. This is further complicated by the unique pharmacological features of a particular medication, such as the poor bioavailability and gastrointestinal irritation of bisphosphonates [27, 28] or of PTH, which requires intermittent administration [29, 30].

2.2 Osteotropic Agents

The anatomical and pathological features of the musculoskeletal system provide unique opportunities for the introduction of specific tissue tropism through rationally designed nanomaterial drug carriers. What distinguish the musculoskeletal system from the other organs and tissues in the body are its mineral composition. The unsaturated Ca^{2+} ions on the surface of bone apatite crystal bind strongly with chelators (e.g., carboxylates and phosphates) that could be used as robust targeting ligands to render nanoformulations osteotropic. Bisphosphonates (BPs) are a major class of drugs used for the treatment of osteoporosis and other musculoskeletal diseases characterized by increased bone resorption. As discussed earlier, BPs have strong bone affinity. They are stable analogs of naturally occurring inorganic pyrophosphate with a general structure of P-C-P (shown in Fig. 2). The P-C-P moiety has a high affinity for calcium crystals. Systemic administration of BPs commonly results in 20–50 % deposition of the molecules at bone tissues with minimal accumulation at other sites [31, 32]. The strong osteotropicity of BPs not only render them preferentially pharmacologically effective in bone but also makes them useful osteotropic ligands that can direct nanomaterial-based formulations to the bone since they retain much of the binding affinity after conjugation to other molecules or carriers. Many nanomedicines decorated with BPs have been developed for treating musculoskeletal diseases, such as osteoporosis and cancers metastasized to the bone [33–36].

Though being very potent bone-binding ligands, the pharmacological nature of BPs may limit this application. As strong inhibitors for osteoclast-mediated bone resorption, long-term use of BPs has been linked to complications such as osteonecrosis of the jaw

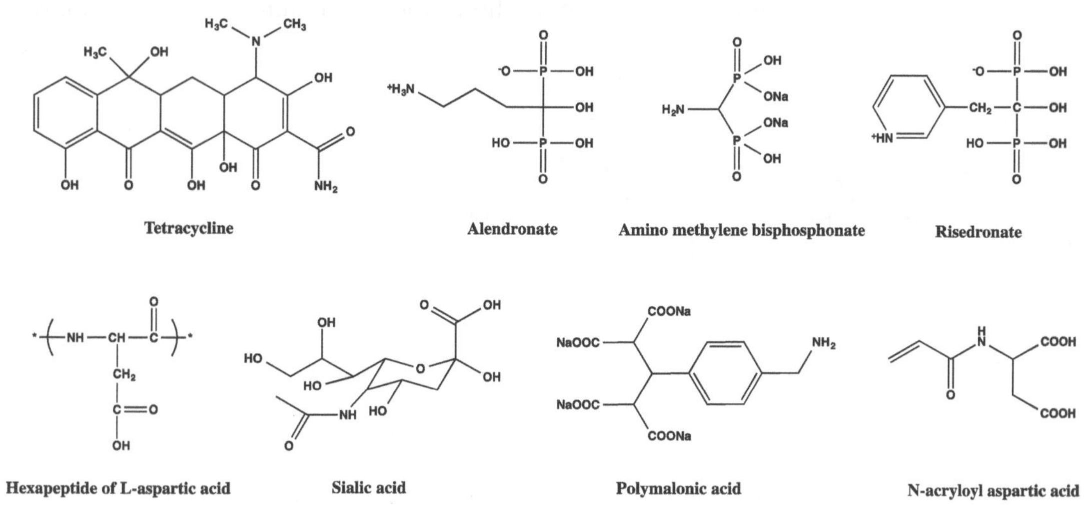

Fig. 2 The structures of representative bone-targeting moieties

(ONJ) [37, 38]. The P-C-P structure in BPs is resistant not only to most chemical reagents but also to enzymatic degradation. As a result, renal excretion is the only route of elimination. The half-life of BPs in the skeleton is very long, ranging among various species from 1 to 10 years, depending largely upon the rate of bone turnover [32]. An understanding of the structure of bone noncollagenous proteins (e.g., osteopontin and bone sialoprotein) with repeating sequences of acidic amino acids inspires the development of novel bone-targeting ligands based on acidic oligopeptides [39]. Studies have proven that acidic amino acid (L-Asp or L-Glu) homopeptides containing six or more residues bind strongly to hydroxyapatite [40]. Small peptides consisting of acidic amino acids may be more practical as osteotropic carriers because they could degrade and be excreted after selectively distributing to the bone and gradually releasing the conjugated drug [39, 41]. Several oligopeptide-conjugated drugs have been developed and shown to successfully target bone [40–43]. Besides BPs and acidic amino acids, a group of other molecules, such as tetracycline and its derivatives [44, 45], polymalonic acid [46], and sialic acid [47], have also been identified as bone targeting moieties.

2.3 Bone Targeting Delivery Systems

2.3.1 Active Targeting

Generally, there are two approaches one may use to direct therapeutic agents to the skeleton using these bone-targeting moieties (Fig. 3). First, the drugs may be chemically conjugated to a carrier, to which bone-targeting moieties can be conjugated to provide the osteotropicity to the prodrug. A good example of this is a *N*-(2-hydroxypropyl)methacrylamide (HPMA) copolymer conjugate containing alendronate (ALN) and potent anti-angiogenic agent TNP-470 [48]. Second, drugs may also be physically entrapped into nanocarriers (e.g., liposomes, nanoparticles, and micelles), their surfaces decorated with bone-binding moieties. These may include liposomes containing a bone-binding

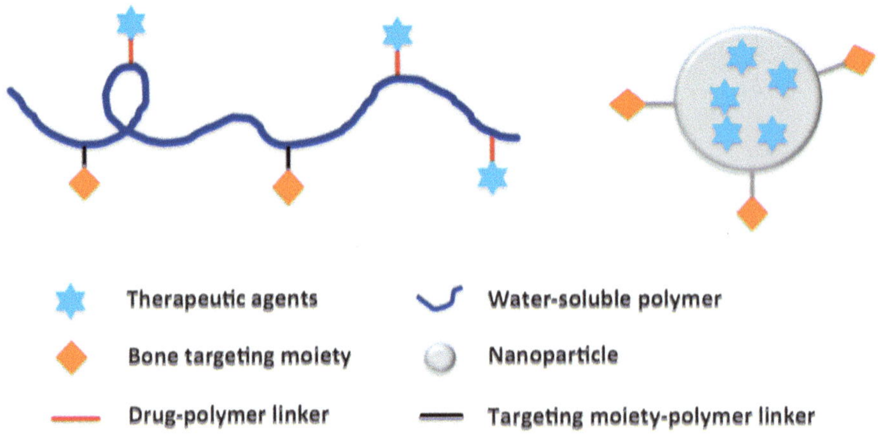

Fig. 3 General structure of bone-target nanomedicines

cholesterol derivative [33] and ALN-functionalized poly(lactic-co-glycolic acid) (PLGA) nanoparticles [49].

As critical is the preferential distribution of the drug to the musculoskeletal system, the proper release/activation of the drug at the targeted pathological site also plays an important role in the development of osteotropic nanomedicine. For drugs encapsulated in nanocarriers, the passive diffusion of the drug from the carrier matrix and the degradation/erosion of the carrier are the major mechanisms of drug release. For chemically conjugated prodrugs, the drug release depends on the cleavage of the drug-carrier linkers. The proper selection of the linker chemistry would enable additional tissue specificity according to local pathology. For example, as a bone specific enzyme, cathepsin K is highly expressed at resorbing osteoclasts. The application of cathepsin K-sensitive linkers would allow bone-specific activation of the prodrug [50]. The acidic environment in the resorption lacuna of osteoclasts (pH 4–4.5) is another unique physiological feature of bone metabolism. Therefore, the use of acid-cleavable linkers may also add bone specificity to chemically conjugated nanomedicine.

2.3.2 Passive Targeting

Many musculoskeletal diseases are accompanied by inflammation. The inflammation process is characterized by a sequence of defined pathophysiological events, including alterations in local vasculature, the recruitment and activation of inflammatory cells, destruction and removal of the initiating stimulus, and subsequent stimulation of repair processes that lead to restoration of tissue homeostasis [51]. The enhanced vasculature fenestration allows nanomedicine to extravasate at the inflammation site. The inflammatory infiltrates and activates local cells then sequesters the drug-containing colloidal systems and gradually activates and releases the drugs. This novel passive inflammation-targeting mechanism is termed the *E*xtravasation through *L*eaky *V*asculature and *I*nflammatory cell-mediated *S*equestration (ELVIS) mechanism (Fig. 4) [52, 53] and has been validated in multiple inflammatory musculoskeletal disease models [52–55]. For example, in adjuvant-induced arthritic rats (a model for rheumatoid arthritis), the vasculature leakage and the accelerated extravasation of the macromolecules (including plasma albumin) have long been proven using Evans Blue and synthetic macromolecular imaging contrast agents for magnetic resonance imaging (MRI) [49, 50]. The sequestration of polymeric prodrugs by local activated inflammatory cells in rat arthritic joints have also been proven by fluorescence-activated cell sorting and immunohistochemical staining [50].

It is also critically important to note that many of the musculoskeletal diseases find their largest patient cohort in the geriatric population. They are mostly of chronic nature, which requires very frequent dosing, probably for the remainder of the patient's

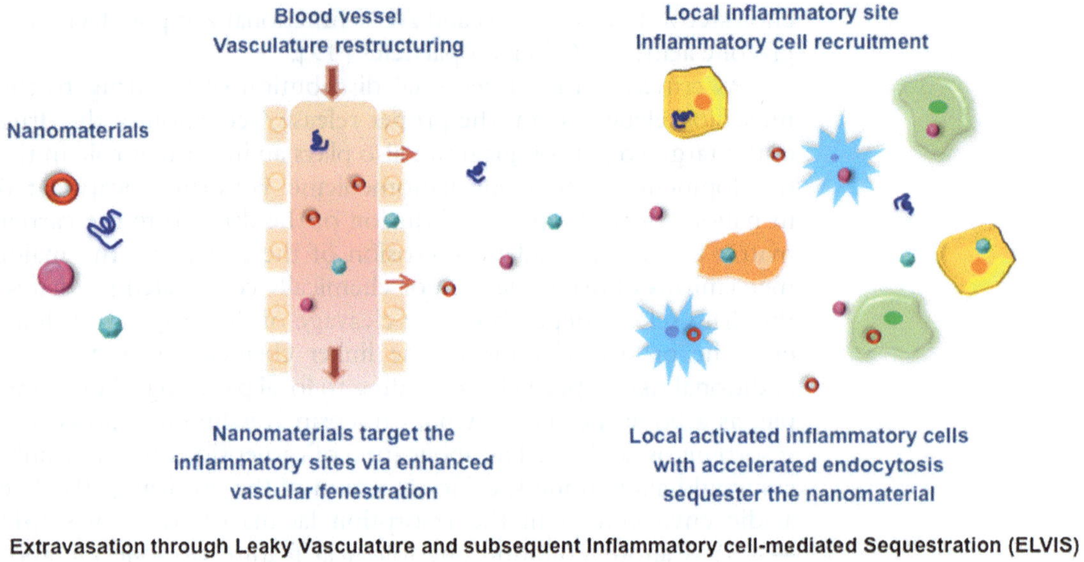

Fig. 4 Passive targeting of nanomedicine to inflammatory site via *E*xtravasation through *L*eaky *V*asculature and *I*nflammatory cell-mediated *S*equestration (ELVIS) mechanism

lifetime. From the pharmaceutical development aspect, this necessitates the development of long-acting dosage forms, such as a daily pill, monthly injection or even yearly injection (e.g., Once-Yearly Zoledronic Acid). For biologics, which mainly requires injections, the oral dosage form would greatly improve the patient compliance. In this case, nanoformulations may have the potential to provide better oral bioavailability for the biologics.

3 Nanomedicine Development for Musculoskeletal Diseases

Based on these unique features of musculoskeletal diseases, many new therapies have been developed using nanomaterial-based carriers. In the following sections, we will highlight their applications in several representative diseases.

3.1 Arthritis

Arthritis is the most common cause of disability among adults in the USA and has significantly higher incidence among patients with multiple chronic conditions [56]. There are two major types of arthritis: rheumatoid arthritis (RA) and osteoarthritis (OA).

3.1.1 Rheumatoid Arthritis

RA is an autoimmune inflammatory disorder that affects many tissues and organs, but primarily synovial joints. It causes significant joint pain, articular bone/cartilage destruction, loss of joint function and premature mortality. The current treatments for RA are generally divided into four categories: glucocorticoids (GC), disease-modifying antirheumatic drugs, nonsteroidal anti-inflammatory drugs, and biologics [57]. While most of these drugs have very well defined molecular targets, they rarely show arthrotropicity (i.e., targeting to the joint). As expected, their off-target distribution often lead to adverse events (e.g., secondary osteoporosis associated with the use of GC), which restrict the treatment duration and the overall dosing level and efficacy of these medications. To overcome these limitations, several unique pathophysiological features of RA can be exploited to enhance the drugs' tissue specificity to the inflamed joints. These include the ELVIS mechanism found in the inflammatory joints discussed above [52], synovial accumulation of inflammatory cells such as T-lymphocytes and macrophages, local tissue hypoxia and metabolic acidosis, and enrichment of inflammatory mediators such as cytokines and chemokines. These features and the discoveries of synovial tissue-specific antigens may allow for the development of nanomedicine that would facilitate the distribution of therapeutic agents to the inflamed joints.

One well-established strategy for the improvement of drug pharmacokinetics and tissue specificity is to develop nanomedicine formulations. The inflammatory features of the synovial tissues facilitate their preferential extravasation and local enrichment. Among the nanoformulation being explored for this purpose, the liposome is one of the most extensively studied formulations. This is mainly attributed to the well-established safety profiles of its excipients and formulation versatility [58]. Several liposomes have been developed for improved RA treatment, incorporating prednisolone, dexamethasone or superoxide dismutase [59–63]. Several formulation factors may be tuned to achieve optimal outcomes for different clinical applications [63–65]. For example, conjugation to polyethylene glycol, or PEGylation, generally increases the liposomal circulation time and reduces the uptake by liver and spleen. Large-sized liposomes show good retention for local intra-articular administration. Small-sized liposomes are better suited to achieve arthritic joint targeting by the ELVIS mechanism. Regardless of the surface modification and the drug encapsulated, all the small-sized liposomes have demonstrated noticeable arthrotropicity to the arthritic joints as opposed to normal joints [59, 62, 66, 67].

In addition to liposomes, other colloidal systems such as nanoparticles and micelles have been explored to improve RA treatment. Among the different materials that have been developed to formulate nanoparticles, PLGA is the most extensively researched. They are biodegradable polymers with good biocompatibility, low toxicity, well-described formulations and methods of production, and have been approved by the US FDA for different clinical applications [68]. For example, betamethasone sodium phosphate has been encapsulated in PLGA nanoparticles coated with lecithin [69], specifically PLGA/poly (D, L-lactic acid) (PLA) homopolymers and polyethylene glycol (PEG)-block-PLGA/PLA copolymers [70]. Both of the designs achieved superior therapeutic effects in an adjuvant-induced arthritis (AA) rat model and a collagen-induced arthritis (CIA) mouse model. For micelle delivery systems, Crielaard et al. developed polymerizable and hydrolytically cleavable dexamethasone (Dex) derivatives that were covalently entrapped in core cross-linked polymeric micelles. The therapeutic efficacy of the Dex-loaded micelles was confirmed in the two aforementioned RA models [71]. Cyclosporine A is a commonly used disease-modifying antirheumatic drug (DMARD) for the clinical management of RA. Due to its known immune suppressant effect, efforts have been made to load it into a polysialic acid grafted polycaprolactone (PCL) system, which self-assembles into micelles. The formulation can be internalized by the synovial fibroblasts through a non-receptor mediated form of endocytosis [72].

The macromolecular prodrug approach is another well-developed delivery strategy for anti-RA drugs. As reviewed by Yuan et al. [52], dextran, human serum albumin (HSA), HPMA copolymer, polyamidoamine (PAMAM) dendrimer, polyvinylpyrrolidone (PVP), and PEG have all been used as carriers. For example, Wang's lab developed an HPMA copolymer-Dex conjugate (P-Dex) using an acid-cleavable hydrazone linker. A single administration of the macromolecular prodrug resulted in sustained amelioration of the joint inflammation for more than 30 days, whereas an equivalent dose of free Dex treatment only provided temporal resolution of the inflammation [73, 74]. Different imaging studies together with immunohistochemistry and fluorescence activated cell-sorting analyses suggest that the superior therapeutic efficacy is due to the ELVIS mechanism as discussed previously [75]. The same lab has also developed a novel linear multifunctional PEG-Dex conjugate (click PEG-Dex) using click polymerization. Dex was conjugated to the click PEG via the acid-labile hydrazone bond to allow the drug release in a pathophysiological environment [76]. The therapeutic effect of click PEG-Dex is similar to P-Dex, but not as potent, which may be explained by the reduced cellular uptake and retention in the synovia due to different cell internalization rates of PEG and HPMA copolymers [77].

Recently, an interesting head-to-head comparison of four Dex-containing nanomedicine formulations was done in an AA rat model with a single equivalent dose (10 mg/kg) of Dex. It was found that the formulations with well-controlled, slow activation mechanisms (core cross-linked micelle and P-Dex-slow) outperform those with faster Dex releasing kinetics (liposome-Dex and P-Dex-fast), suggesting that the sustained local Dex presence in the synovial tissue is critical for ameliorating joint inflammation. As the liposomal formulation is already being explored clinically for improved treatment of RA, we believe other nanomaterials based formulations will have great potential to be translated into clinical application [73].

3.1.2 Osteoarthritis

Osteoarthritis (OA) is the most common cause of chronic joint pain and a leading cause of disability, affecting more than 27 million Americans [78]. It is a primarily non-inflammatory, degenerative joint disease characterized by the progressive loss of articular cartilage, changes in the synovial membrane, and an increased volume of synovial fluid with reduced viscosity, resulting in changed lubrication properties [79, 80]. While inflammation may be present in joints with OA, it is usually mild and involves only the periarticular tissues, which is different from RA [81]. Pain control is the primary goal of OA clinical management. Oral administration of nonsteroidal anti-inflammatory drugs (NSAIDs), aspirin and cyclooxygenase-2 (COX-2) inhibitors are the major therapeutic options for OA, but are often associated with gastrointestinal side effects. Due to the localized pathology of the disease, intra-articular (IA) drug administration is an attractive treatment approach for OA. These IA steroid injections are an effective treatment option, but should not, in most circumstances, be administered more than three to four times per year [82]. A series of weekly IA injections of sodium hyaluronate showed some symptomatic and functional improvement [83]. However, these treatments only provide short-term pain relief. Therefore, there is a large unmet need for novel OA treatments, to which nanomedicine development may contribute.

As early as 34 years ago, Dingle et al. proved that compared to free cortisol, IA injection of a palmitinic acid derivative of cortisol-encapsulated liposomes can provide improved residence time [84]. Foong et al. compared the distribution of free [3H] methotrexate ([3H]MTX) and liposomes containing [3H]MTX with [14C] cholesteryl oleate as a lipid marker in normal and arthritic rabbits. Free [3H]MTX was rapidly cleared from the joint with 79 % being excreted in the urine within 24 h of injection. However, 45.5 % of [3H]MTX liposome was recovered from the joint 24 h after injection. After 24 h, a 40-fold greater amount of [3H]MTX associated with the synovium was observed for the liposome formulation [85].

Numerous biodegradable polymers have been explored as formulation excipients for nanoparticle and microparticle development to be used in IA injections [80, 86]. Albumin and PLGA are the two most commonly used carriers due to their excellent safety profiles. Ratcliffe et al. proved that microparticles with sizes below 6 μm could be readily taken up by synovial macrophages. Radioactively labeled albumin microparticles had a residence time of several weeks in the joint after IA injection [87]. When betamethasone sodium phosphate was encapsulated into PLGA nanospheres, the in vitro releasing study indicated a sustained release of the drug over 3 weeks. When tested in an antigen-induced arthritic rabbit model, a single IA injection of the nanosphere significantly decreased joint swelling, sustained reduced serum antibody to ovalbumin, and prevented cartilage degradation after 21 days. Mechanism studies revealed that the nanospheres were phagocytosed by the activated synovocytes [88]. In addition, microparticular carriers have also been developed by complex coacervation of gelatine and chondroitine sulfate. After intraarticular injection, such a system can be specifically degraded due to its sensitivity to the local gelatinase of the OA joints. Since the preparation of this type of microparticles does not require the use of organic solvents and can be performed at room temperature, it may especially benefit the formulations of peptide and protein drugs when compared to the PLGA particular systems [89].

In summary, the sequestration of the particulate systems into the synovial membrane and subsequent sustained release of the active compound could improve the efficacy and reduce the side effects of drugs injected directly into the joint cavity for OA management. As Lipotalon®, a liposomal formulation of dexamethasone-21-palmitate used for IA injection, is already available on the German market, we believe other IA particulates systems under development may also have the potential to be translated into novel therapy for better clinical management of OA.

3.2 Osteoporosis

Osteoporosis is a progressive systemic skeletal disorder characterized by low bone mass and microarchitectural deterioration of bone tissue, with a consequent increase in bone fragility and susceptibility to fracture [90]. It is estimated that osteoporosis affects over 200 million people worldwide [91]. More than three million osteoporotic fractures are expected in 2025 in the USA alone, with associated costs rising to approximately $25.3 billion [92]. The balance of new bone formation and old bone breakdown is tipped toward resorption for patients with osteoporosis. Therefore, antiresorptive agents have been the major treatment options. Cathepsin K inhibitors, BPs, RANKL inhibitors, calcitonin, estrogen, and estrogen agonists/antagonists are commonly used antiresorptive medications [14]. They inhibit osteoclast-mediated bone resorption and slow down the bone loss through multiple mechanisms [15]. Meanwhile, anabolic agents, such as PTH analogs, are another type of medication that stimulates bone turnover, favoring bone formation [16–18]. As mentioned before, most of these drugs do not have tissue specificity to the skeletal system. Therefore, nanomedicine formulations (e.g., nanoparticles and liposomes) with active targeting mechanisms have been explored to improve their therapeutic potentials [33, 93, 94]. As an example, hormone replacement therapy is a popular management strategy for postmenopausal osteoporosis in women. Due to lack of skeletal specificity, however, long-term clinical use of estrogen may increase the risk of ovarian cancer, stroke, blood clots, etc. To address this issue, Choi et al. encapsulated estrogen in PLGA nanoparticles and modified the particle surface with alendronate, which enables the nanoparticles to have a strong affinity towards HA [49]. In addition, an estradiol/aspartic acid oligopeptide conjugate prodrug was also synthesized. It was found to preferentially distribute to the bone and gradually regenerated the parent drug. As a result, weekly treatment with the prodrug showed comparable pharmacological activities with a once every 3 day estradiol therapy but with less systemic adverse effects [95]. Zhang et al. developed active bone-targeting liposomes decorated with oligopeptides for the delivery of osteogenic siRNAs specifically to bone-formation surfaces. The liposomal formulation was found to markedly promote bone formation, enhance the bone microarchitecture and increase the bone mass in both healthy and osteoporotic rats [96].

Calcitonin (CT) and PTH are important hormones regulating bone metabolism and have both been used for the treatment of osteoporosis. As treatments for a chronic condition, both of them need to be given on a daily basis either as subcutaneous injection or nasal spray. Oral administration, if possible, would be a much more desirable route for better patient compliance. There are many problems associated with peptide and protein drug oral delivery, such as the susceptibility for enzyme degradation and chemical instability in the gastrointestinal tract, poor intrinsic permeability across the intestinal epithelium and rapid post-absorptive clearance. Novel oral nanoformulations have been explored to overcome these limitations. For example, Yoo et al. prepared CT PLGAnanoparticles by loading CT-fatty acid complexes into the nanoparticles [97]. An in vitro study confirmed the dose-dependent transport of the nanoparticles in Caco-2 cell monolayers. Pharmacokinetic studies in rats showed high plasma CT concentration in the nanoparticle-treated group whereas negligible amounts of CT were detected for the free CT group even at a five times higher dosage. In a similar formulation, a PEGylated chitosan nanoparticle system was used to formulate PTH. Another in vivo study found a significant increase of intestinal uptake of PTH [98]. Besides nanoparticles, mucoadhesive liposome formulations have been prepared by coating liposomes with mucoadhesive carbopol or chitosan to achieve better oral delivery of CT [99]. Microspheres containing CT has also been prepared using the pH-sensitive polymer Eudragit P-4135F [100]. Both delivery systems showed an enhanced and prolonged reduction in blood calcium concentration in rats.

As described above, though many nanomaterials-based formulations have been explored to improve the safety profiles or oral bioavailability of osteoporosis drugs [101–104], none have been cleared for clinical application. The additional cost of these new formulations, the chronic nature of the disease and the availability of new drug development may all have to be considered in the future development in this area.

3.3 Cancer Associated with the Musculoskeletal System

3.3.1 Primary Bone Cancer

Primary bone cancers are a specific subtype of cancers known as sarcomas. They start in bone, connective tissue muscle or blood vessels, and can be found anywhere in the body. Primary bone cancer is rare. It accounts for much less than 1 % of all cancers. About 2300 new cases of primary bone cancer are diagnosed in the USA each year [105]. Chondrosarcomas and osteosarcoma are the most common primary malignant bone cancers [106]. Due to the potential benefit of cancer chemotherapeutic agents being passively targeted to the cancer lesions according to EPR effect, several nanomedicine formulations have been developed for the treatment of bone cancer. One of the clinical applications of PEGylated-liposomal doxorubicin (Doxil) [107, 108] is primary bone cancer. Clinical trials in sarcoma patients suggested that Doxil has activity in poor prognosis sarcoma, and is associated with modest toxicity [109, 110]. In addition, studies proved that doxorubicin-loaded calcium carbonate nanocrystals significantly inhibited osteosarcoma bone cancer cells and sustained the slow release of doxorubicin at normal physiological pH but achieved a faster release rate in an acidic environment (pH 4.8) [111]. Susa et al. developed lipid-modified dextran nanoparticles loaded with doxorubicin, which had a curative effect on multidrug resistant osteosarcoma cell lines by increasing the amount of drug accumulation in the nucleus via a Pgp-independent pathway [112]. Federman et al. reported an osteosarcoma-associated cell surface antigen (ALCAM). They engineered an anti-ALCAM-hybrid polymerized liposomal nanoparticle immunoconjugate loaded with doxorubicin. Compared with untargeted nanoparticles and conventional liposomal doxorubicin formulations, the targeted nanoparticles have significantly enhanced cytotoxicity to osteosarcoma cells [113].

3.3.2 Cancer Bone Metastasis

Though primary bone cancer is rare, the skeleton is the most common organ to be affected by metastatic cancer and produces the greatest morbidity [114]. Particularly, bone is the major metastasis site for prostate cancer and approximately 70 % of metastatic breast cancers spread to bone [115]. Therefore, the treatment of cancer bone metastasis is important for patients in providing prolonged survival rates and improved quality of life. One particular class of drug, BPs, has attracted lots of attention. As described in previous sections, BPs are well-established antiresorptive drugs with specific affinity to bone tissues. They have been widely used in treating osteoporosis and as bone targeting moieties for nanomedicine formulations. Emerging data suggest that BPs may also inhibit angiogenesis, tumor cell invasion, adhesion, overall tumor progression and can be used to treat cancer bone metastases [116–119]. Therefore, both BP-loaded nanomedicine formulations and nanomedicine decorated with BPs as the bone-targeting moiety have been developed for improved treatment of cancer bone metastases.

For most cases, BPs have been used to incorporate bone affinity into formulations of anticancer drugs. There are numerous targeted nanomedicines that have been developed based on BPs. It has been demonstrated that zoledronate-conjugated PLGAnanoparticles exhibit increased in-cell cycle arrest, enhanced cell cytotoxicity and more apoptotic activity. In animal studies, technetium-99m (^{99m}Tc)-labeled nanoparticles exhibited a prolong blood circulation half-life, reduced liver uptake, and significantly higher retention in the skeleton [120]. In another case, paclitaxel was conjugated to alendronate-modified HPMA copolymer through a cathepsin B-sensitive linker [121]. The conjugate exhibited significantly improved antitumor efficacy and better tolerance on mCherry-labeled 4T1 mammary adenocarcinoma inoculated into the tibia, as compared with paclitaxel alone or in combination with alendronate [122]. Gemcitabine, a potent anticancer drug, was conjugated with BPs and radiolabeled with ^{99m}Tc. In vitro evaluation proved that the conjugate could bind readily to powdered bone and HA. Biodistribution studies in mice indicated that the conjugate was predominantly distributed in bone with low soft tissue uptake after intravenous dosing. Unbound compound was excreted through the kidneys [36].

There are also nanomedicine formulations of BPs being developed to improve drug efficacy. For example, Daubine et al. employed poly-L-lysine covalently grafted with beta-cyclodextrin to form a polycationic vector for risedronate (third generation BP) delivery. The complexes strongly enhanced the efficacy of risedronate at inhibiting cancer cell invasion in vitro both in solution and while embedded into polyelectrolyte multilayered nanoarchitectures. Moreover, the complexes in solution clearly prevented cancer-induced bone metastasis in animal models [123].

Compared to the relatively low density of vascularization in the normal skeletal tissues, the highly vascularized tumor tissue in bone presents an excellent opportunity for nanomedicine passive targeting according to the EPR effect. Due to the presence of minerals at the cancer lesion, the use of bone targeting moieties in these formulations would provide them with an additional local retention mechanism. It is important to know that different bone cancer lesions, depending on whether they are osteolytic or osteoblastic, may necessitate the use of targeting ligands that favor either a bone formation surface or a resorption surface [96, 124]. Due to their strong affinity to bone apatite, BPs typically could not distinguish between these bone functional domains [124].

3.4 Osteomyelitis

Osteomyelitis is an inflammatory skeletal disorder caused by bacterial infection, leading to necrosis and destruction of bone and perhaps to persistent morbidity. It affects people of all ages and can involve any type of bone. The most common pathogens responsible for osteomyelitis in humans are those of the *Staphylococcus* species [125, 126]. The treatment of chronic osteomyelitis is complicated and is dependent upon disease stage and pathophysiology. There are three commonly used multidisciplinary approaches: surgical debridement, systemic antibiotic therapy and local antibiotic treatment [127–129]. Although intravenous and oral antibiotic therapies are the mainstay of antimicrobial therapy for osteomyelitis, high serum concentrations of the antibiotic and undesired off-target toxicities are generally associated with the systemic drug administration approach. Meanwhile, frequent inaccessibility of the infected zone to blood flow and the resulting low concentration of the antibiotic at the infection site may contribute to pathogenic resistance to antibiotic therapy. Current research focuses on the development of carrier systems that deliver antibiotics directly to the infection site and retain an appropriate antibiotic level.

The carriers for local delivery antibiotic can be classified as nonbiodegradable (non-resorbable) and biodegradable (resorbable) [130]. Poly (methyl methacrylate) (PMMA) beads are the most common type of nonbiodegradable carrier. Septopal®, PMMA beads containing gentamicin at a size of 7 mm, was approved for use in the treatment of osteomyelitis in Europe in the 1970s. Noncommercial beads prepared by surgeons are also in use. These are individually manufactured bead molds made by mixing commercially available PMMA polymer with antibiotics [131]. The sustained release of antibiotics from the PMMA beads has been validated [130, 132]. For example, clindamycin and tobramycin-loaded PMMA beads exhibited release duration as long as 220 days [133]. Placement of these beads is a simple procedure, which is performed at the time of initial debridement for chronic osteomyelitis [125]. However, bead placement generally requires a second operation for removal after the completion of antibiotic release.

In order to address the drawbacks of local delivery with PMMA, such as the need for a second surgery to remove dead space induced by PMMA and limited selection of antibiotics [134], the biodegradable carrier is an attractive alternative and has been actively investigated in recent years. A large number of biodegradable and biocompatible nanomaterials have been developed and tested in vitro and in vivo for local antibiotic therapy of osteomyelitis. For example, calcium phosphates, the natural mineral component of bone, have been developed into nanoparticles. They are bioactive, bioresorptive, and osteo-conductive nanomaterials with great biocompatibility and low toxicity [135, 136]. Uskokovic et al. proved the satisfactory performance of calcium phosphate nanoparticles against *S. aureus* [137, 138]. A sustained release for more than 21 days was observed [139]. To stabilize the surface-bound drug layer, decrease the burst release, and possibly produce multiple-stage release profiles that may additionally boost the antimicrobial activity, polymer-coated calcium phosphate nanoparticles were further developed. Coating calcium phosphate nanoparticles with PLGA suppressed the burst release without diminishing the antibacterial efficacy [140]. Poly(e-caprolactone) coated chitosan/β-tricalcium phosphate composites showed near zero-order release kinetics of vancomycin for 14 days and an overall release period of 42 days [141]. For more information about local delivery systems for osteomyelitis, the readers may refer to reviews [130, 142]. Though these systems are very effective in animal models, to our knowledge, no large human trials have been published. None of the material has been approved by the US FDA for delivering antibiotics to treat osteomyelitis.

3.5 Bone Regeneration

Bone defects and malformation, caused by infection, trauma, tumor resection and pathological degeneration represent a major concern for orthopedic surgeons. With the development of numerous novel nanotechnologies, they have also been explored extensively for applications in bone regeneration. Researchers have been working on developing nanomedicine formulations of bone anabolic agents for skeletal regeneration. Micro- and nano-sized delivery vesicles have been developed to formulate bone anabolic agents. The carrier materials that have been researched include PLGA, hydroxyapatite, collagen, hyaluronic acid, chitosan, and alginate [143–145]. PLGA is the most extensively researched carrier [146]. Porous PLGA-HA scaffolds and fibrous scaffolds have been developed and showed promising bone regeneration effects by loading anabolic drugs [147–149]. Injectable composites composed of PLGA-g-PEG hydrogel and HA presented thermogelling effect and sustainably released encapsulated drug [150]. PLGA-hydroxyapatite microspheres, HA-coated PLGA microspheres, apatite-coated PLGA microspheres are either injectable bone substitute or effective in delivering bone regeneration agents [151–153].

It is important to note that some of the nanocarriers themselves have been found to exhibit positive effects on bone regeneration. For example, Yao et al. demonstrated that gold nanoparticles can promote the proliferation and differentiation of osteoblasts [154]. Sulfated chitosan enhanced bioactivity of BMP-2 by promoting the BMP-2 signaling pathway [154]. These are very important findings, which remind us of the critical need to include proper control groups to more accurately interpret experimental findings. There are many reviews about delivering bone growth factors using nanocarriers [3, 23, 155], which the reader may find to be informative on this particular topic.

Besides nanocarriers, another research focus about bone regeneration is developing bioactive materials for improved bone repair using tissue-engineering approaches. For example, biphasic calcium phosphate nanoparticles were loaded into gelatin-pectin scaffolds. The biodegradable scaffolds showed significantly improved cell adhesion, viability and proliferation in vitro and rapid bone growth in vivo when compared with the scaffold without nanoparticle [156]. Nano-hydroxyapatite was developed and coated to biphasic calcium phosphate ceramics surface. The scaffolds with coating were more conducive for mesenchymal stem cell adhesion, proliferation, and osteogenic differentiation than conventional, uncoated scaffolds, which made this material more suitable for applications in bone tissue engineering [157]. The detail of tissue-engineering is beyond the scope of this chapter. Readers could find more information about this topic in these reviews [158–162].

4 Conclusion

Musculoskeletal disease is an umbrella term for a variety of bone and joint disorders that hinder human mobility and affect quality of life. Although many effective medications have been developed, the balance between their therapeutic efficacy and safety has always been a tricky issue. In this chapter, we first discussed some very unique pathophysiological features of the musculoskeletal system and then focused on how to rationally design and develop nanomedicine according to these features to improve the treatments of musculoskeletal diseases. Local application of nanomedicine for the sustained release of antiresorptive/anabolic agents and antibiotics have been extensively investigated and reviewed. We believe the systemic administration of the newly designed nanomedicine for active targeting using bone-seeking agents and for passive targeting systems based on the ELVIS mechanism are very promising as they are rationally designed and have demonstrated greatly improved therapeutic efficacy and in many cases reduced adverse effects in animal models of musculoskeletal diseases. Additional efforts are needed to further validate and optimize these novel nanomaterial-based therapies in animal models to further accelerate their translation into clinical evaluation and application.

References

1. Boskey AL, Posner AS (1984) Bone structure, composition, and mineralization. Orthop Clin North Am 15(4):597–612
2. Shea JE, Miller SC (2005) Skeletal function and structure: implications for tissue-targeted therapeutics. Adv Drug Deliv Rev 57(7): 945–957
3. Harvey EJ, Henderson JE, Vengallatore ST (2010) Nanotechnology and bone healing. J Orthop Trauma 24(Suppl 1):S25–S30
4. Clarke B (2008) Normal bone anatomy and physiology. Clin J Am Soc Nephrol 3(Suppl 3):S131–S139
5. Hadjidakis DJ, Androulakis II (2006) Bone remodeling. Ann N Y Acad Sci 1092:385–396
6. Feng X, McDonald JM (2011) Disorders of bone remodeling. Annu Rev Pathol 6:121–145
7. Boyle WJ, Simonet WS, Lacey DL (2003) Osteoclast differentiation and activation. Nature 423(6937):337–342

8. Silver IA, Murrills RJ, Etherington DJ (1988) Microelectrode studies on the acid microenvironment beneath adherent macrophages and osteoclasts. Exp Cell Res 175(2):266–276
9. Delaisse JM et al (2003) Matrix metalloproteinases (MMP) and cathepsin K contribute differently to osteoclastic activities. Microsc Res Tech 61(6):504–513
10. Anderson HC (2003) Matrix vesicles and calcification. Curr Rheumatol Rep 5(3): 222–226
11. Boyce BF, Xing L (2007) The RANKL/RANK/OPG pathway. Curr Osteoporos Rep 5(3):98–104
12. Boyce BF, Xing L (2007) Biology of RANK, RANKL, and osteoprotegerin. Arthritis Res Ther 9(Suppl 1):S1
13. Boyce BF, Xing L (2008) Functions of RANKL/RANK/OPG in bone modeling and remodeling. Arch Biochem Biophys 473(2):139–146
14. Takada J (2006) Application of anti-resorptive drugs for the treatment of osteoporosis. Nihon Rinsho 64(2):385–391
15. Stepan JJ et al (2003) Mechanisms of action of antiresorptive therapies of postmenopausal osteoporosis. Endocr Regul 37(4):225–238
16. Honig S, Rajapakse CS, Chang G (2013) Current treatment approaches to osteoporosis - 2013. Bull Hosp Jt Dis 71(3):184–188
17. Blahos J (2011) Current and future options for treatment of osteoporosis. Vnitr Lek 57(11):888–890
18. Baron R, Hesse E (2012) Update on bone anabolics in osteoporosis treatment: rationale, current status, and perspectives. J Clin Endocrinol Metab 97(2):311–325
19. Donahue KE et al (2012) Drug therapy for rheumatoid arthritis in adults: an update. Agency for Healthcare Research and Quality, Rockville, MD
20. John M (2007) Drug therapy for rheumatoid arthritis: comparative effectiveness. In: Comparative effectiveness review summary guides for clinicians. Agency for Healthcare Research and Quality, Rockville, MD
21. Lima AL et al (2014) Recommendations for the treatment of osteomyelitis. Braz J Infect Dis 18:526
22. Tran N, Webster TJ (2009) Nanotechnology for bone materials. Wiley Interdiscip Rev Nanomed Nanobiotechnol 1(3):336–351
23. Stylios G, Wan T, Giannoudis P (2007) Present status and future potential of enhancing bone healing using nanotechnology. Injury 38(Suppl 1):S63–S74
24. Sato M, Webster TJ (2004) Nanobiotechnology: implications for the future of nanotechnology in orthopedic applications. Expert Rev Med Devices 1(1): 105–114
25. Webster TJ, Ahn ES (2007) Nanostructured biomaterials for tissue engineering bone. Adv Biochem Eng Biotechnol 103:275–308
26. Choy EH et al (2005) A two year randomised controlled trial of intramuscular depot steroids in patients with established rheumatoid arthritis who have shown an incomplete response to disease modifying antirheumatic drugs. Ann Rheum Dis 64(9):1288–1293
27. Ruggiero SL et al (2004) Osteonecrosis of the jaws associated with the use of bisphosphonates: a review of 63 cases. J Oral Maxillofac Surg 62(5):527–534
28. McHorney CA et al (2007) The impact of osteoporosis medication beliefs and side-effect experiences on non-adherence to oral bisphosphonates. Curr Med Res Opin 23(12): 3137–3152
29. Uzawa T et al (1995) Comparison of the effects of intermittent and continuous administration of human parathyroid hormone(1-34) on rat bone. Bone 16(4):477–484
30. Lotinun S, Sibonga JD, Turner RT (2002) Differential effects of intermittent and continuous administration of parathyroid hormone on bone histomorphometry and gene expression. Endocrine 17(1):29–36
31. de Ligny CL et al (1990) Bone seeking pharmaceuticals. Int J Rad Appl Instrum B 17(2):161–179
32. Lin JH (1996) Bisphosphonates: a review of their pharmacokinetic properties. Bone 18(2):75–85
33. Hengst V et al (2007) Bone targeting potential of bisphosphonate-targeted liposomes. Preparation, characterization and hydroxyapatite binding in vitro. Int J Pharm 331(2): 224–227
34. El-Mabhouh AA et al (2011) A conjugate of gemcitabine with bisphosphonate (Gem/BP) shows potential as a targeted bone-specific therapeutic agent in an animal model of human breast cancer bone metastases. Oncol Res 19(6):287–295
35. El-Mabhouh AA, Mercer JR (2008) 188Re-labelled gemcitabine/bisphosphonate (Gem/BP): a multi-functional, bone-specific agent as a potential treatment for bone metastases. Eur J Nucl Med Mol Imaging 35(7): 1240–1248
36. El-Mabhouh AA et al (2006) A 99mTc-labeled gemcitabine bisphosphonate drug

conjugate as a probe to assess the potential for targeted chemotherapy of metastatic bone cancer. Nucl Med Biol 33(6):715–722
37. Allen MR, Ruggiero SL (2014) A review of pharmaceutical agents and oral bone health: how osteonecrosis of the jaw has affected the field. Int J Oral Maxillofac Implants 29(1): e45–e57
38. Ryan P, Saleh I, Stassen LF (2009) Osteonecrosis of the jaw: a rare and devastating side effect of bisphosphonates. Postgrad Med J 85(1010):674–677
39. Kasugai S et al (2000) Selective drug delivery system to bone: small peptide (Asp)6 conjugation. J Bone Miner Res 15(5):936–943
40. Takahashi-Nishioka T et al (2008) Targeted drug delivery to bone: pharmacokinetic and pharmacological properties of acidic oligopeptide-tagged drugs. Curr Drug Discov Technol 5(1):39–48
41. Sekido T et al (2001) Novel drug delivery system to bone using acidic oligopeptide: pharmacokinetic characteristics and pharmacological potential. J Drug Target 9(2): 111–121
42. Takahashi T et al (2008) Bone-targeting of quinolones conjugated with an acidic oligopeptide. Pharm Res 25(12):2881–2888
43. Nishioka T et al (2006) Enhancement of drug delivery to bone: characterization of human tissue-nonspecific alkaline phosphatase tagged with an acidic oligopeptide. Mol Genet Metab 88(3):244–255
44. Pierce WM Jr, Waite LC (1987) Bone-targeted carbonic anhydrase inhibitors: effect of a proinhibitor on bone resorption in vitro. Proc Soc Exp Biol Med 186(1):96–102
45. Neale JR et al (2009) Bone selective effect of an estradiol conjugate with a novel tetracycline-derived bone-targeting agent. Bioorg Med Chem Lett 19(3):680–683
46. Thompson WJ, Thompson DD, Anderson PS, Rodan GA (1989) Polymalonic acids as boneaffinity agents. EP 0341961
47. Shimoda Y et al (1994) Calcium ion binding of three different types of oligo/polysialic acids as studied by equilibrium dialysis and circular dichroic methods. Biochemistry 33(5):1202–1208
48. Segal E et al (2009) Targeting angiogenesis-dependent calcified neoplasms using combined polymer therapeutics. PLoS One 4(4):e5233
49. Choi SW, Kim JH (2007) Design of surface-modified poly(D, L-lactide-co-glycolide) nanoparticles for targeted drug delivery to bone. J Control Release 122(1):24–30
50. Pan H et al (2006) Water-soluble HPMA copolymer--prostaglandin E1 conjugates containing a cathepsin K sensitive spacer. J Drug Target 14(6):425–435
51. Henson PM (2005) Dampening inflammation. Nat Immunol 6(12):1179–1181
52. Yuan F et al (2012) Development of macromolecular prodrug for rheumatoid arthritis. Adv Drug Deliv Rev 64(12):1205–1219
53. Ren K et al (2014) Early diagnosis of orthopedic implant failure using macromolecular imaging agents. Pharm Res 31:2086
54. Purdue PE et al (2013) Development of polymeric nanocarrier system for early detection and targeted therapeutic treatment of peri-implant osteolysis. HSS J 9(1):79–85
55. Ren K et al (2014) Macromolecular prodrug of dexamethasone prevents particle-induced peri-implant osteolysis with reduced systemic side effects. J Control Release 175:1–9
56. Centers for Disease Control and Prevention (2009) Prevalence and most common causes of disability among adults—United States, 2005. MMWR Morb Mortal Wkly Rep 58:421–426
57. Quan LD et al (2008) The development of novel therapies for rheumatoid arthritis. Expert Opin Ther Pat 18(7):723–738
58. Tarner IH, Muller-Ladner U (2008) Drug delivery systems for the treatment of rheumatoid arthritis. Expert Opin Drug Deliv 5(9):1027–1037
59. Metselaar JM et al (2003) Complete remission of experimental arthritis by joint targeting of glucocorticoids with long-circulating liposomes. Arthritis Rheum 48(7):2059–2066
60. Khoury M et al (2006) Efficient new cationic liposome formulation for systemic delivery of small interfering RNA silencing tumor necrosis factor alpha in experimental arthritis. Arthritis Rheum 54(6):1867–1877
61. Koning GA et al (2006) Targeting of angiogenic endothelial cells at sites of inflammation by dexamethasone phosphate-containing RGD peptide liposomes inhibits experimental arthritis. Arthritis Rheum 54(4):1198–1208
62. Gaspar MM et al (2007) Enzymosomes with surface-exposed superoxide dismutase: in vivo behaviour and therapeutic activity in a model of adjuvant arthritis. J Control Release 117(2):186–195
63. Kapoor B et al (2014) Application of liposomes in treatment of rheumatoid arthritis: quo vadis. ScientificWorldJournal 2014:978351
64. Vanniasinghe AS, Bender V, Manolios N (2009) The potential of liposomal drug deliv-

ery for the treatment of inflammatory arthritis. Semin Arthritis Rheum 39(3):182–196

65. van den Hoven JM et al (2011) Liposomal drug formulations in the treatment of rheumatoid arthritis. Mol Pharm 8(4): 1002–1015
66. Metselaar JM et al (2004) Liposomal targeting of glucocorticoids to synovial lining cells strongly increases therapeutic benefit in collagen type II arthritis. Ann Rheum Dis 63(4): 348–353
67. Avnir Y et al (2008) Amphipathic weak acid glucocorticoid prodrugs remote-loaded into sterically stabilized nanoliposomes evaluated in arthritic rats and in a Beagle dog: a novel approach to treating autoimmune arthritis. Arthritis Rheum 58(1):119–129
68. Danhier F et al (2012) PLGA-based nanoparticles: an overview of biomedical applications. J Control Release 161(2):505–522
69. Higaki M et al (2005) Treatment of experimental arthritis with poly(D, L-lactic/glycolic acid) nanoparticles encapsulating betamethasone sodium phosphate. Ann Rheum Dis 64(8):1132–1136
70. Ishihara T et al (2009) Treatment of experimental arthritis with stealth type polymeric nanoparticles encapsulating betamethasone phosphate. J Pharmacol Exp Ther 329(2): 412–417
71. Crielaard BJ et al (2012) Glucocorticoid-loaded core-cross-linked polymeric micelles with tailorable release kinetics for targeted therapy of rheumatoid arthritis. Angew Chem Int Ed Engl 51(29):7254–7258
72. Wilson DR et al (2014) Synthesis and evaluation of cyclosporine A-loaded polysialic acid-polycaprolactone micelles for rheumatoid arthritis. Eur J Pharm Sci 51:146–156
73. Quan L et al (2014) Nanomedicines for inflammatory arthritis: head-to-head comparison of glucocorticoid-containing polymers, micelles, and liposomes. ACS Nano 8(1): 458–466
74. Liu XM et al (2008) Synthesis and evaluation of a well-defined HPMA copolymer-dexamethasone conjugate for effective treatment of rheumatoid arthritis. Pharm Res 25(12):2910–2919
75. Quan LD et al (2010) Development of a macromolecular prodrug for the treatment of inflammatory arthritis: mechanisms involved in arthrotropism and sustained therapeutic efficacy. Arthritis Res Ther 12(5):R170
76. Liu XM et al (2010) Syntheses of click PEG-dexamethasone conjugates for the treatment of rheumatoid arthritis. Biomacromolecules 11(10):2621–2628
77. Wang D et al (2002) Inhibition of cathepsin K with lysosomotropic macromolecular inhibitors. Biochemistry 41(28):8849–8859
78. Lawrence RC et al (2008) Estimates of the prevalence of arthritis and other rheumatic conditions in the United States. Part II. Arthritis Rheum 58(1):26–35
79. Felson DT (2014) Osteoarthritis: priorities for osteoarthritis research: much to be done. Nat Rev Rheumatol 10:447
80. Gerwin N, Hops C, Lucke A (2006) Intraarticular drug delivery in osteoarthritis. Adv Drug Deliv Rev 58(2):226–242
81. Hinton R et al (2002) Osteoarthritis: diagnosis and therapeutic considerations. Am Fam Physician 65(5):841–848
82. Hochberg MC et al (1995) Guidelines for the medical management of osteoarthritis. Part II. Osteoarthritis of the knee. American College of Rheumatology. Arthritis Rheum 38(11):1541–1546
83. George E (1998) Intra-articular hyaluronan treatment for osteoarthritis. Ann Rheum Dis 57(11):637–640
84. Dingle JT et al (1978) Novel treatment for joint inflammation. Nature 271(5643): 372–373
85. Foong WC, Green KL (1988) Retention and distribution of liposome-entrapped [3H] methotrexate injected into normal or arthritic rabbit joints. J Pharm Pharmacol 40(7): 464–468
86. Holland TA, Mikos AG (2003) Advances in drug delivery for articular cartilage. J Control Release 86(1):1–14
87. Ratcliffe JH et al (1987) Albumin microspheres for intra-articular drug delivery: investigation of their retention in normal and arthritic knee joints of rabbits. J Pharm Pharmacol 39(4):290–295
88. Horisawa E et al (2002) Prolonged anti-inflammatory action of DL-lactide/glycolide copolymer nanospheres containing betamethasone sodium phosphate for an intra-articular delivery system in antigen-induced arthritic rabbit. Pharm Res 19(4):403–410
89. Brown KE et al (1998) Gelatin/chondroitin 6-sulfate microspheres for the delivery of therapeutic proteins to the joint. Arthritis Rheum 41(12):2185–2195
90. Iwasaki M, Soh M, Kaneko H (1991) Diagnosis, treatment and prophylaxis of catheter related sepsis. Nihon Rinsho 49(Suppl): 182–187
91. Holroyd C, Cooper C, Dennison E (2008) Epidemiology of osteoporosis. Best Pract Res Clin Endocrinol Metab 22(5):671–685

92. Burge R, Dawson-Hughes B, Solomon DH, Wong JB, King A, Tosteson A (2007) Incidence and economic burden of osteoporosis-related fractures in the United States, 2005–2025. J Bone Miner Res 22:465–475
93. Cenni E et al (2008) Biocompatibility of poly(D, L-lactide-co-glycolide) nanoparticles conjugated with alendronate. Biomaterials 29(10):1400–1411
94. Pignatello R et al (2009) A novel biomaterial for osteotropic drug nanocarriers: synthesis and biocompatibility evaluation of a PLGA-ALE conjugate. Nanomedicine (Lond) 4(2): 161–175
95. Wang D et al (2006) Pharmacokinetic and biodistribution studies of a bone-targeting drug delivery system based on N-(2-hydroxypropyl)methacrylamide copolymers. Mol Pharm 3(6):717–725
96. Zhang G et al (2012) A delivery system targeting bone formation surfaces to facilitate RNAi-based anabolic therapy. Nat Med 18(2):307–314
97. Sang Yoo H, Gwan Park T (2004) Biodegradable nanoparticles containing protein-fatty acid complexes for oral delivery of salmon calcitonin. J Pharm Sci 93(2): 488–495
98. Narayanan D et al (2013) In vitro and in vivo evaluation of osteoporosis therapeutic peptide PTH 1-34 loaded PEGylated chitosan nanoparticles. Mol Pharm 10(11):4159–4167
99. Takeuchi H et al (2003) Mucoadhesive properties of carbopol or chitosan-coated liposomes and their effectiveness in the oral administration of calcitonin to rats. J Control Release 86(2-3):235–242
100. Lamprecht A et al (2004) pH-sensitive microsphere delivery increases oral bioavailability of calcitonin. J Control Release 98(1):1–9
101. Narayanan D et al (2014) PTH 1-34 loaded thiolated chitosan nanoparticles for osteoporosis: oral bioavailability and anabolic effect on primary osteoblast cells. J Biomed Nanotechnol 10(1):166–178
102. Saini D, Fazil M, Ali MM, Baboota S, Ali J (2015) Formulation, development and optimization of raloxifeneloaded chitosan nanoparticles for treatment of osteoporosis. Drug Deliv 22:1–14. [Epub ahead of print]
103. Fazil M et al (2013) Exploring drug delivery systems for treating osteoporosis. Expert Opin Drug Deliv 10(8):1123–1136
104. Low SA, Kopecek J (2012) Targeting polymer therapeutics to bone. Adv Drug Deliv Rev 64(12):1189–1204
105. Society AC (2008) Cancer facts and figures 2008. American Cancer Society. Retrieved on March 13, 2008
106. Hughes DP (2009) Strategies for the targeted delivery of therapeutics for osteosarcoma. Expert Opin Drug Deliv 6(12):1311–1321
107. Gabizon A, Martin F (1997) Polyethylene glycol-coated (pegylated) liposomal doxorubicin. Rationale for use in solid tumours. Drugs 54(Suppl 4):15–21
108. Alberts DS, Garcia DJ (1997) Safety aspects of pegylated liposomal doxorubicin in patients with cancer. Drugs 54(Suppl 4):30–35
109. Skubitz KM (2003) Phase II trial of pegylated-liposomal doxorubicin (Doxil) in sarcoma. Cancer Invest 21(2):167–176
110. Judson I et al (2001) Randomised phase II trial of pegylated liposomal doxorubicin (DOXIL/CAELYX) versus doxorubicin in the treatment of advanced or metastatic soft tissue sarcoma: a study by the EORTC Soft Tissue and Bone Sarcoma Group. Eur J Cancer 37(7):870–877
111. Kamba SA et al (2013) In vitro delivery and controlled release of Doxorubicin for targeting osteosarcoma bone cancer. Molecules 18(9):10580–10598
112. Susa M et al (2009) Doxorubicin loaded Polymeric Nanoparticulate Delivery System to overcome drug resistance in osteosarcoma. BMC Cancer 9:399
113. Federman N et al (2012) Enhanced growth inhibition of osteosarcoma by cytotoxic polymerized liposomal nanoparticles targeting the alcam cell surface receptor. Sarcoma 2012:126906
114. Coleman RE (2006) Clinical features of metastatic bone disease and risk of skeletal morbidity. Clin Cancer Res 12(20 Pt 2): 6243s–6249s
115. Guise T (2010) Examining the metastatic niche: targeting the microenvironment. Semin Oncol 37(Suppl 2):S2–S14
116. Clezardin P, Benzaid I, Croucher PI (2011) Bisphosphonates in preclinical bone oncology. Bone 49(1):66–70
117. Coleman R (2011) The use of bisphosphonates in cancer treatment. Ann N Y Acad Sci 1218:3–14
118. Gnant M (2009) Bisphosphonates in the prevention of disease recurrence: current results and ongoing trials. Curr Cancer Drug Targets 9(7):824–833
119. Coleman RE, McCloskey EV (2011) Bisphosphonates in oncology. Bone 49(1): 71–76

120. Ramanlal Chaudhari K et al (2012) Bone metastasis targeting: a novel approach to reach bone using Zoledronate anchored PLGA nanoparticle as carrier system loaded with Docetaxel. J Control Release 158(3):470–478
121. Miller K et al (2009) Targeting bone metastases with a bispecific anticancer and antiangiogenic polymer-alendronate-taxane conjugate. Angew Chem Int Ed Engl 48(16): 2949–2954
122. Miller K et al (2011) Antiangiogenic antitumor activity of HPMA copolymer-paclitaxel-alendronate conjugate on breast cancer bone metastasis mouse model. Mol Pharm 8(4): 1052–1062
123. Daubine F et al (2009) Nanostructured polyelectrolyte multilayer drug delivery systems for bone metastasis prevention. Biomaterials 30(31):6367–6373
124. Wang D et al (2007) Osteotropic Peptide that differentiates functional domains of the skeleton. Bioconjug Chem 18(5):1375–1378
125. Gogia JS et al (2009) Local antibiotic therapy in osteomyelitis. Semin Plast Surg 23(2): 100–107
126. Diana Gomes MP, Bettencourt AF (2013) Osteomyelitis: an overview of antimicrobial therapy. Braz J Pharm Sci 49(1):13–27
127. Verhelle N et al (2003) How to deal with bone exposure and osteomyelitis: an overview. Acta Orthop Belg 69(6):481–494
128. Lang S (1996) Osteomyelitis. A pathomorphologic overview. Radiologe 36(10):781–785
129. Mouzopoulos G et al (2011) Management of bone infections in adults: the surgeon's and microbiologist's perspectives. Injury 42(Suppl 5):S18–S23
130. Kanellakopoulou K, Giamarellos-Bourboulis EJ (2000) Carrier systems for the local delivery of antibiotics in bone infections. Drugs 59(6):1223–1232
131. Holtom PD, Patzakis MJ (2003) Newer methods of antimicrobial delivery for bone and joint infections. Instr Course Lect 52:745–749
132. Nelson CL et al (1992) In vitro elution characteristics of commercially and noncommercially prepared antibiotic PMMA beads. Clin Orthop Relat Res 284:303–309
133. Mader JT, Calhoun J, Cobos J (1997) In vitro evaluation of antibiotic diffusion from antibiotic-impregnated biodegradable beads and polymethylmethacrylate beads. Antimicrob Agents Chemother 41(2):415–418
134. Gitelis S, Brebach GT (2002) The treatment of chronic osteomyelitis with a biodegradable antibiotic-impregnated implant. J Orthop Surg (Hong Kong) 10(1):53–60
135. Desai TA, Uskokovic V (2013) Calcium phosphate nanoparticles: a future therapeutic platform for the treatment of osteomyelitis? Ther Deliv 4(6):643–645
136. Singh N et al (2009) NanoGenotoxicology: the DNA damaging potential of engineered nanomaterials. Biomaterials 30(23-24):3891–3914
137. Uskokovic V, Desai TA (2013) Phase composition control of calcium phosphate nanoparticles for tunable drug delivery kinetics and treatment of osteomyelitis. II. Antibacterial and osteoblastic response. J Biomed Mater Res A 101(5):1427–1436
138. Uskokovic V, Desai TA (2013) Phase composition control of calcium phosphate nanoparticles for tunable drug delivery kinetics and treatment of osteomyelitis. I. Preparation and drug release. J Biomed Mater Res A 101(5):1416–1426
139. Uskokovic V et al (2013) Effect of calcium phosphate particle shape and size on their antibacterial and osteogenic activity in the delivery of antibiotics in vitro. ACS Appl Mater Interfaces 5(7):2422–2431
140. Uskokovic V et al (2013) Osteogenic and antimicrobial nanoparticulate calcium phosphate and poly-(D, L-lactide-co-glycolide) powders for the treatment of osteomyelitis. Mater Sci Eng C Mater Biol Appl 33(6):3362–3373
141. Fang T et al (2012) Poly (epsilon-caprolactone) coating delays vancomycin delivery from porous chitosan/beta-tricalcium phosphate composites. J Biomed Mater Res B Appl Biomater 100(7):1803–1811
142. Samit Kumar Nandi PM, Roy S, Kundu B, De Kumar D, Basu D (2009) Local antibiotic delivery systems for the treatment of osteomyelitis – a review. Mater Sci Eng C 29(8):2478–2485
143. Oldham JB et al (2000) Biological activity of rhBMP-2 released from PLGA microspheres. J Biomech Eng 122(3):289–292
144. Cao L et al (2014) Vascularization and bone regeneration in a critical sized defect using 2-N,6-O-sulfated chitosan nanoparticles incorporating BMP-2. Biomaterials 35(2): 684–698
145. Raftery R, O'Brien FJ, Cryan SA (2013) Chitosan for gene delivery and orthopedic tissue engineering applications. Molecules 18(5):5611–5647
146. Gentile P et al (2014) An overview of poly(lactic-co-glycolic) acid (PLGA)-based

biomaterials for bone tissue engineering. Int J Mol Sci 15(3):3640–3659
147. Puppi D et al (2011) Optimized electro- and wet-spinning techniques for the production of polymeric fibrous scaffolds loaded with bisphosphonate and hydroxyapatite. J Tissue Eng Regen Med 5(4):253–263
148. Nie H, Wang CH (2007) Fabrication and characterization of PLGA/HAp composite scaffolds for delivery of BMP-2 plasmid DNA. J Control Release 120(1-2):111–121
149. Mouthuy PA et al (2010) Physico-chemical characterization of functional electrospun scaffolds for bone and cartilage tissue engineering. Proc Inst Mech Eng H 224(12):1401–1414
150. Lin G et al (2012) Injectable and thermosensitive PLGA-g-PEG hydrogels containing hydroxyapatite: preparation, characterization and in vitro release behavior. Biomed Mater 7(2):024107
151. Lee TJ et al (2010) Apatite-coated porous poly(lactic-co-glycolic acid) microspheres as an injectable bone substitute. J Biomater Sci Polym Ed 21(5):635–645
152. Shi X et al (2009) Enhancing alendronate release from a novel PLGA/hydroxyapatite microspheric system for bone repairing applications. Pharm Res 26(2):422–430
153. Wang Q et al (2013) Hybrid hydroxyapatite nanoparticle colloidal gels are injectable fillers for bone tissue engineering. Tissue Eng Part A 19(23-24):2586–2593
154. Yao Y, Shi X, Chen F (2014) The effect of gold nanoparticles on the proliferation and differentiation of murine osteoblast: a study of MC3T3-E1 cells in vitro. J Nanosci Nanotechnol 14(7):4851–4857
155. Rose FR, Hou Q, Oreffo RO (2004) Delivery systems for bone growth factors - the new players in skeletal regeneration. J Pharm Pharmacol 56(4):415–427
156. Nguyen LT, Min YK, Lee BT (2015) Nanoparticle biphasic calcium phosphate loading on gelatin-pectin scaffold for improved bone regeneration. Tissue Eng Part A 21:1376
157. Hu J et al (2014) Effect of nano-hydroxyapatite coating on the osteoinductivity of porous biphasic calcium phosphate ceramics. BMC Musculoskelet Disord 15:114
158. Kawazoe N, Chen G, Tateishi T (2008) Development of novel biomaterials for bone and cartilage tissue engineering. Clin Calcium 18(12):1713–1720
159. Zhou YN, Xia LG, Xu YJ (2014) Research progress of nano-hydroxyapatite complexes in bone tissue regeneration. Shanghai Kou Qiang Yi Xue 23(2):248–252
160. Matassi F et al (2011) New biomaterials for bone regeneration. Clin Cases Miner Bone Metab 8(1):21–24
161. Perez-Sanchez MJ et al (2010) Biomaterials for bone regeneration. Med Oral Patol Oral Cir Bucal 15(3):e517–e522
162. Allo BA et al (2012) Bioactive and biodegradable nanocomposites and hybrid biomaterials for bone regeneration. J Funct Biomater 3(2): 432–463

Chapter 21

Synthetic Polymeric Nanoparticles for Immunomodulation

Jiaying Liu, Pallab Pradhan, and Krishnendu Roy

Abstract

Synthetic polymeric nanoparticles have gained tremendous attention since the beginning of this century. Their tunable size, shape, and surface properties make them efficient carriers and delivery systems for a vast cohort of drugs into the body, including peptides, proteins, lipid, and nucleic acids. Also, because of their unique and tunable biochemical properties, polymeric nanoparticles are able to modulate immune responses in vivo, either by themselves as adjuvant, or by presenting antigens and/or co-stimulatory/inhibitory signals to the immune system. Therefore, intensive efforts are being devoted to investigating and applying synthetic polymeric nanoparticles in vaccine development and immunotherapy for cancer, infectious diseases and autoimmune disorders. In this book chapter, we first introduce the main targets of particulate systems for immunomodulation, then talk about the factors that influence their function and performance in immunotherapy and lastly discuss the strategies that are currently in use or under investigation to treat immune diseases using synthetic polymeric nanoparticles.

Key words Nanoparticles, Immune response, Vaccine, Immunomodulation, Cancer, Autoimmunity

1 Introduction

Over the past few decades, nanoscale particles synthesized using polymers, lipids, or both have shown great promise in vaccine development and immunotherapy for cancer, infectious and autoimmune diseases. These nanoparticles are usually synthesized using a wide variety of self-assembly and polymerization techniques [1]. Due to their small size and tailored biochemical and surface properties, they can be designed to penetrate physiological barriers and deliver various immunomodulatory molecules (e.g., antigens, adjuvants, immune-evasion molecules) to target organs, tissues, or cells. In this chapter, we focus our attention to polymer-based nanoparticles and briefly introduce the key players of the immune system, crucial factors that influence the performance of engineered particles, and the advances in the design and application of these particles in manipulating innate and adaptive immune responses against various illnesses such as cancer, infectious diseases, and autoimmune disorders.

Zheng-Rong Lu and Shinji Sakuma (eds.), *Nanomaterials in Pharmacology*, Methods in Pharmacology and Toxicology,
DOI 10.1007/978-1-4939-3121-7_21,

1.1 Key Players of Immune System

Our immune system is composed of a complex network of organs and cells, which are critical in the maintenance of physiological homeostasis and act as guards against infectious microbes and the development of tumors or autoimmune diseases. The organs involved are called lymphoid organs, which include primary lymphoid organs, e.g., the thymus and bone marrow, and secondary lymphoid organs, e.g., the spleen, nasal-associated lymphoid tissue, Peyer's patches in the gut, and lymph nodes. The primary lymphoid organs give birth to the immune cells and the secondary ones further provide the cells with appropriate niches to mature and conduct their functions. Immune cells can also be broadly divided into two parts, i.e., innate immune cells (such as macrophages, dendritic cells, neutrophils, and natural killer cells), and the adaptive immune cells (e.g., T cells and B cells) [2]. The former group of cells forms the first set of defense to protect the body from infections at the entry site, i.e., the mucosal surfaces, blood and the skin. The latter group of cells, which mostly reside in the lymphoid organs or tissues, react more slowly with the help of the first group to recognize invading infectious agents (e.g., bacteria or virus) or malignant cells (tumor cells). They would then differentiate into effector cells, which either secrete antibodies to prevent the extracellular pathogen from damaging organs/tissues or kill the cells with intracellular pathogen by cytolytic granules. T and B cells are also able to differentiate into long-lived memory cells that provide faster and stronger protection when the body is exposed to the same pathogen again [3]. On the other hand, dendritic cells, a specialized antigen presenting cell (APC), bridges innate and adaptive immune responses and thus plays a key role in setting up immune responses against pathogens as well as malignant cells [3–5]. Dendritic cells drive T cell activation through three types of signals, i.e., antigens, co-modulatory signals, and cytokines. Absence of the co-modulatory molecules on DCs results in T cell anergy or apoptosis, while presence of co-stimulatory signaling (e.g., CD28/CD86) induces T cell activation and elicits antigen-specific immune responses [4, 5] (Fig. 1). Alternatively, inhibitory signaling, including cell surface receptor-ligands interaction (e.g., PD-1/PD-L1, CTLA-4/CD80) and anti-inflammatory cytokines, prevents the onset of autoimmune diseases and/or triggers immune tolerance by inhibition of T cell activation and directing naïve T cells to differentiate into regulatory T cells [6, 7].

1.2 Cellular and Tissue Targets for Immunotherapy

Antigen-presenting cells (APCs), including dendritic cells, macrophages, and B cells, are the most common targets for immunotherapy. They express a myriad of surface receptors that are capable of recognizing and internalizing antigens from various sources. Among all the different types of APCs, dendritic cells are the most specialized and potent modulator of the immune responses and thus are a promising target in immunotherapy [8]. Immature dendritic

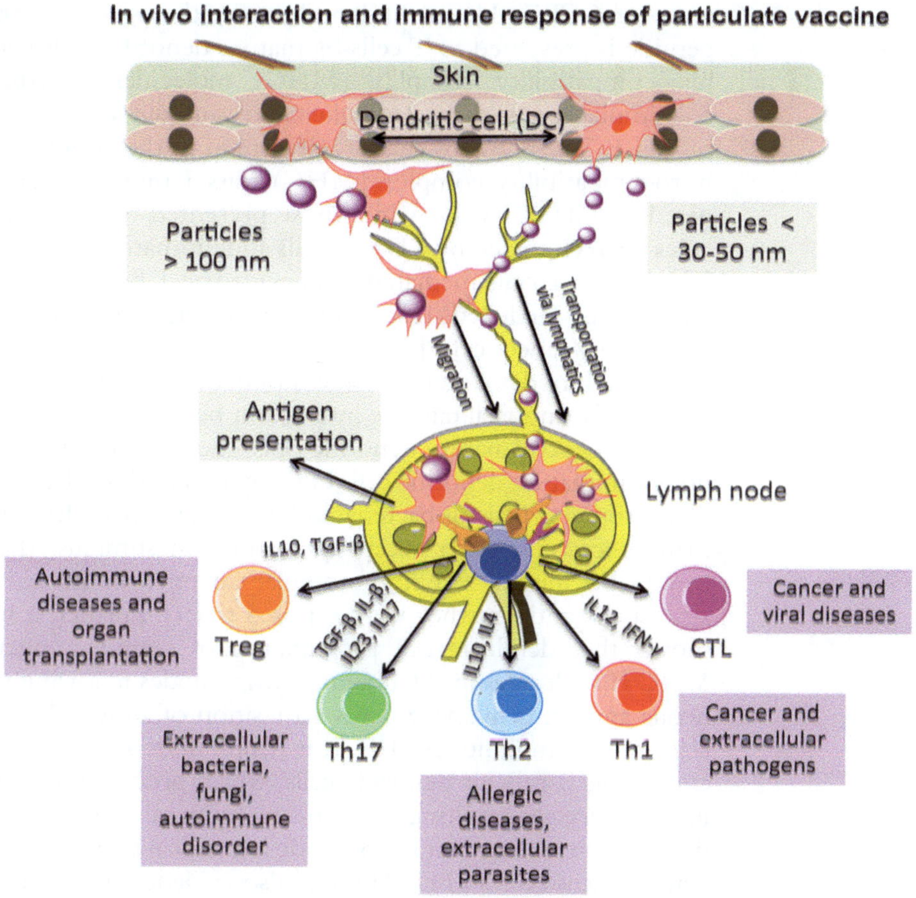

Fig. 1 In vivo interaction and immune responses of particulate vaccines. Upon administration into body through skin (commonly via s.c. injection), the particulate vaccines encounter and are recognized by the resident DCs. They are most likely to be internalized by the encountered cells through receptor-mediated endocytosis. The immature DC patrolling in the tissues are then activated through TLR pathway or other signaling pathways induced by the antigen or adjuvant molecules incorporated on the nanoparticles. Activated DCs will undergo maturation and migrate into local lymph nodes, where they present antigens (first signal) or the costimulatory molecules (second signal) to naïve T cells and guide them to differentiate into effector T cells that are capable of generating various types of antigen-specific immune response (T_H1, T_H2, T_H17. etc.) against intracellular or extracellular pathogens. The interaction between DCs and T cells happens in the context of peptide/major histocompatibility complex (MHC) molecules and can be enhanced by cross-presentation mediated by particulate vaccines. However, in the circumstances of autoimmune diseases, the signals that are delivered by nanoparticles and presented by DCs are usually inhibitory molecules that result in Treg stimulation and T cell anergy. All the immune responses are significantly influenced by the cytokine milieu in the microenvironment, which can also be modulated by the administered particulate vaccines

cells patrol the bloodstream, skin and tissue, sampling for potential risk of infection. In most cases, they present self-antigens to T cells without co-stimulatory molecules in order to maintain self-tolerance. But upon activation by pathogenic or endogenous danger signals and/or adjuvants, they mature and migrate into lymph nodes, an active process facilitated by upregulation of the chemokine receptor CCR7 [1]. In the lymph node, the processed antigenic peptide is presented to T cells by mature dendritic cells (on major histocompatibility complex (MHC) molecules together with co-stimulatory signals) to elicit an antigen-specific immune response. The antigens that are presented in the context of major histocompatibility complex (MHC) class I molecules are recognized by $CD8^+$ T cells, while those presented by MHC II molecules are recognized by $CD4^+$ T cells and ultimately results in T_H1/T_H2 ($CD4^+$ T cells mediated) and cytotoxic T lymphocytic (CTL, $CD8^+$ T cell mediated) responses against intracellular/extracellular pathogens/cancer cells [3, 4] (Fig. 1).

Lymph nodes contain a large number of dendritic cells, B cells, and T cells, and facilitate the interaction between T cells and APCs (Fig. 1). Besides mature dendritic cells, there is also a large population of immature dendritic cells in the lymph nodes. They are better at macropinocytosis of bacteria and larger sized particles (>0.5 μm) than other cells. After receiving maturation stimulus, these cells could also initiate significant cellular adaptive immune response against the antigens they were exposed to [9]. Further, it has been shown that dendritic cell presentation of peptide-antigens with MHC II molecules in the draining lymph nodes following subcutaneous antigen delivery requires acquisition of antigen by dendritic cells in the lymph nodes [10]. It is lymph node B cells, rather than circulating B cells or dendritic cells, which process antigens in the follicles directly resulting in a strong humoral immune response; thus demonstrating that lymph node is a critical target for antibody-generating vaccines [11]. There is also evidence that lymph nodes play a critical role in tolerogenesis, which is important for immunomodulatory therapies against cancer and autoimmune diseases.

Furthermore, epithelial tissues in general can also be targets for immunotherapies because of their strong immuno-surveillance ability. The Langerhans cells and macrophages inside these tissues are all able to recognize multiple types of antigens and induce immune responses (Fig. 1). The mucosal epithelia are another good choice since they encounter a vast number of microorganisms every day and protect the body with specialized humoral response via secretory IgA. Compared to intramuscular injection, vaccination via mucosal routes can induce stronger mucosal immunity in a region-specific manner [12].

1.3 Cytokine and Chemokine Targets in Immunotherapy

The immune response elicited by an antigen is subject to a myriad of factors, among which cytokines and chemokines are of the critical importance. In a microenvironment with different types of cytokines and co-stimulatory molecules, the immune response generated by activated dendritic cells can be driven to different directions, i.e., T_H1-, T_H2-, and T_H17-immune response (Fig. 1). For instance, IL-6 and IL-23 together stimulate naïve $CD4^+$ T cells to differentiate into T_H-17 cells, whereas IL-12, enhanced by IFNγ and CCL3, 4, and 5, promotes T_H1 cell activation. But when T_H1

response occurs, T_H2 and T_H17 cells are inactivated by IFNγ, and the production of tumor-necrosis factorα (TNFα) as well as IL-2 and lymphotoxinα secreted by T_H1 cells can drive B cells to differentiate into opsonizing-antibody-producing plasma cells [1, 4, 7]. On the other hand, anti-inflammatory stimuli, such as IL-4, IL-10, and transforming growth factor β-1(TGFβ1), can drive DCs and macrophages to an alternative activation phenotype rather than an inflammatory phenotype. IL-4 also promotes the expression of CCL17 and CCL22 to recruit inducible ($FoxP3^+$) regulatory T (Treg) cells during tolerogenesis [13]. Treg cells continue to secrete TGFβ1 and IL-10, both of which inhibit T_H1 cell function and suppress the inflammatory response. Hence, vaccines and immunotherapies aiming to deliver or eliminate specific cytokines may have great impact on the immune response.

2 Particulate Immunotherapy

Traditional vaccines are derived from live-attenuated or inactivated whole microorganisms that have strong immunogenicity but are not absolutely safe. During the past several decades, vaccine development efforts have involved recombinant DNA and protein-based vaccines where protein/peptide antigens (or plasmid DNA encoding for those antigens) from those pathogenic microorganisms are used instead of the organism as a whole. However, purified antigens lack the co-stimulatory/adjuvant signals responsible for priming of immune cells, are poor at penetrating tissue barriers, not resistant to enzymes inside human bodies if administered systematically, and thus fail to enhance the antibody and cell-mediated immune response to the extent needed for fighting against diseases. Therefore, significant effort has been put into developing biocompatible carrier systems to either encapsulate or attach the antigen and/or co-stimulatory molecules (adjuvants) to an engineered particle and target it to the site of interest for eliciting a desired antigen-specific immune response (Table 1). In the case of delivering antigens to APCs, nanoparticles, such as those made from poly (lactic-co-glycolic) acid (PLGA), have been reported to have adjuvant properties that can enhance the immune responses against certain antigens [14]. These particulate systems should be able to cross biological barriers and accumulate at the peripheral or lymphoid organs, interact with APCs, direct the immune response towards T_H1 cell response for viral, protozoal and fungal infections as well as cancer, or T_H2 for extracellular pathogens, allergies and helminthic diseases, or induce proliferation and activation of Treg cell response for autoimmune disorders (Fig. 1) [15].

2.1 Rational Design of Particulate Immunotherapy Strategies

The success of immunotherapy relies on the rational design of the particulate system in order to provide sufficient and efficient biological cues for the body to manipulate the direction, strength and duration of the immune response. Rational design refers to the

Table 1
Polymeric nano-sized particulate vaccine

Delivery system	Size (nm)	Adjuvant/Antigen	Study design	Animals	Routes	Outcomes	Reference
PLGA NP	100–400	LPS + OVA	In Vitro	–	–	Stimulation of inflammasome and a $CD8^+$ T cell response	[118]
			Preclinical	C57BL/6 mice	s.c.	Increase in OVA-specific IgG humoral response and IFNγ secretion compared to OVA-nanoparticle group	[118]
PLGA Nanospheres	290,307.9	CpG ODNs + TT	Ex Vivo	–	–	Strong antigen-specific T cell proliferation; Higher levels of interferon γ secretion	[119]
			Preclinical	C57BL/6 mice	s.c.	Higher IgG2b, IgG1, IgG3, IgG titers; Induction of both T_H1 and T_H2 immune responses with bias towards T_H1 type compared to nanosphere-TT alone group	[119]
PLGA NP	200	Poly I:C + R848+ DC-SIGN–specific humanized Abs	In Vitro	–	–	>100-fold more effective induction of CD80 and CD83 expression on human DCs, indicating DC maturation and activation compared to NP-Isotype-TLRL group; Enhanced expression of CTL marker perforin and granzyme B in T cells, suggesting primed $CD8^+$ T cell responses	[71]
			Preclinical	C57Bl/6J mice	i.v.	High levels of IFN-γ and enhanced $CD4^+$ T-cell proliferation and activation are detected; Significant CTL responses were induced in an Ag-dependent manner	[71]
PLGA NP	200–250	Hp91 peptide	In Vitro	–	–	Induction of the secretion of inflammatory cytokines, such IL-6, by DCs; Induction of the expression of CD40, CD80 and MHCII, indicating the phenotypic maturation of BM-DCs; Increased activation of human-DCs and mouse BM-DCs	[120]

PLGA NP	350–410	TRP2 + 7-acyl lipid A	Preclinical	C57BL/6 mice bearing melanoma B16 tumors	s.c.	Induction of therapeutic antitumor effect; Activation of TRP2 specific CD8 T cells capable of IFNγ secretion, Increased level of pro-inflammatory cytokines	[121]
PLGA-CM-TMC NP	~400	BSA–/+IMQ	Preclinical	B6D2F1/J mice	s.c./i.n	Induced a high level of IgG specific for BSA, Addition of IMQ only leads to local adjuvant effects without inducing systemic cytokines	[122]
alginate-PLGA/ Chitosan-PLGA NP	208.1 ± 7.6/ 400.1 ± 13.9	Ac-PLP-BPI-NH_2	Preclinical	SJL/J mice	s.c.	Suppressed and delayed onset of EAE, lower secretion levels of IL-6 and IL-17, suggesting immune response shifted away from T_H17	[123]
PLA NP	500–800	HIV p24 protein	Preclinical	Balb/c mice	s.c.	AMOMKLETI-peptide specific IFN-γ was promoted and IL-2 and IL-6 secretion were increased; Better antibody responses were developed	[57]
				New Zealand White rabbits	s.c.	Lower antibody titers were generated by the PLA group compared to the Freund positive control (both with p24)	[57]
				adult male cynomolgus macaques	s.c.	Considerable levels of IFN-γ secreting T cells were detected	[57]
Folate conjugated and β-cyclodextrin linked PEI NP	100	IL-2 plasmid	Preclinical	C57/BL6 mice	s.c.	Increased secretion of T_H1, T_H2 and T_H17 cytokines; Stimulated activation of $CD8^+$ and $CD4^+$ T cells; Increased density of tumor-infiltrating T cells and NK cells; Reduced tumor growth and prolonged survival of the tumor-bearing mice	[75]
PLL coated polystyrene NP	50 nm	OVA	Preclinical	C57/BL6 mice	i.p.	Induction of high levels of CD8 T cells and OVA-specific antibodies	[124]
Alginate coated chitosan NP	643 ± 171.7 nm	HBsAg + CpG ODNs	Preclinical	BALB/cAnNHsd mice	s.c.	IgG2a/IgG1 ratio increased and IFNγ production by the splenocytes were stimulated	[125]

LPS: Lipopolysaccharide, a type of endotoxin, found in the outer membrane of Gram-negative bacteria, CpG: –C–phosphate–G–, TLR-9 agonist, TT: tetanus toxoid, EAE: Experimental autoimmune encephalomyelitis, TRP2: tyrosinase-related protein 2, 7-acyl lipid A: TLR 4 agonist, Poly I:C: TLR3 agonist, PEI: polyethylenimine, TMC/TPP: *N*-trimethyl chitosan (TMC) cross-linked with tripolyphosphate (TPP), CM-TMC: O-Carboxymethylation of TMC35, IMQ: a hydrophobic TLR7 ligand, QD: quantum dot, PLP-BPI: proteolipid protein bifunctional peptide inhibitors, PLL: poly-L-lysine, R848: resiquimod, TLR7/8 ligand, DC-SIGN–specific humanized Abs: targeting ligands to DCs

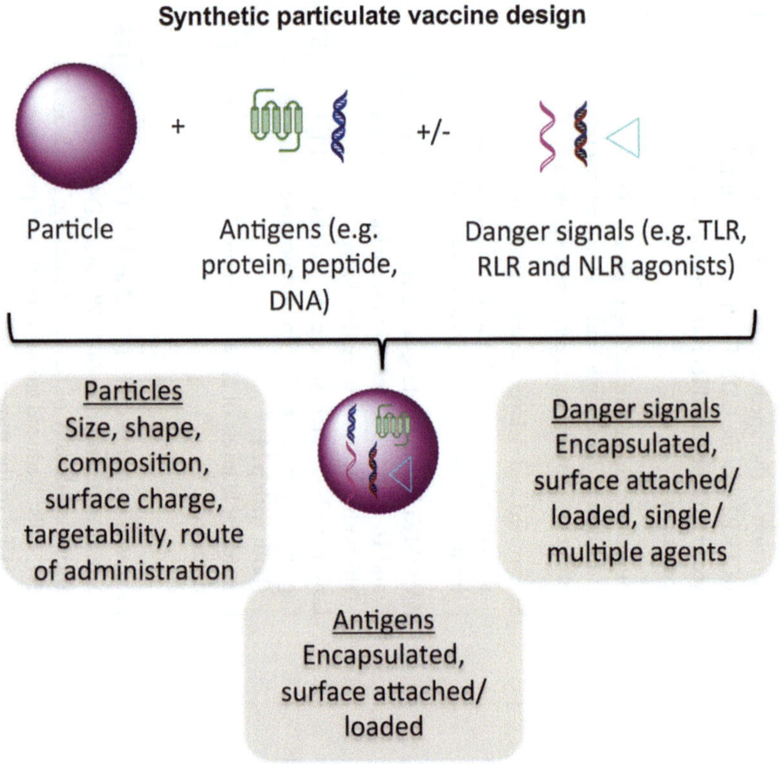

Fig. 2 Synthetic particle vaccine design. Particulate vaccines are usually composed of synthetic particles and antigens (e.g., protein, peptide, or plasmid DNA) encapsulated inside or attached to the surface of the particles. To mimic infectious pathogens and/or enhance the immunomodulation effect, danger signals, such as TLR ligands, can also be incorporated into the particulate systems via surface loading or encapsulation. The therapeutic efficacy of particulate vaccine are significantly influenced by various factors, including the antigens and danger signals they deliver and some important inherent particle characteristics, such as size, shape, composition, and surface properties.

biological, chemical and biophysical properties of the system endowed by fabrication methods, size, geometry, surface and structural properties of nanoparticles (Fig. 2). Moreover, the route of administration will also affect the outcome of immunotherapy using particulate systems.

2.1.1 Fabrication Methods

There are various methods of fabricating nanoparticles. Among them, emulsion polymerization, self-assembly and branched-polymer synthesis are the three most widely used fabrication methods for the generation of small organic nanoparticles in the immunotherapy research field [1], while single- or double emulsion solvent evaporation/extraction type methods as well as complex coacervation between oppositely charged polymers are used to fabricate both nano-sized and micro-sized particles [16–22]. Emulsion polymerization is mainly applied to the formation of surfactant micelles with amphiphilic polymers, e.g., block-copolymers like Pluronics [23]. Generally, these micelles are formed in an aqueous environment with the hydrophobic part inside. The DNA/RNA, peptide-antigen, cytokines and/or other adjuvants can either be encapsulated inside the core of the polymer particles during the polymerization or chemically conjugated outside to the hydrophilic corona [24]. Besides, nanoparticles can also be prepared via single- or double emulsion. Briefly, polymers are usually first emulsified in an organic phase with surfactant or stabilizers, and hydrophobic or hydrophilic cargos are dissolved in either an organic (hydrophobic) or aqueous (hydrophilic) phase. Finally, the polymer/drug emulsion is added to a aqueous phase to form particles [16]. After evaporation of the solvent and particle washing, products are collected by centrifugation or filtration, lyophilized and can be stored for a long period [16, 25]. It is reported that high intensity sonication or homogenization that forms the first emulsion as well as the solvent evaporation and polymer precipitation steps can significantly influence particle morphology, encapsulation and release behaviors [25]. PLGA particulate delivery of antigens prepared through double emulsion has been shown to dramatically enhance cross-presentation of exogenous antigens after endosomal escape compared to other antigen forms (e.g., soluble or latex-bead attached) [26]. A more recent study using lipids as surfactant in double emulsion reported increased loading efficiency of hydrophilic antigenic peptides (hgp100 and p15E) in PLGA nanoparticles (compared to PVA emulsions), high uptake by APC and strong antigen-specific T cell responses which resulted in tumor growth suppression in C57/BL6 mice [27]. Kasturi et al. reported encapsulation of various TLR4 and TLR 7 ligands as well as antigen into PLGA nanoparticles using single and double emulsion methods and demonstrated that the co-delivery of TLR4 and TLR7 ligands along with antigen in nanoparticles synergistically enhanced antigen specific, neutralizing antibody with long lived plasma cell response in mice and further showed immune protection against lethal avian and swine influenza virus challenges in mice and pandemic H1N1 influenza challenge in rhesus macaques [22]. Self-assembly is similar to emulsion but utilizes the difference of solubility of the hydrophobic and hydrophilic part of block-co-polymer in different solvents. Typically, amphiphilic co-polymers are first dissolved in a suitable medium (usually organic solvent) and then forced to form micelles by dropping the solution into water. Because of the inherent unstable nature of the self-assembled micelles, they tend to disassemble after injection into the body. The molecular weight, melting temperature and glass-transition temperature are three main parameters crucial for controlling the equilibrium nature and dissociation rate of the self-assembly process and thus need to be considered in order to improve the design of self-assembly particulate systems [1, 28].

In addition to the three above-mentioned methods, coacervation, which is based on phase separation, is another efficient way to make nanoparticles. Simple coacervation utilizes competition between a more hydrophilic substance or concentration and the original liquid phase for the desolvation of the more colloidal material, while in complex coacervation, polyelectrolytes with opposite charges are complexed together into solid precipitate in a liquid phase at a certain pH [17]. Complex coacervation can also be applied to complexation of polyelectrolytes with proteins or genes, which renders it promising candidate for antigen/adjuvant delivery [17, 18, 29]. It has been reported that the encapsulation efficiencies of IL-12 plasmid DNA by chitosan nanoparticles via complex coacervation were high (73–95 %) and thus led to improved transfection and expression in CT-26 colon carcinoma cells [30, 31]. Roy et al. prepared chitosan-pDNA nanoparticles of 150–300 nm size by complex coacervation using pDNA encoding dominant peanut allergen gene (pCMVArah2) and showed that the oral delivery of these nanoparticles were able to protect against peanut allergen induced anaphylaxis in a murine model of peanut allergy [18]. Parallel to coacervation, phase separation can also be induced by temperature changes or competition for solvent between two nonsolvent organic polymers. These methods are widely applied in the encapsulation of drugs into particles as well [32].

Unlike all other mentioned techniques, branched polymer synthesis is a step-wise strategy starting from a core molecule and growing branches by covalent bonds formation. In this context, dendrimers outweigh other nanoparticles in terms of narrow size distributions and easily tunable surface characteristics. And with each step, the number of branch terminal groups doubles, which provides far more reaction spaces for drug and gene delivery, indicating great potential for its application in vaccine development and immunotherapy. However, amino terminated dendrimers exhibit high generation dependent cytotoxicity due to destructive interaction with cellular membranes [3, 33]. The nondegradable dendrimers can also cause tissue toxicity because of high levels of deposition in the organs (e.g., liver and kidney) before renal excretion, and thus increasing the chance of material-induced inflammation and activation of the complement system [34].

2.1.2 Particle Size and Shape

Size and shape of particles play critical roles in immunomodulation by targeting various immune cells or tissues or organs. Larger nanoparticles are more prone to be phagocytosed by macrophages than their smaller counterparts. Polystyrene particles as large as 1.0 μm in diameter can be easily phagocytosed [35]. And it has been shown that the phagocytic index (particle number per cell) of PEG5000-PHDCA particle increased as the size grew from 80 to 240 nm [36]. On the other hand, small particles (20–40 nm in diameter) can cross tissue barriers, get to the lymph nodes directly via lymphatics and are taken up by the resident DCs more easily [37, 38]. For what little that survives and arrives at the target tissue, size, together with other physical and chemical properties of the particle, also affects how the particles behave inside the tissue and enter the cells. It has been shown that particles between 20 and 100 nm in size (diameter) were most efficiently taken up by LN resident DCs [38]. Another study also demonstrated that 25 nm poly(propylene sulfide) (PPS) nanoparticles are better at entering DCs and promoting T cell expansion [23]. Interestingly, the inflammatory activity by dendritic cells as characterized by IL-1β secretion in response to particle treatment reached maximum when particle sizes were between 400 and 1000 nm [39]. Size of nanoparticles was reported to influence the T_H1/T_H2 balance as well. Larger particles, e.g., 500 nm PLGA, 100 nm nanoemulsions and 95 nm PEG-PHDA, tend to induce the T_H1 responses, while smaller ones, such as 5 nm G5 PAMAM dendrimers, were more associated with T_H2 response [14, 40–43]. And it is also asserted in some studies that small (<100 nm) polystyrene particles elicit stronger CD8 and CD4 type 1T-cell responses, like virus, but less antibody response than larger ones which invoke more bacteria-like responses (>500 nm) [38, 44].

Besides size, particle shape also influences in vivo biodistribution, phagocytosis and subcellular fate as well as the immunological effect of the particles [45–48]. Geng et al. reported that filomicelles stayed in circulation ten times longer than spherical PEGylated "stealth" nanovesicles in rodents after intravenous injection, with a strong dependence on length and more interaction with the lung than spleen [49]. And it was shown in another study that local particle shape determined whether macrophages initiate phagocytosis by altering the complexity of the actin structures, while particle size was primarily involved in the completion of internalization, especially when the particle volume was similar or larger than the cells [47]. Studies have also demonstrated that the internalization was highly cell type-specific as well as shape-dependent. For anionic nanoparticles, mammalian epithelial, endothelial and immune cells all internalized more nanodiscs with higher aspect ratios as compared to lower aspect ratio nanodiscs and rod-shaped particles with similar volume [46]. More importantly, bone marrow dendritic cells (BMDCs) internalized larger particles more efficiently, while HUVEC were more likely to take in intermediately sized disks (220 nm) [46]. Moreover, other researchers have reported that with similar size, charge and hydrophobicity, surface structure and shape become the determinants of whether nanoparticles can transport across the cell membrane and where the destination of the particles inside the cell is [47, 48]. Furthermore, Petersen and his group showed that spherical nanoparticles activate DCs more effectively, with more IL-12 secretion and MHC II expression, than thin films of the same material (polyanhydride) [50].

2.1.3 Surface Properties

Along with size and shape, particle surface properties, such as surface charges, hydrophobicity and surface attachment of ligands have tremendous impact on immunomodulation and thus a tailored particle surface is often necessary for disease specific immune response (Fig. 2). On the one hand, surface properties determine the way in which nanoparticles interact with blood constituents or other body liquids, thus influencing the biodistribution and clearance of the particulate vaccine in vivo. On the other hand, adsorption of some proteins, such as opsonins, outside the particle due to certain surface properties are likely to induce phagocytosis by macrophages resulting in rapid removal of the nanoparticles and significantly reducing the therapeutic effect.

Cationic particles are rather effective for macrophage and DC internalization and can be used to deliver DNA or anionic protein antigens to APCs. Cationic polymers such as poly-L-lysine (PLL), PEI, and Poly (amido amine) (PAMAM) dendrimers have shown great promise in immunomodulation [44, 51]. A recent study showed that PEI conjugated PLGA cationic particles carrying tumor idiotype DNA antigen elicited robust antitumor immunity in mouse model of B-cell lymphoma [52]. Besides presenting antigens on the surface, cationic particles can also co-deliver Toll-like receptor (TLR) ligands, e.g., CpG, polyinosinic:polycytidylic acid (poly I:C), to dendritic cells and lead to strong antitumor immune response. CpG was reported to dampen the function of the immunosuppressive myeloid-derived suppressor cells [53] and poly I: C is rather good at eliciting potent $CD4^+$ T cell responses and low-level CTL responses [54]. In a recent study, cationic PLGA-PEI particles performed efficient delivery of CpG ODN and IL-10 siRNA along with pDNA antigen to dendritic cells and enhanced antitumor immune response in a prophylactic murine model of B cell lymphoma [21]. Cationic particles are also advantageous for delivery of antigen to the anionic epithelial cell layer. Nochi et al. showed that cationic cholesteryl-group bearing pullulan, when administered intranasally, could efficiently deliver antigen to the nasal epithelial layer and generate strong immune response [55]. In addition, anionic particles have also been developed as an alternative method of delivering positively charged antigen and/or adjuvant or avoiding the cytotoxicity issue often encountered with positively charged polymers. Kazza et al. used anionic PLG-SDS particles to adsorb p55 gag protein from HIV-1 and induced cytotoxic T lymphocyte (CTL) response by intramuscular immunization [56]. In another study, it was demonstrated that HIV p24 protein coated anionic poly (D, L-lactide) (PLA) nanoparticles were also able to elicit strong T_H1-oriented response as well as high antibody titers in mice, rabbits and macaques [57]. However anionic G4.5 PAMAM dendrimers alone failed to induce or suppress cytokine release by human peripheral blood mononuclear cells (PBMC) [14, 58] It was also reported that when conjugated with glucosamine, the anionic G3.5 dendrimer even inhibited LPS-mediated induction of chemokines (MIP-1α/β, IL-8) and cytokine (TNFα, IL-1β, IL-6) synthesis by DCs [59]. Besides, due to the high hydrophilicity and low surface potential, a study showed that PVA-coated PLGA nanoparticles had relatively lower cellular uptake and endosomal escape [60]. And the growing negative charge on the surface also affected the APC recognition of PVA-coated PLGA [14, 60]. All these issues need to be further investigated and taken into consideration when developing new anionic particulate vaccines.

Polyethylene glycol (PEG) is widely used to modify particle surfaces so as to endow hydrophilic properties to the particulate systems to increase solubility, avoid protein adsorption and opsonization as well as to prevent phagocytosis and enzymatic degradation in order to enhance delivery to the target tissue or cell population. More importantly, hydrophobic domains of materials might act as a universal danger signal recognized by the TLRs, as suggested by the diverse family of TLR4- and TLR2-ligands (e.g., LPS) [61] and thus resulting in inflammatory response and DC maturation. In contrast, hydrophilic domains are responsible for the activation of alternative complement pathway and induce innate immune response [51].

Surface modification with ligands also helps achieve the targeting goal of the nanoparticles to specific cell population or tissues. For instance, in the case of cancer, conjugation of specific targeting ligands, such as folic acid, transferrin, epidermal growth factor (EGF), or polypeptides, including monoclonal antibodies, on the surface of nanoparticles, have shown significant augmentation in the uptake of these particles by tumor cells, which in turn increased the therapeutic effect [62, 63]. In general, cells internalize nanomaterials relying on various receptor mediated pathways, including mannose receptor (MR-), Fcγ receptor (FcγR-), scavenger receptor (SR-), and complement receptor (CR-), whose intracellular signaling may affect inflammatory responses and associate with TLR signaling [14]. Therefore, it is crucial to understand the mechanism of surface interaction between nanoparticles and cells as well as their immune outcome in order to develop the next generation of safe yet highly effective nanoparticle vaccines.

2.1.4 Route of Administration

Various routes of particle administration, such as intradermal, intranasal, subcutaneous, intraperitoneal and intravenous injection, have been used for vaccine or immunotherapy. Generally, subcutaneous administration of antigen results in the induction of immunity, whereas intravenous administration tends to elicit immuno-tolerance [64]. To trigger robust immune response, T cells should be efficiently primed by antigen-presenting cells. However, due to insufficient resident DCs in peripheral tissues, subcutaneous delivery of antigen is not the optimal way to enhance or suppress immune responses, though it is the most applicable one. Conversely, targeted-delivery of therapeutic agents to lungs, gut and lymph nodes, where a large number of immune cells reside, will lead to more effective immunomodulation. Actually, mucosal immunization was shown to produce both mucosal and systematic antibodies [12]. And chitosan nanoparticle is a promising candidate for intramucosal, intranasal and oral delivery routes because they were demonstrated to be favorably taken up by the M-cells in the Peyer's patches of gut and are good at amplifying mucosal and systemic immune responses. On the other hand, many researchers focused on the development of strategies targeting nanoparticle vaccines directly to lymph nodes where they can activate the resident DCs effectively and prime the T cell response in situ [9]. Last but not least, dsRNA, such as poly I:C, has been indicated to be able to generate aberrant expression of MHC II molecules associated with autoimmune diseases in non-hematopoietic cells [65]. And high dosage of Poly I:C might induce overstimulation. Hence, caution should be exercised when locally administering nanoparticles conjugated with poly I:C.

2.2 Engineered Particles for Immunotherapy of Cancer and Infectious Diseases

Rationally designed nanoparticles modulate the immune response against cancer and infectious diseases through different ways, which can be broadly divided into three basic categories, i.e., targeting antigen-presenting cells, upregulation or targeting of inflammatory cytokines and targeting T regulatory cells and myeloid-derived suppressor cells. Successful immunotherapies usually function in multiple ways in order to fully restore immunity.

2.2.1 Targeting Antigen-Presenting Cells

Although vaccination with live attenuated pathogens has succeeded in preventing many infectious diseases such as small pox and polio, effective vaccines are yet to be developed for various other infectious diseases like HIV and tuberculosis (TB). Similarly, major efforts are currently directed to develop vaccines against cancer to lower its morbidity and mortality. New strategies of vaccination mainly focus on targeting selected antigens to APCs, augmenting the innate and adaptive immunity with molecular adjuvants (e.g., TLR agonists) and directing the immune response towards the desired T cells phenotypes (e.g., Th1/CTL). Incorporation of molecular adjuvants, like CpG, poly I:C, in particulate vaccines, are known to promote the maturation and migration of DCs through toll-like receptors and other signaling pathways [66–68].

Synthetic polymeric particles, including polyester and branched polymers, have been used to encapsulate, adsorb or conjugate antigens with/without adjuvants to form particulate vaccines. These particulate vaccines can be endocytosed and processed by $CD8\alpha^{+}$ DCs resulting in cross-presentation of the antigens [69]. Moreover, particulate vaccines offer more stability and controllability of the formulation as compared to virus-like particles-based vaccines [70] (which is beyond our scope of discussion in this chapter). Paul et al. encapsulated ovalbumin (OVA) as antigen and TLR3 ligand poly I: C and TLR7/8 ligand resiquimod (R848) as adjuvants in 200 nm PLGA nanoparticles targeted to DEC205, a specific C-type lectin receptor (CLR) on DCs to enhance antigen uptake. The experimental results showed that the DC-targeted TLR ligands enhanced DC maturation and activation and also augmented $CD8^+$ T-cell responses against specific OVA antigen [71]. Another study published recently used PLGA nanoparticles with OVA antigen, TLR-7 ligand (imiquimod, R837) and small interfering siRNA for the knockdown of immune-suppressor gene and demonstrated that DCs treated with the nanoparticles can migrate to lymph nodes and present the antigen-peptide to CD8 OVA 1.3T cells through cross-presentation. The OVA-specific cytotoxic T lymphocytes activity against the EF7-OVA tumor model was successfully induced and tumor growth was inhibited efficiently [72].

2.2.2 Targeting Cytokines for Immunomodulation

Cytokines are important cues that can drive naïve lymphocytes towards different fates (e.g., anergy, effector, memory, or deletion) [73]. Also, they play crucial roles in immunomodulation by changing microenvironment during antigen presentation by APCs and effector functions by various lymphocytes including T cells.

Pathogens, such as *Mycobacterium tuberculosis* (Mtb), the causative pathogen of TB, reside in macrophages and paralyze their function by suppressing the antimicrobial response. The mechanisms include the suppression of intracellular generation of bactericidal reactive oxygen and nitrogen species (ROS/RNS) and secretion of pro-inflammatory cytokines such as IL-12 and IFNγ, which are key components of intracellular eradication of mycobacterium. Dube et al. developed 1,2-β-glucan functionalized chitosan shell,·PLGA core nanoparticles which stimulate the production of ROS/RNS, and significantly enhanced the secretion of IL-12p70, TNFα, and IFNγ by human alveolar like macrophages (ALM) by over threefold over 24 h through interaction with the Dectin-1 receptors on ALM surfaces [74]. Therefore, these particles were proved to have potential in eradication of intracellular pathogens, like Mtb and HIV.

Cytokines can also be employed as adjuvants in vaccines. But because of their short half-lives (minutes) following parenteral injection [73] and possible severe side effect if injected repeatedly with high-dose [75], direct administration of cytokine in patients is likely to be unsuccessful and needs to be improved. Nanoparticles again become a great tool to overcome the above-mentioned obstacles by delivery of genes coding the targeted cytokines. One of the strong cytokine candidates as vaccine adjuvant is IL-12, which is known to be able to induce T-cells and natural killer (NK) cells to produce all kinds of inflammatory cytokines (e.g., IFNγ, granulocyte-macrophage colony-stimulating factor (GM-CSF)) and tumor necrosis factor (TNF-α) and also shift $CD4^+$ T cells toward T_H1 response [30, 76, 77]. One group utilized mannosylated chitosan nanoparticles as a gene delivery vehicle to enhance the transfection of IL-12 encoding plasmid via mannose receptor-mediated endocytosis and showed prominent induction of the secretion of mIL-12 p70 and IFN-γfrom dendritic cells, resulting in a retardation or even significant regression of tumor growth in the mice of the treatment group compared to the control group [78]. Similar results have also been achieved by other groups using various types of nanoparticles [30, 79, 80]. Interleukin-2 is another vital cytokine, which induces T cell differentiation and proliferation and amplifies NK cell cytotoxicity, thus eliciting strong antitumor immune activity [30, 81]. Researchers have also reported a polycationic carrier (H1/pIL-2) with folic acid conjugated-PEI and β-cyclodextrin loaded with IL-2 plasmid (pIL-2) and achieved high efficiency and long duration of IL-2 expression in vivo. The subcutaneous inoculation of H1/pIL-2 in tumor bearing mouse model effectively stimulated the activation of effector T cells and NK cells in the peripheral blood, increased the secretion of serum T_H1 cytokines (e.g., IFNγand TNFβ), T_H2 cytokines (IL-4 and IL-6), and IL-17. Also the density of tumor-infiltrating T cells and NK cells are significantly increased, leading to an overall effect of reduced B16-F1 melanoma growth and prolonged survival [75].

2.2.3 Downregulation of Immuno-suppressive Factors

Cancer has long been considered "invincible" due to its strong ability to escape immune surveillance and create a permissible environment. During cancer development, several immunosuppressive factors help cancer cells to evade the immune system. For example, the enzyme, indoleamine-2,3-dioxygenase (IDO), expressed within solid tumors [82] inhibit inflammatory reactions towards tumors by degradation of the essential amino acid tryptophan and recruitment of regulatory T cells. The metabolites generated by IDO activity exert toxic effects on cytotoxic T lymphocytes and T_H1 cells, which shift the immune system towards T_H2 response [83]. IDO also helps to induce proliferation of Treg cells and mediate immune escape driven by myeloid-derived suppressor cell (MDSC) [84, 85]. Besides, tumors also utilize multiple ligands as inhibitory immune checkpoints to defy the specific adaptive immune response, such as cytotoxic T lymphocyte antigen (CTLA) and programmed death ligand 1(PD-L1). In the priming phase of a T cell response, three stimulatory signals are required: MHC–TCR interaction, CD80/CD86:CD28 costimulation, and the appropriate cytokine milieu. Primed T cells up regulate CTLA4 after antigen recognition, which competes with CD28 for interaction with costimulatory B7 family molecules. Another type of overexpressed ligands on DCs or tumor cells in the permissible environment is PD-L1, which interacts with PD1 expressed on activated T cells to restrain TCR-driven proliferation and cytokine production, and results in attenuated T cell response [86]. Also, proteolytic enzymes (e.g., matrix metalloproteinases MMPs) in the extracellular matrix interfere with the activity of multiple growth factors and cytokine receptors (e.g., IL-2 receptor IL-2α) and thereby inhibit proliferation and activation of T cells and increase the resistance of cancer cells to immunologic micromilieu. Several other immunosuppressive cytokines, such as TGFβ, IL-10, contribute to tumor immune escape by reducing the activity of NK cells and the production of the immuno-stimulatory cytokines, like IL-2, IL-6, IFNγ [5, 87, 88].

In order to release cancer immunity from immune suppressive environment and turning tumor itself into vaccines, researchers have developed multiple strategies to eliminate the inhibitory effect of the above-mentioned factor with particulate-based therapies. Jonathan Ellermeier et al. reported that by introducing a bifunctional siRNA combining TGFβ1 silencing with RIG-I activation by JetPEI nanoparticle into Panc02 mouse model of pancreatic cancer, type I IFN and CXCL10 levels in serum were increased, activated $CD8^+$ T cells were recruited to the tumor and a reduced frequency of $CD11B^+$ $Gr1^+$ myeloid suppressor cells were observed together with profound tumor cell apoptosis [89].

In order to reduce the escape of glioblastoma cells to the immunosurveillance, another group developed a type of polybutylcyanoacrylate nanoparticle carrying antisense oligonucleotides blocking TGF. Combined with the vaccination of Newcastle-Disease-Virus modified tumor cells, the tumor-bearing rats were released from immune-suppression with an increased rate of activated $CD25^+$ T cells and reduced concentration of TGFβ2 in plasma, and survived significantly longer than the control group following i.p. administration of nanoparticle formulation [90].

2.2.4 Targeting T Regulatory Cells and Myeloid-Derived Suppressor Cells

Myeloid derived suppressor cells (MDSC) and regulatory T cells (Treg) both play a critical role in maintaining the immune-suppressive microenvironment of tumors. MDSCs are characterized by CD11b and Gr1 expression in mice and they are immunosuppressive precursors of dendritic cells, macrophages, and granulocytes. They infiltrate developing tumors, promote vascularization, disrupt antigen presentation by DCs and hamper T cell activation as well as NK cell cytotoxicity [91]. Regulatory T cells are $CD4^+CD25^+FoxP3^+$ cells responsible for sustaining the homeostasis of innate cytotoxic lymphocytes [92]. Similar to MDSCs, Tregs suppress antigen presentation and cytotoxic T cell function by reducing cytolytic granule release [93]. It was observed that intratumoral presence of Treg cells is associated with poor prognosis in several cancer types [94, 95]. However, strategies aiming at depletion of Tregs are hard to realize because there is a lack of exclusive marker of Tregs to be targeted. Clinical studies of monoclonal antibody studies using the upregulated α-chain of the IL-2 receptor on Tregs as targets have shown conflicting results [96–98] due to the fact that IL-2 receptor is also expressed intensely on other cells, like T effector cells. Similar problems exist for the depletion of MDSCs since they consist of multiple subpopulations of cells with different maturities and plasticities and are able to differentiate into a variety of cell types [91].

Several chemotherapeutic agents have been identified as being able to inhibit the activity of MDSCs, including Gemcitabine and 5-fluorouracil (5-FU), both of which are nucleoside analogs [99, 100]. Studies have demonstrated that encapsulation of 5-FU in nanoparticles, like PLGA and Chitosan exhibit better profile of controlled release and enhanced efficacy and therapeutic effect of the 5-FU cancer chemotherapy [101–103]. Further investigation needs to be carried out on their therapeutic potency in immunomodulation of MDSCs and Treg responses.

2.3 Immunomodulation with Engineered Particles for Autoimmune Disorders

Autoimmune diseases, including multiple sclerosis, psoriasis, rheumatoid arthritis (RA), and type I diabetes, are caused by failure in immune regulation and T cell mediated destruction of self-tissues in most cases. They as a whole contribute a lot to the morbidity and mortality of the world population each year, ranking third in all the diseases [104]. Although global suppression of immune system is highly effective in most of the patients and remains the gold standard in clinic, it often leads to increased susceptibility to life-threatening infections and cancer. In this context, it is of great importance to develop a therapy that induces antigen-specific immunological tolerance while leaving other parts of immunity intact. The success of nanoparticles as platforms of immunostimulatory vaccines has given us sufficient confidence in their potential in immune-regulation to treat the autoimmune disorders. Strategies have been developed using nanoparticles bearing specific antigen peptide to inactivate primed T cells or activate regulatory T cells and showed great potential as better treatment for autoimmune diseases.

Gett, et al. designed encephalitogenic myelin epitope-conjugated particles (500 nm in diameter) and demonstrated their ability to trigger long-term T cell tolerance in mice with relapsing experimental autoimmune encephalomyelitis [104]. Both PLGA and polystyrene particles injected intravenously were able to induce inactivation of myelin-specific $CD4^+$ T cells by a lack of delayed-type hypersensitivity responses, an in vivo measure of $CD4^+$ T cell function. The epitope spreading was also prevented with this treatment strategy together with less T cell proliferation, IFNγ and IL-17 production, indicating T cell anergy. Overall, disease onset was delayed and the course of the disease was completely changed.

Huang and colleagues showed in their recent study that bacterium plasmid DNA conjugated PEI nanoparticle treatment in mice was potent in triggering immuno-tolerance in mice [105]. It was observed that upon DNA/PEI nanoparticle treatment, selective IDO expression in $CD19^+$ DCs and some non-DCs in perifollicular regions of spleen and peripheral LNs were induced. Besides, the treatment also directed splenic DCs and Tregs to acquire stable regulatory phenotype dependent on IDO induction via IFN type I receptor signaling. As a result of IDO activity, DNA/PEI treatment also blocked the in vivo T cell responses to exogenous OVA antigen in B6 (Thy1.2) mice. A following study on a murine model of Ag-induced rheumatoid arthritis demonstrated the efficacy of this DNA/PEI nanoparticle treatment on attenuating destructive autoimmunity.

Researchers have explored various ways to dampen the pathological immune response against self-antigens. One hypothesis is that without costimulatory signal, antigen-recognition by T cell receptor (TCR) will only result in T cell anergy or apoptosis [106]. Therefore, blocking costimulatory pathways is a worthwhile potential strategy to inhibit the activity of self-reactive T cells and attenuate the autoimmune response. In this category, administration of CTLA-4-immunoglobulin (Ig), which competes with the costimulation mediated by CD28, showed great promise in treatment of both rheumatoid arthritis (RA) and psoriatic arthritis, but less in systemic lupus erythematosus, multiple sclerosis and inflammatory bowel disease [106–110]. However, the limitation of this strategy includes the weaker effect on previously activated T cells and the need for continuous administration. Tregs are recognized as the central part of maintaining immune tolerance, indicating an attractive therapy to manipulate autoimmune response. Attempts have been made to isolate Tregs from an autoimmune disease patient, expand in vitro and then inject them back into the individual [111, 112]. Both polyclonal Tregs and autoantigen-specific Treg cells have been tried. Similar to Tregs, marginal zone macrophages (MZ M φ) in the spleen have also been demonstrated to be able to suppress adaptive immune responses to the represented self-antigens when they phagocytose apoptotic cells and debris [53, 113]. To this end, Miller et al. designed ECDI-fixed, antigen-coupled syngeneic splenocytes (Ag-Sp) to induce peripheral immunological tolerance [114]. The ECDI-chemistry by which antigens were conjugated to the surface of splenocytes also led to the apoptosis in the fixed cells after intravenous infusion. MZ Mφ internalized apoptotic cells via scavenger receptors, resulting in a regulatory phenotype, in which IL-10, TGF-β production and PD-L1 expression were upregulated while CD80 and CD86 were reduced. The loss of positive costimulation and increase in inhibitory signals induce the activation of antigen-specific Tregs and mediate Ag-Sp tolerance. Another aspect of immunity which can be modulated to stimulate tolerance is tweaking the balance of cytokines. Blockade of the pro-inflammatory cytokine tumor-necrosis factor (TNF) with TNF-specific antibodies or TNF receptors is now the most widely used immunotherapy for rheumatoid arthritis. However, this therapy causes increased risk of multiple sclerosis and tuberculosis, which renders it unsafe [115]. In addition to this splenocyte therapy, Singh and his coworkers have presented PLGA particles and chitosan nanomicelles carrying plasmid encoding IL-10 for the treatment and prevention of type I diabetes [116, 117], showing promise of particulate immunotherapy of autoimmunity. Both designed particles successfully escaped from endosomal compartment and increased the expression of IL-10 in mice, leading to lower blood glucose and IFNγ levels and reduced islet infiltration. Compared to all the above mentioned cell or antibody based therapies, the particulate system bears the advantage of being cost-effective and less time-consuming, since it does not require the isolation of leukocytes from patients and has more promise in clinical application under good manufacturing practices (GMP).

3 Concluding Remarks

In summary, synthetic polymeric particles in the micro- and nanorange have been successfully employed in the development of immunotherapy against infectious diseases, cancer and autoimmune disorders. These particulate systems have shown advantages in preclinical setting over other immunomodulation strategies since they are able to efficiently deliver multiple cargos to immune cells, are biocompatible and tunable, and some even bear inherent adjuvancy. However, despite preclinical promise, clinical translation and efficacy has been limited. The lessons learned from years of accumulated experience indicate that for particle-based immunotherapy, size, shape, surface properties and route of administration of the particles should be carefully designed since these characteristics are key factors that influence the biodistribution and immunological efficacy of the proposed strategies. Innovative strategies that can precisely tune the balance of Th1 and Th2 immune responses and antigen-specific immune stimulation/tolerance need to be developed. Better strategies to recruit DCs to the site of administration, to break the immune-suppression of the tumor microenvironment and to prevent the immune system from attacking self-antigens need to be developed. Finally, very little work has focused on modeling the human immune system and immune organs in vitro, either through physiome-on-a-chip approaches or through computational modeling. In addition, intra-vital microscopy other imaging based tools must be employed to understand the cellular and molecular interactions, transport kinetics, etc. following nanoparticle administration. These must be critical priorities for the field. Numerous mouse studies showing excellent efficacy has not proven to be predictive in humans. However, with the advancement of novel immunoengineering tools and strategies, we are at the verge of new breakthroughs that can stop the pathological immune response against autoimmune disorders and restore the robust immune-protection against infections and malignancy.

References

1. Hubbell JA, Thomas SN, Swartz MA (2009) Materials engineering for immunomodulation. Nature 462(7272):449–460. doi:10.1038/nature08604
2. Jiao Q, Li L, Mu Q, Zhang Q (2014) Immunomodulation of nanoparticles in nanomedicine applications. BioMed Res Int 2014:426028. doi:10.1155/2014/426028
3. Heegaard PM, Boas U, Sorensen NS (2010) Dendrimers for vaccines and immunostimulatory uses. A Review. Bioconjug Chem 21(3):405
4. Tarik A, Khan STR (2014) Immunological principles regulating immunomodulation with biomaterials. Acta Biomater 10:8
5. Chen DS, Mellman I (2013) Oncology meets immunology: the cancer-immunity cycle. Immunity 39(1):1–10. doi:10.1016/j.immuni.2013.07.012
6. Feldmann M, Steinman L (2005) Design of effective immunotherapy for human autoimmunity. Nature 435(7042):612–619. doi:10.1038/nature03727
7. Steer HJ, Lake RA, Nowak AK, Robinson BW (2010) Harnessing the immune response to treat cancer. Oncogene 29(48):6301–6313. doi:10.1038/onc.2010.437
8. Thiele L, Merkle HP, Walter E (2003) Phagocytosis and phagosomal fate of surface-modified microparticles in dendritic cells and macrophages. Pharm Res 20(2):221–228
9. Thomas SN, Vokali E, Lund AW, Hubbell JA, Swartz MA (2014) Targeting the tumor-draining lymph node with adjuvanted nanoparticles reshapes the anti-tumor immune response. Biomaterials 35(2):814–824. doi:10.1016/j.biomaterials.2013.10.003
10. Itano AA, McSorley SJ, Reinhardt RL, Ehst BD, Ingulli E, Rudensky AY, Jenkins MK (2003) Distinct dendritic cell populations sequentially present antigen to CD4 T cells and stimulate different aspects of cell-mediated immunity. Immunity 19(1):47–57. doi:10.1016/s1074-7613(03)00175-4
11. Pape KA, Catron DM, Itano AA, Jenkins MK (2007) The humoral immune response is initiated in lymph nodes by B cells that acquire soluble antigen directly in the follicles. Immunity 26(4):491–502. doi:10.1016/j.immuni.2007.02.011
12. Holmgren J, Czerkinsky C (2005) Mucosal immunity and vaccines. Nat Med 11(4 Suppl):S45–S53. doi:10.1038/nm1213
13. Boehler RM, Graham JG, Shea LD (2011) Tissue engineering tools for modulation of the immune response. Biotechniques 51(4):239–240. doi:10.2144/000113754, 242, 244 passim
14. Dobrovolskaia MA, McNeil SE (2007) Immunological properties of engineered nanomaterials. Nat Nanotechnol 2:469
15. Abul K, Abbas KMM, Sher A (1996) Functional diversity of helper T lymphocytes. Nature 383:7
16. Rebecca L, McCall RWS (2013) PLGA nanoparticles formed by single- or double-emulsion with vitamin E-TPGS. J Vis Exp 82:8
17. Ebru Kizilay ABK, Dubin PL (2011) Complexation and coacervation of polyelectrolytes with oppositely charged colloids. Adv Colloid Interface Sci 167:14
18. Krishnendu Roy H-Q, Huang S-k, Leong KW (1999) Oral gene delivery with chitosan–DNA nanoparticles generates immunologic protection in a murine model of peanut allergy. Nat Med 5(4):15
19. Sudhir P, Kasturi KS, Roy K (2005) Covalent conjugation of polyethyleneimine on biodegradable microparticles for delivery of plasmid DNA vaccines. Biomaterials 26:11
20. Ankur Singh HN, Ghosn B, Qin H, Kwak LW, Roy K (2008) Efficient modulation of T-cell response by dual-mode, single-carrier delivery of cytokine-targeted siRNA and DNA vaccine to antigen-presenting cells. Mol Ther 16(12):11
21. Pradhan P, Qin H, Leleux JA, Gwak D, Sakamaki I, Kwak LW, Roy K (2014) The effect of combined IL10 siRNA and CpG ODN as pathogen-mimicking microparticles on Th1/Th2 cytokine balance in dendritic cells and protective immunity against B cell lymphoma. Biomaterials 35(21):5491–5504. doi:10.1016/j.biomaterials.2014.03.039
22. Kasturi SP, Skountzou I, Albrecht RA, Koutsonanos D, Hua T, Nakaya HI, Ravindran R, Stewart S, Alam M, Kwissa M, Villinger F, Murthy N, Steel J, Jacob J, Hogan RJ, Garcia-Sastre A, Compans R, Pulendran B (2011) Programming the magnitude and persistence of antibody responses with innate immunity. Nature 470(7335):543
23. Reddy ST, van der Vlies AJ, Simeoni E, Angeli V, Randolph GJ, O'Neil CP, Lee LK, Swartz MA, Hubbell JA (2007) Exploiting lymphatic transport and complement activation in nanoparticle vaccines. Nat Biotechnol 25(10):1159–1164. doi:10.1038/nbt1332
24. Rehor A, Tirelli N, Hubbell JA (2002) A new living emulsion polymerization mechanism-

episulfide anionic polymerization. Macromolecules 35:6

25. Iosif Daniel Roscaa FW, Uob M (2004) Microparticle formation and its mechanism in single and double emulsion solvent evaporation. J Control Release 99:10
26. Hong Shen ALA, Cody V, Giodini A, Hinson ER, Cresswell P, Edelson RL, Mark Saltzman W, Hanlon DJ (2006) Enhanced and prolonged cross-presentation following endosomal escape of exogenous antigens encapsulated in biodegradable nanoparticles. Immunology 117:11
27. Tan S, Sasada T, Bershteyn A, Yang K, Ioji T, Zhang Z (2014) Combinational delivery of lipid-enveloped polymeric nanoparticles carrying different peptides for anti-tumor immunotherapy. Nanomedicine (Lond) 9(5):635–647. doi:10.2217/nnm.13.67
28. Todd CW, Pozzi LA, Guarnaccia JR, Balasubramanianj M, Henkf WG, Youngert LE, Newman MJ (1997) Development of an adjuvant-active nonionic block copolymer for use in oil-free subunit vaccines formulations. Vaccine 15(5):564
29. de Kruif CG, Renko de Vries FW (2004) Complex coacervation of proteins and anionic polysaccharides. Curr Opin Colloid Interface Sci 9:10
30. Somayeh Hallaj-Nezhadi FL, Dass CR (2010) Nanoparticle-mediated interleukin-12 cancer gene therapy. J Pharm Pharm Sci 13(3):14
31. Hallaj-Nezhad S, Valizadeh H, Dastmalchi S, Baradaran B, Jalali MB, Dobakhti F, Lotfipour F (2011) Preparation of chitosan-plasmid DNA nanoparticles encoding interleukin-12 and their expression in CT-26 colon carcinoma cells. J Pharm Pharm Sci 14(2):15
32. Donbrow M (1992) Phase seperation and coacervation. In: Donbrow M (ed) Microcapsules and nanoparticles in medicine and pharmacy. CRC Press, Boca Raton, FL, p 2
33. Landge DA, Shyale SS, Kadam SD, Shah DV, Katare YS, Pawar JB (2014) Dendrimer: an innovative acceptable approach in novel drug delivery system. Pharmacophore 5(1):11
34. Malik N, Wiwattanapatapee R, Klopsch R, Lorenz K, Frey H, Weener JW, Meijer EW, Paulus W, Duncan R (2000) Relationship between structure and biocompatibility in vitro, and preliminary studies on the biodistribution of ^{125}I-labelled dendrimers in vivo. J Control Release 65:133
35. Kimiko Makino NY, Higuchi K, Harada N, Ohshima H, Terada H (2003) Phagocytic uptake of polystyrene microspheres by alveolar macrophages- effects of the size and surface properties of the microspheres. Colloids Surf B Biointerfaces 27:7
36. Fang C, Shi B, Pei YY, Hong MH, Wu J, Chen HZ (2006) In vivo tumor targeting of tumor necrosis factor-alpha-loaded stealth nanoparticles: effect of MePEG molecular weight and particle size. Eur J Pharm Sci 27(1):27–36. doi:10.1016/j.ejps.2005.08.002
37. Manolova V, Flace A, Bauer M, Schwarz K, Saudan P, Bachmann MF (2008) Nanoparticles target distinct dendritic cell populations according to their size. Eur J Immunol 38(5):1404–1413. doi:10.1002/eji.200737984
38. Fifis T, Gamvrellis A, Crimeen-Irwin B, Pietersz GA, Li J, Mottram PL, McKenzie IFC, Plebanski M (2004) Size-dependent immunogenicity: therapeutic and protective properties of nano-vaccines against tumors. J Immunol 173(5):3148–3154. doi:10.4049/jimmunol.173.5.3148
39. Sharp FA, Ruane D, Claass B, Creagh E, Harris J, Malyala P, Singh M, O'Hagan DT, Petrilli V, Tschopp J, O'Neill LA, Lavelle EC (2009) Uptake of particulate vaccine adjuvants by dendritic cells activates the NALP3 inflammasome. Proc Natl Acad Sci U S A 106(3):870–875. doi:10.1073/pnas.0804897106
40. Maaike van Zijverdena BG (2000) Adjuvant activity of particulate pollutants in different mouse model. Toxicology 152:9
41. Lutsiak ME, Kwon GS, Samuel J (2006) Biodegradable nanoparticle delivery of a Th2-biased peptide for induction of Th1 immune responses. J Pharm Pharmacol 58(6):739–747. doi:10.1211/jpp.58.6.0004
42. de Kozak Y, Andrieux K, Villarroya H, Klein C, Thillaye-Goldenberg B, Naud MC, Garcia E, Couvreur P (2004) Intraocular injection of tamoxifen-loaded nanoparticles: a new treatment of experimental autoimmune uveoretinitis. Eur J Immunol 34(12):3702–3712. doi:10.1002/eji.200425022
43. Cui Z, Patel J, Tuzova M, Ray P, Phillips R, Woodward JG, Nath A, Mumper RJ (2004) Strong T cell type-1 immune responses to HIV-1 Tat (1-72) protein-coated nanoparticles. Vaccine 22(20):2631–2640. doi:10.1016/j.vaccine.2003.12.013
44. Xiang SD, Scholzen A, Minigo G, David C, Apostolopoulos V, Mottram PL, Plebanski M (2006) Pathogen recognition and development of particulate vaccines: does size matter? Methods 40(1):1–9. doi:10.1016/j.ymeth.2006.05.016
45. Rachit Agarwal VS, Jurney P, Li S, Sreenivasan SV, Roy K (2012) Scalable imprinting of shape-specific polymeric nano using a release layer of switchable water solubility. ACS Nano 6(3):8
46. Rachit Agarwal VS, Jurney P, Li S, Sreenivasan SV, Roy K (2013) Mammalian cells preferen-

tially internalize hydrogel nanodiscs over nanorods and use shape-specific uptake mechanisms. Proc Natl Acad Sci U S A 110(43):6
47. Champion JA, Mitragotri S (2006) Role of target geometry in phagocytosis. Proc Natl Acad Sci U S A 103(13):4930–4934. doi:10.1073/pnas.0600997103
48. Verma A, Uzun O, Hu Y, Hu Y, Han HS, Watson N, Chen S, Irvine DJ, Stellacci F (2008) Surface-structure-regulated cell-membrane penetration by monolayer-protected nanoparticles. Nat Mater 7(7): 588–595. doi:10.1038/nmat2202
49. Geng Y, Dalhaimer P, Cai S, Tsai R, Tewari M, Minko T, Discher DE (2007) Shape effects of filaments versus spherical particles in flow and drug delivery. Nat Nanotechnol 2:249
50. Petersen LK, Xue L, Wannemuehler MJ, Rajan K, Narasimhan B (2009) The simultaneous effect of polymer chemistry and device geometry on the in vitro activation of murine dendritic cells. Biomaterials 30(28):5131–5142. doi:10.1016/j.biomaterials.2009.05.069
51. Purwada A, Roy K, Singh A (2014) Engineering vaccines and niches for immune modulation. Acta Biomater 10(4):1728 1740. doi:10.1016/j.actbio.2013.12.036
52. Pai Kasturi S, Qin H, Thomson KS, El-Bereir S, Cha SC, Neelapu S, Kwak LW, Roy K (2006) Prophylactic anti-tumor effects in a B cell lymphoma model with DNA vaccines delivered on polyethylenimine (PEI) functionalized PLGA microparticles. J Control Release 113(3):261–270. doi:10.1016/j.jconrel.2006.04.006
53. Zoglmeier C, Bauer H, Norenberg D, Wedekind G, Bittner P, Sandholzer N, Rapp M, Anz D, Endres S, Bourquin C (2011) CpG blocks immunosuppression by myeloid-derived suppressor cells in tumor-bearing mice. Clin Cancer Res 17(7):1765–1775. doi:10.1158/1078-0432.CCR-10-2672
54. Kastenmuller W, Kastenmuller K, Kurts C, Seder RA (2014) Dendritic cell-targeted vaccines - hope or hype? Nat Rev Immunol 14(10):705–711. doi:10.1038/nri3727
55. Nochi T, Yuki Y, Takahashi H, Sawada S, Mejima M, Kohda T, Harada N, Kong IG, Sato A, Kataoka N, Tokuhara D, Kurokawa S, Takahashi Y, Tsukada H, Kozaki S, Akiyoshi K, Kiyono H (2010) Nanogel antigenic protein-delivery system for adjuvant-free intranasal vaccines. Nat Mater 9(7):572–578. doi:10.1038/nmat2784
56. Kazzaz J, Neidleman J, Singh M, Ott G, O'Hagan DT (2000) Novel anionic microparticles are a potent adjuvant for the induction of cytotoxic T lymphocytes against recombinant p55 gag from HIV-1. J Control Release 67:347
57. Ataman-Onal Y, Munier S, Ganee A, Terrat C, Durand PY, Battail N, Martinon F, Le Grand R, Charles MH, Delair T, Verrier B (2006) Surfactant-free anionic PLA nanoparticles coated with HIV-1 p24 protein induced enhanced cellular and humoral immune responses in various animal models. J Control Release 112(2):175–185. doi:10.1016/j.jconrel.2006.02.006
58. Nanotechnology Characterization Laboratory (2006) Dendrimer-based MRI contrast agents, NCL200612A, December 2006. As of November 17, 2008. http://ncl.cancer.gov/120406.pdf
59. Shaunak S, Thomas S, Gianasi E, Godwin A, Jones E, Teo I, Mireskandari K, Luthert P, Duncan R, Patterson S, Khaw P, Brocchini S (2004) Polyvalent dendrimer glucosamine conjugates prevent scar tissue formation. Nat Biotechnol 22(8):977–984. doi:10.1038/nbt995
60. Sanjeeb K, Sahoo JP, Prabha S, Labhasetwar V (2002) Residual polyvinyl alcohol associated with poly(D, L-lactide-co-glycolide) nanoparticles affects their physical properties and cellular uptake. J Control Release 82:10
61. Seong S-Y, Matzinger Y (2004) Hydrophobicity: an ancient damage-associated molecular pattern that initiates innate immune responses. Nat Rev Immunol 4:10
62. Marcucci F, Lefoulon F (2004) Active targeting with particulate drug carriers in tumor therapy: fundamentals and recent progress. Drug Discov Today 9(5):219–228. doi:10.1016/s1359-6446(03)02988-x
63. Brannon-Peppas L, Blanchette JO (2012) Nanoparticle and targeted systems for cancer therapy. Adv Drug Deliv Rev 64:206–212. doi:10.1016/j.addr.2012.09.033
64. McCarthy DP, Hunter ZN, Chackerian B, Shea LD, Miller SD (2014) Targeted immunomodulation using antigen-conjugated nanoparticles. Wiley Interdiscip Rev Nanomed Nanobiotechnol 6(3):298–315. doi:10.1002/wnan.1263
65. Hafner AM, Corthesy B, Merkle HP (2013) Particulate formulations for the delivery of poly(I:C) as vaccine adjuvant. Adv Drug Deliv Rev 65(10):1386–1399. doi:10.1016/j.addr.2013.05.013
66. Thibaut De Smedt BP, Muraille E, Lespagnard L, Heinen E, De Baetselier P, Urbain J, Leo O, Moser M (1996) Regulation of dendritic cell numbers and maturation by lipopolysaccharide in vivo. J Exp Med 184:12
67. Hiroaki Hemmi OT, Kawai T, Kaisho T, Sato S, Sanjo H, Matsumoto M, Hoshino K,

Wagner H, Takeda K, Akira S (2000) A Toll-like receptor recognizes bacterial DNA. Nature 408:6

68. Takeda K, Kaisho T, Akira S (2003) Toll-like receptors. Annu Rev Immunol 21:335–376. doi:10.1146/annurev.immunol.21.120601.141126
69. Oliver Schiulz CRES (2002) Cross-presentation of cell-associated antigens by CD8α+dendritic cells is attributable to their ability to internalize dead cells. Immunology 107:7
70. Anita Gamvrellis DL, Hanley JC, Xiang SD, Mottram P, Plebanski M (2004) Vaccines that facilitate antigen entry into dendritic cells. Immunol Cell Biol 82:11
71. Tacken PJ, Zeelenberg IS, Cruz LJ, van Hout-Kuijer MA, van de Glind G, Fokkink RG, Lambeck AJ, Figdor CG (2011) Targeted delivery of TLR ligands to human and mouse dendritic cells strongly enhances adjuvanticity. Blood 118(26):6836–6844. doi:10.1182/blood-2011-07-367615
72. Heo MB, Lim YT (2014) Programmed nanoparticles for combined immunomodulation, antigen presentation and tracking of immunotherapeutic cells. Biomaterials 35(1):590–600. doi:10.1016/j.biomaterials.2013.10.009
73. Irvine DJ, Swartz MA, Szeto GL (2013) Engineering synthetic vaccines using cues from natural immunity. Nat Mater 12(11):978–990. doi:10.1038/nmat3775
74. Dube A, Reynolds JL, Law WC, Maponga CC, Prasad PN, Morse GD (2014) Multimodal nanoparticles that provide immunomodulation and intracellular drug delivery for infectious diseases. Nanomedicine 10(4):831–838. doi:10.1016/j.nano.2013.11.012
75. Yao H, Ng SS, Huo LF, Chow BK, Shen Z, Yang M, Sze J, Ko O, Li M, Yue A, Lu LW, Bian XW, Kung HF, Lin MC (2011) Effective melanoma immunotherapy with interleukin-2 delivered by a novel polymeric nanoparticle. Mol Cancer Ther 10(6):1082–1092. doi:10.1158/1535-7163.MCT-10-0717
76. Heffernan MJ, Zaharoff DA, Fallon JK, Schlom J, Greiner JW (2011) In vivo efficacy of a chitosan/IL-12 adjuvant system for protein-based vaccines. Biomaterials 32(3):926–932. doi:10.1016/j.biomaterials.2010.09.058
77. Zaharoff DA, Hoffman BS, Hooper HB, Benjamin CJ Jr, Khurana KK, Hance KW, Rogers CJ, Pinto PA, Schlom J, Greiner JW (2009) Intravesical immunotherapy of superficial bladder cancer with chitosan/interleukin-12. Cancer Res 69(15):6192–6199. doi:10.1158/0008-5472.CAN-09-1114
78. Kim TH, Jin H, Kim HW, Cho MH, Cho CS (2006) Mannosylated chitosan nanoparticle-based cytokine gene therapy suppressed cancer growth in BALB/c mice bearing CT-26 carcinoma cells. Mol Cancer Ther 5(7):1723–1732. doi:10.1158/1535-7163.MCT-05-0540
79. Yockman JW, Maheshwari A, S-o H, Kim SW (2003) Tumor regression by repeated intratumoral delivery of water soluble lipopolymers/p2CMVmIL-12 complexes. J Control Release 87(1-3):177–186. doi:10.1016/s0168-3659(02)00362-0
80. Diez S, Navarro G, de ILarduya CT (2009) In vivo targeted gene delivery by cationic nanoparticles for treatment of hepatocellular carcinoma. J Gene Med 11(1):38–45. doi:10.1002/jgm.1273
81. Yang Y, Chen J, Li H, Wang Y, Xie Z, Wu M, Zhang H, Zhao Z, Chen Q, Fu M, Wu K, Chi C, Wang H, Gao R (2007) Porcine interleukin-2 gene encapsulated in chitosan nanoparticles enhances immune response of mice to piglet paratyphoid vaccine. Comp Immunol Microbiol Infect Dis 30(1):19–32. doi:10.1016/j.cimid.2006.09.006
82. Godin-Ethier J, Hanafi LA, Piccirillo CA, Lapointe R (2011) Indoleamine 2,3-dioxygenase expression in human cancers: clinical and immunologic perspectives. Clin Cancer Res 17(22):6985–6991. doi:10.1158/1078-0432.CCR-11-1331
83. Platten M, Wick W, Van den Eynde BJ (2012) Tryptophan catabolism in cancer: beyond IDO and tryptophan depletion. Cancer Res 72(21):5435–5440. doi:10.1158/0008-5472.CAN-12-0569
84. Smith C, Chang MY, Parker KH, Beury DW, DuHadaway JB, Flick HE, Boulden J, Sutanto-Ward E, Soler AP, Laury-Kleintop LD, Mandik-Nayak L, Metz R, Ostrand-Rosenberg S, Prendergast GC, Muller AJ (2012) IDO is a nodal pathogenic driver of lung cancer and metastasis development. Cancer Discov 2(8):722–735. doi:10.1158/2159-8290.CD-12-0014
85. Andersen MH (2012) The specific targeting of immune regulation: T-cell responses against Indoleamine 2,3-dioxygenase. Cancer Immunol Immunother 61(8):1289–1297. doi:10.1007/s00262-012-1234-4
86. Freeman GJ, Long AJ, Iwai Y, Bourque K, Chernova T, Nishimura H, Fitz LJ, Malenkovich N, Okazaki T, Byrne MC, Horton HF, Fouser L, Carter L, Ling V, Bowman MR, Carreno BM, Collins M, Wood CR, Honjo T (2000) Engagement of the PD-1 immunoinhibitory receptor by a novel B7 family member leads to negative regulation of lymphocyte activation. J Exp Med 192(7):1027

87. Pickup M, Novitskiy S, Moses HL (2013) The roles of TGFbeta in the tumour microenvironment. Nat Rev Cancer 13(11):788–799. doi:10.1038/nrc3603
88. Motz GT, Coukos G (2013) Deciphering and reversing tumor immune suppression. Immunity 39(1):61–73. doi:10.1016/j.immuni.2013.07.005
89. Ellermeier J, Wei J, Duewell P, Hoves S, Stieg MR, Adunka T, Noerenberg D, Anders HJ, Mayr D, Poeck H, Hartmann G, Endres S, Schnurr M (2013) Therapeutic efficacy of bifunctional siRNA combining TGF-beta1 silencing with RIG-I activation in pancreatic cancer. Cancer Res 73(6):1709–1720. doi:10.1158/0008-5472.CAN-11-3850
90. Schneider T, Becker A, Ringe K, Reinhold A, Firsching R, Sabel BA (2008) Brain tumor therapy by combined vaccination and antisense oligonucleotide delivery with nanoparticles. J Neuroimmunol 195(1-2):21–27. doi:10.1016/j.jneuroim.2007.12.005
91. Quail DF, Joyce JA (2013) Microenvironmental regulation of tumor progression and metastasis. Nat Med 19(11):1423–1437. doi:10.1038/nm.3394
92. Whiteside TL, Schuler P, Schilling B (2012) Induced and natural regulatory T cells in human cancer. Expert Opin Biol Ther 12(10):1383–1397. doi:10.1517/14712598.2012.707184
93. von Boehmer H, Daniel C (2013) Therapeutic opportunities for manipulating T(Reg) cells in autoimmunity and cancer. Nat Rev Drug Discov 12(1):51–63. doi:10.1038/nrd3683
94. Curiel TJ, Coukos G, Zou L, Alvarez X, Cheng P, Mottram P, Evdemon-Hogan M, Conejo-Garcia JR, Zhang L, Burow M, Zhu Y, Wei S, Kryczek I, Daniel B, Gordon A, Myers L, Lackner A, Disis ML, Knutson KL, Chen L, Zou W (2004) Specific recruitment of regulatory T cells in ovarian carcinoma fosters immune privilege and predicts reduced survival. Nat Med 10(9):942–949. doi:10.1038/nm1093
95. Bates GJ, Fox SB, Han C, Leek RD, Garcia JF, Harris AL, Banham AH (2006) Quantification of regulatory T cells enables the identification of high-risk breast cancer patients and those at risk of late relapse. J Clin Oncol 24(34):5373–5380. doi:10.1200/JCO.2006.05.9584
96. Dannull J, Su Z, Rizzieri D, Yang BK, Coleman D, Yancey D, Zhang A, Dahm P, Chao N, Gilboa E, Vieweg J (2005) Enhancement of vaccine-mediated antitumor immunity in cancer patients after depletion of regulatory T cells. J Clin Invest 115(12):3623–3633. doi:10.1172/JCI25947
97. Rech AJ, Vonderheide RH (2009) Clinical use of anti-CD25 antibody daclizumab to enhance immune responses to tumor antigen vaccination by targeting regulatory T cells. Ann N Y Acad Sci 1174:99–106. doi:10.1111/j.1749-6632.2009.04939.x
98. Jacobs JF, Punt CJ, Lesterhuis WJ, Sutmuller RP, Brouwer HM, Scharenborg NM, Klasen IS, Hilbrands LB, Figdor CG, de Vries IJ, Adema GJ (2010) Dendritic cell vaccination in combination with anti-CD25 monoclonal antibody treatment: a phase I/II study in metastatic melanoma patients. Clin Cancer Res 16(20):5067–5078. doi:10.1158/1078-0432.CCR-10-1757
99. Vincent J, Mignot G, Chalmin F, Ladoire S, Bruchard M, Chevriaux A, Martin F, Apetoh L, Rebe C, Ghiringhelli F (2010) 5-Fluorouracil selectively kills tumor-associated myeloid-derived suppressor cells resulting in enhanced T cell-dependent antitumor immunity. Cancer Res 70(8):3052–3061. doi:10.1158/0008-5472.CAN-09-3690
100. Suzuki E, Kapoor V, Jassar AS, Kaiser LR, Albelda SM (2005) Gemcitabine selectively eliminates splenic Gr-1+/CD11b+myeloid suppressor cells in tumor-bearing animals and enhances antitumor immune activity. Clin Cancer Res 11(18):6713–6721. doi:10.1158/1078-0432.CCR-05-0883
101. Tigli Aydin RS, Pulat M (2012) 5-fluorouracil encapsulated chitosan nanoparticles for pH-stimulated drug delivery: evaluation of controlled release kinetics. J Nanomater 2012:1–10. doi:10.1155/2012/313961
102. Shenoy VS, Gude RP, Ramachandra Murthy RS (2013) In vitro anticancer evaluation of 5-fluorouracil lipid nanoparticles using B16F10 melanoma cell lines. Int Nano Lett 3:9
103. Nair KL, Jagadeeshan S, Nair SA, Kumar GS (2011) Biological evaluation of 5-fluorouracil nanoparticles for cancer chemotherapy and its dependence on the carrier, PLGA. Int J Nanomedicine 6:1685–1697. doi:10.2147/IJN.S20165
104. Getts DR, Martin AJ, McCarthy DP, Terry RL, Hunter ZN, Yap WT, Getts MT, Pleiss M, Luo X, King NJ, Shea LD, Miller SD (2012) Microparticles bearing encephalitogenic peptides induce T-cell tolerance and ameliorate experimental autoimmune encephalomyelitis. Nat Biotechnol 30(12):1217–1224. doi:10.1038/nbt.2434
105. Huang L, Lemos HP, Li L, Li M, Chandler PR, Baban B, McGaha TL, Ravishankar B, Lee JR, Munn DH, Mellor AL (2012) Engineering DNA nanoparticles as immunomodulatory reagents that activate regulatory T cells. J Immunol 188(10):4913–4920. doi:10.4049/jimmunol.1103668

106. Michael D, Rosenblum IKG, Paw JS, Abbas AK (2012) Treating human autoimmunity-current practice and future prospects. State Art Rev 4(125):10
107. Maxwell LJ, Singh JA (2010) Abatacept for rheumatoid arthritis: a Cochrane systematic review. J Rheumatol 37(2):12
108. Viglietta V, Bourcier K, Buckle GJ, Healy B, Weiner HL, Hafler DA, Egorova S, Guttmann CR, Rusche JR, Khoury SJ (2008) CTLA4Ig treatment in patients with multiple sclerosis: an open-label, phase 1 clinical trial. Neurology 71(12):8
109. Felix NJ, Suri A, Salter-Cid L, Nadler SG, Gujrathi S, Corbo M, Aranda R (2010) Targeting lymphocyte co-stimulation: from bench to bedside. Autoimmunity 43(7):13
110. Mease P, Genovese MC, Gladstein G, Kivitz AJ, Ritchlin C, Tak PP, Wollenhaupt J, Bahary O, Becker JC, Kelly S, Sigal L, Teng J, Gladman D (2011) Abatacept in the treatment of patients with psoriatic arthritis: results of a six-month, multicenter, randomized, double-blind, placebo-controlled, phase II trial. Arthritis Rheum 63(4):939–948. doi:10.1002/art.30176
111. Marek-Trzonkowska N, Mysliwec M, Siebert J, Trzonkowski P (2013) Clinical application of regulatory T cells in type 1 diabetes. Pediatr Diabetes 14(5):322–332. doi:10.1111/pedi.12029
112. Tang Q, Bluestone JA (2013) Regulatory T-cell therapy in transplantation: moving to the clinic. Cold Spring Harb Perspect Med 3(11):pii: a015552. doi:10.1101/cshperspect.a015552
113. McGaha TL, Chen Y, Ravishankar B, van Rooijen N, Karlsson MC (2011) Marginal zone macrophages suppress innate and adaptive immunity to apoptotic cells in the spleen. Blood 117(20):5403–5412. doi:10.1182/blood-2010-11-320028
114. Millers SD, Henry RPW, Claman N (1979) The induction of cell-mediated immunity and tolerance with protein antigens coupled to syngeneic lymphoid cells. J Exp Med 149:16
115. Caspi RR (2008) Immunotherapy of autoimmunity and cancer: the penalty for success. Nat Rev Immunol 8(12):970–976. doi:10.1038/nri2438
116. Mandke R, Singh J (2012) Cationic nanomicelles for delivery of plasmids encoding interleukin-4 and interleukin-10 for prevention of autoimmune diabetes in mice. Pharm Res 29(3):883–897. doi:10.1007/s11095-011-0616-1
117. Basarkar A, Singh J (2009) Poly (lactide-co-glycolide)-polymethacrylate nanoparticles for intramuscular delivery of plasmid encoding interleukin-10 to prevent autoimmune diabetes in mice. Pharm Res 26(1):72–81. doi:10.1007/s11095-008-9710-4
118. Demento SL, Eisenbarth SC, Foellmer HG, Platt C, Caplan MJ, Mark Saltzman W, Mellman I, Ledizet M, Fikrig E, Flavell RA, Fahmy TM (2009) Inflammasome-activating nanoparticles as modular systems for optimizing vaccine efficacy. Vaccine 27(23):3013–3021. doi:10.1016/j.vaccine.2009.03.034
119. Manish Diwan MT, Samuel J (2002) Enhancement of immune responses by co-delivery of a CpG oligodeoxynucleotide and tetanus toxoid in biodegradable nanospheres. J Control Release 85:16
120. Clawson C, Huang CT, Futalan D, Seible DM, Saenz R, Larsson M, Ma W, Minev B, Zhang F, Ozkan M, Ozkan C, Esener S, Messmer D (2010) Delivery of a peptide via poly(D, L-lactic-co-glycolic) acid nanoparticles enhances its dendritic cell-stimulatory capacity. Nanomedicine 6(5):651–661. doi:10.1016/j.nano.2010.03.001
121. Hamdy S, Molavi O, Ma Z, Haddadi A, Alshamsan A, Gobti Z, Elhasi S, Samuel J, Lavasanifar A (2008) Co-delivery of cancer-associated antigen and Toll-like receptor 4 ligand in PLGA nanoparticles induces potent CD8+ T cell-mediated anti-tumor immunity. Vaccine 26(39):5046–5057. doi:10.1016/j.vaccine.2008.07.035
122. Primard C, Poecheim J, Heuking S, Sublet E, Esmaeili F, Borchard G (2013) Multifunctional PLGA-based nanoparticles encapsulating simultaneously hydrophilic antigen and hydrophobic immunomodulator for mucosal immunization. Mol Pharm 10(8):2996–3004. doi:10.1021/mp400092y
123. Buyuktimkin B, Wang Q, Kiptoo P, Stewart JM, Berkland C, Siahaan TJ (2012) Vaccine-like controlled-release delivery of an immunomodulating peptide to treat experimental autoimmune encephalomyelitis. Mol Pharm 9(4):979–985. doi:10.1021/mp200614q
124. Minigo G, Scholzen A, Tang CK, Hanley JC, Kalkanidis M, Pietersz GA, Apostolopoulos V, Plebanski M (2007) Poly-L-lysine-coated nanoparticles: a potent delivery system to enhance DNA vaccine efficacy. Vaccine 25(7):1316–1327. doi:10.1016/j.vaccine.2006.09.086
125. Borges O, Silva M, de Sousa A, Borchard G, Junginger HE, Cordeiro-da-Silva A (2008) Alginate coated chitosan nanoparticles are an effective subcutaneous adjuvant for hepatitis B surface antigen. Int Immunopharmacol 8(13–14):1773–1780. doi:10.1016/j.intimp.2008.08.013

Chapter 22

Nanomedicine and Infection

Takami Akagi and Mitsuru Akashi

Abstract

Nanomedicine is the medical application of nanotechnology and related study to the prevention and treatment of disease in the human body. In recent years, significant effort has been directed to develop nanotechnology for drug delivery devices since it offers a suitable means of delivering small-molecule drugs, as well as biomacromolecules such as proteins, peptides, or oligonucleotides by either localized or targeted delivery to cells and tissues of interest. Until now, lipid-, polymer-, or nano-/microparticle-based drug delivery systems (DDS) have been developed to improve the efficacy and reduce the systemic toxicity of a wide range of drugs. Several DDS formulations of anticancer drugs, antifungal drugs, and vaccines are approved for clinical use. In this chapter, we will mainly focus on the clinical use of DDS on therapy and prevention of infectious diseases.

Key words Drug delivery system, Liposome, PEGylation, Vaccine adjuvant

1 Introduction

Nanomedicine is the application of nanotechnology to a given therapy; it also encompasses the prevention and diagnosis of disease in the human body and has the potential to change medical sciences significantly [1–5]. Nano-engineered and nanostructured drug carriers allow for the delivery of small-molecule hydrophobic drugs and the delivery of proteins and nucleic acids in a targeted fashion. Delivery of these molecules to specific sites within the body can be achieved to reduce systemic toxicity and allow for more efficient use of the drugs. The designing of an effective drug-targeting system is based on therapeutic efficacy, appropriate concentrations, and a longer circulation time in the blood. The drug needs to be released by the targeting system over a desired period of time with targeted specificity. This specific drug targeting is derived by taking advantage of the pathophysiological changes that take place in the course of diseases [6–8].

Nanotechnology focuses on formulating therapeutic agents in biocompatible and biodegradable nanocomposites such as

Zheng-Rong Lu and Shinji Sakuma (eds.), *Nanomaterials in Pharmacology*, Methods in Pharmacology and Toxicology,
DOI 10.1007/978-1-4939-3121-7_22, © Springer Science+Business Media New York 2016

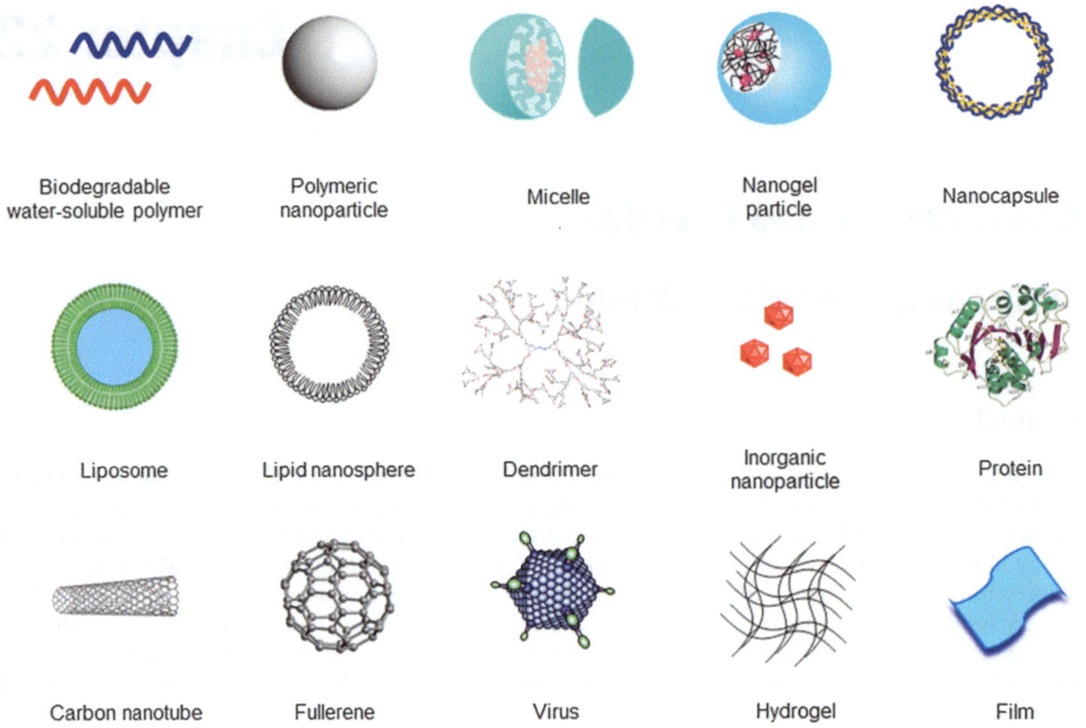

Fig. 1 Schematic illustration of carriers for drug delivery

nanoparticles, micelles, liposomes, emulsions, and conjugates consisting of polymers, lipids, inorganic compounds, and biological materials (Fig. 1). Since these systems are often polymeric and submicron in size, they have multiple advantages in drug delivery applications. In general, these systems can be used to provide targeted cellular and tissue delivery of drugs, to improve oral bioavailability, to sustain drug effect in target tissues, to solubilize drugs for intravascular delivery, and to improve the stability of drugs against enzymatic degradation by nucleases and proteases, especially for proteins and nucleic acids [9–11]. In addition, water-soluble polymers are most simple and attractive as potential carrier systems for targeted drug delivery. Though many different kinds of polymers are available, it was the development of polyethylene glycol (PEG) conjugation technology, generally known as PEGylation, that provided the real breakthrough to overcome the problems associated with peptides, proteins, and drugs [12, 13]. PEGylation (i.e., the attachment of PEG to proteins, drugs, and liposome) as a tool to drastically improve the pharmacokinetics and pharmacodynamic properties of the administered drugs is well established and is clinically used in the field of drug delivery [14, 15]. PEGylation can drastically enhance circulating time of administrated drugs in blood.

Recent advances in nanobiotechnology, pharmaceutical sciences, molecular biology, and polymer chemistry are now opening up exciting possibilities in the field of DDS. However, it is also perceived that there are several key issues to overcome such approaches into routine clinical use. The safety and efficacy of DDS-related drugs can be influenced by minor variations in multiple parameters and need to be carefully explored in preclinical and clinical studies, particularly relating to the stability, biodistribution, targeting to intended sites, and potential immune toxicities [16]. Liposomes are typical nano-sized DDS and the first of these received clinical approval in 1990. DOXIL®, liposomal doxorubicin, was the first commercially available liposomal anticancer drug (1995) [17]. It has an enhanced circulation half-life compared to the free drug because of its surface-grafted PEG coating. Liposomes can act as sustained release delivery systems. Recently, several types of DDS formulations containing antifungal, antiviral drugs, and vaccines for therapy and prevention of infectious diseases have been approved for clinical use. In this chapter, we will address the clinical use of DDS in the field of infectious disease. Vaccines are the most important preventive measure against infectious diseases. Nanotechnology-based DDS provides multiple platforms that can be used as vaccine adjuvants in the clinic and in the next generation of subunit vaccines.

2 Antifungal Drugs

Opportunistic fungal infections are a major problem for public health. Amphotericin B (AMB), a polyene antibiotic with broad spectrum antifungal activity, is considered the first-line therapy for systemic fungal infections. For over 50 years, AMB deoxycholate (AMBD), the conventional colloidal dispersion formulation known as Fungizone®, has been the treatment of choice for these infections. In spite of its high toxicity, it is still widely employed for the treatment of systemic fungal infections and parasitic diseases. One reason for this toxicity is the formation of self-aggregates as a result of low water solubility. In the last 10–15 years, new formulations of AMB that incorporate the drug into liposomes (AmBisome®) have been developed to overcome its toxic effects (Fig. 2) [18].

Liposomes are spherical vesicles where an aqueous core is surrounded by a phospholipid layer and cholesterol. Liposomes have several important properties like uniform particle size in the range of 50–700 nm and special surface characteristics. Water-soluble drugs can be entrapped in the interior of liposome-enclosed aqueous cores, and the encapsulating bilayer can be used to load hydrophobic drugs. Liposomal drug delivery systems have been widely studied since the 1970s to increase the solubility and therapeutic effect of chemotherapeutic compounds. They can be classified on the basis of size and the number of layers as small unilamellar, large unilamellar, small multilamellar, and large multilamellar [19].

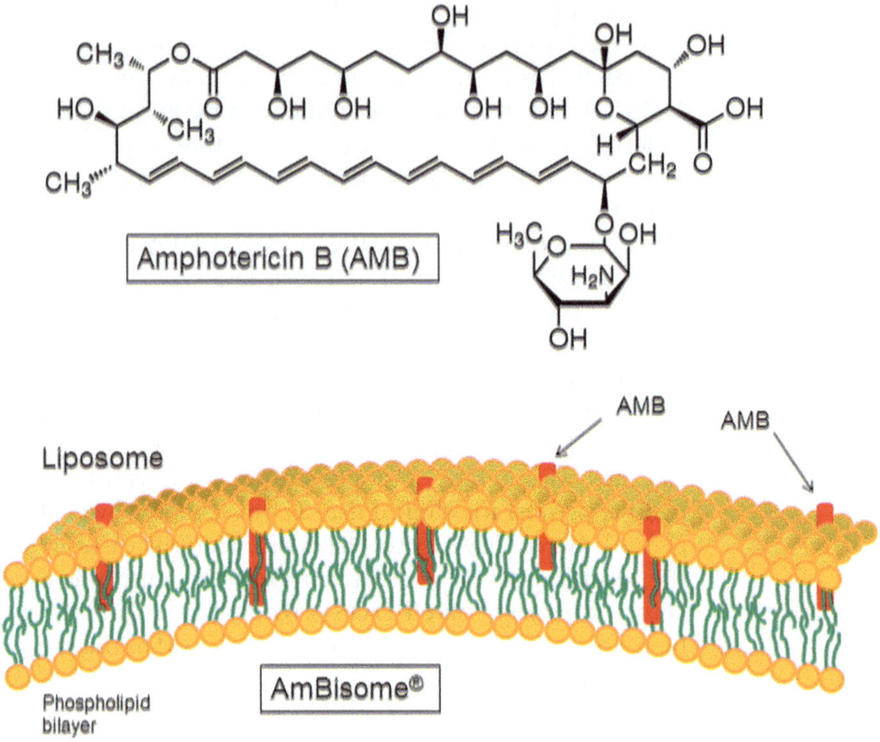

Fig. 2 Chemical structure of amphotericin B (AMB) and illustration of liposomal AMB (AmBisome®). AmBisome® is designed as unilamellar liposomes (<100 nm) with AMB present within the lipid bilayer membrane

The circulating time of liposomes in the blood can be modified by attaching PEG molecules on their surface. These molecules protect liposomes and prevent protein adsorption and clearance. Some of the important application of liposomes can be identified in the field of drug delivery and imaging [20, 21].

In order to improve the therapeutic effect of AMB and reduce its related toxicity, lipid-based formulations have been developed for intravenous administration. The liposomal formulation AmBisome®, a small unilamellar liposome (diameter 45–80 nm) containing AMB in the bilayer composed of hydrogenated soy phosphatidylcholine, distearoyl phosphatidylglycerol, and cholesterol, showed reduced toxicity and elevated peak plasma levels compared with conventional AMB without loss of the broad spectrum antifungal activity of AMB. After intravenous injection, AmBisome® can result in higher concentrations of AMB in the liver and spleen, but lower concentrations in the kidney and lungs, thereby decreasing its toxicity. Moreover, liposomal systems can enhance the drug accessibility to organs and tissues (e.g., bone marrow) otherwise inaccessible to free drug. In clinical trials, AmBisome® has demonstrated efficacy comparable to that of AMBD while reducing the incidence of treatment-related nephrotoxicity, electrolyte-wasting, and infusion-related reactions [22, 23]. In aqueous solutions, AmBisome® is quite stable, less than 5 % of the drug releases from the liposomes during extended incubation periods in human plasma. This stability is a key factor, accounting for the ability of AmBisome® to significantly reduce the acute and chronic toxicities associated with AMB. Numerous animal and clinical studies have documented the therapeutic efficacy of AmBisome® for a wide range of fungal infections. Mechanism of action studies show that AmBisome® liposomes specifically bind to fungal cell surfaces, damage the cell membrane, and kill the fungus [24, 25].

Despite the improvement in the therapeutic index for liposomal AMB, their use still remains limited due to higher cost, difficult route of administration, and ongoing concerns about toxicity [26]. There have been extensive studies to develop new AMB formulations on the basis of polymers, lipids, or physical aggregates of AMB to replace costly lipid-based formulations [23]. However, non-liposomal AMB delivery systems have not yet reached the clinic. Moreover, although the liposome delivery system has been tried for several drugs, only a few have been used in patients due to the slow development of the large-scale production technologies of pharmaceutical grade products.

3 Pegylated Interferons

Cytokine or antibody therapies have received widespread attention for their use as advanced drug therapies. Indeed, attempts are being made to develop a wide variety of therapeutic proteins for diseases including cancer, viral infections, and chronic autoimmune disorders. The potential value of bioactive proteins as therapeutics has been recognized for years. Unfortunately, many therapeutic proteins have disadvantages of short circulating half-life period ($t_{1/2}$) and low stability in the body. Therefore, these drugs are required the use of high and repeated doses to maintain therapeutic efficacy. This may increase the chance for the development of an adverse immune response [27]. Abuchowski et al. first described a method to covalently bond methoxy PEG (mPEG) to proteins in 1977 [28], called PEGylation. PEG is a hydrophilic polymer that has been widely used for the development of polymer-drug conjugates because it can improve protein solubility, stability, and pharmacokinetic parameters. The PEG conjugate obtained had the properties of a significantly increased circulating $t_{1/2}$, reduced immunogenicity and antigenicity, and retention of a circus-large portion of bioactivity. It has been postulated that these effects are due to a shell of PEG molecules around the protein that sterically hinders immunoreactions with immune cells (stealth effect) and protects the drug from proteolytic degradation. The discovery that PEGylation could greatly enhance the circulation time of nanocarriers such as polymeric nanoparticles and liposomes has greatly advanced the clinical translation of nanomedicines [29–31].

Chronic infection with hepatitis C virus (HCV) has an estimated prevalence of 1.6–2.0 % worldwide and is a major cause of liver-related diseases. The first attempts to halt the progression of infection relied on the empirical use of interferon (IFN), a naturally occurring cytokine that is implicated in antiviral innate immunity. The first studies of this treatment in the early 1990s, however, led to disappointing response rates. To improve the effectiveness and tolerability of the three times per week therapeutic schedule of IFN, two forms of pegylated interferon (PEG-IFN) were developed in the early 2000s, PEG-IFNα-2a and PEG-IFNα-2b [32]. Two PEG-IFNα molecules are commercially available for the treatment of chronic hepatitis C, and these differ in the size and nature of the covalently attached PEG molecule, with resulting differences in pharmacokinetics and in dosing regimens. PEG-IFNα-2b (PEGINTRON®) has a linear 12 kDa PEG chain covalently attached primarily to histidine-34 (about 50 % of all positional isomers) of IFNα-2b ($M_w = 19$ kDa) via an unstable urethane bond that is subject to hydrolysis once injected, releasing native IFNα-2b (Fig. 3). PEGINTRON® has a prolonged serum

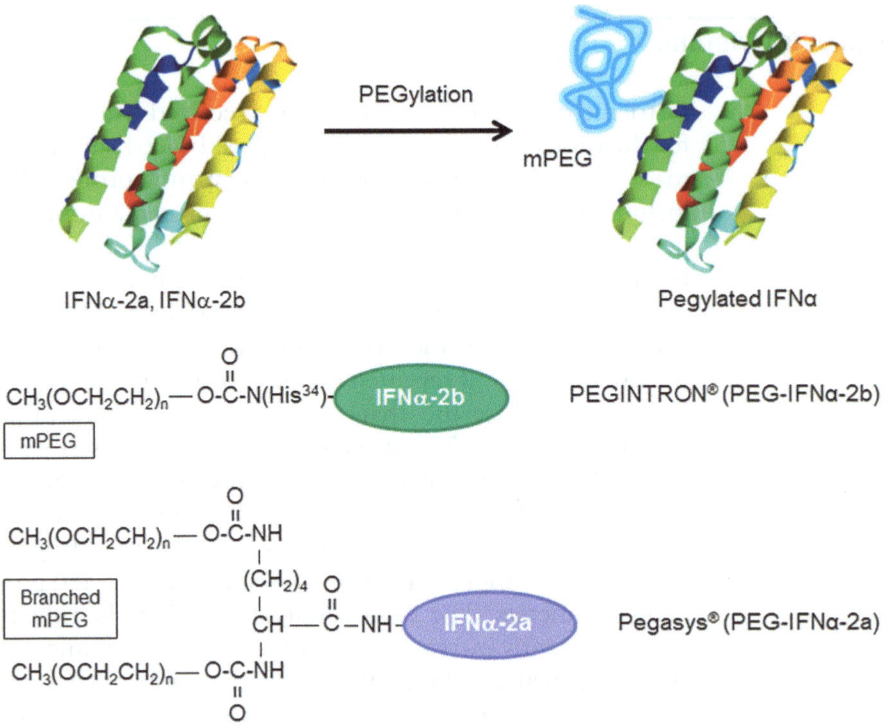

Fig. 3 Conjugation of mPEG (PEGylation) to interferon (IFN). PEG-IFNα-2b (PEGINTRON®) is produced by forming a covalent bond between a 12 kDa mPEG and IFNα-2b core protein using succinimidyl carbonate pegylation chemistry. PEG-IFNα-2a with 40 kDa-branched mPEG (Pegasys®) is synthesized using *N*-hydroxysuccinimid pegylation chemistry

half-life (40 h) relative to standard IFNα-2b (7–9 h). The branched, 40 kDa PEG molecule of PEG-IFNα-2a (Pegasys®) is covalently attached via stable amide bonds to lysine residues of IFNα-2a and circulates as an intact molecule. Consequently, Pegasys® has a very restricted volume of distribution, longer half-life and reduced clearance compared with native IFNα-2a, and can be administrated once weekly independently of bodyweight. PEGINTRON® has a shorter half-life in serum than Pegasys® and requires bodyweight-based dosing. The greater polymer size of Pegasys® works to reduce glomerular filtration, remarkably prolonging its serum half-life (72–96 h) compared with standard IFNα-2a (6–9 h). In clinical studies, once-weekly dosing of the PEG-IFNs was associated with a sustained virological response in patients infected with HCV. Once-weekly dosing with either of the PEG-IFNs was more effective than the respective thrice-weekly regimen of IFNα, with a comparable safety profile [33–35].

PEG-IFNα in combination with ribavirin (guanosine analog) is currently recommended as a standard-of-care treatment for chronic HCV infection [36]. This combination therapy has drastically improved the rate of sustained virological response, specifically in difficult-to-treat patients. PEGylation is now established as the method of choice for improving the pharmacokinetics and pharmacodynamics of protein pharmaceuticals. Applications of PEG-based hydrogels and PEG-modified liposomes have become increasingly important. New frontiers for the technology are now emerging, for example, in small-molecule modification, and it is certain that PEGylation will play an increasingly important role in pharmaceutical science and technology.

PEG is nontoxic and eliminated by a combination of renal and hepatic pathways. In fact, PEG has been approved for human intravenous, oral, and dermal applications. However, it has been reported that repeated parenteral administration of PEGylated proteins to animals is associated with cellular vacuolation in macrophages and/or histiocytes in various organs. Further understanding of the pharmacokinetics, metabolism, and biodistribution of PEG in PEGylated proteins will lead to develop safer PEGylated drugs [37].

4 Vaccines

4.1 Role of Adjuvants in Vaccine Development

The purpose of vaccination is to generate a strong immune response, thus providing long-term protection against infection. Vaccines have traditionally consisted of live attenuated pathogens, whole inactivated organisms, or inactivated toxins. Live vaccines typically induce potent immune responses (both humoral and cellular immunity) and complete protection against infection. However, live vaccines have been associated with a number of safety concerns, including reversion to virulence, resulting in disease and other adverse effects. The most recently licensed vaccines are typically recombinant products and are well defined at the molecular level. Unfortunately, these component vaccines generate a weaker immune response and typically require multiple doses. Indeed, the limited immunogenicity and difficulties in inducing antibodies of the appropriate specificity are major limitations of modern vaccine development. With the development of these new types of vaccines, there exists a critical need for additional delivery carriers as well as new adjuvants as immunostimulants. In many cases, the antigen itself is only very weakly immunogenic; therefore, an adjuvant is needed to induce optimal immune responses [38–42].

Adjuvants are compounds that enhance the immune response against co-inoculated antigens. The word "adjuvant" is derived from the Latin word "*adjuvare*" which means "to help" or "to enhance." In the past, many kinds of adjuvants have been developed, and they can be divided into two classes on the basis of their mechanism of action: vaccine delivery systems and immunostimulants [43]. Vaccine delivery systems generally have a particulate form (e.g., emulsions, liposomes, micelles, and polymeric nano/microparticles) and function mainly to target associated antigens into antigen-presenting cells (APCs) such as dendritic cells (DCs) and macrophages [41, 44–46]. In contrast, immunostimulants mostly consist of pathogen-associated molecules (e.g., lipopolysaccharide, monophosphoryl lipid A, cholera toxin, CpG ODN), which activate cells of the innate immune system via specific receptors, such as Toll-like receptors (TLRs). TLRs are critical in sensing infections and are therefore common targets of various adjuvants used in immunological studies [47–49].

4.2 Aluminum Adjuvants

Until recently, hydroxide and phosphate salts of aluminum (commonly called alum) and calcium were the only adjuvants licensed for human use. The adjuvant effects of alum were first discovered in the 1920s [50]. The mechanism of action of alum adjuvant is complex and not yet fully understood. It likely involves various mechanisms including the formation of depot, increasing targeting of antigens to APCs and (non-) specific activation of immune systems. Antigen depots enhance immunogenicity of antigens by concentrating the antigens and extending the time antigen resides in the body, thus increasing the probability of interaction with immune cells [51, 52]. Recently, it was proposed that alum adjuvants activate an intracellular innate immune response system called the NALP3 inflammasome. Several research groups have implicated components of the inflammasome in the adjuvant activity of alum [53–55]. The inflammasome is a large multi-protein complex which plays a key role in innate immunity by participating in the production of the pro-inflammatory cytokines interleukin-1β

(IL-1β) and IL-18. NALP3 activation is induced by phagocytosis of aluminum salt or silica crystals, and this uptake subsequently lead to lysosomal damage and rupture. The NALP3 inflammasome senses lysosomal damage as an endogenous danger signal [56]. Recently, Marichal et al. proposed that alum adjuvant activity is related to the production of another danger signal derived from DNA released from necrotic cells exposed to alum [57].

Most adjuvant formulation development focuses on micro- and nanoparticulate platforms, including alum, liposomes, and emulsions. Alum has been employed as adjuvants in human vaccines for many decades, and they consist of crystalline nanoparticles that aggregate to form a heterogeneous dispersion of several micron-sized particles. They are highly charged and conducive to the adsorption of antigens or immunomodulatory molecules. Alum adjuvants have primarily been used in tetanus, diphtheria, pertussis, and poliomyelitis vaccines as part of standard child vaccination programs in many countries for approximately 50 years. Alum adjuvants have also been introduced into hepatitis A and hepatitis B virus (HBV) vaccines [50]. However, the use of alum-type adjuvant for vaccination has some disadvantages. They induce local reactions, induce IgE antibody responses, and generally fail to induce cell-mediated immunity, particularly cytotoxic T lymphocyte (CTL) responses. Therefore, the development of more efficient and safe adjuvants to obtain high and long-lasting immune responses is of primary importance.

Limitations of single-adjuvant vaccine formulations are driving the need to explore combination adjuvants. For example, alum or monophosphoryl lipid A (MPL), a derivative of lipopolysaccharide (LPS), alone induce only modest immune responses to a human papillomavirus (HPV) vaccine, but when these two adjuvants are combined, they induce potent immune responses [58]. Indeed, it has been demonstrated that the use of combination adjuvants can be highly beneficial by significantly improving immune responses induced by a vaccine. The adjuvant combination of MPL (TLR4 ligand) and aluminum hydroxide (named AS04) was approved for use in HBV (Fendrix®) and HPV (Cervarix®) vaccines [59].

4.3 Emulsion-Based Adjuvants

Emulsions have a long history of adjuvant development, although they were not approved as vaccines until the 1990s. Modern emulsion adjuvants for human vaccines consist of oil-in-water (O/W), with nano-sized oil droplets emulsified with biocompatible surfactants in an aqueous phase. MF59® is a submicron O/W emulsion of a squalene oil, polyoxyethylene sorbitan monooleate (Tween 80), and sorbitan trioleate (Span 85) (Fig. 4) [60]. Squalene is a natural organic compound originally obtained from shark liver oil and a biochemical precursor to steroids. The oil droplets, which have a mean diameter of about 160 nm, are stabilized by two non-ionic surfactants. MF59® is an effective vaccine adjuvant which was

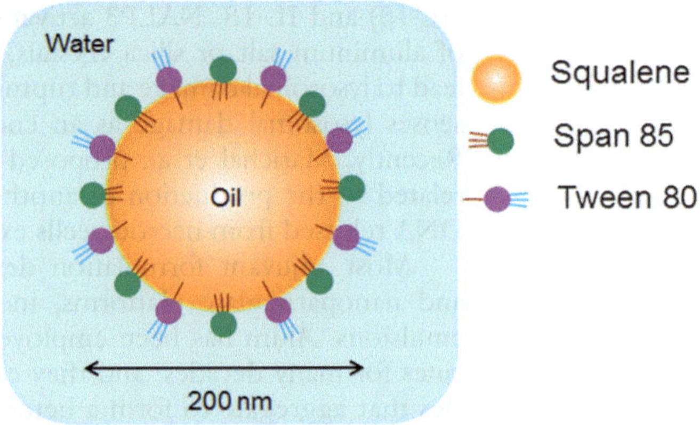

Fig. 4 The composition of MF59® O/W emulsion. Squalene droplets (4.3 %) are stabilized by two nonionic surfactants, polyoxyethylene sorbitan monooleate (Tween 80) (0.5 %) and sorbitan triolate (Span 85) (0.5 %) in water

originally approved to be included in a licensed influenza vaccine to be used in the elderly in Europe in 1997. The MF59® containing influenza vaccine (Fluad®) is now licensed in more than 20 countries worldwide [61]. More recently, MF59® has also been shown to enhance immune responses against both homologous and heterologous influenza virus strains in young children and infants with safety. In a subsequent study, MF59® was shown to increase the efficacy of an influenza vaccine from 43 to 89 % in young children. Moving beyond seasonal influenza vaccines, MF59® has also significantly improved the immunogenicity of pandemic influenza vaccines with relatively low-antigen content and with fewer doses [62].

The mechanism of action of O/W emulsions is still not completely understood. Initially it was thought to be due to a depot effect. However, the depot effect of the MF59® was subsequently disputed. A soluble gD2 antigen from herpes simplex virus (HSV) and MF59® injected intramuscularly in mice had different clearance kinetics, and the presence of MF59® did not alter the clearance kinetics of the antigen [63]. The O/W emulsions did not form a long-lived depot at the injection site. Both the antigen and the emulsion were cleared relatively rapidly. Using a similar model, it has been reported that the intracellular colocation of antigen and MF59® was observed after intramuscular injection. MF59® acted mainly as a delivery system of co-injected antigen to activated local cells. The antigen-internalized cells at the injection site were positive for DEC205 and for MHC class II molecule, suggesting that they were DCs [64]. In addition, using peripheral blood mononuclear cells from healthy blood donors, it has been found that MF59® induces the production of chemokines involved in cell recruitment to the tissues such as MCP-1, MIP-1α, MIP-1β, and

IL-8 and the expression of surface markers of differentiation to a DC phenotype [65]. From these results, it was confirmed that MF59 could directly increase phagocytosis and pinocytosis and promote antigen uptake by antigen-presenting cells (APCs). Furthermore, it was shown that MF59® induced extensive changes in the mouse muscle transcriptome and promoted the production of immune mediators in muscle tissues, which activated resident DCs and initiated cell recruitment. It is suggested that the MF59® creates a transient immunocompetent environment at the injection site (muscles), resulting in the recruitment of different immune cells, which are able to take up antigen and adjuvant and transport them to the draining lymph nodes, where the immune response is induced [66–68].

AS03 is an adjuvant system composed of DL-α-tocopherol (vitamin E), squalene, and polysorbate 80 in an O/W emulsion, essentially increasing the oil content in AS03 as compared with MF59®. The size of the emulation droplet is lower than 200 nm [69]. In various nonclinical and clinical studies, high titers of antigen-specific antibodies were obtained after injection of an AS03 containing vaccine, permitting antigen-sparing strategies. AS03 is able to enhance the vaccine antigen-specific adaptive response by activating the innate immune system locally and by increasing antigen uptake in local lymph nodes. In nonclinical (animal) models of the AS03 containing prepandemic H5N1 influenza vaccine, increased levels of anti-influenza antibodies showed protection against disease and against virus replication of influenza strains homologous/heterologous to the vaccine strain [70]. By incorporating AS03 in the pandemic H1N1/2009 vaccine, vaccine immunogenicity was increased compared with H1N1 vaccines without adjuvant. High H1N1/2009/AS03 vaccine effectiveness was demonstrated in several assessments in a wide range of human populations. Altogether, the nonclinical and clinical data illustrate the ability of AS03 to induce superior adaptive responses against the vaccine antigen, principally in terms of antibody levels and immune memory. Recently, AS03, O/W emulsion, was approved as a component of a prepandemic H5N1 vaccine (Prepandrix®) [71].

4.4 Polymeric Particle-Based Adjuvants

Antigen-loaded polymeric nano- and microparticles are being investigated as vaccine adjuvant alternatives to the currently used alum [42, 72–74]. Poly(lactide-*co*-glycolide) (PLGA) particles are extensively investigated for developing particulate vaccines in controlled release applications [75]. Other formulations using nanoparticles composed of biodegradable polymers have undergone extensive research and development, but no approved vaccine products are on the horizon.

In order to develop new particulate adjuvants, we designed a novel vaccine delivery system with self-assembled amphiphilic polymeric nanoparticles (NPs) [76–78]. We prepared amphiphilic NPs consisting of hydrophilic poly(γ-glutamic acid) (γ-PGA) and hydrophobic L-phenylalanine ethylester (Phe) as the side chain. The γ-PGA-*graft*-Phe copolymer (γ-PGA-Phe) formed monodispersed NPs in water due to their amphiphilic characteristics. The size of the γ-PGA-Phe NPs could be easily controlled from 30 to 200 nm by varying the preparative conditions [79, 80]. Antigen-encapsulated γ-PGA-Phe NPs could be successfully used to enhance the antigen delivery to DCs. The NPs also had adjuvant activity via TLR for DC maturation [81–84]. Thus, the NPs have significant potential as antigen carriers and adjuvants for DCs (Fig. 5). It has been demonstrated that the antigen-conjugated γ-PGA-Phe NPs are also effective for induction of antigen-specific cellular immunity and for vaccines against viral infections such as influenza virus [85, 86] but also reduce the toxicity associated with inflammatory reactions compared to other common vaccine adjuvants. In addition, the efficacy of γ-PGA-Phe NPs as vaccine adjuvants against

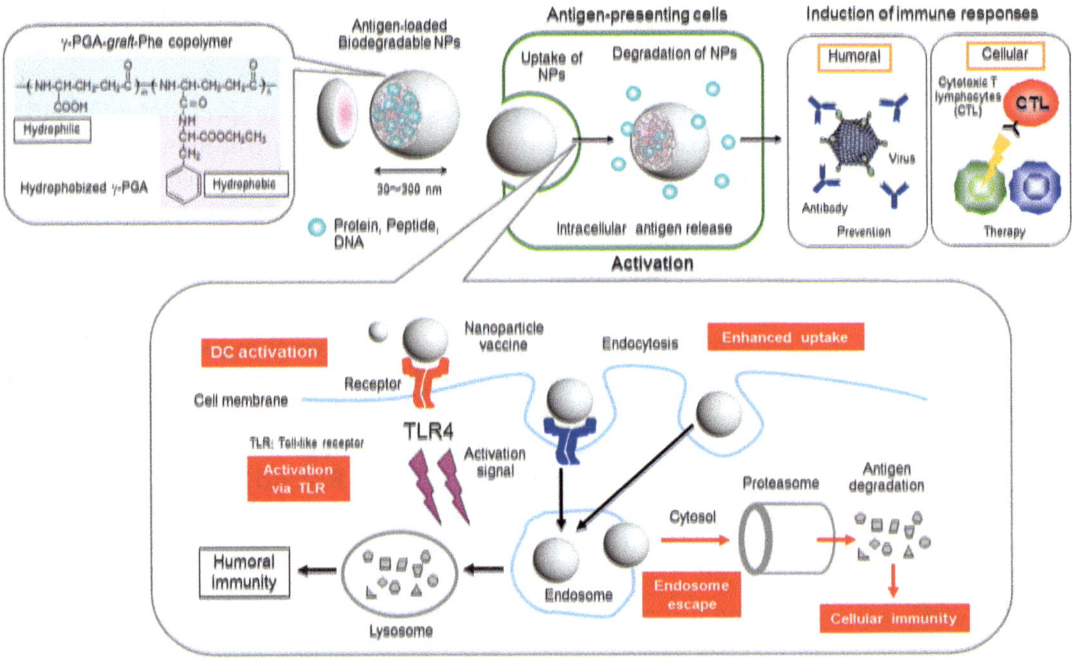

Fig. 5 Induction of adaptive immune responses (humoral and cellular immunity) by particulate adjuvant (γ-PGA-Phe NPs). Antigen-loaded γ-PGA-Phe NPs can be internalized into dendritic cells (DCs) via endocytosis, depending on their sizes. The NPs activate DCs through TLR. The NPs taken up by DCs can disrupt or destabilize the endosomal membrane and release antigen into the cytoplasm. Polymer hydrophobicity is also important factor for endosome escape of antigens. Antigens taken up by DCs are processed into peptide epitopes and directed through two discrete pathways to MHC classes I and II, which present peptide for interaction with either $CD8^+$ or $CD4^+$ T cells, respectively. Antigen-loaded γ-PGA-Phe NPs induces potent antigen-specific cellular and humoral immune responses

human immunodeficiency virus (HIV), Japanese encephalitis virus, human T-cell leukemia virus type-I (HTLV-I), or cancers has been demonstrated using mouse immunization study [78]. This strategy will provide novel immune therapies for infectious diseases. In the near future, the platform technology for the practical application and commercialization of vaccines using γ-PGA-Phe NPs as next-generation adjuvants is under way.

Polymeric NPs are promising adjuvants, and they have various physicochemical characteristics that can regulate immune responses, including size, morphology, surface properties (charge and hydrophobicity), and rigidity, but how it affects particle adjuvanticity remains unknown [87]. Particle size is the most important particulate physicochemical factor and plays crucial roles in the interaction between particles and APCs. For instance, Kanchan et al. reported that polylactide (PLA) NPs (200–600 nm) were efficiently taken up by macrophages compared to microparticles (2–8 μm) [88]. The particle uptake by APCs is affected by their sizes. Particle shape is also an important factor for cellular uptake. Champion et al. observed that the cellular uptake of particles strongly depends on the shape of particles. The wormlike particles with high aspect ratios showed negligible phagocytosis when compared to traditional spherical particles [89]. The result indicates that uptake of particles by APCs strongly depends on the local geometry at the interface of particle and the cells. Recently, it has been reported that the hydrophobicity of particulate materials is one of the dominant factors for the initiation of immune responses. It has been showed that the hydrophobicity of gold NPs significantly affected cytokine gene expression of spleen cells in vitro. The cytokine expression correlated with the surface hydrophobicity of gold NPs with different functional groups [90]. The capability to manipulate physiochemical properties of particles strongly holds up the continuing promise of target-oriented particles for a range of biomedical applications. Understanding the biological interactions controlled by the physicochemical properties of particles will be essential for the design of next-generation adjuvants and particle delivery systems and for continued progress in translational research.

5 Future Prospects

Nanomedicine is the biomedical application of nanoscale materials for the prevention, therapy, and diagnosis of disease. Nano-engineered DDS have been successfully used as clinical tools, not only for the regulation of pharmacological drug release profiles but also for specific targeting of cells and diseased tissues. Moreover, nanotechnology is currently being used to manipulate specific immune responses for prophylactic and therapeutic effects. In the future, the use of nanoparticles with unique immunological properties and various physicochemical characteristic (size, degradability, stimulus-responsibility, and so on) will enable to customize immune responses in new strategies. In the years to come, it is expected that the emergence of nanotechnology platforms and progress in pharmaceutics, biology, and polymer science will further promote the development of multifunctional nanoparticulate systems to meet the ultimate goal of controlled drug delivery, which is to maximize therapeutic activity while minimizing the negative side effects of the drugs.

References

1. Moghimi SM, Hunter AC, Murray JC (2005) Nanomedicine: current status and future prospects. FASEB J 19:311–330
2. Singh S (2010) Nanomedicine-nanoscale drugs and delivery systems. J Nanosci Nanotechnol 10:7906–7918
3. Duncan R, Gaspar R (2011) Nanomedicine(s) under the microscope. Mol Pharm 8: 2101–2141
4. Smith DM, Simon JK, Baker JR Jr (2013) Applications of nanotechnology for immunology. Nat Rev Immunol 13:592–605
5. Sosnik A, Carcaboso AM (2014) Nanomedicines in the future of pediatric therapy. Adv Drug Deliv Rev 73C:140–161
6. Torchilin VP (2006) Multifunctional nanocarriers. Adv Drug Deliv Rev 58:1532–1555
7. Petros RA, DeSimone JM (2010) Strategies in the design of nanoparticles for therapeutic applications. Nat Rev Drug Discov 9:615–627
8. Aslan B, Ozpolat B, Sood AK, Lopez-Berestein G (2013) Nanotechnology in cancer therapy. J Drug Target 21:904–913
9. Nishiyama N, Kataoka K (2006) Nanostructured devices based on block copolymer assemblies for drug delivery: designing structures for enhanced drug function. Adv Polym Sci 193:67–101
10. Doshi N, Mitragotri S (2009) Designer biomaterials for nanomedicine. Adv Funct Mater 19:3843–3854
11. Musyanovych A, Landfester K (2014) Polymer micro- and nanocapsules as biological carriers with multifunctional properties. Macromol Biosci 14:458–477
12. Greenwald RB, Choe YH, McGuire J, Conover CD (2003) Effective drug delivery by PEGylated drug conjugates. Adv Drug Deliv Rev 55:217–250
13. Harris JM, Chess RB (2003) Effect of pegylation on pharmaceuticals. Nat Rev Drug Discov 2:214–221
14. Parveen S, Sahoo SK (2006) Nanomedicine: clinical applications of polyethylene glycol conjugated proteins and drugs. Clin Pharmacokinet 45:965–988
15. van der Meel R, Vehmeijer LJ, Kok RJ, Storm G, van Gaal EV (2013) Ligand-targeted particulate nanomedicines undergoing clinical evaluation: current status. Adv Drug Deliv Rev 65:1284–1298
16. Desai N (2012) Challenges in development of nanoparticle-based therapeutics. AAPS J 14: 282–295
17. Slingerland M, Guchelaar HJ, Gelderblom H (2012) Liposomal drug formulations in cancer therapy: 15 years along the road. Drug Discov Today 17:160–166
18. Gibbs WJ, Drew RH, Perfect JR (2005) Liposomal amphotericin B: clinical experience and perspectives. Expert Rev Anti Infect Ther 3:167–181
19. Akbarzadeh A, Rezaei-Sadabady R, Davaran S, Joo SW, Zarghami N, Hanifehpour Y, Samiei M, Kouhi M, Nejati-Koshki K (2013) Liposome: classification, preparation, and applications. Nanoscale Res Lett 8:102
20. Petersen AL, Hansen AE, Gabizon A, Andresen TL (2012) Liposome imaging agents in personalized medicine. Adv Drug Deliv Rev 64:1417–1435
21. Cullis PR (2013) Liposomal drug delivery systems: from concept to clinical applications. Adv Drug Deliv Rev 65:36–48
22. Wong-Beringer A, Jacobs RA, Guglielmo BJ (1998) Lipid formulations of amphotericin B: clinical efficacy and toxicities. Clin Infect Dis 27:603–618
23. Torrado JJ, Espada R, Ballesteros MP, Torrado-Santiago S (2008) Amphotericin B formulations and drug targeting. J Pharm Sci 97:2405–2425
24. Adler-moore JP, Proffitt RT (1993) Development, characterization, efficacy and mode of action of AmBisome, a unilamellar

liposomal formulation of amphotericin B. J Liposome Res 3:429–450

25. Boswell GW, Buell D, Bekersky I (1998) Am Bisome (liposomal amphotericin B): a comparative review. J Clin Pharmacol 38:583–592
26. Egger SS, Meier S, Leu C, Christen S, Gratwohl A, Krahenbuhl S, Haschke M (2010) Drug interactions and adverse events associated with antimycotic drugs used for invasive aspergillosis in hematopoietic SCT. Bone Marrow Transplant 45:1197–1203
27. Nucci ML, Shorr R, Abuchowski A (1991) The therapeutic value of poly(ethylene glycol)-modified proteins. Adv Drug Deliv Rev 6: 133–151
28. Abuchowski A, McCoy TJR, Palczuk NC, van Es T, Davis FF (1977) Effect of covalent attachment of polyethylene glycol on immunogenicity and circulating life of bovine liver catalase. J Biol Chem 252:3582–3586
29. Fishburn CS (2008) The pharmacology of PEGylation: balancing PD with PK to generate novel therapeutics. J Pharm Sci 97:4167–4183
30. Joralemon MJ, McRae S, Emrick T (2010) PEGylated polymers for medicine: from conjugation to self-assembled systems. Chem Commun 46:1377–1393
31. Vllasaliu D, Fowler R, Stolnik S (2014) PEGylated nanomedicines: recent progress and remaining concerns. Expert Opin Drug Deliv 11:139–154
32. Grace MJ, Cutler DL, Bordens RW (2005) Pegylated IFNs for chronic hepatitis C: an update. Expert Opin Drug Deliv 2:219–226
33. Kozlowski A, Harris JM (2001) Improvements in protein PEGylation: pegylated interferons for treatment of hepatitis C. J Control Release 72:217–224
34. Luxon BA, Grace M, Brassard D, Bordens R (2002) Pegylated interferons for the treatment of chronic hepatitis C infection. Clin Ther 24:1363–1383
35. Wang YS, Youngster S, Grace M, Bausch J, Bordens R, Wyss DF (2002) Structural and biological characterization of pegylated recombinant interferon alpha-2b and its therapeutic implications. Adv Drug Deliv Rev 54:547–570
36. Tsubota A, Fujise K, Namiki Y, Tada N (2011) Peginterferon and ribavirin treatment for hepatitis C virus infection. World J Gastroenterol 17(4):419–432
37. Baumann A, Tuerck D, Prabhu S, Dickmann L, Sims J (2014) Pharmacokinetics, metabolism and distribution of PEGs and PEGylated proteins: quo vadis? Drug Discov Today 19: 1623–1631
38. Singh M, O'Hagan DT (1999) Advances in vaccine adjuvants. Nat Biotechnol 17:1075–1081
39. Singh M, O'Hagan DT (2002) Recent advances in vaccine adjuvants. Pharm Res 19:715–728
40. Peek LJ, Middaugh CR, Berkland C (2008) Nanotechnology in vaccine delivery. Adv Drug Deliv Rev 60:915–928
41. Rice-Ficht AC, Arenas-Gamboa AM, Kahl-McDonagh MM, Ficht TA (2010) Polymeric particles in vaccine delivery. Curr Opin Microbiol 13:106–112
42. De Koker S, Lambrecht BN, Willart MA, van Kooyk Y, Grooten J, Vervaet C, Remon JP, De Geest BG (2011) Designing polymeric particles for antigen delivery. Chem Soc Rev 40:320–339
43. O'Hagan DT, Valiante NM (2003) Recent advances in the discovery and delivery of vaccine adjuvants. Nat Rev Drug Discov 2:727–735
44. Reddy ST, Swartz MA, Hubbell JA (2006) Targeting dendritic cells with biomaterials: developing the next generation of vaccines. Trends Immunol 27:573–579
45. Klippstein R, Pozo D (2010) Nanotechnology-based manipulation of dendritic cells for enhanced immunotherapy strategies. Nanomedicine 6:523–529
46. Salvador A, Igartua M, Hernández RM, Pedraz JL (2011) An overview on the field of micro- and nanotechnologies for synthetic peptide-based vaccines. J Drug Deliv 2011:181646
47. Ishii KJ, Akira S (2007) Toll or toll-free adjuvant path toward the optimal vaccine development. J Clin Immunol 27:363–371
48. Duthie MS, Windish HP, Fox CB, Reed SG (2011) Use of defined TLR ligands as adjuvants within human vaccines. Immunol Rev 239:178–196
49. Steinhagen F, Kinjo T, Bode C, Klinman DM (2011) TLR-based immune adjuvants. Vaccine 29:3341–3355
50. Marrack P, McKee AS, Munks MW (2009) Towards an understanding of the adjuvant action of aluminium. Nat Rev Immunol 9:287–293
51. Gupta RK (1998) Aluminum compounds as vaccine adjuvants. Adv Drug Deliv Rev 32: 155–172
52. Brewer JM (2006) (How) do aluminium adjuvants work? Immunol Lett 102:10–15
53. Eisenbarth SC, Colegio OR, O'Connor W, Sutterwala FS, Flavell RA (2008) Crucial role

for the Nalp3 inflammasome in the immunostimulatory properties of aluminium adjuvants. Nature 453:1122–1126

54. Franchi L, Núñez G (2008) The Nlrp3 inflammasome is critical for aluminium hydroxide-mediated IL-1beta secretion but dispensable for adjuvant activity. Eur J Immunol 38: 2085–2089

55. Reed SG, Orr MT, Fox CB (2013) Key roles of adjuvants in modern vaccines. Nat Med 19:1597–1608

56. Hornung V, Bauernfeind F, Halle A, Samstad EO, Kono H, Rock KL, Fitzgerald KA, Latz E (2008) Silica crystals and aluminum salts activate the NALP3 inflammasome through phagosomal destabilization. Nat Immunol 9: 847–856

57. Marichal T, Ohata K, Bedoret D, Mesnil C, Sabatel C, Kobiyama K, Lekeux P, Coban C, Akira S, Ishii KJ, Bureau F, Desmet CJ (2011) DNA released from dying host cells mediates aluminum adjuvant activity. Nat Med 17: 996–1002

58. Didierlaurent AM, Morel S, Lockman L, Giannini SL, Bisteau M, Carlsen H, Kielland A, Vosters O, Vanderheyde N, Schiavetti F, Larocque D, Van Mechelen M, Garçon N (2009) AS04, an aluminum salt- and TLR4 agonist-based adjuvant system, induces a transient localized innate immune response leading to enhanced adaptive immunity. Immunology 183:6186–6197

59. Mutwiri G, Gerdts V, van Drunen Littel-van den Hurk S, Auray G, Eng N, Garlapati S, Babiuk LA, Potter A (2011) Combination adjuvants: the next generation of adjuvants? Expert Rev Vaccines 10:95–107

60. Calabro S, Tritto E, Pezzotti A, Taccone M, Muzzi A, Bertholet S, De Gregorio E, O'Hagan DT, Baudner B, Seubert A (2013) The adjuvant effect of MF59 is due to the oil-in-water emulsion formulation, none of the individual components induce a comparable adjuvant effect. Vaccine 31:3363–3369

61. Pellegrini M, Nicolay U, Lindert K, Groth N, Della Cioppa G (2009) MF59-adjuvanted versus non-adjuvanted influenza vaccines: integrated analysis from a large safety database. Vaccine 27:6959–6965

62. O'Hagan DT, Ott GS, De Gregorio E, Seubert A (2012) The mechanism of action of MF59 - an innately attractive adjuvant formulation. Vaccine 30:4341–4348

63. Dupuis M, McDonald DM, Ott G (2000) Distribution of adjuvant MF59 and antigen gD2 after intramuscular injection in mice. Vaccine 18:434–439

64. Dupuis M, Murphy TJ, Higgins D, Ugozzoli M, van Nest G, Ott G, McDonald DM (1998) Dendritic cells internalize vaccine adjuvant after intramuscular injection. Cell Immunol 186:18–27

65. Seubert A, Monaci E, Pizza M, O'Hagan DT, Wack A (2008) The adjuvants aluminum hydroxide and MF59 induce monocyte and granulocyte chemoattractants and enhance monocyte differentiation toward dendritic cells. J Immunol 180:5402–5412

66. Tritto E, Mosca F, De Gregorio E (2009) Mechanism of action of licensed vaccine adjuvants. Vaccine 27:3331–3334

67. Lambrecht BN, Kool M, Willart MA, Hammad H (2009) Mechanism of action of clinically approved adjuvants. Curr Opin Immunol 21:23–29

68. El Sahly H (2010) MF59™ as a vaccine adjuvant: a review of safety and immunogenicity. Expert Rev Vaccines 9:1135–1141

69. Garçon N, Vaughn DW, Didierlaurent AM (2012) Development and evaluation of AS03, an adjuvant system containing α-tocopherol and squalene in an oil-in-water emulsion. Expert Rev Vaccines 11:349–366

70. Baras B, Stittelaar KJ, Simon JH, Thoolen RJ, Mossman SP, Pistoor FH, van Amerongen G, Wettendorff MA, Hanon E, Osterhaus AD (2008) Cross-protection against lethal H5N1 challenge in ferrets with an adjuvanted pandemic influenza vaccine. PLoS One 3, e1401

71. Vogel FR, Caillet C, Kusters IC, Haensler J (2009) Emulsion-based adjuvants for influenza vaccines. Expert Rev Vaccines 8:483–492

72. Dey AK, Srivastava IK (2011) Novel adjuvants and delivery systems for enhancing immune responses induced by immunogens. Expert Rev Vaccines 10:227–251

73. Mamo T, Poland GA (2012) Nanovaccinology: the next generation of vaccines meets 21st century materials science and engineering. Vaccine 30:6609–6611

74. Gregory AE, Titball R, Williamson D (2013) Vaccine delivery using nanoparticles. Front Cell Infect Microbiol 3:13

75. Mundargi RC, Babu VR, Rangaswamy V, Patel P, Aminabhavi TM (2008) Nano/micro technologies for delivering macromolecular therapeutics using poly(d,l-lactide-co-glycolide) and its derivatives. J Control Release 125:193–209

76. Akagi T, Wang X, Uto T, Baba M, Akashi M (2007) Protein direct delivery to dendritic cells using nanoparticles based on amphiphilic poly(amino acid) derivatives. Biomaterials 28:3427–3436

77. Akagi T, Baba M, Akashi M (2007) Preparation of nanoparticles by the self-organization of polymers consisting of hydrophobic and hydrophilic segments: potential applications. Polymer 48:6729–6747
78. Akagi T, Baba M, Akashi M (2012) Biodegradable nanoparticles as vaccine adjuvants and delivery systems: regulation of immune responses by nanoparticle-based vaccine. Adv Polymer Sci 247:31–64
79. Kim H, Akagi T, Akashi M (2009) Preparation of size tunable amphiphilic poly(amino acid) nanoparticles. Macromol Biosci 9:842–848
80. Kim H, Uto T, Akagi T, Baba M, Akashi M (2010) Amphiphilic poly(amino acid) nanoparticles induce size-dependent dendritic cell maturation. Adv Funct Mater 20:3925–3931
81. Uto T, Wang X, Sato K, Haraguchi M, Akagi T, Akashi M, Baba M (2007) Targeting of antigen to dendritic cells with poly(γ-glutamic acid) nanoparticles induce antigen-specific humoral and cellular immunity. J Immunol 178:2979–2986
82. Broos S, Lundberg K, Akagi T, Kadowaki K, Akashi M, Greiff L, Borrebaeck CAK, Lindstedt M (2010) Immunomodulatory nanoparticles as adjuvants and allergen delivery system to human dendritic cells: Implications for specific immunotherapy. Vaccine 28:5075–5085
83. Uto T, Akagi T, Yoshinaga K, Toyama M, Akashi M, Baba M (2011) The induction of innate and adaptive immunity by biodegradable poly(γ-glutamic acid) nanoparticles via a TLR4 and MyD88 signaling pathway. Biomaterials 32:5206–5212
84. Shima F, Uto T, Akagi T, Baba M, Akashi M (2013) Size effect of amphiphilic poly(γ-glutamic acid) nanoparticles on cellular uptake and maturation of dendritic cells in vivo. Acta Biomater 9:8910–8920
85. Okamoto S, Matsuura M, Akagi T, Akashi M, Tanimoto T, Ishikawa T, Takahashi M, Yamanishi K, Mori Y (2009) Poly(γ-glutamic acid) nano-particles combined with mucosal influenza virus hemagglutinin vaccine protects against influenza virus infection in mice. Vaccine 27:5896–5905
86. Okamoto S, Matsuoka S, Takenaka N, Haredy A, Tanimoto T, Gomi Y, Ishikawa T, Akagi T, Akashi M, Okuno Y, Mori Y, Yamanishi K (2012) Intranasal immunization with formalin-inactivated human influenza A whole-virion vaccine alone or split-virion vaccine with mucosal adjuvants show similar cross-protection. Clin Vaccine Immunol 19:979–990
87. Yan Y, Such GK, Johnston AP, Best JP, Caruso F (2012) Engineering particles for therapeutic delivery: prospects and challenges. ACS Nano 6:3663–3669
88. Kanchan V, Panda AK (2007) Interactions of antigen-loaded polylactide particles with macrophages and their correlation with the immune response. Biomaterials 28:5344–5357
89. Champion JA, Mitragotri S (2006) Role of target geometry in phagocytosis. Proc Natl Acad Sci U S A 103:4930–4934
90. Moyano DF, Goldsmith M, Solfiell DJ, Milo DL, Miranda OR, Peer D, Rotello VM (2012) Nanoparticle hydrophobicity dictates immune response. J Am Chem Soc 134:3965–3967

Chapter 23

Cancer Therapy with Nanotechnology-Based Drug Delivery Systems: Applications and Challenges of Liposome Technologies for Advanced Cancer Therapy

Ryo Suzuki*, Daiki Omata*, Yusuke Oda, Johan Unga, Yoichi Negishi, and Kazuo Maruyama

Abstract

Nanotechnologies have the potential to improve cancer therapy. In particular, liposomes and micelles serve as nano-sized drug delivery carriers for the administration of cancer drugs. Although micelles have not been approved by the Food and Drug Administration (FDA) in USA, some liposomal drugs have been already approved for use in anticancer therapy. In most cases, these liposomal drugs have improved pharmacokinetics and reduced side effects due to the encapsulation of the drug. Also, passive targeting to the tumor can be achieved due to physiological properties that lead to the enhanced permeability and retention (EPR) effect in tumor tissue. More recently, modification of the liposomal surface with active targeting molecules such as antibodies or natural receptor ligands has been investigated in clinical trials. Moreover, novel strategies for drug release, activation, and delivery with physical stimuli have been developed. There is a plethora of preclinical and clinical data about liposomal drugs for cancer therapy because they have been utilized as commercially available drugs for a long time. In the present review, we summarize the use of tumor-targeting technologies and approved liposomal antitumor drugs, describe their properties, and assess applications and challenges of liposome technologies for advanced cancer therapy.

Key words Liposome, Cancer therapy, Nanomedicine, Enhanced permeability and retention (EPR) effect, Targeting, Drug delivery system, Theranostics

1 Introduction

Chemotherapy, radiotherapy, and immunotherapy are commonly used in the treatment of cancer, and are continuously being developed as individual therapies. These advances in noninvasive cancer therapies have gradually improved the quality of life (QOL) for cancer patients by suppressing cancer growth, recurrence, and metastasis. Recently, various antitumor drugs consisting of antibodies and molecular targeting agents have been developed and

*Author contributed equally with all other contributors.

Zheng-Rong Lu and Shinji Sakuma (eds.), *Nanomaterials in Pharmacology*, Methods in Pharmacology and Toxicology,
DOI 10.1007/978-1-4939-3121-7_23, © Springer Science+Business Media New York 2016

applied as cancer therapies. Anticancer chemotherapies are usually developed with the aim of producing a "magic bullet" that travels through the body and selectively kills cancer cells without harming healthy cells [1], as first proposed by the German bacteriologist Paul Ehrich in the late nineteenth century. To develop such a "magic bullet" would require that components of drug delivery systems (DDS)—that is the drugs, targeting moieties and drug carrier components—must be coordinated so that drug can be delivered with appropriate timing and dose and to the right site in the body. Achieving complete coordination of these factors may lead to the discovery of ideal antitumor agents. Although no current drugs fully satisfy these properties, much progress has been made during the past few decades and recent antitumor drugs with nanotechnology-based carriers show significant potential.

Applications of nanotechnologies for drug delivery have been investigated for half a century, resulting in numerous nanotechnology-based carriers, some of which have been approved for clinical use. Liposomes were investigated in the 1960s as the first nanotechnology-based drug delivery carriers [2]. As membranous vesicles of phospholipids, liposomes mimic cellular membranes and can be used to encapsulate both hydrophilic agents into the inner aqueous cores, as well as hydrophobic agents into the amphiphilic phospholipid bilayers. In addition, surface charge, membrane hardness, and sensitivity to external stimuli, such as temperature and pH, can be adjusted by altering which phospholipids are incorporated. Moreover, liposomal surfaces can be modified using polymers, peptides, and proteins such as antibodies, allowing sustained circulation and targeting to specific sites in vivo. Thus, liposomes can be designed as an intelligent drug delivery carrier. Liposomal therapeutics have had preclinical and commercial success, with more than 46,000 publications, 850 patents, and 13 clinically approved liposome agents, producing >$750 million in revenue in 2011 [3]. Table 1 shows approved liposome formulations that have been intensively characterized [4, 5].

Liposomes improve pharmacokinetic profiles and tissue distribution of incorporated drugs. Pharmacokinetic parameters of liposomes reflect their physicochemical characteristics, such as size, surface charge, surface modification, lipid composition, and stability; both dose and route of administration alter such parameters [6, 7]. These characteristics can be manipulated to reduce side effects and enhance antitumor effects by, for example, introducing surface-bound molecules that target tumor tissues. Accordingly, liposome encapsulation of antitumor drugs dramatically changes their biodistribution through passive targeting, leading to their accumulation in tumor tissues. Additional modifications of liposome surfaces using targeting molecules can produce active targeting, further improving delivery of antitumor drugs. Currently, various liposomal antitumor drugs with passive and active targeting have been developed toward clinical use.

Table 1
Liposome-based drugs on market [4, 5]

Product name	Drug	Particle type	Approved indication	Approved year
AmBisome	Amphotericin B	Liposome	Severe fungal infections	1990
Amphotec	Amphotericin B	Lipid complex	Severe fungal infections	1993
Abelect	Amphotericin B	Lipid complex	Severe fungal infections	1995
DaunoXome	Daunorubicin	Liposome	Blood tumors	1995
Doxil	Doxorubicin	PEGylated liposome	Kaposi's sarcoma, ovarian/breast cancer	1995
Inflexal V	Inactivated hemagglutinin of Influenza virus strains A and B	Liposome	Influenza	1997
Depocyt	Cytarabine	Liposome	Neoplastic meningitis and lymphomatous meningitis	1999
Lipo-dox	Doxorubicin	PEGylated liposome	Kaposi's sarcoma, ovarian/breast cancer	2001
Myocet	Doxorubicin	Liposome	Combination therapy with cyclophosphamide in metastatic breast cancer	2001
Visudyne	Verteporfin	Liposome	Age-related molecular degeneration, pathologic myopia, ocular histoplasmosis	2001
DepoDur	Morphine sulfate	Liposome	Pain management	2004
Epaxal	Inactivated hepatitis A virus	Liposome	Hepatitis A	2011
Marqibo	Vincristine	Liposome	Metastatic malignant uveal melanoma	2012

Like other drug carrier systems that utilize nanotechnologies, self-assembled polymeric micelles are well characterized. Since the late 1980s, Kataoka et al. have been developing micelle-based cancer chemotherapies [8], which are prepared by self-assembly of poly(ethylene glycol)-b-poly(amino acid) copolymers into core–shell nanostructures [9]. The core is formed by the hydrophobic poly(amino acids) after self-aggregation of the block polymers and hydrophobic antitumor drugs are incorporated into this core mainly through hydrophobic association. The drugs are protected from interaction with plasma proteins and cells by the core, and thus achieve long circulation in the bloodstream by avoiding recognition by macrophages of the reticuloendothelial system. The diameter of the micelles can be tuned between 10 and 100 nm, which is smaller than that of most liposomal drug carriers. This small diameter reduces the accumulation of micelles to the organs of the reticuloendothelial system and enhances extravasation and deep penetration of them into tumor tissue. Recently, polymeric micelles that incorporate antitumor drugs such as paclitaxel, SN-38, doxorubicin, cisplatin, oxaliplatin, or epirubicin have been developed and passed on to clinical evaluation. While these micelles have gone to clinical trial, they have yet to be approved by the FDA. However, liposomal drugs have already been approved, and clinical data in patients has been gathered. Liposome technologies precede micelle-based drug carrier development and discussion of a generic brand liposome for medicines like doxorubicin has already begun. In short, liposomal drugs are the pioneer of nanotechnology DDS. Because they represent the foundation of nanotechnology DDS, we focus on recent studies of liposomal DDS in this review, and discuss current data, trends, prospective achievements, and challenges.

2 Properties of Liposomes as Drug Carriers

Liposome-encapsulated antitumor drugs have multiple advantages over non-encapsulated drugs, including improved pharmacokinetics, selective tumor tissue targeting, reduced side effects, and controlled drug release. In general, side effects of antitumor drugs are caused by distribution of drugs that exceed a toxic threshold to undesired tissues. For example, liposome-encapsulated doxorubicin (Doxil) was approved as an antitumor drug, with average half-lives ($T_{1/2}$) in blood of 0.041 h (α), 0.79 h (β), and 25.8 h (γ), and a distribution volume (V_d) of 24.0 L/kg (700–1100 L/m^2) after intravenous injections of 50 mg/m^2 into humans [10]. Doxorubicin causes acute and cumulative cardiotoxicity and the frequency of abnormal electrocardiograms following systemic injections of doxorubicin is about 12 %. In brief, it is expected that doxorubicin is quickly eliminated from blood and widely distributed to various tissues and that toxic levels of drug are distributed to the heart. In contrast, according to 1-compartment model analyses, the average $T_{1/2}$ in blood and V_d of Doxil are 95.3 h and 1.47 L/m^2, respectively, after intravenous injection of 50 mg/m^2 into humans [11]. Moreover, the area under the concentration-time curve (AUC) after 50 mg/m^2 doses is about 300-fold greater with Doxil compared with doxorubicin. Cardiac toxicity is also decreased with Doxil and occurs in less than 1 % and 5 % of cases after 20- and 50-mg/m^2 injections, respectively, although precise cardiotoxicity rates at both doses are unknown. The reduced frequency of side effects is thought to reflect the pharmacokinetic effects of liposomes with improved half-lives and low distribution volumes. The pharmacokinetics of doxorubicin-loaded liposomes have been investigated in clinical trials [12, 13], and Huwyler et al. have compared pharmacokinetic properties of the polyethylene glycol (PEG)-modified liposomal formulations of Doxil/Caelyx, the conventional liposomal formulation of Myocet and free doxorubicin in humans [14]. The development of Doxil is the subject of a recent review [15].

Most conventional liposomes that lack surface modification with hydrophilic polymers are rapidly cleared from circulation by the reticuloendothelial system such as in the spleen and liver [7], which plays a role in host defense by removing foreign molecules [16–18]. Sterically stabilized liposomes with hydrophilic polymer-modified surfaces have decreased protein adsorption to lipid membranes; their escape from opsonization leads to reduced liposome adhesion to cell surfaces, increased stability in the blood and prolonged circulation times. Distribution of such surface-modified liposomes in tumor tissues is also improved by the passive targeting activity, which is due to the enhanced permeability and retention (EPR) effect as described by Matsumura and Maeda in 1986 [19]. This basic concept has been used to facilitate the distribution of large molecules, such as albumin and IgG, and nano-sized particles, such as liposomes and micelles, into tumor tissues. Excessive growth of tumors requires the formation of neovasculature and increased nutrient supply. Neovessels have incomplete endothelial barriers compared with normal tissue and consequently have high permeability. Moreover, tumor tissues have dysfunctional lymphatic drainage, leading to an ineffective clearance of extravascular proteins and particles [20]. Accordingly, sustained circulation of liposomes increases the chances of extravasation and retention in tumor tissues.

Liposome stability in the circulation was originally improved using glycolipids, such as GM1 ganglioside, cerebroside sulfate and phosphatidylinositol [21, 22]. After that there was a significant breakthrough: liposome modification with PEG, which is a synthetic polymer [23]. PEG is multi-potent for modification of the liposome surface since it is possible to use PEG with different chain lengths and PEG-lipids can act as anchors for virtually any functional group. Doxil, which contains PEG-2000-1,2-distearoyl-*sn*-glycero 3-phosphoethanolamine (PEG2000–DSPE), was the first PEG-liposome approved by the FDA in 1995 (Table 1).

On the other hand, it was reported that PEG-liposomes are rapidly eliminated from the circulation following a second injection under certain conditions, including injection volume and interval. This is called the accelerated blood clearance (ABC) effect [24] and it reflects immune responses to PEG-modified materials. Moreover, PEG-liposomes elicited an anti-PEG IgM response with the first injection [25], indicating that the ABC effect may influence the utility of PEG-liposomes. Recently, other synthetic polymer-modified lipids have been designed for sustained circulation [26–43], and future studies may lead to polymers that are resistant to the ABC effect. Properties of various polymer-modified liposomes are the subject of a recent review [3].

3 Passive Targeting for Tumor Tissues

Tumor-specific liposomal DDS are categorized as passive or active targeting. As mentioned above, passive targeting is based on the EPR effect and enhanced permeability of tumor neovasculature is a key factor for the accumulation of liposomal drugs. Tumor neovasculature is more permeable than normal blood vessels, which have inter-endothelial junctions or clefts with an effective size of 6–7 nm [44]. Matsumura and Maeda showed that Evans blue-bound albumin was extravasated in tumor tissues, and we confirmed this in experiments using fluorescence-labeled liposomes, which extravasated in tumor tissues but not in normal tissues (Fig. 1a) [45]. Additionally, the optimal liposome diameter for extravasation was around 120 nm in various tumors of 1000–1500 mm^3 (Fig. 1b) [45]. Yuan et al. showed that gaps between tumor blood vessels were 100–600 nm [46]. Moreover, Hobbs et al.

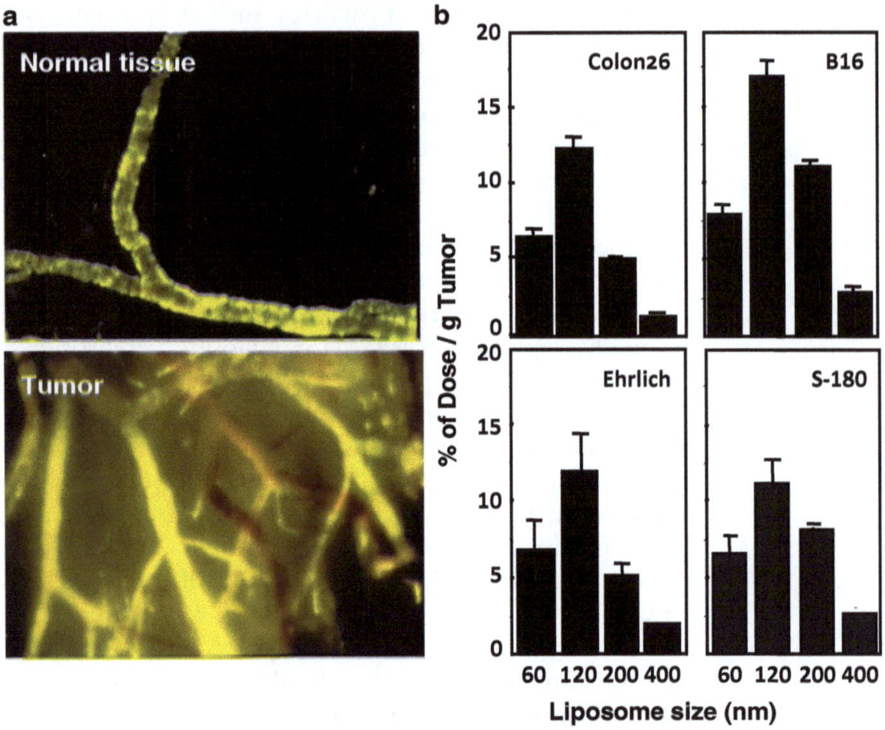

Fig. 1 Accumulation of PEG-liposomes based on EPR effect [176]. (**a**): Extravasation of DiI-labeled PEG-liposomes; Tumor-bearing mice were generated by subcutaneous inoculation of mouse neuroblastoma C-1300 cells into A/J mice. DiI-labeled PEG-liposomes with mean diameters of 100–150 nm were injected into tail veins; normal tissue (*upper panel*) and tumor (*lower panel*) were observed using a microscope. (**b**): Effects of liposome size on the extravasation of PEG-liposomes into various types of tumor tissues; Liposomes were injected into tumor-bearing mice via the tail vein, and biodistribution was investigated at 6 h after injection. Tumor-bearing mice were prepared by subcutaneously inoculating tumor cells (approximately 1×10^7), and were tested when tumor volumes reached 1000–1500 mm^3

reported that whereas long-circulating liposomes of 100–200 nm widely extravasated along vessels in tumor tissue, particles of 380–780 nm partially extravasated in a more focal manner. Therefore, they also concluded that a vascular pore size cutoff of 380–780 nm in most tumors [47]. The authors suggested that heterogeneity of pore sizes along vessels led to the observed differences in extravasation, although the diffusion of smaller-sized particles through the interstitium may have also contributed. Nonetheless, this data indicates that smaller liposomes that remain in the circulation for longer have higher extravasation efficiency and diffuse widely in tumor tissue. We demonstrated an optimal liposome size for extravasation and retention in tumor tissue with decreased tumor accumulation of 60 nm liposomes, despite a smaller vascular pore size cut-off (Fig. 1b). Thus, much smaller liposomes can return to the circulation after extravasation into tumor tissue, leading to reduced accumulation. Accordingly, numerous liposomal drugs that were designed for passive targeting with the EPR effect are between 100 and 200 nm in diameter. The discovery of passive targeting systems based on the EPR effect led to the development of various antitumor liposomal drugs. In addition, combinations of factors were shown to enhance the EPR effect by mediating inflammatory responses and increasing vessel permeability in tumors. Specifically, bradykinin, prostaglandin, nitric oxide (NO), NO-releasing factor, and tumor necrosis factor-alpha (TNF-α) improved the accumulation efficiencies of liposomes by enhancing the EPR effect [48, 49].

4 Active Targeting for Tumor Tissue

Active targeting with site-selective DDS can be achieved by exploiting interactions between ligands incorporated on the surfaces of the liposomes and the receptors or molecules that are overexpressed on the membranes of target cells. Thus, the specificity and delivery efficiency of liposomal drugs can be markedly enhanced by surface modification with tumor-targeting ligands. Liposomes with modified monoclonal antibodies on their surfaces (immunoliposomes) were originally developed in 1980 [50, 51]. Tumor cells and tumor endothelial cells overexpress specific membrane molecules, such as folate receptors [52], transferrin receptors (TfRs) [53–58], CD44 [59], asialoglycoprotein receptors [60–65], vascular endothelial growth factor receptors (VEGFR) [66–68], CD13 (aminopeptidase N) [69–71], integrins (such as $\alpha_v\beta_3$ and $\alpha_5\beta_1$) [68], endothelial growth factor receptor (EGFR) [72], somatostatin receptor [73–75], CD19 [76–79], CD20 [80, 81], intercellular cell adhesion molecule-1 (ICAM-1), vascular cell adhesion molecule-1 (VCAM-1), and endothelial-leukocyte adhesion molecule-1 (E-selectin) [82, 83]. These receptors can be used to target tumors using surface modification of liposomes with receptor ligands, antibodies, and peptides. Whereas tumor endothelial cell-targeting ligands need to extravasate to bind to tumor cells or leak their drug load outside tumor vessels, active targeting liposomes do not. With the exception of circulating cancers, such as leukemia, active tumor-targeting liposomes first exploit passive targeting based on the EPR effect so that they come in the vicinity of the cancer cells and then active targeting based on cell-specific binding. Thus, active targeting liposomes should be stable in the circulation and retained in the target site due to binding and internalization into target cells.

4.1 Natural Ligand-Modified Liposomes

Active targeting liposomes initially were prepared by modification of ligands for receptors of nutrition transport and adhesion, such as folate receptors and TfRs. As candidates for active targeting, these receptors are generally expressed on normal cells and are overexpressed on some tumor cells. In particular, folate receptors are highly upregulated in many human tumors and increase with the progression of cancer stages. As a natural ligand, folic acid has a high affinity (K_d = approximately 10^{-10} mol/L) [84] and no toxicity or immunogenicity; it is inexpensive and small and can be incorporated into liposomes with ease. Lee et al. were the first to report folic acid-conjugated liposomes with tumor cell-targeting activities [85], and multiple folic acid-modified liposomes have since been developed [86–88].

TfRs are also overexpressed in cancer cells, offering an effective therapeutic target. After binding iron-containing transferrin (Tf), TfRs are endocytosed as a mechanism of cellular iron uptake, and their expression on rapidly growing cancer cells [89, 90] is increased by 10–100-fold due to high iron requirements [55, 91]. TfR-mediated active targeting strategies have been developed using Tf [45, 53, 55–58, 92–95], anti-TfR antibodies [91, 96, 97], and TfR-binding peptides [98–100]. Because Tf is a natural ligand for TfRs, it exhibits no toxicity and low immunogenicity and is therefore a candidate for active tumor-targeting liposomes. Previously, we developed an intracellular drug delivery using Tf coupled to the distal termini of PEG chains (Tf-PEG-liposome) [57]. Tf-PEG-liposomes, bearing approximately 20–25 Tf molecules per liposome, readily bound mouse Colon-26 cells in vitro and were internalized by receptor-mediated endocytosis [56]. Tf-PEG-liposomes exhibited desirable biodistribution, tumor accumulation, and internalization in vivo.

Oxaliplatin (trans-L-diaminocyclohexane oxalatoplatinum; L-OHP) is the third generation of platinum drugs, after cisplatin and carboplatin, and has antitumor effect against cisplatin-resistant murine leukemia cells [101]. Although L-OHP has no renal toxicity, it often induces adverse drug reactions, such as peripheral sensory neuropathy and thrombocytopenia [102]. L-OHP is rapidly eliminated by the kidney and also goes to the erythrocytes [103],

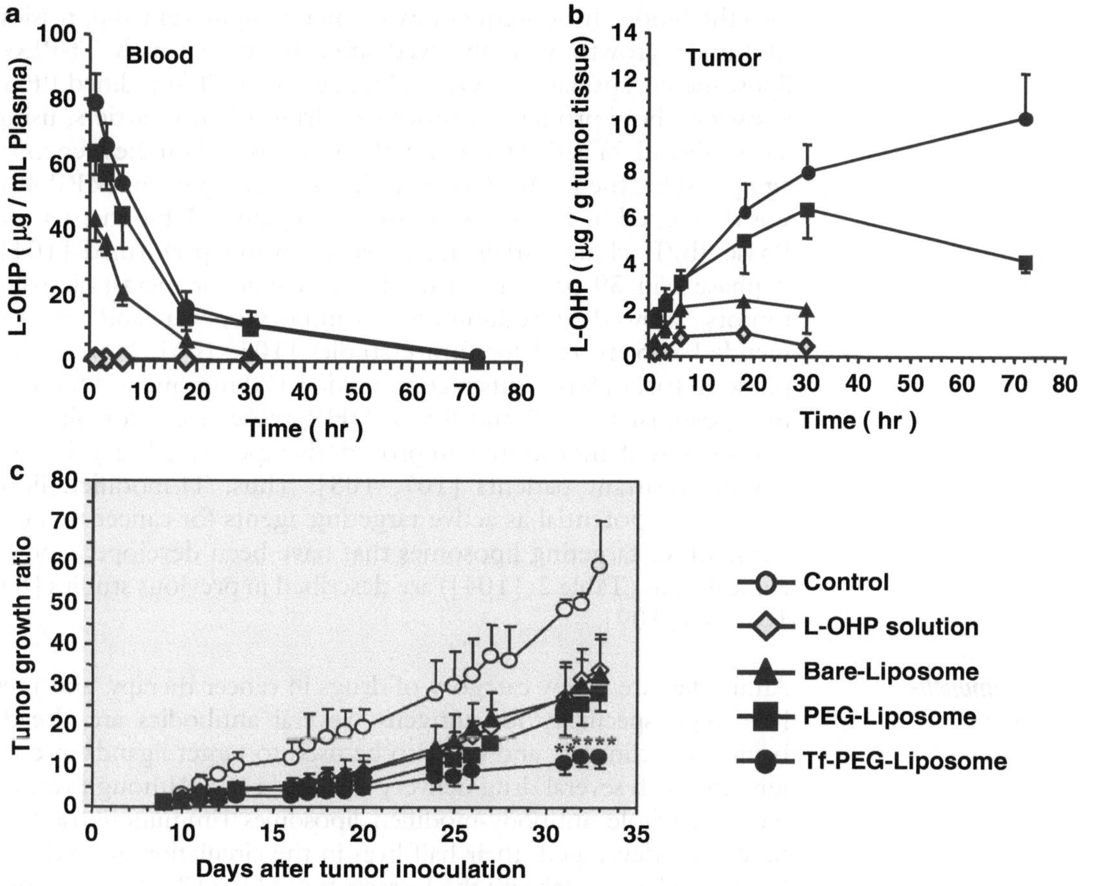

Fig. 2 L-OHP delivery by Tf-PEG-liposomes [57]. Mouse colon carcinoma (Colon-26) cells were subcutaneously inoculated into BALB/c mice. L-OHP solution or L-OHP encapsulated in Bare, PEG-, or Tf-PEG-liposomes (L-OHP: 5 mg/kg) were administered via tail veins, and blood concentrations (**a**) and tumor accumulation of L-OHP (**b**) were determined. Antitumor effects were evaluated by measuring tumor volumes after treatment with L-OHP-encapsulated Tf-PEG-liposomes (**c**). L-OHP formulations were injected on days 9 and 12 after tumor cell inoculation; $^{**}P < 0.01$, PEG-liposomes vs. Tf-PEG-liposomes

but it can be efficiently delivered with enhanced antitumor effects by reducing the fraction that goes to the erythrocytes. Thus, L-OHP-encapsulating Tf-PEG-liposomes were developed to efficiently deliver L-OHP to tumor tissues [57]. Tf-PEG-liposome-encapsulated L-OHP remained in the circulation in tumor-bearing mice with a similar profile to that of PEG-liposomes (Fig. 2a). In addition, the distribution of L-OHP in tumor tissues was enhanced after treatment with PEG-liposome and Tf-PEG-liposome-encapsulated L-OHP (Fig. 2b). Notably, the concentration of L-OHP in tumors treated with Tf-PEG-liposome-encapsulated L-OHP was higher than in those treated with PEG-liposome-encapsulated L-OHP at 72 h after intravenous injection. Hence, Tf-PEG-liposomes are internalized into cancer cells, leading to the accumulation of L-OHP and diminished repartitioning into the blood. In subsequent experiments, significant suppression of tumor growth was observed after treatment with Tf-PEG-liposome-encapsulated L-OHP (Fig. 2c). Thus, Tf-modified PEG-liposomes hold promise as anticancer drug delivery carriers, using Tf as a ligand for active targeting of tumors. Based on these encouraging results, the L-OHP-loaded, Tf-modified liposome MBP-426 was developed by a Japanese venture company (Mebiopharm) and Phase Ib/II clinical trials are currently being performed [104]. A phase I in 39 patients with advanced solid or metastatic solid tumors showed dose-limiting thrombocytopenia and recommended 226 mg/m^2 for future studies [105, 106]. Moreover, a phase Ib trial of 9 patients recommended 170 mg/m^2 and 85 mg/m^2 liposomal L-OHP and free L-OHP, respectively, for phase II studies and demonstrated improved therapeutic efficacy in two L-OHP-resistant patients [107, 108]. Thus, Tf-modified liposomes have potential as active targeting agents for cancer therapy. Some other targeting liposomes that have been developed and in clinical trials (Table 2; [104]) are described in previous studies [84, 101, 104, 109].

4.2 Immunoliposomes

Antibodies are a new category of drugs in cancer therapy, and they have high specificity for antigens. Several antibodies are already being used clinically and can also be used to target ligands in conjunction with several drug delivery carriers [110]. Although various types of whole antibody-modified liposomes (immunoliposomes) have been developed, their half-lives in the circulation are reduced by macrophage uptake via the Fc receptor [111–113]. The sustained circulation of immunoliposomes is required for sufficient tumor-targeting. To improve this point, new types of immunoliposomes modified with a Fab′ fragments that lack the Fc fragment were developed [45]. Fab′-modified PEG-liposomes showed improved circulation times in the blood and low accumulation in the liver compared with IgG-modified PEG-liposomes with intact Fc fragments. The accumulation of Fab′-modified PEG-liposomes in tumor tissue was higher than that of IgG-modified liposomes. Although the accumulation of Fab′-modified PEG-liposomes was similar to that of PEG-liposomes, it was demonstrated that Fab′-modified PEG-liposomes attached more readily to cancer cells compared with PEG-liposomes in vitro [45]. Therefore, upon extravasation into tumor tissues by the EPR effect, Fab′-modified PEG-liposomes bind and are internalized into cancer cells, leading to an enhanced anticancer effect compared with that of PEG-liposomes. Similarly, other recent reports show that Fab′-modified liposomes have higher anticancer effects than PEG-liposomes [114, 115].

Although numerous studies report the development of immunoliposomes, they have not been approved for clinical use because of insufficient therapeutic efficacy. Moreover, due to steric hindrance between antibodies, therapeutic efficiency was not improved

Table 2
Overview of ligand-targeted lipid-based nanomedicines in development [104]

Product name	Company	Approx. size (nm)	Payload	Ligand	Target	Clinical indication	Clinical phase
MBP-426	Mebiopharm	50–200	Oxaliplatin	Protein	Transferrin receptor	Metastatic gastric, gastroesophageal junction, esophageal adenocarcinoma	Phase II
SGT-53	SynerGene Therapeutics	90	p53 plasmid DNA	Antibody fragment (scFv)	Transferrin receptor	Solid tumors	Phase Ib
SGT-94	SynerGene Therapeutics	90	BR94 plasmid DNA	Antibody fragment (scFv)	Transferrin receptor	Solid tumors	Phase I
MM-302	Merrimack Pharmaceuticals	75–110	Doxorubicin	Single domain antibody (dAb) fragment (VH)	ErbB (HER2)	Brest cancer	Phase I
Lipovaxin-MM	Lipotek		Melanoma antigens and IFNγ	Protein	DC-SIGN	Melanoma vaccine	Phase I
Anti-EGFR ILs-DOX	University Hospital Basel	85	Doxorubicin	Antibody fragment (Fab′)	EGFR	Solid tumors	Phase I
283-101	to-BBB technologies		Doxorubicin	Protein	Glutathione transporters	Solid tumors	Phase I/lia
MCC-465	Mitsubishi Pharma corporation	140	Doxorubicin	Antibody fragment (F(ab)′2)	Not characterized	Advanced gastric cancer	Phase I (Discontinued)

by increasing the concentrations of the liposome-modified antibody [81]. Manufacturing costs also hamper the development of immunoliposomes. In particular, the production of Fab′ from whole antibody is time consuming and costly. However, the cost of production may be dramatically reduced by single-chain antibody fragment (scFv) technology, because they are small compared to Fab′ antibodies and scFv, have similar high affinity for the antigen, and can be produced without hybridomas. Accordingly, anti-TfR scFv-modified liposomes have been developed and are under assessment in a Phase I study [116].

5 External Stimuli Responsive Therapies

Although various systems that deliver drugs to target tissues have been developed, many deliver insufficient quantities of drug to cure the disease. Insufficient release of drug from the drug delivery carrier may underlie this issue [117, 118], necessitating that DDS remain stable and intact until they reach the targeted tissues, where they would then release sufficient quantities of drug. To address this requirement, some studies have demonstrated the utility of drug delivery carriers that respond to biological stimuli, such as comparing differences in the pH between target tissues and non-target tissues or blood [119, 120]. Such external stimulation may also enhance the release of drugs and improve treatment efficacy.

5.1 Thermosensitive Liposomes

Hyperthermia is one of several strategies that exploit the sensitivity of cancer cells to temperature. Accordingly, cancer cells die more rapidly than normal cells following increases in temperature. To take advantage of this and to future exploit the temperature increase, thermosensitive liposomes that release drugs into tumor cells with changes in temperature were developed. In subsequent experiments, the concentration of doxorubicin in tumors was assessed after treatment with doxorubicin-encapsulated thermosensitive PEG-liposomes under conditions of hyperthermia [121]. In these experiments, thermosensitive PEG-liposomes delivered higher concentrations of doxorubicin to tumors than under normal temperature conditions. While hyperthermia suppressed tumor growth, it did not improve survival time. In contrast, treatment with doxorubicin-encapsulated thermosensitive PEG-liposomes and hyperthermia significantly suppressed tumor growth and increased survival times (Table 3). These observations suggest that doxorubicin-encapsulating thermosensitive PEG-liposomes combined with hyperthermia enhance therapeutic efficacy by increasing the release of doxorubicin into tumor tissues. It should be noted that Tagami et al. also developed a novel thermosensitive liposome [122–124]. It is the physical external stimulation of drug carriers that holds promise as a useful tool for controlled drug release to targeted tissues and enhanced treatment efficacy (Fig. 3).

Table 3
Antitumor effects of doxorubicin (DXR)-encapsulated thermosensitive PEG-liposomes under conditions of hyperthermia (42 °C, 20 min) in Colon-26 solid tumor-bearing mice [121]

	Tumor volume (cm^3)[a]		Survival time[a]	
Treatments	Day 7	Day 14	Mean (day)	%ILS[b]
Control	3.0 (0.7)	6.9 (1.5)	29.4 (4.2)	–
Heat	1.7 (0.4)	4.8 (0.7)**	30.1 (4.5)	2.4
DXR solution + Heat	1.6 (0.4)	3.0 (1.0)	31.5 (5.6)	7.1
DXR-TSL + Heat	0.9 (0.2)	1.3 (0.8)*	39.8 (8.4)	35.4
DXR-PEG1K-TSL + Heat	0.6 (0.1)	0.7 (0.1)*,***	46.0[c]	56.6
DXR-PEG5K-TSL + Heat	0.7 (0.2)	0.7 (0.2)*,***	44.3[d]	50.7

Data are presented as the mean and standard deviation (SD) of 10 mice per group; *Significant difference from DXR solution + Heat, $P < 0.01$; **No significant difference from DXR solution + Heat; ***Significant difference from DXR-TSL + Heat, $P < 0.05$

[a]Tumor volume and survival time post-treatment (day 0)

[b]Increased life span (ILS) was calculated as %ILS = ((Mean survival of treated group)/(Mean survival of control group) − 1) × 100

[c]Three mice survived for over 70 days

[d]One mouse survived for over 79 days

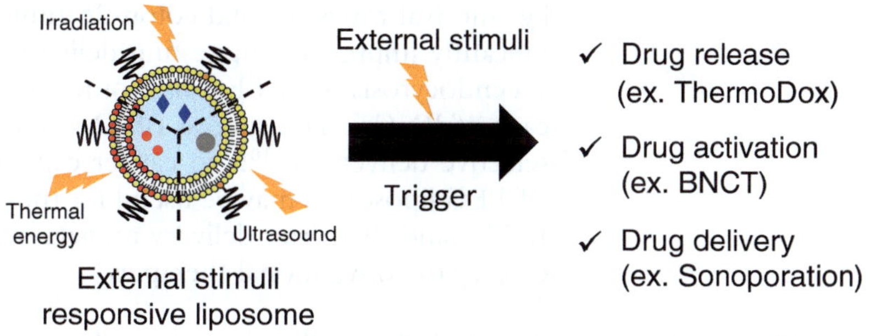

Fig. 3 Strategies of external stimuli responsive liposome. External stimuli, such as radio irradiation, and thermal and ultrasound energies activate drug delivery and release

Recent trials of thermosensitive, liposome-encapsulated doxorubicin (ThermoDox) [125] demonstrate significant improvements in drug release rates and drug uptake in heated tumors (approximately 41 °C). Moreover, ThermoDox has been considered in phase III clinical trials for liver cancer and phase II trials for breast cancer recurrent at the chest wall [126–128].

Other physical energy sources may also have potential, such as photo-energy and ultrasound [128]. Accordingly, magnetic resonance-guided focused ultrasound (MRgFUS) has been combined with thermosensitive liposome-based drug delivery to provide localized chemotherapy and simultaneous quantification of drug release within tumors [129]. Current state-of-the-art, image-guided heating technologies that utilize this combination strategy are presented with examples of real-time monitoring of drug delivery and prediction of efficacy in the following sections.

5.2 Liposomal Boron Neutron Capture Therapy (BNCT)

As described above, physical external stimulation can be used in conjunction with drug carriers to improve drug delivery to target tissues and cells. DDS may also enhance the efficacy of conventional therapies and improve the accuracy of diagnosis using techniques such as magnetic resonance and ultrasound imaging. The BNCT technique was designed to suppress tumor growth [130, 131]. Cancer cells take up the stable boron isotope ^{10}B; when these cells are subsequently irradiated with low energy neutrons, and lithium ions and α-particles are produced. These α-particles only affect cells within approximately 10 μm of the site of production [132]. Therefore, selective delivery of ^{10}B to cancer cells may enhance the therapeutic effect of BNCT (Fig. 3). Accordingly, we developed a cancer cell-selective ^{10}B delivery carrier using Tf-PEG-liposomes that exhibit internalization by cancer cells and selective drug delivery [131, 133]. Subsequent experiments showed that mercaptoundecahydrododecaborate-^{10}B (BSH)-encapsulating Tf-PEG-liposomes delivered BSH to tumor tissues more effectively than PEG-liposomes. When BSH-encapsulated Tf-PEG-liposomes were administered to mice at doses of 5- or 20-mg ^{10}B/kg, survival times of solid colon-26 tumor-bearing mice were significantly improved, suggesting delivery of BSH to tumor tissues via endocytosis of Tf-PEG-liposomes and enhanced treatment efficacy of BNCT. The success of BNCT treatment depends on the selective delivery of ^{10}B to cancer cells. Our studies suggest that Tf-PEG liposomes may be useful for the selective delivery of ^{10}B in BNCT and that drug delivery carriers may improve the treatment efficacy of conventional therapies.

5.3 Ultrasound Responsive Liposomes

The clinical use of various physical energy forms for treatment and diagnosis is widespread. In particular, ultrasound (US) is used as a noninvasive diagnostic tool and a high energy cancer therapy. Microbubbles, which are contrast agents that are used in US imaging can be used to improve gene transfection efficiency [134–137], and submicron-sized bubbles (nanobubbles) have also been developed and applied as drug and gene delivery systems. We developed echo-contrast gas (perfluoropropane) entrapping PEG-liposomes (Bubble liposomes; BL) of approximately 500 nm (Fig. 4) [138–140] for drug and gene delivery. Later, a doxorubicin delivery system involving concomitant use of BL and US demonstrated marked inhibition of osteosarcoma cell proliferation in vitro and in vivo. Furthermore, this system achieved an equivalent antitumor effect at about 1/5th of the dose of antitumor agents employed in monotherapy with doxorubicin, suggesting reductions in adverse

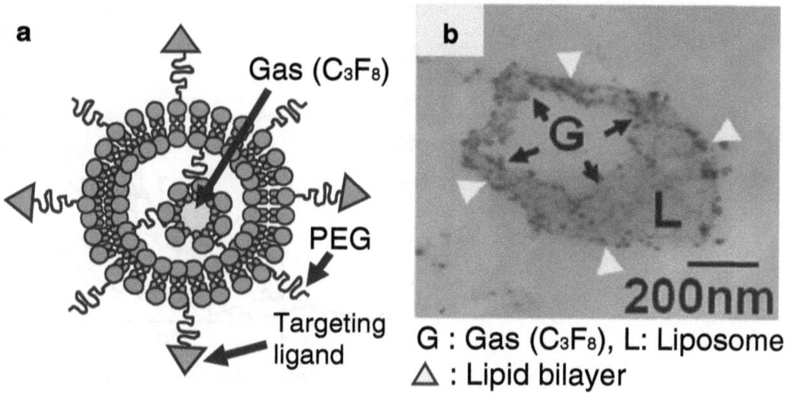

Fig. 4 Structure of Bubble liposome [140]. (**a**): A cartoon of a Bubble liposome; (**b**): Transmission electron microscopy of a Bubble liposome negatively stained at 80 °C. The distance between the two lines in the microscopic field was 5.6 nm, indicating a single lipid bilayer. Original magnification, ×50,000; JEOL JEM2000EX operated at 100 kV

events [141]. In addition, we demonstrated antitumor effects using therapeutic gene delivery with BL and US, which delivered plasmid DNA (pDNA) into cells without significant toxicity in vitro and in vivo.

Gene therapy with interleukin-12 (IL-12) has been shown to produce immunomodulatory antitumor effects and is considered an effective antitumor agent. However, the short half-life and systemic toxicity of IL-12 following intravenous injections is a major obstacle to its therapeutic use. Thus, delivery of IL-12 encoding pDNA (pCMV-IL-12) into tumor tissues using local tumor injections of pCMV-IL-12 and BL was examined. Subsequent US treatment suppressed tumor growth more in pCMV-IL-12-treated tissues than in control tissues (Fig. 5). Therefore, BL with US may be a useful tool for efficient and safe delivery of genes to cancer cells. Delivery of various molecules such as oligonucleotides, siRNA [142, 143], miRNA [144], and antigens [145, 146] has also been studied using BL with US (Fig. 3). Furthermore, active-targeting BL-modified liposomes containing ligands such as peptides and sugars have been developed [147–155].

Recently, the eLiposome formulation was developed with a similar liposome structure containing perfluoropentene nanodroplets (Fig. 6a, b) [156, 157]. Initially, nanodroplets of perfluoropentane were prepared. They were then encapsulated by sonication with liposomes or by hydration of lipid films with nanodroplet suspensions. Finally, nanodroplet-encapsulated liposomes were purified using stepwise density gradient centrifugation [157]. Calcein-encapsulating eLiposomes were sensitive to US, and released calcein after the liquid droplets were changed to gas by the US [158]. Folate-modified eLiposomes were also developed and

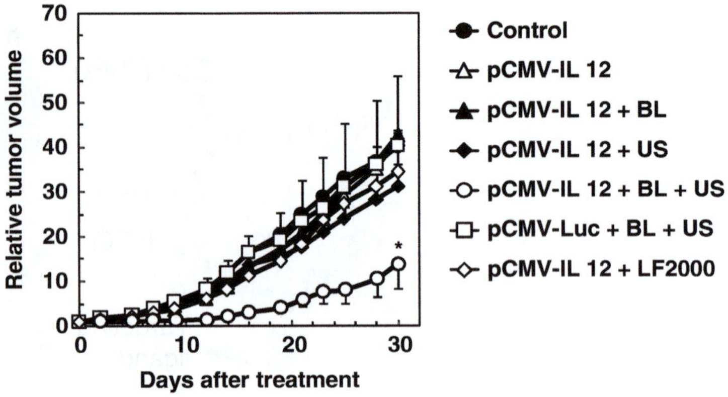

Fig. 5 Antitumor effects of treatment with pCMV-IL 12, Bubble liposomes, and ultrasound [177]. B6C3F1 mice were inoculated intradermally with murine ovarian carcinoma (OV-HM) cells, and pCMV-IL 12 (10 μg) or pCMV-Luc (which expresses the luciferase protein) were transfected using BL (2.5 μg) and ultrasound (1 MHz, 0.7 W/cm^2, 1 min), or using Lipofectamine 2000. Tumor volumes were measured after treatment, and data represent tumor volumes relative to those on the first day. Points represent the mean ± SD ($n = 5$); *$P < 0.05$ compared to other groups

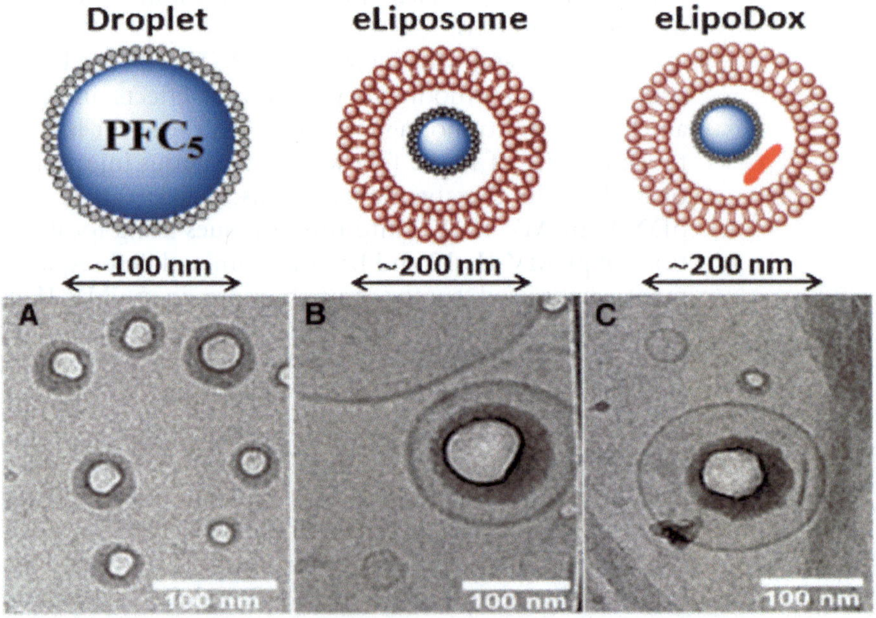

Fig. 6 Cryo-TEM and illustrations of nanodroplet-encapsulated liposomes (eLiposome) [160]. (**a**): C_5F_{12} nanodroplet, (**b**): C_5F_{12} nanodroplet-encapsulated liposome (eLiposome), and (**c**): Doxorubicin-loaded eLiposome (eLipoDox)

were shown to deliver calcein and plasmid DNA into Hela cells following exposure to US [159]. Moreover, folate-modified, doxorubicin-encapsulating eLiposomes (Fig. 6c) reportedly delivered doxorubicine into Hela cells and enhanced cytotoxicity against Hela cells in vitro [160]. Taken together, these results indicate that liposomal bubbles and liposomes containing gas-forming liquid can be used as ultrasound imaging agents and as US-sensitive drug and gene delivery systems for both diagnostic and therapeutic applications. Recently, a strategy known as theranostics was proposed for simultaneous or sequential therapy and diagnosis [161], and the promise of liposomal bubbles as theranostic candidates was shown, with safety, versatility, and proven clinical effectiveness.

6 Problems and Perspectives

One of problems in liposomal drug development is drug loading or encapsulating efficiency. Although various drugs such as anthracyclines can be effectively loaded into liposomes using remote loading techniques, most drugs are inefficiently encapsulated in liposomes. For example, the encapsulation efficiency of water soluble L-OHP was less than 30 % [162], which was much lower than remote loading of doxorubicin (more than 95 %). Most antitumor drugs are very expensive; thus, low loading efficiency is a serious problem for clinical development and directly influences antitumor effects. However, the loading efficiency of L-OHP was reportedly increased to 58 % by optimizing the preparation technique [163], indicating that loading efficiency can be improved even for water soluble drugs. Moreover, hydrophobic drugs that are not suitable for remote loading were preloaded into modified cyclodextrins, and drug preloaded cyclodextrins were remotely loaded into liposomes [164]. These methods for improved loading efficiency will encourage the development of liposomal antitumor drug formulations.

As another concern, there is a problem of liposome-specific adverse effects. Although liposomal formulations of antitumor drugs have improved therapeutic effects and reduced side-effects compared with non-liposomal drugs, some liposomal formulations induce liposome-specific adverse effects such as skin reactions and hypersensitivity reactions. Lotem et al. reported skin toxicity and hand–foot syndrome following the injection of doxorubicin loaded PEG-liposomes [165], reflecting sustained circulation and high stability of the liposome rather than effects of doxorubicin. Accordingly, it has been suggested that long circulating liposomes may accumulate in palms, soles, and areas of repeated friction or trauma, and that doxorubicin is released from liposomes under these conditions [166]. In addition, Chan et al. reported acute hypersensitivity associated with infusions of liposomal doxorubicin in an ovarian cancer patient during the first cycle of chemotherapy [167]. In other studies, up to 30.8 % of patients experienced hypersensitivity reactions such as hypotension and hypertension; hemodynamic, respiratory, and cutaneous reactions; and subjective manifestations, such as dyspnea, flushing, rash, and choking feelings [166, 168–174]. These reactions likely arise from the activation of complement immunity [166]. At present, it is required to elucidate a mechanism about the induction of liposome-specific adverse effects and to develop the methods to avoid the adverse effects.

To enhance therapeutic effect of liposomal drugs, active targeting liposomes have been developed. There are several clear aims when using ligand-mediated tumor targeting of drug-loaded liposomes compared to more traditional dosage forms. Ideally, drugs in liposomes should not only accumulate in the interstitial space inside tumors but also be internalized by the target cells creating high intracellular drug concentration and allowing multidrug resistance to be bypassed. To achieve these goals, certain considerations should be taken into account: (1) a target should be identified which is present (overexpressed) on the surface of tumor cells in sufficient quantity to provide good opportunity for the targeted liposomes to tightly bind with cancer cells; (2) the specific ligand should be attached to the surface of the drug-loaded liposomes in a way which does not affect its specific binding properties and long circulating activity in blood; (3) the targeting ligand is internalizable and facilitates the internalization of the carrier and carrier-incorporated anticancer drug; (4) drug release from the carrier inside the tumor or inside the tumor cell should deliver the therapeutic concentration of the drug and maintain it for a reasonable period of time.

As mentioned above, numerous liposomal antitumor drugs have been studied in clinical trials and some have been approved for clinical use. In addition, various active targeting strategies have been explored. However, no FDA-approved platforms exist, indicating difficulties in reliably improving accumulation at tumor sites using active targeting [175]. Thus, external-stimuli-responsive liposomes have been developed, and combinations of passive and active-targeting liposomal technologies have been used to achieve drug activation or controlled release following external stimulation. These technologies may ultimately lead to breakthroughs in effective and site-specific drug delivery. More recently, the application of physical energies to DDS has been reported, and in combination with liposome technologies, this may improve the release, drug targeting, and drug activation at specific sites. Moreover, fusion of DDS with liposomes and imaging technologies offers significant diagnostic and therapeutic potential as an ideal "theranostics".

7 Conclusion

Since the development of the first liposomal antitumor drug, numerous preclinical and clinical studies of antitumor effects and side-effects have accumulated, nano-sized drug carriers have been developed, and the limitations of the EPR effect in human tumor tissues have been investigated. Hypovascular tumors, in particular, have limited passive targeting based on the EPR effect. Thus, a lot of problems to overcome still remain. On the other hand, this information about liposomal drugs, including problems associated with them, would be a very important asset to development of ideal liposomal antitumor drugs. Moreover, these preclinical and clinical experiences in liposomal drugs development would be useful for the development of other nano-sized drug carriers. Anyway, nanotechnology-based DDS would be an ideal antitumor therapeutic system in terms of enhancement of therapeutic effects and reduction of adverse effects.

Acknowledgements

We are grateful to Dr. Alexander Klibanov (Robert M. Berne Cardiovascular Research Center, University of Virginia, USA) for his technical advice on liposome technologies. The authors would like to thank Ms. Lindsey Brinton (Department of Biomedical Engineering, University of Virginia) for the English language review. This study was supported by JSPS KAKENHI (Grant Number 21700511, 23300192, 24650299, and 23500567), the MEXT-Supported Program for the Strategic Research Foundation at Private Universities 2013–2017, the Programs for Promotion of Fundamental Studies in Health Sciences of the National Institute of Biomedical Innovation (NIBIO), and the Third Term Comprehensive Control Research for Cancer from the Ministry of Health, Labour and Welfare of Japan.

References

1. Strebhardt K, Ullrich A (2008) Paul Ehrlich's magic bullet concept: 100 years of progress. Nat Rev Cancer 8:473–480
2. Bangham AD, Standish MM, Watkins JC (1965) Diffusion of univalent ions across the lamellae of swollen phospholipids. J Mol Biol 13:238–252
3. Kohli AG, Kierstead PH, Venditto VJ, Walsh CL, Szoka FC (2014) Designer lipids for drug delivery: from heads to tails. J Control Release 190:274
4. Kikuchi H (2013) Current aspect and future perspective of DDS medicines. Pharma Med Dev Regulat Sci 44:602–611
5. Chang HI, Yeh MK (2012) Clinical development of liposome-based drugs: formulation, characterization, and therapeutic efficacy. Int J Nanomedicine 7:49–60
6. Drummond DC, Meyer O, Hong K, Kirpotin DB, Papahadjopoulos D (1999) Optimizing liposomes for delivery of chemotherapeutic agents to solid tumors. Pharmacol Rev 51:691–743
7. Allen TM, Hansen C (1991) Pharmacokinetics of stealth versus conventional liposomes: effect of dose. Biochim Biophys Acta 1068:133–141
8. Cabral H, Kataoka K (2014) Progress of drug-loaded polymeric micelles into clinical studies. J Control Release 190:465–476
9. Nishiyama N, Kataoka K (2006) Current state, achievements, and future prospects of polymeric micelles as nanocarriers for drug and gene delivery. Pharmacol Ther 112:630–648
10. Mross K, Maessen P, van der Vijgh WJ, Gall H, Boven E, Pinedo HM (1988)

Pharmacokinetics and metabolism of epidoxorubicin and doxorubicin in humans. J Clin Oncol 6:517–526

11. Fujisaka Y, Horiike A, Shimizu T, Yamamoto N, Yamada Y, Tamura T (2006) Phase 1 clinical study of pegylated liposomal doxorubicin (JNS002) in Japanese patients with solid tumors. Jpn J Clin Oncol 36:768–774
12. Harris L, Batist G, Belt R et al (2002) Liposome-encapsulated doxorubicin compared with conventional doxorubicin in a randomized multicenter trial as first-line therapy of metastatic breast carcinoma. Cancer 94:25–36
13. O'Brien ME, Wigler N, Inbar M et al (2004) Reduced cardiotoxicity and comparable efficacy in a phase III trial of pegylated liposomal doxorubicin HCl (CAELYX/Doxil) versus conventional doxorubicin for first-line treatment of metastatic breast cancer. Ann Oncol 15:440–449
14. Huwyler J, Drewe J, Krahenbuhl S (2008) Tumor targeting using liposomal antineoplastic drugs. Int J Nanomedicine 3:21–29
15. Barenholz Y (2012) Doxil(R)--the first FDA-approved nano-drug: lessons learned. J Control Release 160:117–134
16. Frank MM (1993) The reticuloendothelial system and bloodstream clearance. J Lab Clin Med 122:487–488
17. Daemen T, Hofstede G, Ten Kate MT, Bakker-Woudenberg IA, Scherphof GL (1995) Liposomal doxorubicin-induced toxicity: depletion and impairment of phagocytic activity of liver macrophages. Int J Cancer 61:716–721
18. Scherphof GL, Dijkstra J, Spanjer HH, Derksen JT, Roerdink FH (1985) Uptake and intracellular processing of targeted and non-targeted liposomes by rat Kupffer cells in vivo and in vitro. Ann N Y Acad Sci 446:368–384
19. Matsumura Y, Maeda H (1986) A new concept for macromolecular therapeutics in cancer chemotherapy: mechanism of tumoritropic accumulation of proteins and the antitumor agent smancs. Cancer Res 46:6387–6392
20. Mattheolabakis G, Rigas B, Constantinides PP (2012) Nanodelivery strategies in cancer chemotherapy: biological rationale and pharmaceutical perspectives. Nanomedicine (Lond) 7:1577–1590
21. Gabizon A, Papahadjopoulos D (1988) Liposome formulations with prolonged circulation time in blood and enhanced uptake by tumors. Proc Natl Acad Sci U S A 85:6949–6953
22. Gabizon A, Papahadjopoulos D (1992) The role of surface charge and hydrophilic groups on liposome clearance in vivo. Biochim Biophys Acta 1103:94–100
23. Klibanov AL, Maruyama K, Torchilin VP, Huang L (1990) Amphipathic polyethyleneglycols effectively prolong the circulation time of liposomes. FEBS Lett 268:235–237
24. Abu Lila AS, Kiwada H, Ishida T (2013) The accelerated blood clearance (ABC) phenomenon: clinical challenge and approaches to manage. J Control Release 172:38–47
25. Ishida T, Wang X, Shimizu T, Nawata K, Kiwada H (2007) PEGylated liposomes elicit an anti-PEG IgM response in a T cell-independent manner. J Control Release 122:349–355
26. Duncan R, Vicent MJ (2010) Do HPMA copolymer conjugates have a future as clinically useful nanomedicines? A critical overview of current status and future opportunities. Adv Drug Deliv Rev 62:272–282
27. Duncan R (2009) Development of HPMA copolymer-anticancer conjugates: clinical experience and lessons learnt. Adv Drug Deliv Rev 61:1131–1148
28. Etrych T, Kovar L, Strohalm J, Chytil P, Rihova B, Ulbrich K (2011) Biodegradable star HPMA polymer-drug conjugates: biodegradability, distribution and anti-tumor efficacy. J Control Release 154:241–248
29. Immordino ML, Dosio F, Cattel L (2006) Stealth liposomes: review of the basic science, rationale, and clinical applications, existing and potential. Int J Nanomedicine 1: 297–315
30. Zelikin AN, Such GK, Postma A, Caruso F (2007) Poly(vinylpyrrolidone) for bioconjugation and surface ligand immobilization. Biomacromolecules 8:2950–2953
31. Gaertner FC, Luxenhofer R, Blechert B, Jordan R, Essler M (2007) Synthesis, biodistribution and excretion of radiolabeled poly(2-alkyl-2-oxazoline)s. J Control Release 119:291–300
32. Zalipsky S, Hansen CB, Oaks JM, Allen TM (1996) Evaluation of blood clearance rates and biodistribution of poly(2-oxazoline)-grafted liposomes. J Pharm Sci 85:133–137
33. Torchilin VP, Trubetskoy VS, Whiteman KR, Caliceti P, Ferruti P, Veronese FM (1995) New synthetic amphiphilic polymers for steric protection of liposomes in vivo. J Pharm Sci 84:1049–1053
34. Drotleff S, Lungwitz U, Breunig M et al (2004) Biomimetic polymers in pharmaceutical and biomedical sciences. Eur J Pharm Biopharm 58:385–407
35. Torchilin VP, Shtilman MI, Trubetskoy VS, Whiteman K, Milstein AM (1994)

Amphiphilic vinyl polymers effectively prolong liposome circulation time in vivo. Biochim Biophys Acta 1195:181–184

36. Abu Lila AS, Nawata K, Shimizu T, Ishida T, Kiwada H (2013) Use of polyglycerol (PG), instead of polyethylene glycol (PEG), prevents induction of the accelerated blood clearance phenomenon against long-circulating liposomes upon repeated administration. Int J Pharm 456:235–242
37. Takeuchi H, Kojima H, Toyoda T, Yamamoto H, Hino T, Kawashima Y (1999) Prolonged circulation time of doxorubicin-loaded liposomes coated with a modified polyvinyl alcohol after intravenous injection in rats. Eur J Pharm Biopharm 48:123–129
38. Takeuchi H, Kojima H, Yamamoto H, Kawashima Y (2001) Evaluation of circulation profiles of liposomes coated with hydrophilic polymers having different molecular weights in rats. J Control Release 75:83–91
39. Roux E, Stomp R, Giasson S, Pezolet M, Moreau P, Leroux JC (2002) Steric stabilization of liposomes by pH-responsive N-isopropylacrylamide copolymer. J Pharm Sci 91:1795–1802
40. Riche EL, Erickson BW, Cho MJ (2004) Novel long-circulating liposomes containing peptide library-lipid conjugates: synthesis and in vivo behavior. J Drug Target 12:355–361
41. Romberg B, Metselaar JM, Baranyi L et al (2007) Poly(amino acid)s: promising enzymatically degradable stealth coatings for liposomes. Int J Pharm 331:186–189
42. Romberg B, Oussoren C, Snel CJ, Hennink WE, Storm G (2007) Effect of liposome characteristics and dose on the pharmacokinetics of liposomes coated with poly(amino acid)s. Pharm Res 24:2394–2401
43. Metselaar JM, Bruin P, de Boer LW et al (2003) A novel family of L-amino acid-based biodegradable polymer-lipid conjugates for the development of long-circulating liposomes with effective drug-targeting capacity. Bioconjug Chem 14:1156–1164
44. Lum H, Malik AB (1994) Regulation of vascular endothelial barrier function. Am J Physiol 267:L223–L241
45. Maruyama K, Ishida O, Takizawa T, Moribe K (1999) Possibility of active targeting to tumor tissues with liposomes. Adv Drug Deliv Rev 40:89–102
46. Yuan F, Dellian M, Fukumura D et al (1995) Vascular permeability in a human tumor xenograft: molecular size dependence and cutoff size. Cancer Res 55:3752–3756
47. Hobbs SK, Monsky WL, Yuan F et al (1998) Regulation of transport pathways in tumor vessels: role of tumor type and microenvironment. Proc Natl Acad Sci U S A 95:4607–4612
48. Fang J, Nakamura H, Maeda H (2011) The EPR effect: unique features of tumor blood vessels for drug delivery, factors involved, and limitations and augmentation of the effect. Adv Drug Deliv Rev 63:136–151
49. Maeda H (2012) Macromolecular therapeutics in cancer treatment: the EPR effect and beyond. J Control Release 164:138–144
50. Leserman LD, Barbet J, Kourilsky F, Weinstein JN (1980) Targeting to cells of fluorescent liposomes covalently coupled with monoclonal antibody or protein A. Nature 288:602–604
51. Heath TD, Fraley RT, Papahdjopoulos D (1980) Antibody targeting of liposomes: cell specificity obtained by conjugation of F(ab')2 to vesicle surface. Science 210:539–541
52. Yamada A, Taniguchi Y, Kawano K, Honda T, Hattori Y, Maitani Y (2008) Design of folate-linked liposomal doxorubicin to its antitumor effect in mice. Clin Cancer Res 14:8161–8168
53. Doi A, Kawabata S, Iida K et al (2008) Tumor-specific targeting of sodium borocaptate (BSH) to malignant glioma by transferrin-PEG liposomes: a modality for boron neutron capture therapy. J Neurooncol 87:287–294
54. Hatakeyama H, Akita H, Maruyama K, Suhara T, Harashima H (2004) Factors governing the in vivo tissue uptake of transferrin-coupled polyethylene glycol liposomes in vivo. Int J Pharm 281:25–33
55. Iinuma H, Maruyama K, Okinaga K et al (2002) Intracellular targeting therapy of cisplatin-encapsulated transferrin-polyethylene glycol liposome on peritoneal dissemination of gastric cancer. Int J Cancer 99:130–137
56. Ishida O, Maruyama K, Tanahashi H et al (2001) Liposomes bearing polyethyleneglycol-coupled transferrin with intracellular targeting property to the solid tumors in vivo. Pharm Res 18:1042–1048
57. Suzuki R, Takizawa T, Kuwata Y et al (2008) Effective anti-tumor activity of oxaliplatin encapsulated in transferrin-PEG-liposome. Int J Pharm 346:143–150
58. Yanagie H, Ogura K, Takagi K et al (2004) Accumulation of boron compounds to tumor with polyethylene-glycol binding liposome by using neutron capture autoradiography. Appl Radiat Isot 61:639–646
59. Park JH, Cho HJ, Yoon HY et al (2014) Hyaluronic acid derivative-coated nanohybrid liposomes for cancer imaging and drug delivery. J Control Release 174:98–108

60. Hara T, Kuwasawa H, Aramaki Y et al (1996) Effects of fusogenic and DNA-binding amphiphilic compounds on the receptor-mediated gene transfer into hepatic cells by asialofetuin-labeled liposomes. Biochim Biophys Acta 1278:51–58
61. Hara T, Aramaki Y, Takada S, Koike K, Tsuchiya S (1995) Receptor-mediated transfer of pSV2CAT DNA to mouse liver cells using asialofetuin-labeled liposomes. Gene Ther 2:784–788
62. Hara T, Aramaki Y, Takada S, Koike K, Tsuchiya S (1995) Receptor-mediated transfer of pSV2CAT DNA to a human hepatoblastoma cell line HepG2 using asialofetuin-labeled cationic liposomes. Gene 159:167–174
63. Koike K, Hara T, Aramaki Y, Takada S, Tsuchiya S (1994) Receptor-mediated gene transfer into hepatic cells using asialoglycoprotein-labeled liposomes. Ann N Y Acad Sci 716:331–333
64. Zhou X, Zhang M, Yung B et al (2012) Lactosylated liposomes for targeted delivery of doxorubicin to hepatocellular carcinoma. Int J Nanomedicine 7:5465–5474
65. Xiao Y, Zhang H, Zhang Z et al (2013) Synthesis of novel tetravalent galactosylated DTPA-DSPE and study on hepatocyte-targeting efficiency in vitro and in vivo. Int J Nanomedicine 8:3033–3050
66. Oku N, Asai T, Watanabe K et al (2002) Anti-neovascular therapy using novel peptides homing to angiogenic vessels. Oncogene 21:2662–2669
67. Maeda N, Takeuchi Y, Takada M, Sadzuka Y, Namba Y, Oku N (2004) Anti-neovascular therapy by use of tumor neovasculature-targeted long-circulating liposome. J Control Release 100:41–52
68. Sugiyama T, Asai T, Nedachi YM et al (2013) Enhanced active targeting via cooperative binding of ligands on liposomes to target receptors. PLoS One 8:e67550
69. Luo LM, Huang Y, Zhao BX et al (2013) Anti-tumor and anti-angiogenic effect of metronomic cyclic NGR-modified liposomes containing paclitaxel. Biomaterials 34: 1102–1114
70. Pastorino F, Brignole C, Marimpietri D et al (2003) Vascular damage and anti-angiogenic effects of tumor vessel-targeted liposomal chemotherapy. Cancer Res 63:7400–7409
71. Negussie AH, Miller JL, Reddy G, Drake SK, Wood BJ, Dreher MR (2010) Synthesis and in vitro evaluation of cyclic NGR peptide targeted thermally sensitive liposome. J Control Release 143:265–273
72. Park JW, Hong K, Kirpotin DB, Meyer O, Papahadjopoulos D, Benz CC (1997) Anti-HER2 immunoliposomes for targeted therapy of human tumors. Cancer Lett 118:153–160
73. Iwase Y, Maitani Y (2011) Octreotide-targeted liposomes loaded with CPT-11 enhanced cytotoxicity for the treatment of medullary thyroid carcinoma. Mol Pharm 8:330–337
74. Iwase Y, Maitani Y (2012) Dual functional octreotide-modified liposomal irinotecan leads to high therapeutic efficacy for medullary thyroid carcinoma xenografts. Cancer Sci 103:310–316
75. Zhang J, Jin W, Wang X, Wang J, Zhang X, Zhang Q (2010) A novel octreotide modified lipid vesicle improved the anticancer efficacy of doxorubicin in somatostatin receptor 2 positive tumor models. Mol Pharm 7:1159–1168
76. Allen TM, Mumbengegwi DR, Charrois GJ (2005) Anti-CD19-targeted liposomal doxorubicin improves the therapeutic efficacy in murine B-cell lymphoma and ameliorates the toxicity of liposomes with varying drug release rates. Clin Cancer Res 11:3567–3573
77. Cheng WW, Allen TM (2008) Targeted delivery of anti-CD19 liposomal doxorubicin in B-cell lymphoma: a comparison of whole monoclonal antibody, Fab′ fragments and single chain Fv. J Control Release 126:50–58
78. Cheng WW, Das D, Suresh M, Allen TM (2007) Expression and purification of two anti-CD19 single chain Fv fragments for targeting of liposomes to CD19-expressing cells. Biochim Biophys Acta 1768:21–29
79. Harata M, Soda Y, Tani K et al (2004) CD19-targeting liposomes containing imatinib efficiently kill Philadelphia chromosome-positive acute lymphoblastic leukemia cells. Blood 104:1442–1449
80. Sapra P, Allen TM (2004) Improved outcome when B-cell lymphoma is treated with combinations of immunoliposomal anticancer drugs targeted to both the CD19 and CD20 epitopes. Clin Cancer Res 10:2530–2537
81. Laginha K, Mumbengegwi D, Allen T (2005) Liposomes targeted via two different antibodies: assay, B-cell binding and cytotoxicity. Biochim Biophys Acta 1711:25–32
82. Gunawan RC, Auguste DT (2010) The role of antibody synergy and membrane fluidity in the vascular targeting of immunoliposomes. Biomaterials 31:900–907
83. Gunawan RC, Auguste DT (2010) Immunoliposomes that target endothelium in vitro are dependent on lipid raft formation. Mol Pharm 7:1569–1575

84. Wang X, Li S, Shi Y et al (2014) The development of site-specific drug delivery nanocarriers based on receptor mediation. J Control Release 193:139
85. Lee RJ, Low PS (1995) Folate-mediated tumor cell targeting of liposome-entrapped doxorubicin in vitro. Biochim Biophys Acta 1233:134–144
86. Zhang Z, Yao J (2012) Preparation of irinotecan-loaded folate-targeted liposome for tumor targeting delivery and its antitumor activity. AAPS PharmSciTech 13:802–810
87. Musacchio T, Torchilin VP (2011) Recent developments in lipid-based pharmaceutical nanocarriers. Front Biosci (Landmark Ed) 16:1388–1412
88. Kularatne SA, Low PS (2010) Targeting of nanoparticles: folate receptor. Methods Mol Biol 624:249–265
89. Mehra NK, Mishra V, Jain NK (2013) Receptor-based targeting of therapeutics. Ther Deliv 4:369–394
90. Nakase I, Lai H, Singh NP, Sasaki T (2008) Anticancer properties of artemisinin derivatives and their targeted delivery by transferrin conjugation. Int J Pharm 354:28–33
91. Dufes C, Al Robaian M, Somani S (2013) Transferrin and the transferrin receptor for the targeted delivery of therapeutic agents to the brain and cancer cells. Ther Deliv 4:629–640
92. Kakudo T, Chaki S, Futaki S et al (2004) Transferrin-modified liposomes equipped with a pH-sensitive fusogenic peptide: an artificial viral-like delivery system. Biochemistry 43:5618–5628
93. Miyata S, Kawabata S, Hiramatsu R et al (2011) Computed tomography imaging of transferrin targeting liposomes encapsulating both boron and iodine contrast agents by convection-enhanced delivery to F98 rat glioma for boron neutron capture therapy. Neurosurgery 68:1380–1387, discussion 1387
94. Omori N, Maruyama K, Jin G et al (2003) Targeting of post-ischemic cerebral endothelium in rat by liposomes bearing polyethylene glycol-coupled transferrin. Neurol Res 25:275–279
95. Okazaki F, Matsunaga N, Okazaki H et al (2010) Circadian rhythm of transferrin receptor 1 gene expression controlled by c-Myc in colon cancer-bearing mice. Cancer Res 70:6238–6246
96. Xu L, Huang CC, Huang W et al (2002) Systemic tumor-targeted gene delivery by anti-transferrin receptor scFv-immunoliposomes. Mol Cancer Ther 1:337–346
97. Gosk S, Vermehren C, Storm G, Moos T (2004) Targeting anti-transferrin receptor antibody (OX26) and OX26-conjugated liposomes to brain capillary endothelial cells using in situ perfusion. J Cereb Blood Flow Metab 24:1193–1204
98. Han L, Huang R, Liu S, Huang S, Jiang C (2010) Peptide-conjugated PAMAM for targeted doxorubicin delivery to transferrin receptor overexpressed tumors. Mol Pharm 7:2156–2165
99. Oh S, Kim BJ, Singh NP, Lai H, Sasaki T (2009) Synthesis and anti-cancer activity of covalent conjugates of artemisinin and a transferrin-receptor targeting peptide. Cancer Lett 274:33–39
100. Liu S, Guo Y, Huang R et al (2012) Gene and doxorubicin co-delivery system for targeting therapy of glioma. Biomaterials 33:4907–4916
101. Yang C, Fu ZX (2014) Liposomal delivery and polyethylene glycol-liposomal oxaliplatin for the treatment of colorectal cancer (Review). Biomed Rep 2:335–339
102. Extra JM, Espie M, Calvo F, Ferme C, Mignot L, Marty M (1990) Phase I study of oxaliplatin in patients with advanced cancer. Cancer Chemother Pharmacol 25:299–303
103. Pendyala L, Creaven PJ (1993) In vitro cytotoxicity, protein binding, red blood cell partitioning, and biotransformation of oxaliplatin. Cancer Res 53:5970–5976
104. van der Meel R, Vehmeijer LJ, Kok RJ, Storm G, van Gaal EV (2013) Ligand-targeted particulate nanomedicines undergoing clinical evaluation: current status. Adv Drug Deliv Rev 65:1284–1298
105. Mebiopharm Co., Ltd. A phase I, open label study of MBP-426 given by intravenous infusion in patients with advanced or metastatic solid tumors. In: Clinical Trials.gov [Internet], Bethesda, MD: National Library of Medicine. Accessed on July, 2013. Available from http://www.clinicaltrials.gov/ct2/show/NCT00355888?term=NCT00355888&rank=1. NLM Identifier: NCT00355888
106. Sankhala KK, Mita AC, Adinin R et al. A phase I pharmacokinetic (PK) study of MBP-426, a novel liposome encapsulated oxaliplatin. [abstract]. ASCO Annual Meeting, June 2009, ASCO, Orlando, FL, 2009. 2009:Abstract nr 2535
107. Mebiopharm Co., Ltd. A phase Ib/II study of MBP-426 in patients with second line gastric, gastro esophageal, or esophageal adenocarcinoma. In: ClinicalTrials.gov [Internet], Bethesda, MD: National Library of Medicine.

Accessed on July, 2013. Available from http://www.clinicaltrials.gov/ct2/show/NCT00964080. NLM Identifier: NCT00964080

108. Senzer NN, Matsuno K, Yamagata N et al. MBP-426, a novel liposome-encapsulated oxaliplatin, in combination with 5-FU/leucovorin (LV): phase I results of a phase I/II study in gastro-esophageal adenocarcinoma, with pharmacokinetics. [Abstract]. Molecular targets and cancer therapeutics, AACR-NCI-EORTC, Boston, MA, 2009. 2009:Abstract nr C36
109. Kamaly N, Xiao Z, Valencia PM, Radovic-Moreno AF, Farokhzad OC (2012) Targeted polymeric therapeutic nanoparticles: design, development and clinical translation. Chem Soc Rev 41:2971–3010
110. Maruyama K, Holmberg E, Kennel SJ, Klibanov A, Torchilin VP, Huang L (1990) Characterization of in vivo immunoliposome targeting to pulmonary endothelium. J Pharm Sci 79:978–984
111. Aragnol D, Leserman LD (1986) Immune clearance of liposomes inhibited by an anti-Fc receptor antibody in vivo. Proc Natl Acad Sci U S A 83:2699–2703
112. Derksen JT, Morselt HW, Scherphof GL (1988) Uptake and processing of immunoglobulin-coated liposomes by subpopulations of rat liver macrophages. Biochim Biophys Acta 971:127–136
113. Papahadjopoulos D, Gabizon A (1987) Targeting of liposomes to tumor cells in vivo. Ann N Y Acad Sci 507:64–74
114. Iden DL, Allen TM (2001) In vitro and in vivo comparison of immunoliposomes made by conventional coupling techniques with those made by a new post-insertion approach. Biochim Biophys Acta 1513:207–216
115. Sapra P, Shor B (2013) Monoclonal antibody-based therapies in cancer: advances and challenges. Pharmacol Ther 138:452–469
116. Senzer N, Nemunaitis J, Nemunaitis D et al (2013) Phase I study of a systemically delivered p53 nanoparticle in advanced solid tumors. Mol Ther 21:1096–1103
117. Bandak S, Goren D, Horowitz A, Tzemach D, Gabizon A (1999) Pharmacological studies of cisplatin encapsulated in long-circulating liposomes in mouse tumor models. Anticancer Drugs 10:911–920
118. Ta T, Porter TM (2013) Thermosensitive liposomes for localized delivery and triggered release of chemotherapy. J Control Release 169:112–125
119. Bibi S, Lattmann E, Mohammed AR, Perrie Y (2012) Trigger release liposome systems: local and remote controlled delivery? J Microencapsul 29:262–276
120. Yatvin MB, Kreutz W, Horwitz BA, Shinitzky M (1980) pH-sensitive liposomes: possible clinical implications. Science 210:1253–1255
121. Unezaki S, Maruyama K, Takahashi N et al (1994) Enhanced delivery and antitumor activity of doxorubicin using long-circulating thermosensitive liposomes containing amphipathic polyethylene glycol in combination with local hyperthermia. Pharm Res 11:1180–1185
122. Tagami T, Ernsting MJ, Li SD (2011) Optimization of a novel and improved thermosensitive liposome formulated with DPPC and a Brij surfactant using a robust in vitro system. J Control Release 154:290–297
123. Tagami T, Foltz WD, Ernsting MJ et al (2011) MRI monitoring of intratumoral drug delivery and prediction of the therapeutic effect with a multifunctional thermosensitive liposome. Biomaterials 32:6570–6578
124. Tagami T, Ernsting MJ, Li SD (2011) Efficient tumor regression by a single and low dose treatment with a novel and enhanced formulation of thermosensitive liposomal doxorubicin. J Control Release 152:303–309
125. Landon CD, Park JY, Needham D, Dewhirst MW (2011) Nanoscale drug delivery and hyperthermia: the materials design and preclinical and clinical testing of low temperature-sensitive liposomes used in combination with mild hyperthermia in the treatment of local cancer. Open Nanomed J 3:38–64
126. Celsion. Phase 3 study of ThermoDox with radiofrequency ablation (RFA) in treatment of hepatocellular carcinoma (HCC). [Internet]. Bethesda, MD: National Library of Medicine. Accessed on June 15, 2012. Available from http://www.clinicaltrials.gov/ct2/show/NCT00617981. NLM Identifier: NCT00617981
127. Celsion. Phase 1/2 study of ThermoDox with approved hyperthermia in treatment of breast cancer recurrence at the chest wall (DIGNITY). [Internet]. Bethesda, MD: National Library of Medicine. Accessed on June 15, 2012. Available from http://www.clinicaltrials.gov/ct2/show/NCT00826085. NLM Identifier: NCT0826085 2000
128. Kheirolomoom A, Lai CY, Tam SM et al (2013) Complete regression of local cancer using temperature-sensitive liposomes combined with ultrasound-mediated hyperthermia. J Control Release 172:266–273
129. May JP, Li SD (2013) Hyperthermia-induced drug targeting. Expert Opin Drug Deliv 10:511–527

130. Suzuki M, Kato I, Aihara T et al (2014) Boron neutron capture therapy outcomes for advanced or recurrent head and neck cancer. J Radiat Res 55:146–153
131. Nakamura H (2013) Boron lipid-based liposomal boron delivery system for neutron capture therapy: recent development and future perspective. Future Med Chem 5:715–730
132. Barth RF, Soloway AH, Fairchild RG (1990) Boron neutron capture therapy of cancer. Cancer Res 50:1061–1070
133. Maruyama K, Ishida O, Kasaoka S et al (2004) Intracellular targeting of sodium mercaptoundecahydrododecaborate (BSH) to solid tumors by transferrin-PEG liposomes, for boron neutron-capture therapy (BNCT). J Control Release 98:195–207
134. Greenleaf WJ, Bolander ME, Sarkar G, Goldring MB, Greenleaf JF (1998) Artificial cavitation nuclei significantly enhance acoustically induced cell transfection. Ultrasound Med Biol 24:587–595
135. Shohet RV, Chen S, Zhou YT et al (2000) Echocardiographic destruction of albumin microbubbles directs gene delivery to the myocardium. Circulation 101:2554–2556
136. Taniyama Y, Tachibana K, Hiraoka K et al (2002) Development of safe and efficient novel nonviral gene transfer using ultrasound: enhancement of transfection efficiency of naked plasmid DNA in skeletal muscle. Gene Ther 9:372–380
137. Newman CM, Bettinger T (2007) Gene therapy progress and prospects: ultrasound for gene transfer. Gene Ther 14:465–475
138. Suzuki R, Takizawa T, Negishi Y et al (2007) Gene delivery by combination of novel liposomal bubbles with perfluoropropane and ultrasound. J Control Release 117:130–136
139. Suzuki R, Takizawa T, Negishi Y et al (2008) Tumor specific ultrasound enhanced gene transfer in vivo with novel liposomal bubbles. J Control Release 125:137–144
140. Kodama T, Tomita N, Horie S et al (2010) Morphological study of acoustic liposomes using transmission electron microscopy. J Electron Microsc (Tokyo) 59:187–196
141. Ueno Y, Sonoda S, Suzuki R et al (2011) Combination of ultrasound and bubble liposome enhance the effect of doxorubicin and inhibit murine osteosarcoma growth. Cancer Biol Ther 12:270–277
142. Endo-Takahashi Y, Negishi Y, Kato Y, Suzuki R, Maruyama K, Aramaki Y (2012) Efficient siRNA delivery using novel siRNA-loaded Bubble liposomes and ultrasound. Int J Pharm 422:504–509
143. Negishi Y, Endo Y, Fukuyama T et al (2008) Delivery of siRNA into the cytoplasm by liposomal bubbles and ultrasound. J Control Release 132:124–130
144. Endo-Takahashi Y, Negishi Y, Nakamura A et al (2014) Systemic delivery of miR-126 by miRNA-loaded Bubble liposomes for the treatment of hindlimb ischemia. Sci Rep 4:3883
145. Oda Y, Suzuki R, Otake S et al (2012) Prophylactic immunization with Bubble liposomes and ultrasound-treated dendritic cells provided a four-fold decrease in the frequency of melanoma lung metastasis. J Control Release 160:362–366
146. Suzuki R, Oda Y, Utoguchi N et al (2009) A novel strategy utilizing ultrasound for antigen delivery in dendritic cell-based cancer immunotherapy. J Control Release 133:198–205
147. Un K, Kawakami S, Suzuki R, Maruyama K, Yamashita F, Hashida M (2010) Development of an ultrasound-responsive and mannose-modified gene carrier for DNA vaccine therapy. Biomaterials 31:7813–7826
148. Un K, Kawakami S, Suzuki R, Maruyama K, Yamashita F, Hashida M (2010) Enhanced transfection efficiency into macrophages and dendritic cells by a combination method using mannosylated lipoplexes and bubble liposomes with ultrasound exposure. Hum Gene Ther 21:65–74
149. Un K, Kawakami S, Suzuki R, Maruyama K, Yamashita F, Hashida M (2011) Suppression of melanoma growth and metastasis by DNA vaccination using an ultrasound-responsive and mannose-modified gene carrier. Mol Pharm 8:543–554
150. Un K, Kawakami S, Yoshida M et al (2011) The elucidation of gene transferring mechanism by ultrasound-responsive unmodified and mannose-modified lipoplexes. Biomaterials 32:4659–4669
151. Un K, Kawakami S, Yoshida M et al (2012) Efficient suppression of murine intracellular adhesion molecule-1 using ultrasound-responsive and mannose-modified lipoplexes inhibits acute hepatic inflammation. Hepatology 56:259–269
152. Negishi Y, Hamano N, Tsunoda Y et al (2013) AG73-modified Bubble liposomes for targeted ultrasound imaging of tumor neovasculature. Biomaterials 34:501–507
153. Negishi Y, Omata D, Iijima H et al (2010) Enhanced laminin-derived peptide AG73-mediated liposomal gene transfer by bubble liposomes and ultrasound. Mol Pharm 7:217–226

154. Negishi Y, Tsunoda Y, Hamano N et al (2013) Ultrasound-mediated gene delivery systems by AG73-modified bubble liposomes. Biopolymers 100:402–407
155. Hagisawa K, Nishioka T, Suzuki R et al (2013) Thrombus-targeted perfluorocarbon-containing liposomal bubbles for enhancement of ultrasonic thrombolysis: in vitro and in vivo study. J Thromb Haemost 11:1565–1573
156. Lattin JR, Belnap DM, Pitt WG (2012) Formation of eLiposomes as a drug delivery vehicle. Colloids Surf B Biointerfaces 89:93–100
157. Javadi M, Pitt WG, Belnap DM, Tsosie NH, Hartley JM (2012) Encapsulating nanoemulsions inside eLiposomes for ultrasonic drug delivery. Langmuir 28:14720–14729
158. Lattin JR, Pitt WG, Belnap DM, Husseini GA (2012) Ultrasound-induced calcein release from eLiposomes. Ultrasound Med Biol 38:2163–2173
159. Javadi M, Pitt WG, Tracy CM et al (2013) Ultrasonic gene and drug delivery using eLiposomes. J Control Release 167:92–100
160. Lin CY, Javadi M, Belnap DM, Barrow JR, Pitt WG (2014) Ultrasound sensitive eLiposomes containing doxorubicin for drug targeting therapy. Nanomedicine 10:67–76
161. Chen XS (2011) Introducing theranostics journal - from the editor-in-chief. Theranostics 1:1–2
162. Abu Lila AS, Doi Y, Nakamura K, Ishida T, Kiwada H (2010) Sequential administration with oxaliplatin-containing PEG-coated cationic liposomes promotes a significant delivery of subsequent dose into murine solid tumor. J Control Release 142:167–173
163. Yang C, Liu HZ, Fu ZX, Lu WD (2011) Oxaliplatin long-circulating liposomes improved therapeutic index of colorectal carcinoma. BMC Biotechnol 11:21
164. Sur S, Fries AC, Kinzler KW, Zhou S, Vogelstein B (2014) Remote loading of preencapsulated drugs into stealth liposomes. Proc Natl Acad Sci U S A 111:2283–2288
165. Lotem M, Hubert A, Lyass O et al (2000) Skin toxic effects of polyethylene glycol-coated liposomal doxorubicin. Arch Dermatol 136:1475–1480
166. Slingerland M, Guchelaar HJ, Gelderblom H (2012) Liposomal drug formulations in cancer therapy: 15 years along the road. Drug Discov Today 17:160–166
167. Chan A, Shih V, Tham Chee K (2007) Liposomal doxorubicin-associated acute hypersensitivity despite appropriate preventive measures. J Oncol Pharm Pract 13:105–107
168. Stathopoulos GP, Antoniou D, Dimitroulis J et al (2010) Liposomal cisplatin combined with paclitaxel versus cisplatin and paclitaxel in non-small-cell lung cancer: a randomized phase III multicenter trial. Ann Oncol 21:2227–2232
169. Szebeni J (2005) Complement activation-related pseudoallergy caused by amphiphilic drug carriers: the role of lipoproteins. Curr Drug Deliv 2:443–449
170. Veal GJ, Griffin MJ, Price E et al (2001) A phase I study in paediatric patients to evaluate the safety and pharmacokinetics of SPI-77, a liposome encapsulated formulation of cisplatin. Br J Cancer 84:1029–1035
171. White SC, Lorigan P, Margison GP et al (2006) Phase II study of SPI-77 (sterically stabilised liposomal cisplatin) in advanced non-small-cell lung cancer. Br J Cancer 95:822–828
172. Alexopoulos A, Karamouzis MV, Stavrinides H et al (2004) Phase II study of pegylated liposomal doxorubicin (Caelyx) and docetaxel as first-line treatment in metastatic breast cancer. Ann Oncol 15:891–895
173. Katsaros D, Oletti MV, Rigault de la Longrais IA et al (2005) Clinical and pharmacokinetic phase II study of pegylated liposomal doxorubicin and vinorelbine in heavily pretreated recurrent ovarian carcinoma. Ann Oncol 16:300–306
174. Katsumata N, Fujiwara Y, Kamura T et al (2008) Phase II clinical trial of pegylated liposomal doxorubicin (JNS002) in Japanese patients with mullerian carcinoma (epithelial ovarian carcinoma, primary carcinoma of fallopian tube, peritoneal carcinoma) having a therapeutic history of platinum-based chemotherapy: a Phase II Study of the Japanese Gynecologic Oncology Group. Jpn J Clin Oncol 38:777–785
175. Dawidczyk CM, Kim C, Park JH et al (2014) State-of-the-art in design rules for drug delivery platforms: lessons learned from FDA-approved nanomedicines. J Control Release 187C:133–144
176. Maruyama K (2011) Intracellular targeting delivery of liposomal drugs to solid tumors based on EPR effects. Adv Drug Deliv Rev 63:161–169
177. Suzuki R, Namai E, Oda Y et al (2010) Cancer gene therapy by IL-12 gene delivery using liposomal bubbles and tumoral ultrasound exposure. J Control Release 142:245–250

Index

Zheng-Rong Lu and Shinji Sakuma (eds.), *Nanomaterials in Pharmacology*, Methods in Pharmacology and Toxicology, DOI 10.1007/978-1-4939-3121-7, © Springer Science+Business Media New York 2016

I

L

M

N

O

P

MIX
Papier aus verantwortungsvollen Quellen
Paper from responsible sources
FSC® C105338

If you have any concerns about our products,
you can contact us on
ProductSafety@springernature.com

In case Publisher is established outside the EU,
the EU authorized representative is:
Springer Nature Customer Service Center GmbH
Europaplatz 3, 69115 Heidelberg, Germany

Printed by Libri Plureos GmbH
in Hamburg, Germany